Handbook of Experimental Pharmacology

Continuation of Handbuch der experimentellen Pharmakologie

Vol. 67/I

Antibiotics

Containing the Beta-Lactam Structure

Part I

Contributors

E. P. Abraham · Y. Aharonowitz · C. Ball · B. G. Christensen
A. L. Demain · R. P. Elander · R. Kirby . J. F. Martin · R. D. Miller
D.-G. Mou · N. Neuss · T. N. Salzmann · E. O. Stapley · A. Tomasz
S. B. Zimmerman

Editors

A. L. Demain and N. A. Solomon

Springer-Verlag Berlin Heidelberg New York Tokyo 1983

Professor Dr. ARNOLD L. DEMAIN
Ms. NADINE A. SOLOMON
Fermentation Microbiology Laboratory
Department of Nutrition and Food Science
Massachusetts Institute of Technology
Cambridge, MA 02139/USA

With 83 Figures

ISBN 3-540-12107-2 Springer-Verlag Berlin Heidelberg New York Tokyo
ISBN 0-387-12107-2 Springer-Verlag New York Heidelberg Berlin Tokyo

Library of Congress Cataloging in Publication Data. Main entry under title: Antibiotics containing the beta-lactam structure. (Handbook of experimental pharmacology; v. 67, pt. 1–) Includes index. 1. Antibiotics – Synthesis. 2. Beta-lactamases. 3. Fungi – Genetics. [DNLM: 1. Antibiotics – Pharmacodynamics. 2. Beta-lactamases – Pharmacodynamics. W1 HA51L v. 67/QV 350 A62935] QP905.H3 vol. 67, pt. 1, etc. 615'.1s 82-19689 [QD375] [547.7'6]

Typesetting, printing, and bookbinding: Brühlsche Universitätsdruckerei Giessen
2122/3130-543210

Preface

It is quite amazing that the oldest group of medically useful antibiotics, the β-lactams, are still providing basic microbiologists, biochemists, and clinicians with surprises over 50 years after Fleming's discovery of penicillin production by *Penicillium*. By the end of the 1950s, the future of the penicillins seemed doubtful as resistant strains of *Staphylococcus aureus* began to increase in hospital populations. However, the development of semisynthetic penicillins provided new structures with resistance to penicillinase and with broad-spectrum activity. In the 1960s, the discovery of cephalosporin C production by *Cephalosporium* and its conversion to valuable broad-spectrum antibiotics by semisynthetic means excited the world of chemotherapy. In the early 1970s, the 40-year-old notion that β-lactams were produced only by fungi was destroyed by the discovery of cephamycin production by *Streptomyces*. Again this basic discovery was exploited by the development of the semisynthetic cefoxitin, which has even broader activity than earlier β-lactams. Later in the 1970s came the discoveries of nocardicins from *Nocardia*, clavulanic acid from *Streptomyces*, and the carbapenems from *Streptomyces*. Now in the 1980s we learn that β-lactams are produced even by unicellular bacteria and that semisynthetic derivatives of these monobactams may find their way into medicine. Indeed, the future of the prolific β-lactam family seems brighter with each passing decade.

Considering the level of excitement in this area, we felt that this would be the right time for the leaders in the field to survey past and present research, development, and clinical applications of β-lactams and prospects for future progress. We were pleasantly surprised that so many busy people agreed to give up their time to contribute to this project. The result is this volume in two parts describing all aspects of β-lactam antibiotics.

Cambridge

ARNOLD L. DEMAIN
NADINE A. SOLOMON

List of Contributors

Sir E. P. ABRAHAM, Sir William Dunn School of Pathology, University of Oxford, South Parks Road, Oxford OX1 3RE, Great Britain

Dr. Y. AHARONOWITZ, Department of Microbiology, The George S. Wise Faculty of Life Sciences, Tel-Aviv University, Tel-Aviv, Israel

Dr. C. BALL, Squibb Institute for Medical Research, Biological Process Development, E.R. Squibb & Sons, Inc., Georges Road, New Brunswick, NJ 08903/USA

Dr. B.G. CHRISTENSEN, Merck Sharp & Dohme Research Laboratories, P.O. Box 2000, Rahway, NJ 07065/USA

Professor Dr. A. L. DEMAIN, Fermentation Microbiology Laboratory, Department of Nutrition and Food Science, Massachusetts Institute of Technology, Cambridge, MA 02139/USA

Dr. R. P. ELANDER, Fermentation Research and Development, Bristol-Myers Co., Industrial Division, P.O. Box 657, Syracuse, NY 13201/USA

Dr. R. KIRBY, University of Cape Town, Department of Microbiology, Rondebosch 7700, South Africa

Professor Dr. J. F. MARTIN, Department of Microbiology, Faculty of Biology, University of León, León, Spain

Dr. R. D. MILLER, Eli Lilly & Co., P.O. Box 685, Lafayette, IN 47902/USA

Dr. D.-G. MOU, Research Laboratories, Eastman Kodak Company, Kodak Park, Rochester, NY 14650/USA

Dr. N. NEUSS, Lilly Research Laboratories, Eli Lilly & Co., Indianapolis, IN 46205/USA

Dr. T.N. SALZMANN, Merck Sharp & Dohme Research Laboratories, Rahway, NJ 07065/USA

Dr. E. O. STAPLEY, Merck Sharp & Dohme Research Laboratories, Department of Basic Macrobiological Research, P.O. Box 2000, Rahway, NJ 07065/USA

Dr. A. TOMASZ, The Rockefeller University, 1230 York Avenue, New York, NY 10021/USA

Dr. S. B. ZIMMERMAN, Merck Sharp & Dohme Research Laboratories, Department of Basic Macrobiological Research, P.O. Box 2000, Rahway, NJ 07065/USA

Contents

CHAPTER 3

Strain Improvement and Preservation of β-Lactam-Producing Microorganisms.
R. P. ELANDER. With 9 Figures

CHAPTER 4

Genetics of β-Lactam-Producing Fungi. C. BALL. With 4 Figures

CHAPTER 5

Genetics of β-Lactam-Producing Actinomycetes. R. KIRBY. With 4 Figures

CHAPTER 6

Biosynthesis of β-Lactam Antibiotics. A. L. DEMAIN. With 6 Figures

CHAPTER 7

Regulation of Biosynthesis of β-Lactam Antibiotics. J. F. MARTIN and Y. AHARONOWITZ. With 5 Figures

CHAPTER 8

Biochemical Engineering and β-Lactam Antibiotic Production
D.-G. MOU. With 13 Figures

CHAPTER 9

Screening for New β-Lactam Antibiotics. S. B. ZIMMERMAN and E. O. STAPLEY. With 7 Figures

CHAPTER 10

High-Performance Liquid Chromatography of β-Lactam Antibiotics.
R. D. Miller and N. Neuss. With 18 Figures

CHAPTER 11

Strategy in the Total Synthesis of β-Lactam Antibiotics.
B. G. CHRISTENSEN and T. N. SALZMANN

Contents of Companion Volume 67, Part II

CHAPTER 1

History of β-Lactam Antibiotics

E. P. ABRAHAM

A. The Past Fifty Years

I. Fleming's Discovery

During the second half of the nineteenth century observations of the antagonism of fungi of the genus *Penicillium* to the growth of bacteria were recorded by JOHN TYNDALL, JOHN BURDON-SANDERSON, JOSEPH LISTER, T.H. HUXLEY, ERNEST DUCHESNE, who was a French medical student, and others. Whether any of these examples of microbial antagonism was due to the presence of penicillin is unknown. However that may be, they bore no fruit. It was not until 1929 that ALEXANDER FLEMING, in a paper from St. Mary's Hospital, London, introduced the term "penicillin" for an entity with well-defined antibacterial properties (FLEMING 1929).

While looking at plates that had been seeded with staphylococci and left on a laboratory bench during a vacation, Fleming noticed that one plate had been contaminated by a mold and that in the vicinity of this contaminant the bacteria were apparently undergoing lysis. He grew the mold *(Penicillium notatum)* in broth and showed that the resulting culture filtrate powerfully inhibited the growth of a number of gram-positive pathogenic bacteria and gram-negative cocci, but not that of gram-negative bacilli; and he decided to use the name penicillin for the more cumbersome phrase "mold broth filtrate."

The phenomenon seen by FLEMING is not easily reproducible in the laboratory, because penicillin brings about the lysis of growing staphylococci but not that of staphylococci in cultures that have reached the end of their growth. It appears that a period of cool weather allowed the *Penicillium* to form a large colony and produce penicillin before growth of the bacteria was completed as a result of a rise in the ambient temperature. FLEMING's great achievement lay in his flair for seizing on the unexpected, which he had revealed earlier in his discovery of lysozyme. He found that his penicillin was no more toxic than ordinary broth to a rabbit, a mouse, or the leukocyte and he tried it as a local antiseptic. But there is nothing to indicate that he ever envisaged that it could be injected into the blood stream to act as a chemotherapeutic agent in systemic infections. His interest focused on its use as a selective antibacterial agent in differential cultures.

FLEMING's two assistants, F. RIDLEY and S.R. CRADDOCK, prepared crude extracts of penicillin. In 1932 CLUTTERBUCK, LOVELL and RAISTRICK made an attempt to isolate penicillin, but abandoned it after finding that the antibacterial activity of the substance could readily be lost. Clearly no one imagined, at this time, that penicillin was of outstanding medical value. It must be remembered that the therapeutic properties of the sulfonamides were then unknown and that the possibility of finding chemical substances that could cope with bacterial septicaemia was viewed with pessismism. Nevertheless, when the successful use of prontosil and sulfanilamide was revealed in 1935, no interest in penicillin was rekindled.

II. Discovery of the Therapeutic Power of Penicillin in Systemic Infections

A second chapter in the history of penicillin began in 1938, when Professor H. W. FLOREY and Dr. E. B. CHAIN, in the Sir William Dunn School of Pathology at Oxford University, decided to make a systematic survey of the antibacterial substances known to be produced by microorganisms. This project was suggested by CHAIN during the course of discussions on these substances with FLOREY and it arose out of FLOREY's interest in lysozyme. It was motivated by scientific interest and not by the hope that such substances would prove to have medical value. Nevertheless, in 1939, after attempts to purify bactericidal substances produced by *P. notatum* and *Pseudomonas pyocyanea* had begun, the possibility that such substances might have clinical application was noted in a successful request to the Rockefeller Foundation for support.

The use of a solvent-transfer process for the purification of penicillin, suggested independently in Oxford by N. G. HEATLEY following its earlier unpublished use by L. B. HOLT at St. Mary's Hospital, led to the preparation of material that was not more than 1% pure. Between May and July 1940 FLOREY showed conclusively that this crude penicillin, given subcutaneously, could protect mice from otherwise fatal infections with the streptococcus or the staphylococcus. By this time, A. D. GARDNER, A. G. SANDERS, E. P. ABRAHAM and others had also begun to work on the penicillin project and a major effort was made to purify it further and produce enough material for a small clinical trial. The treatment in Oxford of five patients who were gravely ill with streptococcal or staphylococcal infections was carried out by FLOREY and C. M. FLETCHER early in 1941. The purity of the penicillin used varied from 0.3% to 7% and the supply was inadequate, even though it was supplemented by material recovered from the urine. Nevertheless, the results of this trial indicated that penicillin was not toxic to man and could control very severe infections.

III. Large-Scale Production

In view of the wartime situation in Britain FLOREY and HEATLEY went to the United States in June 1941, with FLEMING's strain of *P. notatum* and in the hope that penicillin could be made there in larger quantities. Their visit was facilitated by the Medical Research Council and supported by the Rockefeller Foundation. Work on penicillin at Columbia University was already being done by DAWSON, HOBBY, MEYER and CHAFFEE. At the Northern Regional Research Laboratory (NRRL) in Peoria Dr. COGHILL suggested that the use of deep fermentation, rather than stationary surface culture, might facilitate commercial production. A. J. MOYER, who worked with HEATLEY, introduced the use of corn-steep liquor (which contained phenylacetic acid) in the fermentation and this led to an increase in yield and to the production of benzylpenicillin (penicillin G) instead of the 2-pentenylpenicillin (penicillin F) produced in England. NRRL also became involved in a search for higher yielding cultures, organized by the Office of Production Research and Development of the War Production Board and examined samples from widespread sources. But one of the best isolates was a strain of *Penicillium chrysogenum* (NRRL 1951) from the stem of a cantaloupe found in Peoria itself. A succession of mutants was obtained from NRRL 1951 and led to the isolation at Madison, Wisconsin of strain Q176, which produced nearly 20 times as much penicillin as the parent in deep culture.

Before returning to England in September 1941 FLOREY saw a former acquaintance, Dr. A. N. RICHARDS, who had recently become Chairman of a Committee on Medical Research of the Office of Scientific Research and Development. Dr. RICHARDS decided to recommend the expenditure of American government money on the penicillin project and in October and December meetings were held, under the Chairmanship of Dr. VANNEVAR BUSH, at which representatives of pharmaceutical companies were present. Merck & Co, Inc., E. R. Squibb & Sons and Charles Pfizer & Co, Inc. were the first major companies to become involved. From December 1941 to June 1942 HEATLEY worked at Merck, where there had been some interest in penicillin before his arrival with FLOREY in the United States.

In 1942 penicillin was produced on a small scale by Imperial Chemical Industries Limited and by Kemball Bishop & Co. Ltd. in the United Kingdom and production was continued in Oxford. The British effort enabled enough crude penicillin to be obtained for FLOREY and ETHEL FLOREY to carry out a second clinical trial. In this, 15 cases were treated by systemic, and 172 by local application and further information was obtained about methods of administration and dosage of the drug. By 1943 supplies of penicillin had become sufficient for a small study to be made in North Africa of the use of penicillin in war surgery and in October the favorable results of this trial were made known by Professor FLOREY and Brigadier HUGH CAIRNS to the Medical Research Council.

During this time larger amounts of penicillin were becoming available in the United States, where clinical trials were carried out on a larger scale. These trials amply confirmed the earlier conclusions that penicillin was a substance of great value for the treatment of streptococcal and staphylococcal infections and showed that pneumococcal and gonococcal infections also responded to it. In addition they confirmed and extended previous observations on its absorption, excretion and destruction. In December 1943 American surgeons began a study of the treatment of war wounds with penicillin. At the time of the invasion of Normandy in 1944 enough penicillin was available to treat all British and American battle casualties. For this much credit was due to pharmaceutical companies in the United States, where deep fermentation in large tanks supplanted surface cultures.

IV. Wartime Interest in Penicillin in Europe and Japan

Accounts of the work at Oxford on penicillin appeared in *The Lancet* in 1940 and 1941. Although World War II had then begun, these publications became known in Germany and Switzerland in 1942 and an account of them reached Japan by submarine in 1943. In January 1944 the members of an Anglo-American Scientific Mission to Moscow were shown a penicillin-producing strain of *Penicillium* that had been recovered from a Moscow air raid shelter by Dr. KAPLAN, who was awarded a Stalin Prize for her discovery. Another strain which apparently produced penicillin was presented to the Mission at the Pasteur Institute in Teheran. Both fungi were identified later as *P. notatum*. However, despite this interest, substantial amounts of penicillin did not become available in Europe and Japan until after the war.

V. Isolation, Structure, and Synthesis

In parallel with wartime efforts to produce penicillin in large amounts by fermentation, which succeeded beyond all expectations, there developed a major project whose aim was the determination of the structure of penicillin and its production in quantity by total synthesis. CHAIN and ABRAHAM began attempts to purify penicillin in June 1940, using filtrates from surface cultures of FLEMING'S *P. notatum* which contained about 4 units per milliliter. The material obtained by solvent transfer was purified further by chromatography on alumina, which fortunately removed a pyrogenic impurity. This crude penicillin, which was used in the first clinical trial in 1941, had an activity of around 50 units per milligram and was about 3% pure. By 1942, the purity of the penicillin obtained had been increased to nearly 50%.

At this stage it was decided to begin chemical investigations. ABRAHAM and CHAIN then began a collaboration with Sir ROBERT ROBINSON and Dr. WILSON BAKER of the Dyson Perrins Laboratory, Oxford, and were later joined by Dr. J. W. CORNFORTH (now Sir JOHN CORNFORTH) and others. The penicillin was shown to be nitrogenous and to yield carbon dioxide on hydrolysis, but the presence of sulfur was at first missed, because the purified material was unaccountably reported by microanalysts to be sulfur-free. However, the isolation and properties of the characteristic degradation product, penicillamine, showed in July 1943 that this was a β-thiol-α-amino acid and its synthesis by CORNFORTH demonstrated that it was D-β-thiolvaline. In 1943 a further degradation product of penicillin, penilloaldehyde, was characterized in Oxford and at the Imperial College of Science in London. It then became clear that the removal of the elements of water from the thiazolidine formed by condensation of penicillamine with a β-aldehydocarboxylic acid would lead to the structure of the penicillin.

In October 1943 Sir ROBERT ROBINSON proposed a thiazolidine-oxalone structure while ABRAHAM, BAKER and CHAIN favored a β-lactam structure, partly because no basic nitrogen had been detected in the molecule. One-and-a-half years elapsed before the β-lactam structure was shown conclusively to be correct.

Because of the potential value of penicillin in war medicine and the possibility of producing it by chemical synthesis a ban on the publication of the results of chemical studies was imposed in the United Kingdom early in 1943. A similar ban operated in the United States and an agreement was made later in the year whereby the findings of British and American chemists were transmitted to each other trough the Medical Research Council in London and the Committee on Medical Research in Washington. The first reports reached their respective destinations early in 1944. They made it clear that some of the findings in England during 1943 had been duplicated independently in the United States and that the American penicillin contained sulfur but differed from the British product in having a benzyl group instead of a 2-pentenyl group in its side chain. Before this, in August 1943, the Medical Research Council had been notified by telegram that the sodium salt of penicillin had been crystallized by MACPHILLAMY and WINTERSTEINER at Squibb. Penicillin had been purified at Oxford as a barium salt, but on receipt of the telegram it was converted to a sodium salt and the latter was found to crystallize spontaneously.

The wartime chemical research on the degradation and synthesis of penicillin developed into a great Anglo-American enterprise in which hundreds of chemists in more than 30 major institutions were involved. Degradation and transformation products were obtained which pointed in some cases to a thiazolidine-oxazolone and in others to a β-lactam structure. By the end of 1944 R. B. Woodward had reached the conclusion that only the β-lactam structure was consistent with the properties of penicillin and had provided a rational explanation for the reactivity of its β-lactam ring. But it was not until May 1945, when DOROTHY (CROWFOOT) HODGKIN and BARBARA LOW completed a successful x-ray crystallographic analysis, that the β-lactam structure was shown beyond question to be correct.

Between 1944 and January 1, 1946, when the official ban on publication was lifted, great efforts to synthesize penicillin were made on both sides of the Atlantic. In many cases the procedures were designed to produce the thiazolidine-oxazolone structure and expectations were at first high. Trace amounts of antibacterial activity which were undoubtedly due to penicillin were obtained on several occasions, but nothing approaching a satisfactory synthesis was ever achieved. With the end of the war the great Anglo-American collaborative enterprise came to an end and for some years it seemed that attempts to devise a rational synthesis of penicillin had been abandoned.

In the early 1950s the challenge presented by the fused β-lactam-thiazolidine structure to synthetic organic chemists was taken up by JOHN SHEEHAN and his colleagues at the Massachusetts Institute of Technology. By the avoidance of conditions which might favor cyclization to an oxazolone and by the introduction of carbodiimides for the formation of peptide bonds, phenoxymethylpenicillin and the nucleus of the penicillin molecule, 6-aminopenicillanic acid (6-APA), were synthesized in a rational manner. Nevertheless, the production of penicillin by fermentation had by then become so efficient that total chemical synthesis remained commercially unattractive.

VI. Penicillin-Resistant Bacteria

FLEMING had recorded the selective action of his penicillin which showed only low activity against gram-negative bacilli. The later discovery of the difference between penicillin F (2-pentenylpenicillin) and penicillin G (benzylpenicillin) was followed by the finding of penicillins with related side chains, and a systematic study by O. K. BEHRENS and his colleagues showed that a variety of monosubstituted acetic acids, in which the substituent contained no ionizable group, could function as side-chain precursors in *P. notatum*. None of the resulting penicillins were markedly superior to benzylpenicillin in their antibacterial activities, although it was shown in 1954 that phenoxymethylpenicillin (penicillin V) was relatively stable in dilute acid and was well absorbed when given by mouth.

By this time a serious addition to the limitations of benzylpenicillin had become evident. In 1940 the first penicillinase had been discovered in *Escherichia coli* by ABRAHAM and CHAIN, who suggested that it was one cause of bacterial resistance. For some years afterwards the staphylococci commonly encountered in patients were penicillin sensitive. But penicillinase-producing strains of staphylococci, which were resistant to benzylpenicillin and had grown while sensitive strains were suppressed, then became prevalent in hospitals. Later, the resistance of penicillinase-producing gram-negative bacteria became a problem of increasing importance.

During the 1950s, however, two events provided the starting points for developments which were to greatly improve the outlook for the usefulness of β-lactam antibiotics in medicine. One was the discovery of methods for obtaining 6-APA in quantity and the other was the discovery of cephalosporin C and its nucleus, 7-aminocephalosporanic acid (7-ACA).

VII. 6-Aminopenicillanic Acid and New Penicillins

The suggestion that the penicillin nucleus was present in fermentations of *P. chrysogenum* was made in 1953 in Japan by K. KATO, who found that culture fluids gave higher values for penicillin in a chemical assay than would have been expected on the basis of their antibacterial activities. Three years earlier K. SAKAGUCHI and S. MURAO had reported that an amidase produced by *P. chrysogenum* removed the *N*-acyl side-chain from penicillin to yield its nucleus. These reported findings were not explored further at the time, but in 1956 observations similar to those of KATO were made independently by two members of the Beecham Laboratories. G. N. ROLINSON and F. R. BATCHELOR had been sent by Beecham to work on *p*-aminobenzylpenicillin in the International Research Centre of Chemical Microbiology at the Istituto Superiore di Sanita in Rome, of which CHAIN had become the Director in 1948. They found that the discrepancy between the results of chemical and antibacterial assays was most obvious with fermentations to which no side-chain precursor had been added. On their return to England they collaborated with F. P. DOYLE and J. H. C. NAYLER. It was then shown, in May 1957, that a compound was present in the fermentation fluids which behaved like 6-APA, since it could be acylated to yield benzylpenicillin. Early in 1958, 6-APA was isolated in crystalline form.

The production of 6-APA in quantity, which was subsequently carried out by the use of bacterial acylases to remove the side chain of benzylpenicillin, opened the way to the semisynthesis of a series of new penicillins that could not be obtained by fermentation. Among them were methicillin, which was resistant to staphylococcal penicillinase; ampicillin, which had a higher activity than benzylpenicillin against a variety of gram-negative organisms; and carbenicillin, whose range of useful activity included strains of *Pseudomonas aeruginosa*.

VIII. 7-Aminocephalosporanic Acid and the Cephalosporins

Cephalosporin C was discovered by G. G. F. NEWTON and E. P. ABRAHAM in 1953, while they were studying the antibiotics of a strain of *Cephalosporium acremonium* that had been isolated by Professor GUISEPPE BROTZU from the sea near a sewage outfall at Cagliari in Sardinia. The first substances isolated in Oxford from culture fluids of this organism were acidic steroids which showed significant activity only against gram-positive bacteria and differed in this respect from BROTZU's crude material. These substances were named collectively cephalosporin P. A search for a second antibiotic revealed a hydrophilic substance which had activity against gram-negative as well as gram-positive bacteria and was named cephalosporin N. This substance was undoubtedly the antibiotic whose activity had been observed by BROTZU. It was shown to be a new penicillin with a δ-(D-α-aminoadipyl) side chain. The free amino group in its side chain was associated with its broad range of activity, because acylation of this group resulted in a decrease in activity against gram-negative bacteria but an increase in activity against gram-positive organisms. Like benzylpenicillin, however, it was readily hydrolyzed by penicillinase.

Because penicillin N was difficult to purify a partially purified preparation of the antibiotic was transformed into its isomeric penillic acid with a view to conforming its apparent molecular formula. Chromatography of the penillic acid revealed the presence of a small amount of a second compound with an absorption maximum in UV light at 260 nm. This compound, named cephalosporin C, was the first of the cephalosporins as they are known today. It was soon found to resemble penicillin N in containing sulfur, a δ-(D-α-aminoadipyl) side chain, and apparently a β-lactam ring, but it clearly did not have the characteristic thiazolidine-β-lactam ring system of the penicillins. Its antibacterial activity was low and similar in range to that of penicillin N, but, unlike the latter, it was not hydrolyzed by a penicillinase. These properties gave it a potential clinical interest.

The amount of cephalosporin C that was first isolated was extremely small, but somewhat larger quantities became available when a higher yielding mutant of the wild strain of *C. acremonium* was isolated in an Antibiotics Research Station of the Medical Research Council at Clevedon, near Bristol, which was under the direction of Mr. B. K. KELLY. The results of chemical degradations and physicochemical studies led Abraham and Newton to propose a fused β-lactam-dihydrothiazine structure for the molecule in 1959 and this structure was soon confirmed by an x-ray crystallographic analysis by Professor DOROTHY HODGKIN and Dr. E. N. MASLEN.

In the meantime FLOREY had demonstrated that cephalosporin C showed an even lower acute toxicity to mice than benzylpenicillin and that it could protect mice from infections with penicillinase-producing staphylococci that did not respond to penicillin. Cephalosporin C might well have been used clinically for the treatment of such infections had not methicillin been produced in 1960 from 6-APA in the Beecham Laboratories. This semisynthetic penicillin was more active than cephalosporin C against the staphylococcus in vitro and proved to be effective in patients.

Analogy with penicillin N and other penicillins indicated that more active cephalosporins might be obtained by exchanging the α-aminoadipyl side chain of cephalosporin C for other side chains. Moreover, the finding that the dihydrothiazine ring of cephalosporin C had an acetoxymethyl substituent at C-3 whose acetoxy group could readily be displaced by nucleophiles to yield compounds with significantly different activities suggested that the effects of changes in this part of the molecule could profitably be studied further. In 1960 P. B. Loder, Newton, and Abraham obtained small amounts of 7-ACA by acid hydrolysis of cephalosporin C under controlled conditions. They then confirmed the expectation that a penicillinase-resistant cephalosporin with high activity, at least against gram-positive bacteria, would be obtained from 7-ACA by acylation with substances such as phenylacetyl chloride. However, a method for the production of 7-ACA in much higher yield was required before the potential value of this compound as a source of semisynthetic cephalosporins could be adequately explored.

Before this, two pharmaceutical companies, Glaxo in the United Kingdom and Eli Lilly in the United States, had become seriously interested in the cephalosporin problem. Patents arising from work in Oxford and at Clevedon were assigned to the National Research Development Corporation (NRDC), which had been set up by the British Government after the war to foster the development of inventions in the national interest. By the end of 1961 the NRDC had negotiated agreements relating to the cephalosporins with five companies in the United States, with two in Europe and with one in Japan, as well as with Glaxo.

Although extensive searches were made for an enzyme that would remove the α-aminoadipyl side chain from cephalosporin C, no such enzyme was found. But a chemical procedure by which the side chain could be removed to produce 7-ACA in good yield was discovered in 1962 by Morin and his colleagues in the Lilly Research Laboratories and subsequently an improved procedure was devised at Ciba-Geigy. This enabled the properties of large numbers of different cephalosporins to be evaluated. In 1964 cephalothin and cephaloridine were introduced into medicine and were followed by cefazolin. These antibiotics were active against the penicillinase-producing staphylococcus and, unlike methicillin, they also showed significant activity against a number of gram-negative bacilli.

A further major advance in the cephalosporin field, which came from the Lilly Research Laboratories in 1963, was the chemical conversion of a penicillin sulfoxide to a deacetoxycephalosporin. All the early cephalosporins had failed to be adsorbed from the gut, despite their relative acid stability. But the deacetoxycephalosporin, cephalexin, with a D-phenylglycyl side chain, proved, unpredictably, to be effective when given by mouth.

At the beginning of the 1970s reports appeared from the Lilly and Merck laboratories that certain species of *Streptomyces* produced 7α-methoxycephalosporins (cephamycins). The presence of a 7α-methoxy group in the cephalosporin (cephem) ring system was found to be associated with an unusually high resistance to many β-lactamases and chemical methods for the attachment of this group to the β-lactam ring were then devised.

In 1970, more than 10 years after the first total synthesis of phenoxymethylpenicillin by John Sheehan, a remarkable total synthesis of cephalosporin C was accomplished by R. B. Woodward and his colleagues at Harvard and at the Woodward Institute in Basel. This was followed by other syntheses, in the Merck and the Smith Kline and French laboratories, of nuclear analogues of the cephalosporins in which sulfur was replaced by oxygen or CH_2, or in which sulfur was moved to a different position in the dihydrothiazine ring. Later, a synthesis of 7α-methoxy-1-oxacephems from penicillins was achieved in the Shionogi Research Laboratory. The properties of these synthetic compounds showed that the sulfur atom in the cephalosporin ring system was not a unique requirement for high antibacterial activity.

IX. New β-Lactam Compounds

Screening of strains of *Streptomyces* spp. for inhibitors of β-lactamases, and for β-lactam antibiotics that might be revealed by the use of supersensitive strains of *E. coli* and *P. aeruginosa* as test organisms, led to the discovery of further β-lactam compounds that were neither penicillins nor cephalosporins. They included the β-lactamase inhibitors, clavulanic acid and olivanic acid, from the Beecham laboratories, a monocyclic β-lactam, nocardicin, from the Fujisawa Pharmaceutical Company and a highly active β-lactamase-resistant antibiotic, thienamycin, from Merck. Following the discovery of these compounds a new monocyclic β-lactam antibiotic, sulfazecin, was obtained in Takeda Chemical Industries from a bacterium of the genus *Pseudomonas*. This substance and several related antibiotics were also obtained from cultures of a variety of bacteria at the Squibb Institute for Medical Research and were named monobactams. Members of the monobactam family can be obtained in good yield by chemical synthesis. In addition R. B. WOODWARD and his colleagues synthesized active penems, which shared features of the penicillin (penam) and the cephalosporin (cephem) ring systems respectively.

X. Biosynthesis

The production and testing of many thousands of semisynthetic β-lactam antibiotics during the last 20 years has been accompanied by a growing body of research on the biosynthesis of the naturally occurring β-lactam antibiotics, on β-lactamases and on the enzymes with which the β-lactam antibiotics react in bacterial cell membranes.

The early work on side-chain precursors of the classic penicillins produced by *Penicillium* spp. indicated that the incorporation of the side-chain was catalyzed by an enzyme that would accept a limited number of different but chemically related substrates. Sir ROBERT ROBINSON stated later that the formation of the penicillin ring system from cysteine and valine had always been sun-clear, but it was largely the work of H. R. V. ARNSTEIN and his colleagues in the 1950 s that established experimentally the nature of the amino acid precursors. They also showed that a tripeptide, δ-(α-aminoadipyl)cysteinylvaline, was present in the mycelium of *P. chrysogenum* and suggested that it was a precursor of penicillin N. In later studies at Oxford we found this peptide in *Cephalosporium* and showed that it had the LLD configuration and was incorporated intact by cell-free extracts into a penicillin. We and DEMAIN'S group at MIT then found independently that the penicillin was isopenicillin N. The latter penicillin, with an L-α-aminoadipyl side chain, had been discovered in *P. chrysogenum* in 1962 and 1963 in the Lilly and Beecham laboratories.

By the end of the 1970s contributions to our present knowledge of the interrelated pathways of penicillin and cephalosporin biosynthesis had come from biochemical and genetic researches in laboratories at many institutions, including MIT, Ciba-Geigy, Eli Lilly, Glaxo, Takeda, and the Universities of Oxford and Wisconsin. The results of studies with mutants of antibiotic-producing organisms and with cell-free systems indicated that both penicillins and cephalosporins were derived from the same tripeptide and that isopenicillin N had a central rôle, being a precursor of penicillin N and cephalosporins in the *Cephalosporium* and *Streptomyces* spp. and of the classic penicillins in *P. chrysogenum*. A. L. DEMAIN and J. E. BALDWIN and their colleagues first demonstrated a biochemical conversion of penicillin N into deacetoxycephalosporin C.

XI. Mode of Action and Resistance

FLEMING'S observation of the bactericidal effect of penicillin was confirmed and extended by G. L. HOBBY, K. MEYER, and M. H. DAWSON in 1942. Before that, A. D. GARDNER had reported that striking morphological changes occurred in bacteria grown in the presence of subinhibitory concentrations of the antibiotic. By 1946 it was widely accepted that both the bactericidal and lytic effects of penicillin were dependent on the ability of the cells to grow. In 1949 P. D. COOPER and D. ROWLEY showed that small amounts of penicillin were bound irreversibly by sensitive bacteria. In 1956 JOSHUA LEDERBERG demonstrated that rod-shaped *E. coli* growing in a hypertonic medium in the presence of penicillin were converted into spherical protoplasts and he concluded that the antibiotic interfered with the biosynthesis of bacterial cell walls. Twenty years later work by A. TOMASZ indicated that the action of bacterial enzymes able to hydrolyze the cell wall could contribute to the bactericidal and bacteriolytic effects of penicillin.

Towards the end of the 1940s J. T. PARK began a study of the biochemical consequences of the antibacterial action of penicillin, and in 1965 E. M. WISE and PARK and D. J. TIPPER and J. L. STROMINGER showed that the antibiotic inhibited the cross-linking of peptidoglycan strands which normally occurred during wall synthesis. TIPPER and STROMINGER then proposed that penicillin reacted with a transpeptidase to form a penicilloyl derivative because of its structural resemblance to one of the conformations of the terminal *N*-acyl-D-alanyl-D-alanine portion of the natural substrate for the enzyme. During the following decade, investigations by STROMINGER, J. M. GHUYSEN, B. G. SPRATT and others showed that families of enzymes that are inactivated by β-lactam antibiotics occur in the cell membranes of prokaryotes and that inactivation of different members of a family may have different morphological consequences.

Penicillinase was at first regarded as a single enzyme, but with the advent of cephalosporin C and then of the semisynthetic penicillins and cephalosporins it became evident that there were many enzymes of this type, distinguishable from each other by their substrate profiles. All these enzymes catalyzed the hydrolysis of a β-lactam ring and thus they became known as β-lactamases. Evidence accumulated for their widespread importance among the factors determining bacterial resistance to β-lactam antibiotics.

Some of the early contributions to our knowledge of the production and properties of the inducible and constitutive β-lactamases from *Bacillus cereus* and the inducible enzyme from *Bacillus licheniformis* were made in the 1950s by MARTIN POLLOCK at the National Institute for Medical Research in the United Kingdom. Subsequent studies of the staphyloccal β-lactamase by M. H. RICHMOND and R. P. NOVICK showed that this enzyme was the product of a gene carried on a plasmid. Between 1960 and 1980 extensive investigations were made of cell-bound β-lactamases mediated by genes in R-plasmids that could be transferred from one gram-negative bacterium to another by conjugation, and by genes forming part of a transposon that could move from one plasmid to another.

A number of β-lactamases were isolated in a virtually homogeneous form and a study of their amino acid sequences was begun by R. P. AMBLER. In four different β-lactamases the sequences were so similar that these enzymes could be assumed to have evolved from a single ancestral gene. On the other hand, a zinc-requiring β-lactamase from *B. cereus*, characterized by SABATH and ABRAHAM in 1966, appeared to be an enzyme of a different class.

Our finding in 1956 that cephalosporin C inhibited the hydrolysis of benzylpenicillin by β-lactamase I from *B. cereus* was the first example of the ability of certain β-lactam antibiotics to act as competitive inhibitors of β-lactamases for which they are poor substrates. This led to the suggestion that synergism between such inhibitors and other β-lactam antibiotics against β-lactamase-producing organisms might have practical application. In 1962 we observed that certain β-lactam antibiotics brought about the inactivation of certain β-lactamases while the antibiotics were undergoing hydrolysis. More recently substances such as clavulanic acid have proved to be powerful inactivators and synergistic agents. A partial understanding of the mechanisms by which such suicide phenomena may occur has come from the work of S. G. WALEY, PRATT and LOOSEMORE, J. R. KNOWLES and others, and it has been established that some β-lactamases, at least, contain an active serine residue with which a β-lactam substrate reacts to yield an acyl-enzyme intermediate.

The earlier finding that penicillin reacted with a serine residue in a penicillin-sensitive membrane enzyme and the reported homology between the amino sequences of membrane enzymes and β-lactamases gave support to the suggestion that these two groups of enzymes had an evolutionary relationship.

B. The Future

The development of the β-lactam antibiotics could not have been envisaged by FLEMING in 1929, or by FLOREY and CHAIN when they initiated a further study of penicillin 10 years later. Even in 1940 FLEMING wrote, "Penicillin has not yet been tried in war surgery and it will not be tried until some chemist comes along and finds out what it is and if possible manufactures it." In the event it was the microbiologists who were largely responsible for transforming what at that time seemed to be an almost impossible project – the economic production of penicillin by fermentation on a large scale.

With this lesson from the past, it would be hazardous to predict the future. The one thing that is virtually certain is that growth in this field has not come to an end, as it appeared to have done for some years after World War II. The outstanding clinical value of non-toxic β-lactam antibiotics, together with their limitations in the face of changing patterns of bacterial resistance, provided a powerful incentive to continued research. This incentive remains. And the scientific interest of problems relating to the biosynthesis and mode of action of such substances should alone continue to stimulate many investigators. But it is scarcely possible to say whether future generations of β-lactam antibiotics will be notable for compounds with ever wider ranges of activity or for compounds with high activity against selected organisms, and whether synergistic mixtures will become more important in chemotherapy than they have been hitherto.

In the past, acute and fortunate observations, sometimes but not always made in the course of systematic screening programmes, provided leads from which new penicillins and cephalosporins emerged. Screening for compounds with new properties, and the use of more sensitive methods of detection, later revealed β-lactams of new types. In consequence, almost the sole common feature in the range of known β-lactams with potential medical value is the presence of a β-lactam ring. There is no reason to believe that further β-lactams with new biological properties will not be discovered by such procedures. Moreover, a knowledge of the nature and location of the DNA required for the biosynthesis of β-lactam antibiotics and the use of new genetic techniques that are more sophisticated than mutagenesis could lead eventually to the production by eukaryotic and prokaryotic microorganisms of substances that cannot now be obtained by fermentation. The use of bacteria as producing organisms has become a possibility. Further understanding of the mechanisms by which biosynthesis is controlled could lead to further increases in efficiency. Immobilized cell-free enzymes could also find increasing application.

It was the determination of the structure of β-lactam compounds obtained by fermentation and the achievements of synthetic organic chemists that enabled the discoveries of these compounds to bear such remarkable fruit. Total chemical syntheses of useful β-lactam antibiotics, although outstanding academic achievements, showed little sign of being economically competitive, although semisynthesis from natural products proved to be highly rewarding. But, with the increasing opportunities provided by new knowledge of the structural features which allow a compound containing a β-lactam to show high biological activity, total chemical synthesis may sometimes become commercially feasible. Furthermore, it is conceivable that the highly efficient mechanisms by which the biosynthesis of β-lactam compounds is accomplished in microorganisms will be understood at the molecular level within the next 30 years and will suggest new chemical approaches to synthetic problems.

Unlike screening programmes, in which compounds produced by microorganisms are first revealed by their biological activity, chemical syntheses produce compounds whose activities are only known after the synthesis is complete. The possession of a β-lactam ring that is reactive, but not so reactive that the compound containing it is highly unstable and nonspecific in its effect on living cells, is only one of many properties required of valuable β-lactam antibiotics. One impediment to our understanding of this complex situation is a lack of knowledge of the three-dimensional structures of the active sites in the families of enzymes which inactivate, or are inactivated by, the antibiotics of this group.

Several β-lactamases are now being studied by x-ray crystallography. The structures of one or more of them may be known within the next decade and it is reasonable to hope that the structures of some of the penicillin-binding enzymes of bacterial membranes will be determined within the foreseeable future. In that event, a step will have been taken towards the rational design of β-lactam antibiotics. But further knowledge of the factors that govern the penetration of such antibiotics to the active sites in bacterial cell membranes will be needed before their activities in vitro can be predicted with confidence. And much more must be learned about the mechanisms of absorption, distribution, and excretion of these antibiotics in the patient before predictions can be extended with confidence to their behavior in vivo.

References

Abraham EP (1949) The chemistry of penicillin. Historical introduction. In: Antibiotics, vol 2, Chapter 20. Oxford Univ Press, Oxford, pp 768–784

Abraham EP (1977) β-Lactam antibiotics and related substances. J Antibiotics [Suppl] 30:1–36

Abraham EP (1979) A glimpse of the early history of the cephalosporins. Rev Infect Dis 1:99–105

Abraham EP, Loder PB (1972) Cephalosporin C. In: Flynn EH (ed) Cephalosporins and penicillins chemistry and biology, Chapter 1. Academic Press, London New York, pp 1–24

Abraham EP, Chain E, Fletcher CM, Florey HW, Gardner AD, Heatley NG, Jennings MA (1941) Further observations on penicillin. Lancet II:177–211

Abraham EP, Baker W, Chain E, Robinson R (1949a) Chemical nature of 2-pentenyl penicillin. In: Clarke HT, Johnson JR, Robinson R (eds) The chemistry of penicillin. Princeton Univ Press, Princeton, pp 11–34

Abraham EP, Chain E, Florey HW, Florey ME, Heatley NG, Jennings MA, Sanders AG (1949b) Penicillin. Historical introduction. In: Antibiotics, vol 2, Chapter 15. Oxford Univ Press, Oxford, pp 631–671

Baddiley J, Abraham EP (Organisers) (1980) Penicillin fifty years after penicillin. A Royal Society discussion. The Royal Society, London

Batchelor FR, Doyle FP, Nayler JHC, Rolinson GN (1959) Synthesis of penicillin: 6-aminopenicillanic acid in penicillin fermentations. Nature 183:257–258

Clarke HT, Johnson JR, Robinson R (1949) Brief history of the chemical study of penicillin. In: Clarke HT, Johnson JR, Robinson R (eds) The chemistry of penicillin. Princeton Univ Press, Princeton, pp 3–9

Fleming A (1929) On the antibacterial action of cultures of a penicillium, with special reference to their use in the isolation of *B. influenzae*. Br. J Exp Pathol 10:226–236

Hamilton-Miller JMT, Smith JT (eds) (1979) Beta-lactamases. Academic Press, London New York

Hare R (1970) The birth of penicillin. Allen & Unwin, London

Helfand WH, Woodruff HB, Coleman KMH, Cowen DL (1980) Wartime industrial development of penicillin in the United States. In: Parascandola J (ed) The history of antibiotics a symposium. American Institute of Pharmacy, Madison, Wisconsin, pp 31–56

Hopwood DA, Merrick MJ (1977) Genetics of antibiotic production. Bacteriol Rev 41:595–635

O'Callaghan CH (1975) Description and classification of the newer cephalosporins and their relationship with the established compounds. J Antimicrob Chemother 5:655–671

Park JT, Strominger JL (1957) Mode of action of penicillin. Biochemical basis for the mechanism of action and for its selective toxicity. Science 125:99–101

Selwyn S (1979) Pioneer work on the "Penicillin phenomenon" 1870–1876. J Antimicrob Chemother 5:249–255

Sheehan JC, Henery-Logan KR (1959) The total synthesis of penicillin V. J Am Chem Soc 81:3089–3094

Spratt BG (1977) Penicillin-binding proteins of *E. coli:* General properties and characterisation of mutants. In: Schlessinger D (ed) Microbiology. American Society for Microbiology, Washington D.C., pp 209–215

Woodward RB, Heusler K, Gosteli J, Naegeli P, Oppolzer W, Ramage R, Ranganathan S, Vorgrüggen H (1966) The total synthesis of cephalosporin C. J Am Chem Soc 88:852–853

CHAPTER 2

Mode of Action of β-Lactam Antibiotics – A Microbiologist's View

A. TOMASZ

A. Introduction

I. Mode of Action Studies: Benefits for Basic and Applied Sciences

Curiosity about how and why certain substances are toxic to man or microbes has traditionally been one of the major guiding forces of biological research, and it would be easy to document how much of our basic understanding of biochemical mechanisms, cell structure and physiology has been generated in the context of drug mode-of-action studies. This remains true for many contemporary branches of biology, and particularly so in the case of the β-lactam antibiotics. While the academically oriented scientist has benefited tremendously from the availability of various β-lactams, the clinician or pharmaceutical chemist interested in developing new antibiotics of improved efficacy against disease-causing microbes has received relatively little benefit from mode-of-action studies. In fact, until recently, most of the new β-lactams with improved spectrum and biological activity were developed more or less by trial and error using bacterial minimal inhibitory concentration (MIC) values as the main criteria of evaluation. It seems, however, that this area is headed for change. During the past five to seven years, mode-of-action studies began producing information that has the potential to be translated into practical use for more selective screening and perhaps eventually for more rational drug design. The tremendous revival of interest in these antibiotics during the past few years documents this recognition.

Indeed, interesting discoveries have been made in virtually every aspect of this field. Use of more sophisticated screening methods led to the isolation of β-lactams of novel chemical structure – and novel antibacterial properties – such as the thienamycins (ALBERS-SCHONBERG et al. 1978) and the monocyclic β-lactams (monobactams) (IMADA et al. 1981; SYKES et al. 1981 b). Of particular interest is the fact that the latter compounds are produced by eubacteria.

Major advances were made concerning the permeability barrier function of the gram-negative outer membrane and the role of porins in the uptake of β-lactam antibiotics (NIKAIDO 1981). The proposal that β-lactams are active site-directed acylating agents received striking support from the demonstration that penicillin and a model natural substrate both acylated a serine residue within the same polypeptide chain (YOCUM et al. 1979; WAXMAN and STROMINGER 1980). Much detailed information about the nature of antibiotic and substrate binding sites should be available soon, now that crystallization of several carboxypeptidases has been reported (KNOX et al. 1979; DIDEBERG et al. 1979).

A further development of major importance was the introduction of SDS-gel electrophoresis and labeling with radioactive penicillin for the identification of penicillin binding proteins (PBPs) (SPRATT 1975). Perhaps the most important aspect of the introduction of this rapid and sensitive method has been that it opened the field of cell wall synthesis for genetic investigation. The combination of the technique of PBP labeling with genetic and morphological methods has been primarily responsible for the recognition that bacteria contain multiple target proteins for β-lactam antibiotics; furthermore, these proteins were shown to perform distinct physiological functions and have selective affinities for β-lactams of varying chemical structure. Finally, a variety of different types of experiments indicated that the ultimate physiological consequences of β-lactam action – namely, the inhibition of bacterial growth and cell division, and dissolution of the bacterial cell – are often only indirectly related to the biochemical interference with cell wall synthesis (TOMASZ 1979a, b). In addition, these antibacterial effects may depend on bacterial factors that do not directly react with the penicillin molecule (e.g., autolytic enzymes) and these effects can be modulated by factors in the bacterial environment (TOMASZ et al. 1979).

II. Mode of Action of Penicillin: A Multilevel Problem

A full understanding of the mode of action of any drug requires clarification of all levels of interaction between the drug molecules and the target cell. This includes: (1) elucidation of the pathway by which the drug molecule reaches its biochemical target(s); (2) identification of the biochemical target(s); (3) recognition of the cell's physiological response to the inhibition of the drug-sensitive reaction; (4) an understanding of exactly how and why inhibition of the target reaction leads to inhibition of the whole cell; and finally, (5) in the case of β-lactam antibiotics, one also has to reconsider some of these questions as a function of the environment of the target bacterium, particularly in the complex milieu of an invaded host, since it has been shown that the chemical and physical nature of the bacterial medium can profoundly influence the outcome of the encounter between the antibiotic and the target cell.

The structure of this review will roughly follow these five levels of discussion. No attempt is made to give a lexically complete account of the activities in any one area of this enormous and rapidly growing field. Instead, I shall try to provide an overview of how the different levels of interactions between the bacterium and the penicillin molecule interlock to give a complex multistep inhibitory pathway that begins with the penetration of the bacterial surface by the drug molecules, followed by their attachment to the membrane-bound PBPs, and the metabolic disturbances that, ultimately, lead to the halt of growth, then death and dissolution of the bacterial cell. One purpose of this review is to illustrate the gradually increasing complexity of drug action as one moves from target enzyme to target cell, and from target cell in a culture tube to target pathogen in the complex environment of an infected host.

β-Lactamases, despite their obvious importance, will not be discussed since recent reviews cover advances in this field (see Chap. 12; AMBLER 1980; FISCHER et al. 1980). More specific details of various aspects of the mode of action of penicillin have also been published in reviews recently: on the biochemistry of penicillin binding proteins (YOCUM et al. 1980b; SPRATT 1979); on the enzymology of penicillin sensitive enzymes (GHUYSEN et al. 1981); several genetic and biochemical studies on the penicillin binding proteins (YOCUM et al. 1980b; SPRATT 1979; SUZUKI et al. 1978); the mechanism of β-lactam penetration through the gram-negative outer membrane (NIKAIDO 1981); and various findings and ideas concerning the mechanism of the cell physiological effects of β-lactams (TOMASZ 1979a, b; SHOCKMAN et al. 1981).

B. Journey of the Extracellular Antibiotic to the Intracellular Targets

I. Extracellular Barriers

The biochemical targets of β-lactam molecules are located on the plasma membrane and, depending on the particular bacterium and on its special environment, the antibiotic molecules have to traverse a variety of chemical and/or physical barriers en route to their targets.

Several pathogenic microorganisms (e.g., *Chlamydia*, *Listera* or *Legionella*) multiply intracellularly in their natural hosts. Little is known about the permeability properties of eucaryotic membranes to β-lactam antibiotics. Some data indicate that lysosomal membranes are impermeable to penicillin (BROWN and PERCIVAL 1978; VEALE et al. 1976).

The mucous polysaccharide capsules or matrices produced by many pathogenic bacteria may present a chemical barrier to the diffusion of β-lactams, particularly in the cases of antibiotics carrying a net charge, since many of these extracellular polysaccharides are anionic. The resistance to carbenicillin or flucloxacillin demonstrated by mucoid strains of *Pseudomonas aeruginosa* isolated from cystic fibrosis patients was attributed in part to such an entrapment of the antibiotic molecules (GOVAN 1975; COSTERTON 1979). No clear evidence exists concerning other bacterial capsules. It should be remembered, as pointed out by NIKAIDO (1981), that any such structure, be it capsule, murein or outer membrane, and irrespective of its particular chemistry, is expected to decrease tremendously the free diffusion rate of solutes (e.g., the permeability coefficient for cephaloridine, a compound capable of most rapidly penetrating the *Escherichia coli* outer membrane, was calculated to be 4×10^{-4} cm/s, i.e., almost 10^4-fold lower than the free diffusion coefficient for the same compound). Whether or not such barriers actually influence the antibacterial effectiveness (MIC) depends largely on the fate of the antibiotic molecule after it has passed these barriers (NIKAIDO 1981).

II. Barriers in the Bacterial Envelope

The penetration of the bacterial surface by β-lactam molecules does not seem to involve active transport, and the various surface structures of bacteria may present barriers to the free diffusion of the antibiotic molecules. The inner and outer forespore membranes of sporulating *Bacillus subtilis* or *Bacillus megaterium* were claimed to partially hinder the access of radioactive penicillin to the penicillin-binding proteins (PBPs) (Lawrence and Strominger 1970). Little information is available about the possible barrier function of the cell walls of gram-positive bacteria. Generally, the more lipophilic β-lactams were found to have lower MIC values in lactamase-negative staphylococci (Smith et al. 1969). The possibility that the high cephalosporin MIC values in most strains of *Streptococcus faecalis* and *Streptococcus faecium* (Williamson et al. 1980a) and the high methicillin MIC in intrinsically resistant *Staphylococcus aureus* (Hartman and Tomasz 1980) might be due to a permeability barrier in the cell walls of these bacteria was tested with negative results. In these studies, live cells and equivalent numbers of protoplasts prepared from the same cells (by a rapid enzymatic method) were compared in PBP competition assays using cephalothin and tritium-labeled penicillin as the reagent. Identical titration profiles were obtained in both cells and protoplasts and the same very high concentrations ($> 100\ \mu g/ml$) of cephalothin and/or methicillin were necessary to achieve saturation of the relevant PBPs.

The gram-positive cell wall is composed of as many as 50–100 molecular sheets of peptidoglycan which often contain anionic polymers, such as teichoic acids; some entrapment of β-lactam molecules in such a structure would not be surprising. Nevertheless, a report describing some evidence for this in *B. megaterium* appeared only recently (Reynolds and Chase 1981).

III. The Outer Membrane of Gram-Negative Bacteria

Extensive studies performed mainly with *E. coli*, *Salmonella*, *Neisseria gonorrhoeae*, and *Pseudomonas aeruginosa* (Nikaido and Nakae 1979; Nikaido 1979; Nakae 1976; Hancock and Nikaido 1978) clearly indicate that the outer membrane of gram-negative bacteria may present a barrier to the diffusion of β-lactam antibiotics so that this effect may appear as a major determinant of the antibacterial effectiveness (MIC value). An accurate method for the measurement of diffusion rates has been developed by introducing a plasmid-borne β-lactamase into the bacterial strains to be assayed. As long as the lactamase molecules remain located in the periplasmic space (i.e., the cells are not "leaky"), the in vivo rate of hydrolysis of various β-lactams may be used to calculate the rate of diffusion of these molecules through the outer membrane (Zimmerman and Rosselet 1977). Such measurements and in vitro assays of β-lactam penetration into artificial vesicles has allowed the establishment of some of the correlates between antibiotic structure and penetration rates (Nakae and Nikaido 1975).

There seem to be two major routes available for the penetration through the gram-negative outer membrane: direct dissolution in the lipid phase of the membrane, or diffusion through the water-filled holes composed of aggregates of a special group of membrane proteins called porins (Nakae and Nikaido 1975; Nixdorff et al. 1977). This class of protein molecules (molecular mass: 34,000–38,000) forms channels of varying diameter (about 1.2 nm in *E. coli*) across the outer membrane, with a water-filled luminal space. Mutants defective in porins were shown to have very poor permeability (and elevated MIC values) for several β-lactam antibiotics, indicating that diffusion through porins is the major route of antibiotic entry in these bacteria. Entry via dissolution in the lipid phase by the more lipophilic β-lactams appears to be less important, presumably because in most wild-type bacteria the outer surface of the outer membrane contains hydrophilic lipopolysaccharide chains. Evidence for the entry of nafcillin via the lipid phase has been presented in deep-rough mutants of *E. coli* (NIKAIDO 1976).

Two types of major variables seem to influence β-lactam diffusion through the porins. The first represents structural features of the antibiotic, such as molecular size (decreased uptake above a critical size, because of the pore diameter), relative hydrophilicity, and net charge (NIKAIDO 1981). The second major variable seems to be in the bacterial cell: certain anomalies in the observed diffusion rates suggest that *Pseudomonas* (and probably other bacteria as well) can regulate (i.e., open or close) the available number of pores.

Abundant evidence in the literature clearly indicates that in gram-negative bacteria, access of the β-lactam antibiotics to their targets may be a rate-limiting factor in their antibacterial effectiveness (NIKAIDO 1981; ZIMMERMAN and ROSSELET 1977; RICHMOND 1981; CURTIS and ROSS 1980). In several types of hypersensitive mutants, the lower MIC values could be correlated with increased access of the antibiotic to the plasma membrane. Nikaido has called attention to an important (and often overlooked) paradox in the quantitative aspect of these findings: it may be calculated that even with a slow-diffusing (relatively hydrophobic) β-lactam, equilibration across an average outer membrane would occur within a few seconds; this would, at least in theory, provide sufficient concentration of antibiotic at the plasma membrane surface to exert antibacterial effects. The fact that the MIC values are still dependent on diffusion rates is explicable only if one assumes an extremely rapid removal of the antibiotic at the inner surface of the outer membrane (NIKAIDO 1981). Processes potentially responsible for this would be β-lactamases or some as yet undefined side reactions that may lower the effective concentration of the antibiotic, possibly by some noncovalent binding (perhaps analogous to serum binding). These considerations underline the importance of viewing drug permeability as a quantitative phenomenon, and in the context of the fate of the molecules subsequent to the crossing of cellular boundaries (NIKAIDO 1981).

IV. The End of the Journey: Arrival at the Plasma Membrane

β-Lactam molecules that have traveled across the various outer boundaries surrounding the bacterium and crossed the outer membrane and murein layers of the cell (and also managed to survive periplasmic β-lactamases) arrive at the outer surface of the bacterial plasma membrane. There they react and form covalent complexes with a group of membrane proteins called penicillin-binding proteins (PBPs) (SPRATT 1975) that vary in number from few (e.g., three in gonococci) (DOUGHERTY et al. 1980) to as many as ten (in *E. coli*), and represent a quantitatively minor fraction of the total membrane protein (an estimated 2,000 molecules per cell in *E. coli* and about 10,000–20,000 molecules per gram-positive cell). The stability of the penicillin–PBP complexes varies. The complex of gonococcal PBP 1 and penicillin has a half life of > 200 min (DOUGHERTY et al. 1980). In contrast, the complex of PBP 4 of *Proteus mirabilis* rapidly loses the antibiotic (half-life 10 s) through the enzymatic activity of the PBP (MARTIN and GMEINER 1979). The degradation products (penicilloic acid or fragmentation products) have no antibacterial activity and are, presumably, released into the medium.

In our current view, the reaction with the PBPs represents the end of the physical journey of the antibiotic molecule into the bacterial cell. Virtually nothing is known about possible further penetration across the plasma membrane except that covalent complexes (i.e., complexes capable of surviving boiling with hot SDS used in the PBP technique) between radioactive penicillin and cytoplasmic components could not be detected in *E. coli* (Spratt 1977b).

What are these penicillin binding proteins? What are their natural substrates and how are they related to the antibacterial effects of β-lactam molecules? In order to provide a proper discussion of these questions, we must first briefly survey the various lines of study that led to the identification of the penicillin-sensitive reactions in the bacterial cell.

C. The Biochemical Targets of β-Lactam Antibiotics

Within about a decade after the isolation of penicillin, much of the chemistry of this class of compounds has been elucidated. However, this did not offer much help in the search for the targets of these drugs. The first important clues concerning the nature of the biochemical targets of penicillin in the bacterial cell came from findings concerning the selective toxicity of β-lactams to procaryotic cells, the localization of radioactively labeled penicillin in bacteria, and the morphological and biochemical effects of penicillin.

I. Selective Toxicity of β-Lactams

One of the remarkable features of the β-lactam antibiotics is that in their structure they combine powerful antibacterial properties and a generally low toxicity against eucaryotic cells. Table 1 illustrates the scope and degree of sensitivity to some representative types of β-lactam antibiotics among various groups of bacteria.

The extreme sensitivity of bacteria to β-lactam antibiotics may be further illustrated by the fact that at the lowest concentration of penicillin capable of inhibiting the growth of a pneumococcal culture (about 6 ng of antibiotic and 10^8 bacteria per milliliter), the ratio of drug to drug-sensitive target may be as low as about 10 molecules of penicillin per molecule of penicillin binding protein.

In contrast, the extreme insensitivity of eucaryotic cells may be best illustrated by some figures on the recommended therapeutic doses of β-lactam antibiotics: 40 g per day of carbenicillin or 3–10 g per day (parenteral route).

Sensitivity of microorganisms to β-lactam antibiotics parallels the presence of the rigid murein (or peptidoglycan) material in the bacterial cell envelope. Mycoplasma or stable L-forms of bacteria (lacking most or all of the murein material) are insensitive to penicillin. Similarly, *Halobacteria* and certain *Archaebacteria* (Woese et al. 1978) in which the maintenance of defined cellular shape appears to depend on a structural protein (Konig and Kandler 1978) or a sulfonated heteropolysaccharide (Steber and Schleifer 1975), rather than a murein "sacculus," are not sensitive to β-lactam antibiotics.

A recent interesting addition to this list of penicillin-insensitive microorganisms are certain methane-forming bacteria. These gram-negative microbes contain a rig-

Table 1. The minimal inhibitory concentrations of some β-lactam antibiotics against a variety of bacteria

Organism	MIC (µg/ml)						Reference
	Penicillin		Cephalothin	Cefoxitin	Thienamycin MK 0787	SQ 26776 [a]	
	MIC	MBC					
S. pneumoniae R36A	0.006	0.006	0.03	1.6	0.01	> 100	ZIGLEHBOIM and TOMASZ (1979)
S. pneumoniae SA8249 *pen*^{R}	6.2	–	12.5	50.0	0.1	–	
S. pyogenes T4/56	0.006	0.006	0.05	1.0	0.0035	> 100	GUTMANN and TOMASZ (1982)
S. pyogenes T4/56 P23 *pen*^{R}	0.2	–	–	2.0	0.06	–	
S. pyogenes T4/56 To123 TOL$^+$	0.006	≧1.0	–	1.0	0.0035	–	
S. faecalis	1–4	–	> 100	100	0.4	> 100	SHOCKMAN et al. (1981)
S. mutans GS-5 TOL$^+$	0.01	> 1.0	–	–	–	–	SHOCKMAN et al. (1981)
S. sanguis (Wicky) TOL$^+$	0.05	100.0	10	3	0.2	–	HORNE and TOMASZ (1977)
Staph. aureus 209P							
grown at pH 7.0	0.02	0.04	0.05	0.4	0.2	> 100	HARTMAN and TOMASZ (1980)
grown at pH 5.2	0.02	0.06	0.05	0.5	0.03	–	
Staph. aureus RUCUS 1112 Meth^R							
grown at pH 7.0	50.0	50.0	50 (200)	100 (400)	0.08	–	
grown at pH 5.2	50.0	50.0	0.05 (100)	0.4 (> 100)	–	–	
Staph. aureus TOL$^+$	0.02	5.0	0.05	0.5	0.02	–	
E. coli DCO L^-	16.0		2–8	4	0.5	0.1	CURTIS and ROSS (1980)
E. coli DCO RP1$^+$ L^+	10,000.0		–	4	0.8	0.1	
E. coli DC2 permeab. mutant L^-	1.6		–	2	–	–	
E. coli DC2 RP1 permeab. mutant L^+	2,500.0		–	3	–	–	
Pseudomonas aeruginosa K 799 L^+	250		250	125	1–5	0.8–12	CURTIS and ROSS (1980)
P. aeruginosa K 799/61 permeab. mutant L$^+$	0.08		–	0.16	–	–	
Serratia	> 300		300	25	3–5	0.2–12	HOOVER and DUNN (1979)
Enterobacter cloaceae	> 200		100	0.5–50	0.5	0.1–10	HOOVER and DUNN (1979)
Legionella pneumophyla L$^+$	8		4–30	0.1	–	–	PASCULLE et al. (1982)

[a] SYKES et al. 1981a

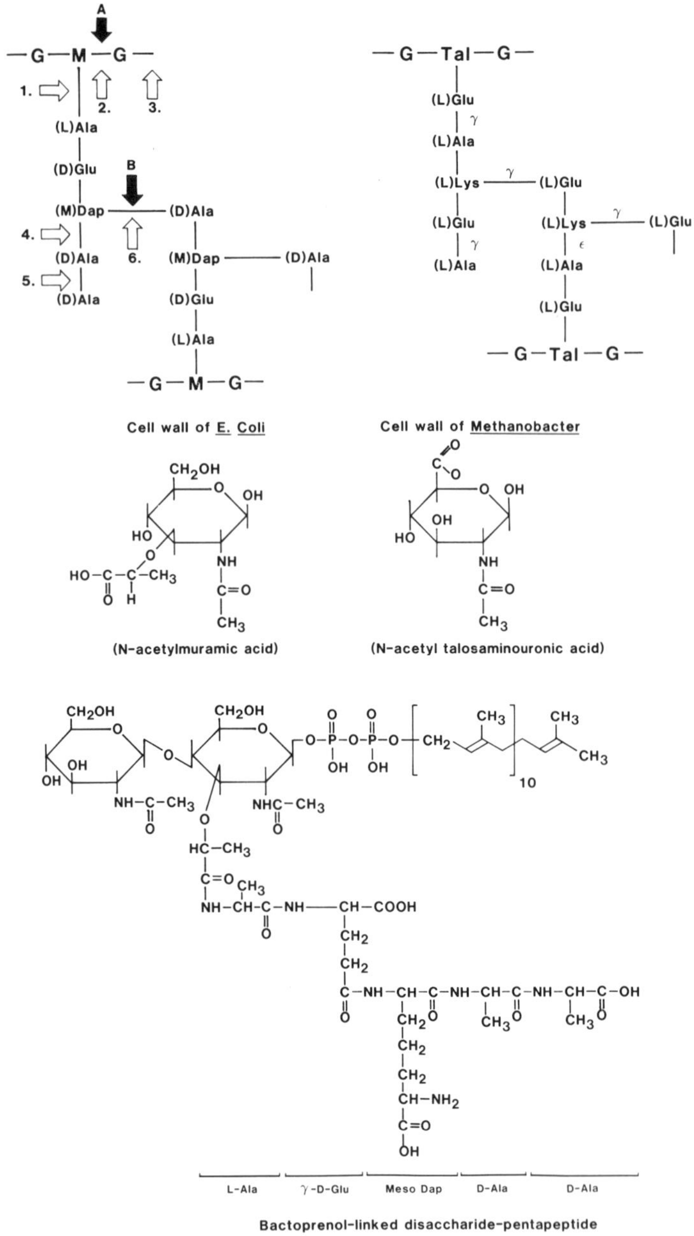

Fig. 1. Some features of the cell walls of *E. coli* and an *Archaebacterium*. *Upper part* of figure shows a segment of the repeating structures of the cell wall of *E. coli* (*left side*) and an *Archaebacterium*. *M*, *N*-acetylmuramic acid; *G*, *N*-acetylglucosamine; *Tal*, *N*-acetyl talosaminouronic acid. *Black arrows* indicate the two main repeating chemical bonds in the cell wall of *E. coli:* the β-1,4 glycosidic bonds (*A*) and the transpeptide bonds (*B*). The *white arrows* indicate the sites of attack of hydrolytic enzymes identified in *E. coli:* amidase (*1*); transglycosylase (*2*); glucosaminidase (*3*); L,D carboxypeptidase (*4*); D,D carboxypeptidase (*5*); and endopeptidase (*6*). The *bottom part* of the figure shows the structure of the bactoprenol-linked disaccharide-pentapeptide cell wall precursor. The tentative structure of the murein of the *Archaebacterium* is from Hammes and Kandler (1976)

id cell wall that can be isolated and can be shown to retain the size and shape of the original bacterium (HAMMES et al. 1979). In contrast to these anatomical similarities to real murein, the cell walls of these archebacteria contain a "pseudomurein": a glycopeptide network that contains *N*-acetylglucosamine; the L-isomers of glutamic acid, lysine, and alanine; lysine to glutamic acid cross-links; but no D-amino acids, and the muramic acid component of the glycan chain is replaced by *N*-acetyltalosamine uronic acid (Fig. 1).

As expected, these bacteria are not only inert to penicillin but are also insensitive to several other inhibitors of cell wall synthesis, such as phosphonomycin (inhibitor of muramic acid synthesis), D-cycloserine and vancomycin (drugs that interfere with the biosynthesis and metabolism of D-alanyl-D-alanine, respectively) (HAMMES et al. 1979).

II. Localization of Radioactively Labeled Penicillin in Bacteria

The notion that the biochemical targets of penicillin action lie somewhere within the general area of the metabolism of murein (peptidoglycan) (i.e., the unique bacterial surface component) has been supported not only by the selective toxicity of penicillin against procaryotes but also by several lines of evidence presented in the literature by the mid-1950 s.

In 1956, Cooper reviewed the results of experiments in which the intracellular localization of radioactively labeled penicillin was studied (COOPER 1956). Virtually all the cell-associated penicillin could be recovered with a protein- and lipid-rich fraction, presumably the plasma membrane. The binding of antibiotic was strong enough to withstand washings with salt solutions, and extraction of the radioactivity required the use of NH_2OH or alkali (i.e., reagents capable of breaking covalent bonds).

III. Morphological and Biochemical Effects of Penicillin

The importance of cell walls for the maintenance of shape and structure of bacteria has been established (SALTON 1964). It was recognized that the penicillin-induced formation of osmotically sensitive protoplasts involved loss of the cell wall material (LEDERBERG 1956, 1957). Microscopic observation of bacteria during penicillin treatment revealed further striking antibiotic-induced changes in cell morphology, such as formation of filaments, bulging at the cellular equator, appearance of "rabitt ear"-like forms, etc. (GARDNER 1940; DUGUID 1946). All these suggested some interference with the metabolism of cell walls.

After several erroneous leads concerning the general biochemical nature of penicillin action, it was shown in a series of critically important studies (PARK and JOHNSON 1949; PARK 1952) that the unusual uridine-diphosphate (UDP)-linked peptides accumulating in penicillin-treated staphylococci also contained *N*-acetylmuramic acid, the unique component of cell wall murein. Further similarities between the composition and structure of these muramyl-peptides and that of the cell wall murein led to the proposition that the UDP-linked muramylpeptides were biosynthetic precursors of cell wall material and that penicillin in some way interfered with their utilization for cell wall synthesis (PARK and STROMINGER 1957).

By the mid-1950s extensive studies with many bacterial species led to the understanding of the basic chemical features of bacterial cell wall structure (Ghuysen 1968; Kandler et al. 1968; Schleifer and Kandler 1972). It was recognized that the polymerization of the disaccharide-pentapeptide murein building blocks involved the formation of essentially two kinds of covalent bonds: the glycosidic linkages connecting the C1 positions of the *N*-acetyl-muramic acid of one disaccharide-peptide to the C4 positions of *N*-acetylglucosamine units of another disaccharide-peptide unit, thus forming a continuous β-1,4 linked glycan chain (the length of which is now known to vary from 30–40 up to several hundred units). The other regular linkages apparent in the cell walls were the transpeptide bonds connecting the carboxy terminal D-alanine of one side chain to the free amino group of the R3 position in the peptide side chain of a neighboring murein building block (see Fig. 17.1). A peculiar difference between the composition of mature cell walls and the supposed, precursor disaccharide-peptide was noted: the peptide side chains in the former were mostly tetrapeptides missing the second D-alanine residue that was present in the uridine diphosphate-linked disaccharide-pentapeptide monomers accumulating in penicillin-treated staphylococci (Tipper and Berman 1969).

By the early 1960s the multistep biosynthetic pathway leading to the formation of the activated disaccharide-pentapeptide (complete with the oligopeptide substituents on the R3 amino-group) was elucidated. Sites of inhibition for a variety of antibacterial agents were identified (e.g., phosphonomycin; D-cycloserine; bacitracin, etc.) but none of the reactions were found to be sensitive to penicillin (Strominger 1970).

Furthermore, it was shown in staphylococci that the incorporation of radioactively labeled precursors continued, at a slower rate, into cell wall material in the presence of moderate concentrations of penicillin (Tipper and Strominger 1968). A somewhat analogous situation was noted by Martin in 1964, while studying the cell walls of an unstable L-form of *Proteus* that seemed to produce, in the continued presence of penicillin, a cell wall of grossly normal composition, despite the osmotic instability of such cells. He proposed that penicillin may inhibit the formation of some special cross-linkages within the murein (Martin 1964).

All these observations directed attention to the two terminal reactions in cell wall synthesis: the formation of glycosidic and transpeptide bonds. This set the stage for two extremely important experiments.

In 1965, the observation was made simultaneously by Wise and Park (1965) and by Tipper and Strominger (1965) that the murein produced by staphylococci during treatment with low concentrations of penicillin contained an increased amount of D-alanine per cell wall subunit as compared to the composition of cell walls prepared from nontreated cells which contained one mole of D-alanine per mole of subunit. Indeed, enzymatic digests of the murein made in the presence of penicillin contained mostly disaccharide pentapeptide monomers (Tipper and Strominger 1965), thus closely resembling the peptide structure of the uridine diphosphate-linked muramyl pentapeptide that accumulated in penicillin-treated bacteria. In contrast, lysozyme digests of walls from normal cells yielded mostly cross-linked disaccharide tetrapeptides.

On the basis of these observations, it was suggested that penicillin inhibits a step in cell wall biosynthesis that involves loss of the carboxy terminal D-alanine residue from the precursor disaccharide pentapeptide. It was further suggested that this loss is coupled to the formation of transpeptide cross-links between the carbonyl group of the penultimate D-alanine of the precursor pentapeptide and a free amino group (lysine, diaminopimelic acid or glycine) on a neighboring peptide side chain in the cell wall (WISE and PARK 1965; TIPPER and STROMINGER 1965).

These experiments narrowed down the nature of the penicillin-sensitive process to the formation of transpeptide bonds, and the search for the penicillin-sensitive enzyme catalyzing this process was begun.

In retrospect, one must recognize the lucky coincidence involved with these revealing and by now classic experiments. They were performed in a bacterium that has very low carboxypeptidase activity and that also responds to penicillin treatment by the accumulation of UDP-disaccharide-peptides (in contrast to many other bacteria).

IV. Penicillin-Sensitive Enzymes

The first in vitro demonstration of murein transpeptidase activity was achieved in *E. coli:* when UDP-disaccharide-pentapeptide labeled with radioactive D-alanine was incubated with a particulate fraction from *E. coli* plus appropriate cofactors, the formation of *bis*-disaccharide-tetrapeptides could be detected, accompanied by the release of free D-alanine (IZAKI et al. 1966). Unexpectedly, in the same experiments it was also noted that along with the transpeptidation two more reactions were also taking place: removal of the carboxy terminal D-alanine uncoupled to the formation of peptide bonds (i.e., a D,D carboxypeptidase reaction) and hydrolysis of the transpeptide bonds (i.e., an endopeptidase reaction). All three reactions were sensitive to penicillin (IZAKI et al. 1966). Subsequently, the same types of penicillin-sensitive enzyme reactions were detected in a large number of other bacterial species (IZAKI et al. 1968; ARAKI et al. 1966; LINNETT and STROMINGER 1974a, b; PELLON et al. 1976; WICKUS and STROMINGER 1972a; WICKUS and STROMINGER 1972b).

The basic similarity between the carboxypeptidase and transpeptidase reactions has been recognized: in both cases the carbonyl of the penultimate D-alanine is transferred to an exogenous nucleophile. If the latter is water, hydrolysis is the result; if, however, it is an amino group of another peptide, the product is a cross-linked dimer of the two peptides. Endopeptidase activity can hydrolyse such dimers (Fig. 2).

These developments signaled the beginning of several important and somewhat divergent lines of investigation aimed at more precisely defining the biochemical targets of penicillin action:

1. A plausible model for the molecular basis of the selectivity of β-lactam action was proposed (TIPPER and STROMINGER 1965).
2. Enzymological studies were initiated on three different water-soluble carboxypeptidase-transpeptidase proteins secreted into the culture medium by two strains of *Streptomyces* and an *Actinomadura*. The solubility and varying degrees of penicillin sensitivity of these enzymes appeared to provide an ideal model system for mechanistic studies using a variety of model peptides as substrates and a number of β-lactams as inhibitors (GHUYSEN et al. 1980).

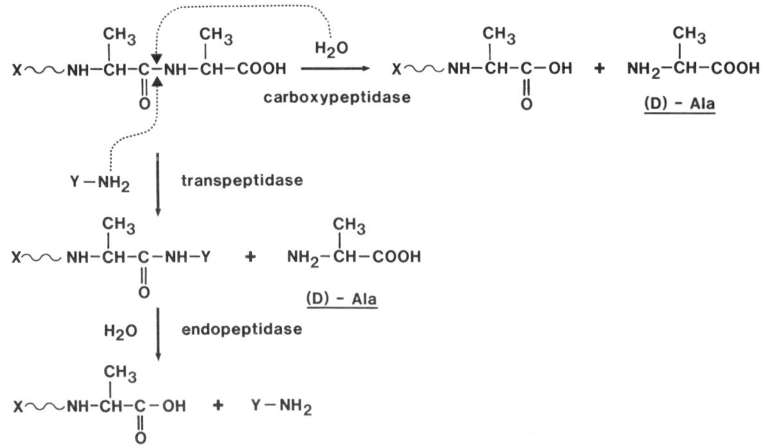

Fig. 2. Model reactions catalyzed by the D,D carboxypeptidase, transpeptidase, and endopeptidase

3. Another direction of study (primarily that of Strominger et al.) concentrated on the purification and biochemical characterization of the penicillin-sensitive enzymes from a number of bacteria (STROMINGER et al. 1974).
4. One major finding which emerged from these studies was the realization that penicillin formed covalent complexes with those enzymes (BLUMBERG and STROMINGER 1974). This, together with the earlier localization of cell-bound penicillin molecules to the bacterial plasma membrane (COOPER 1956), has prepared the ground work for the introduction of radioactive penicillin labeling for the visualization of bacterial proteins capable of covalently binding penicillin (PBPs). The sensitivity and relative simplicity of this approach, pioneered by SPRATT (1975), has become perhaps the most important and productive line of current investigation, substantially narrowing or even bridging the gap between enzymological and physiological approaches to the mode of action of penicillin. In addition, this technique has greatly simplified and increased the sensitivity of biochemical efforts in purifying the penicillin sensitive enzymes from bacteria.
5. Still another direction of research involved a number of laboratories studying the effects of penicillin and other β-lactam antibiotics on the biosynthesis of cell wall material in various strains of bacteria, using essentially in vivo or semi-in vivo labeling techniques (MIRELMAN et al. 1976; TYNECKA and WARD 1975; WARD 1974; TAKU and FAN 1976; SCHRADER and FAN 1974; ELLIOTT et al. 1975; WARD and PERKINS 1974; MIRELMAN et al. 1972).

The next sections of this review will attempt to briefly summarize some of the salient findings of these different approaches. The interested reader may find more detailed coverage and extensive lists of references in recent reviews specifically dealing with these various types of studies (WAXMAN and STROMINGER 1980 and YOCUM et al. 1980b – for (1); GHUYSEN et al. 1980 and GHUYSEN 1977 – for (2); STROMINGER et al. 1974 and BLUMBERG and STROMINGER 1974 – for (3); YOCUM et al. 1980b and SPRATT 1979 – for (4); and TIPPER and WRIGHT 1979 for (5).

1. Molecular Basis of Specificity

One of the major guiding forces of these studies has been the model proposed in 1965 by TIPPER and STROMINGER to explain the molecular basis of the selective inhibitory action of penicillin. On the basis of comparisons of molecular models, these authors proposed that penicillin may be a structural analog of a conformational isomer of D-alanyl-D-alanine, i.e., the carboxyterminal portion of the cell wall precursor disaccharide-pentapeptide. It was further suggested that penicillin may be an active-site directed inhibitor capable of acylating (and, thus, inactivating) bacterial transpeptidases. This model predicts three main kinds of requirements for biological activity: structural similarity to the natural substrate to allow recognition by the transpeptidase; sufficient chemical reactivity to perform acylation of the active site; and some structural feature to assure a long half-life for the antibiotic–enzyme complex.

Through the synthesis and chemical modification of thousands of structurally different β-lactam antibiotics, the pharmaceutical industry has accumulated an enormous body of information on the correlation between chemical structure and antibacterial potency (for recent reviews, see HOOVER and DUNN 1979, NAYLER 1973, FLYNN 1972). Most of the structure–activity relationships have been evaluated on the basis of the practically important and technically simple MIC determination vis-à-vis various clinically important pathogens. Unfortunately, these data are of little use in testing the predictions of the structural analogy model, since many of the chemical modifications significantly affecting the drugs' antimicrobial effectiveness occurred in the acyl side chains or in the substituents of the fused ring systems, i.e., in parts of the β-lactam structure that bear no structural analogy to the D-alanyl-D-alanine residue. Nevertheless, a set of specific structural features both in the penicillins and in the cephalosporins seems to represent the absolute requirements for antibiotic activity; these features are likely to reflect a combination of requirements for chemical reactivity and structure recognizable by some target enzyme(s).

In all conventional penicillins the four-membered ring is fused to another five-membered heterocyclic ring (thiazolidine in penicillins, pyrroline in carbopenems, and oxazolidine in clavulanic acid). At similar positions the cephalosporins contain the 5,6 fused six-membered dihydrothiazine ring. This arrangement has been shown to introduce steric constraints giving rise to pyramidal nitrogen. Within a certain range, the degree of deviation from coplanarity in this nitrogen could be correlated with both chemical reactivity and antibacterial activity in synthetic penems (WOODWARD 1980; GENSMANTEL et al. 1980). Another factor that was thought to increase reactivity of the β-lactam ring to nucleophile atack was attributed to the electron withdrawing effect of sulfur at position 1. In cephalosporins, electron-negative substituents at C3 may further contribute to this effect.

Some of the common structural features of the major, therapeutically useful β-lactams are shown in Fig. 3.

All of the compounds shown contain the four-membered β-lactam ring, have a carboxyl group on the carbon atom attached to the lactam nitrogen with the stereochemistry as shown. In the monobactams, the sulfonate oxygen atoms are in the same positions as the carboxylate oxygens in the conventional β-lactams. All of the structures shown (except clavulanic acid and thienamycin) have an acylated aminogroup on the carbon atom diagonally across from the lactam nitrogen (i.e., on the C6 of penicillins or C7 of cephalosporins).

In penicillins and cephalosporins, the two fused rings are not coplanar. Their stereochemistry is such that the H-atoms on C5 and C6 of penicillins (C6 and C7

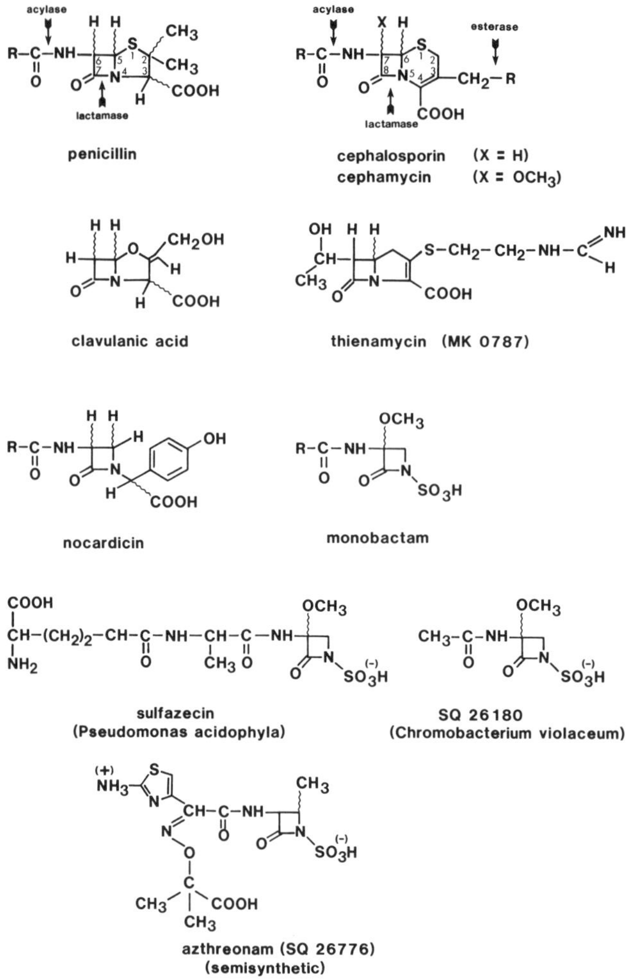

Fig. 3. Structures of some important β-lactam antibiotics

of cephalosporins) are on the *same* side of the ring system, while the C3 carboxyl and the acylated amide group on C6 are on the opposite sides, in penicillins. More of the characteristic stereochemical features of these compounds are shown in Fig. 3.

The simple monocyclic structure of monobactams (IMADA et al. 1981; SYKES et al. 1981 b) presents a challenge to structure–activity relationships based on features of the conventional β-lactams. Clearly, with the monocyclic structure there is no steric activation and the sulfonate residue is coplanar with the four-membered ring. It seems that the reactivity of the β-lactam ring in the monobactams is solely due to the electron withdrawal by the sulfonate group.

The availability of synthetic methods to modify the simple basic structure of monobactams will provide an excellent tool for testing the specificity of penicillin-sensitive enzymes and structure-affinity relationships in PBPs. Data concerning the antimicrobial activities and PBP affinities have begun to appear in the literature (SYKES et al. 1981 a).

As mentioned above, the fused rings (thiazolidine or dihydrothiazine) of penicillins and cephalosporins, and the side-chain (C6 and C7) substituents have no structural analogy with the D-alanyl-D-alanine dipeptide. Yet, the antibacterial activity of β-lactams can be dramatically altered by variations in the substituents of ring and side-chain structure. Although some of these effects may be explained in terms of modulation of the chemical reactivity of the β-lactam ring, the major cause of these variations in biological activity seems to originate in the fact that a number of different bacterial components (porins, β-lactamases, various PBPs) recognize more than just the basic β-lactam structure. In fact, penicillin-sensitive enzymes may have several recognition sites, in addition to the active site, and interaction of the antibiotic molecule with these may have a profound influence upon reactivity with the active site. Various lines of evidence supporting this view have emerged from enzymological studies with several water-soluble carboxypeptidase/transpeptidase enzymes; these observations will be reviewed next.

2. Studies with Model Substrates and Model Enzymes

Although the existence of penicillin-sensitive carboxypeptidase, transpeptidase, and endopeptidase activities has been demonstrated in many bacterial species, detailed kinetic and enzymological analysis of these reactions has been performed with only a limited number of enzymes. GHUYSEN (1976, 1977) and GHUYSEN et al. (1974, 1981) have performed extensive studies on three water-soluble enzymes secreted spontaneously into the medium of *Streptomyces albus* G, an *Actinomadura* species (strain R39), and a *Streptomyces* (strain R61). Model peptide substrates of varying structure have been prepared and tested, permitting recognition of specificity for substrate. These and other studies with enzymes solubilized and purified from several bacteria (primarily in the laboratory of Strominger) have yielded a large body of information about the kinetics and molecular mechanism of the reactions catalyzed by penicillin sensitive enzymes. Some of the salient findings of these studies may be summarized as follows.

a) Kinetics

All the enzymes studied catalyze hydrolysis or transpeptidation with substrates having the general carboxyterminal structure of L-R-D-Ala-D-Ala; reaction with water gives L-R-D-Ala + D-Ala; reaction with peptides containing a free amino-group (Y-NH_2) yields L-R-D-Ala-NH-Y + D-Ala. In the presence of a β-lactam, the antibiotic may be considered a substrate analog competing with the substrate peptide for the enzyme.

The kinetics of the reactions with substrate or with the β-lactam antibiotic may both be described in the following mechanism:

$$\text{A)}\ \text{E}+\text{peptide} \underset{k_2}{\overset{k_1}{\rightleftharpoons}} \text{E}\cdot\text{peptide} \xrightarrow{k_3} \text{E}\sim\text{peptide} \xrightarrow{k_4} \text{E}+\text{products},$$

$$\text{B)}\ \text{E}+\text{antibiotic}(a) \underset{k_2}{\overset{k_1}{\rightleftharpoons}} \text{E}\cdot a \xrightarrow{k_3} \text{E}\sim a \xrightarrow{k_4} \text{E}+\text{degraded}\ a,$$

where E represents enzyme; E·peptide or E·*a* are enzyme-substrate (or inhibitor) complexes; E ~ peptide or E ~ *a* represent acylated enzyme. With good substrates, formation of products is rapid (high k_4) and the half life of E peptide is short ($k_4 \gg k_3$). In contrast, good inhibitors tie up the enzyme in an antibiotic–enzyme complex for a long time (low k_4) and the rate of formation of these complexes is fast (high k_3).

b) Poor Affinity of Model Substrates and β-Lactams for the Model Enzymes

Under appropriate conditions, the dissociation constant for the enzyme peptide complex

$$\left(\text{in reaction A}; \frac{k_2}{k_1} = K\right)$$

may be considered equivalent to the K_m value. Interestingly, evaluation of these for a number of model substrates resulted in the finding that the observed K_m values were high (mM) and showed only relatively minor (about 10-fold) variation even though the substrates differed greatly in their overall qualities. Similarly, the K-values measured for the binding of various β-lactams were all high and showed no parallel variation with the effectiveness of the β-lactam as inhibitor of the enzyme reactions. These observations indicate that the recognition of either model substrate or β-lactam inhibitor by the enzymes is not very efficient and shows no selective, high affinities.

The surprisingly low affinities for model peptides may reflect differences between the structure of these model substrates and that of the unknown in vivo substrates of these enzymes. Alternatively, in situ in the bacterial membrane, the local substrate concentration in the vicinity of the enzyme may be sufficiently high to not require high affinities. The high K value for β-lactams may also explain, in part, the relatively long incubation times needed to achieve saturation of PBPs exposed to low concentrations (1–4 times the MIC value) of penicillin in vivo.

c) Effect of Substrate Structure on Reaction Rate

The effect of structural variations in the carbonyl donor substrate on the rate of the carboxypeptidase reaction was determined.

i) There was found to be an absolute requirement for D-alanine in the penultimate position. ii) The carboxyterminal D-alanine could be replaced by other D-amino acids, but *not* by L-amino acids. iii) Variation in the side chain structure of the L-amino acid, preceding the penultimate D-alanine, caused substantial variation in activity. As mentioned above, these variations in rate had relatively little effect on the K values, but were paralleled by variation in the V_{max} values.

d) Effect of β-Lactam Structure

Similarly, the quality of β-lactams as inhibitors depended on the chemical nature of the substituents attached to the N atom at the C-6 position in penicillins (and C-7 on cephalosporins). Similarly to the case with substrates, there was relatively little difference between enzyme-affinities (K) of the various β-lactams, but great variations (ranging over 3–5 orders of magnitude) could be observed both in the

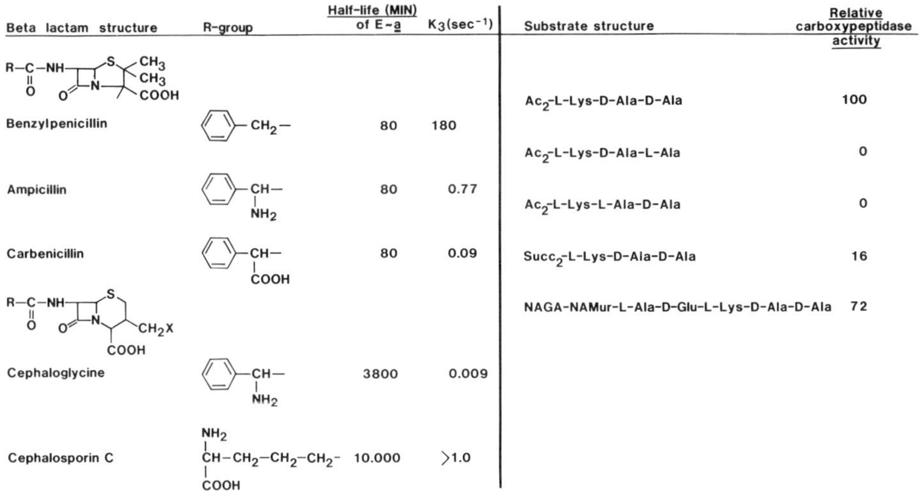

Fig. 4. Influence of β-lactam and peptide substrate structure on the kinetic parameters of interaction with a D,D carboxypeptidase model enzyme. Data from GHUYSEN (1977)

rates of acylation (k3 values that paralleled inhibitory activity) and in the stability of the antibiotic enzyme complexes (increase in the half-lives of the complexes (Fig. 4).

e) Specificity in the Type of Cross-link Formed

Additional specificity for substrate structure was recognized when the chemistry of model peptides used as acceptors in transpeptidation was varied. In short, it was found that the R61 and R39 enzymes preferentially catalyzed transpeptidations that resulted in the formation of cross-linkages resembling those present in the cell walls of the parent R61 and R39 strains. The cell wall of strain R61 is an A3 type murein containing L,L diaminopimelic acid and cross-bridges made of a single glycine residue. The R39 strain has A1α type murein and contains direct cross-bridges between its meso-diaminopimelic acid and neighboring D-alanyl residues (see Fig. 1).

Correspondingly, the optimal substrates with the R61 enzyme contained the free amino group on a glycine, while good acceptors for the R39 enzyme contained the aminogroup on a meso-diaminopimelic acid residue (Fig. 5).

f) Differences Among the Model Enzymes

The various penicillin-sensitive enzymes studied could be grouped into a series of proteins representing a gradually increasing specificity for the structure of the acceptor nucleophile. Thus, the *S. albus* G enzyme had exclusively hydrolytic (D,D carboxypeptidase and endopeptidase) activities. Other *Streptomyces* enzymes could catalyze both carboxypeptidase and transpeptidase activities, the latter with a variety of simple amino acids and peptides. The R39 and R61 enzymes, while still potentially bifunctional enzymes, nevertheless showed specific structural prefer-

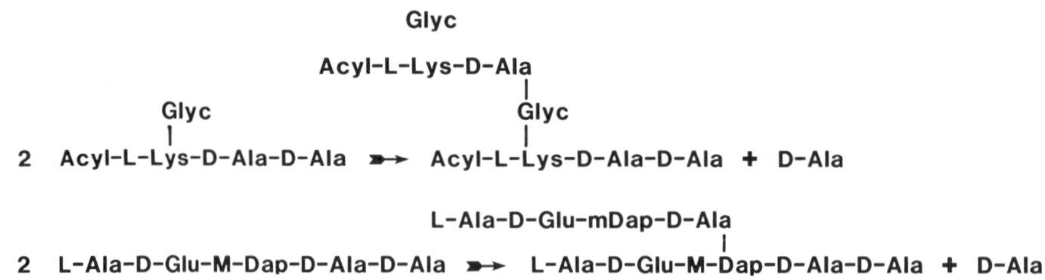

Fig. 5. Preferred peptide substrates in the transpeptidase model reactions. The *upper part* of figure shows the substrate preferred by the R61, the *lower part* the substrate preferred by the R36 enzyme. Data from GHUYSEN (1977)

ences, both for the carbonyl donor and for the acceptor peptides. Finally, a membrane-bound protein of *Streptomyces* R61 catalyzed transpeptidations exclusively. It has been suggested that this gradually increasing specificity may reflect the appearance of more complex acceptor sites on the enzyme protein.

In the case of the enzymes capable of catalyzing both the hydrolytic and the transpeptidase reaction, these two reactions competed with one another. The relative hydrolase or transpeptidase activities were found to depend also on the chemical structure and concentration of the amino group containing peptide and on the physicochemical characteristics of the medium (e.g., a decrease in water concentration caused a relative increase in transpeptidation). Since the in vivo microenvironment of these enzymes is not known, one should exercise caution in drawing conclusions as to the nature of the in vivo activity of an enzyme solely on the basis of a demonstration of in vitro carboxypeptidase or transpeptidase activity.

g) Acyl Enzymes

Several lines of evidence indicate the formation of acyl-enzyme intermediates in carboxypeptidase catalyzed reactions and also the formation of covalent acyl linkage between the penicillin-sensitive enzymes and the antibiotic molecule (NISHINO et al. 1977). However, there has been disagreement with respect to both the chemical nature of the bond and its precise site within the enzyme protein. While the original proposal by TIPPER and STROMINGER (1965) implied that penicillin was an active site-directed acylating agent, another view holds that the antibiotic interacted with a site on the enzyme (allosteric site) which was different from the active site for the substrate (GHUYSEN et al. 1974). In striking support of the original proposal, it has recently become possible to show that both penicillin (and cefoxitin) as well as a model natural substrate – the D-lactic ester of *N*-diacyl-lysyl-D-alanine-D-alanine – acylated the same serine residue (number 36 from the amino terminus) in the same polypeptide chain in the purified carboxypeptidases of *Bacillus subtilis* and *Bacillus stearothermophilus* (RASMUSSEN and STROMINGER 1978; YOCUM et al. 1980a). Comparable results were also obtained with the *Streptomyces* R61 enzyme and with carboxypeptidases from *E. coli* and *S. aureus* (YOCUM et al. 1979; WAXMAN and STROMINGER 1980). Since in most carboxypeptidases the kinetic parameters do not favor accumulation of the acyl-enzyme intermediate ($k_4 \gg k_3$), a substrate had to be developed that had a sufficiently high relative rate of acylation to allow the entrapment of such an intermediate. This was achieved using the D-lactic ester of the model peptide.

The ultimate fate of the acyl-enzyme intermediate with the substrate was found to depend on the specificity of the protein, physicochemical conditions, etc. Depending on whether or not the enzyme has an acceptor site to accommodate the amino group containing acceptor peptide, transpeptidation or hydrolysis will occur, the altered substrate molecules will be released, making the enzyme active site, and other postulated recognition sites, free again.

h) Fate of the Antibiotic Molecule

In contrast to the molecules of natural substrates, the antibiotic molecules that reacted with the active sites of model enzymes are released only slowly; this fact is as important a criterion of a good β-lactam inhibitor as are the structural resemblance to the D-alanyl-D-alanine substrate and the chemical reactivity to assure rapid acylation of their active site. It has been speculated that the stability of the penicilloyl-enzyme complex may be due to the interaction of the thiazolidine (or dihydrothiazine) ring with some hypothetical tertiary enzyme site causing a conformational change in the protein such that nucleophilic attack on the active site becomes difficult (WAXMAN and STROMINGER 1980; GHUYSEN et al. 1980).

Nevertheless, the penicilloyl complexes of both model enzymes and enzymes isolated from bacterial membranes do undergo deacylation eventually, with greatly varying rates that are dependent on both the enzyme and the particular β-lactam. In addition, decomposition of the penicilloyl enzyme can follow two routes, which again depend on the particular enzyme, on the nature of the β-lactam, and also on the physicochemical conditions of the reaction. For instance, penicilloyl complexes of PBPs 5 and 6 of *E. coli* decompose the antibiotic to penicilloic acid (TAMURA et al. 1976). On the other hand, the *Streptomyces* carboxypeptidase R61 (FRERE et al. 1975a, b) and the carboxypeptidase of *B. stearothermophilus* (HAMMARSTROM and STROMINGER 1975) decomposes bound penicillin to phenylacetylglycine and a thiazoline derivative. The first reaction is obviously identical to that catalyzed by β-lactamases. The physiological significance of the second type of fragmentation (Fig. 6) is not known although fragmentation products might be utilized and the

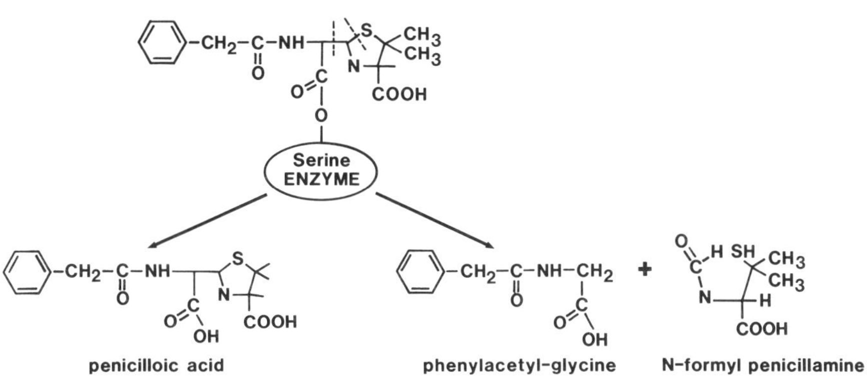

Fig. 6. Alternative pathways for the degradation of the β-lactam acyl-enzyme complexes

reported incorporation of radioactivity from a cephamycin (MT 141) into the bacterial cell wall may represent such a process (Yamada et al. 1981).

i) Multiple Sites on the Enzymes

The presence of secondary, tertiary, etc. binding sites for substrate (and for antibiotic) has been postulated as a way to interpret the very substantial effect of structural variation (in the side chain of the L-amino acid of substrate peptides and in the substituents on the C-6 acyl group on the thiazolidine ring of the penicillin molecule) on the kinetic parameters of these reactions. However, comparison of the chemical structure of recognized portions of model peptide substrates and β-lactams showed no similarities. Thus, one has to assume the existence of distinct secondary, etc., sites for peptide substrates and a separate set of these for the β-lactam antibiotics.

It has also been proposed that an initial interaction of the substrate with some of these sites leads to conformational change in the protein, resulting in the repositioning of the substrate so as to facilitate interaction with the active site. The temporal order of interactions between the carbonyl-donor and -acceptor peptides and the corresponding recognition sites in the protein is not settled yet. Neither is the nature and number of these sites and their precise interaction with the substrate (or antibiotic) known at the present time.

The existence of secondary sites is consistent with biochemical data suggesting that in some carboxypeptidases chemical groups other than serine residues (e.g., thiol) may also participate in enzyme catalysis (Curtis and Strominger 1978; Umbreit and Strominger 1973). Clearly, for proper functioning of these enzymes in the bacterial cell, a high degree of precision is required in the alignment of donor and acceptor sites, and it may also be necessary, at least for some transpeptidases, to recognize relatively large, oligomeric substrates (see later).

j) Inhibition of Enzyme Vs. Inhibition of the Cell

While much valuable information concerning the general enzymology of penicillin-sensitive enzymes has been learned from studies on those model enzymes, the relationship between the β-lactam sensitivity of the enzyme activities and the antimicrobial effectiveness of the same drugs against the parent *Streptomyces* strains remains an open question. In the case of the membrane-bound form of the R61 enzyme, it was shown that as the concentrations (μM) of various antibiotics needed to inhibit 50% of the transpeptidase increased from 8 (ampicillin) through 39 (cloxacillin) to 540 (cephalosporin C), the concentrations of the same antibiotics needed for inhibition of a *Streptomyces* bioassay also increased from 5 through 50–112 μM (Ghuysen 1977). The meaning of similar comparisons is questionable in the case of the water-soluble R61 and R39 enzymes, which have been so valuable as models in studies on the enzymology of β-lactam inhibition. While the parent organisms release these enzymes into the growth medium, the membranes of the same organisms also contain three additional penicillin-binding proteins which have molecular weights different from those of the released enzymes and which do not react with antibodies against the soluble enzymes (Dusart et al. 1981). The membrane-bound PBPs are more likely to represent the antibacterial targets of penicillin.

V. Penicillin-Binding Proteins (PBPs)

Exposure of plasma membrane preparations to radioactively labeled penicillin results in the formation of covalently linked complexes between the antibiotic molecule and a number of proteins. The link between antibiotic molecules and these proteins is strong enough to withstand being boiled in sodium dodecyl sulphate (SDS). Although the formation of weak, or reversible, complexes between β-lactams and cellular proteins cannot be excluded, reports of such weak interactions have so far been described only for the monocyclic β-lactam, nocardicin A (KUNUGITA et al. 1981).

All bacterial membranes examined so far gave rise to such labeled proteins, which could be detected by SDS-gel electrophoretic separation and detection of the radioactively labeled proteins by autoradiography. The binding reactions were found to be specific in that they were specifically prevented by preincubation of the membranes with nonradioactive penicillin or by denaturation of the proteins (by detergent or heating). Furthermore, hydroxylamine treatment resulted in the release of radioactivity, in the form of penicilloic acid, from native protein complexes. No such radioactively labeled proteins were detected when membranes prepared from *Mycoplasma* or eucaryotic cells were exposed to moderate concentrations of labeled penicillin.

The procedure, first developed for *E. coli* membranes by Spratt (SPRATT 1975) and then adapted to various bacteria by others, resulted in the detection of a number of bacterial proteins capable of binding penicillin, their number, molecular size, the relative and absolute amounts of penicillin bound by them and the stability of the penicilloyl complexes varying from one bacterium to another. However, the number of PBPs and their molecular sizes appear to be reproducible characteristics of the bacterial species (GEORGOPAPADAKOU and LIU 1980). In fact, the PBP pattern may provide corroborating evidence for the taxonomic classification of bacteria. One should note that the numerical connotation of PBPs is strictly a reference to their relative molecular size within the group of PBPs detected in a microorganism (PBP 1 being the slowest moving, i.e., highest molecular size on the gel). Thus PBP 1 of *E. coli* need not have anything in common with PBP 1 of gonococci. Nevertheless, a more detailed comparison of PBPs, by a variety of functional criteria, suggests that within the group of *Enterobacteriaceae*, at least some of the PBPs of comparable molecular size may have similar physiological functions as well (GEORGOPAPADAKOU and LIU 1980; NOGUCHI et al. 1979; CURTIS et al. 1979 a, b).

The quantitative distribution of bound penicillin among the PBPs differs from one bacterium to another. Assuming monovalent binding, one can estimate the approximate number of molecules of various PBPs per cell and also the fraction of total membrane protein represented by the PBPs. The latter figure indicates that PBPs are minor components of the plasma membrane (representing up to 1% of total membrane proteins in *E. coli*). About 2,000 molecules of penicillin are bound per *E. coli* cell (SPRATT 1979) and the figure is 10–15 times higher in the case of the gram-positive *B. subtilis* or pneumococcus.

1. Enzymatic Activity of PBPs with Model Substrates

Several of the PBPs have already been identified as carboxypeptidases, and weak transpeptidase (and transglycosylase) activity has also been detected in some others. Nevertheless, considering all the bacterial PBPs detected by the binding protein assay, the biochemical activity of the overwhelming majority of these remains to be elucidated. It is conceivable that all the PBPs will eventually be shown to possess transpeptidase and/or carboxypeptidase activities, once problems of protein concentration, instability and proper reaction conditions are established. However, the number of PBPs detected in several bacteria (e.g., 9–11 in *E. coli*) is certainly far too high to match them with the number of known, or even of postulated, murein-related enzyme activities. Thus, at present, one should not exclude the possibility that some of the PBPs may turn out to have truly novel (e.g., regulatory) functions. On the basis of the structural analogy model one may assume, however, that whatever the natural substrates of those proteins may turn out to be, they (the substrates) would contain the D-alanyl-D-alanine structure.

The precise relationship which individual PBPs have to one another is not clear yet. In the case of *E. coli*, precursor–product relationships among the PBPs are unlikely since each of the major PBPs has distinct genetic determinants, and antibodies prepared against individual PBPs did not show cross-reactivity (SPRATT 1977a; BUCHANAN et al. 1977). On the other hand, in vivo penicillin labeling experiments in *Streptococcus pyogenes* indicated a transient increase in the intensity of labeling in PBP 3, parallel with the decrease in PBP 2, and it was suggested that PBP 2 may be a precursor of PBP 3 in this organism (GUTMANN et al. 1980).

2. Penicillin Binding and Inactivation of Enzyme Activity

For several purified bacterial carboxypeptidases, experimental evidence indicates that the binding of radioactive penicillin to the protein registers the formation of the catalytically inactive acyl-enzyme complex. After exposure to radioactive penicillin, several of the PBP-penicillin complexes could be isolated (NISHINO et al. 1977) and the gradual loss of enzymatic (carboxypeptidase) activity paralleled the formation of penicillin complex (KOZARICH and STROMINGER 1978; LAWRENCE and STROMINGER 1970). For these enzymes (and, presumably, for some other PBPs as well), the binding (and release) of penicillin to the PBPs follows a kinetic pattern similar to that of the well-studied carboxypeptidase/transpeptidase model enzymes:

$$\text{PBP}+\text{pen} \underset{k_2}{\overset{k_1}{\rightleftharpoons}} \text{pen PBP} \xrightarrow{k_3} \underline{\text{pen}\sim\text{PBP}} \xrightarrow{k_4} \text{PBP (active)}+\text{antibiotic (inactive)},$$

where the underlined $\underline{\text{pen}\sim\text{PBP}}$ represents the radioactive penicillin labeled PBP, as visualized on the fluorogram. Individual PBPs differ in the rate of formation of these $\underline{\text{pen}\sim\text{PBP}}$ complexes and also in the stability of the complexes. It follows from these kinetics that β-lactams with either slow rates of acylation ($k_3 < k_2$) or with very fast deacylation rates (k_4 high) will both appear to have "poor" binding to the PBPs. The three gonococcal PBPs each form complexes of very long half lives (> 100 min) with penicillin (DOUGHERTY et al. 1981). In contrast, the half lives of the penicillin complexes of PBPs 1 a and b of *B. subtilis* (BLUMBERG et al. 1974) and of *B. megaterium* (CHASE et al. 1977) are 10 min and 35 min respectively. As expected from the experience with model enzymes, the stability of the binding protein complexes also depends on the chemical nature of the β-lactam. For instance, the half-life of the complex of the *E. coli* PBP 5 (and 6) with the cephamycin CS 1170 is several hundred minutes, while the same PBPs form rapidly deacylating complexes (half-life 10 min) with benzylpenicillin (OHYA et al. 1978). This finding raises the possibility, already considered in the literature (SPRATT 1977b; REYNOLDS and CHASE 1981), that proteins might exist for which the kinetic parameters of binding benzylpenicillin make the detection of acylproteins difficult although, if using a structurally different β-lactam, these binding proteins might be detectable. The overwhelming majority of data in the literature of PBPs is based on the use of radioactively labeled benzylpenicillin. Tests in *B. megaterium* (CHASE et al. 1977) and *E. coli* with some radioactively labeled cephalosporins, mecillinam, and thienamycin (SPRATT 1977c) yielded no evidence for binding proteins other than the ones detectable with radioactive benzylpenicillin. On the other hand, studies with an iodinated ampicillin derivative have apparently yielded evidence for additional binding proteins not detectable by radioactive benzylpenicillin (SCHWARZ et al. 1981).

Little information is available about enzymatic activities of the higher molecular weight PBPs, although detection of transpeptidase and transglycosylase activities in PBPs 1b and 3 of *E. coli* has been reported and transpeptidase activity has also been claimed in PBP 2 of *E. coli*, assayed by a modified procedure (ISHINO et al. 1980; NAKAGAWA and MATSUHASHI 1980; SUZUKI et al. 1981).

The higher molecular weight PBPs are usually present only in small quantities. It is likely that the problem of low yield could soon be overcome since through gene cloning techniques it has already been possible to increase the cellular concentration of several PBPs at least 20–30 fold (NISHIMURA et al. 1977; TAMURA et al. 1980; SPRATT 1980). Other problems with detecting in vitro enzymatic activities in the high molecular weight PBPs may have to do with either the inappropriate assay conditions (these proteins may perform their in vivo functions in a lipid environment) or the fact that these proteins may have more stringent requirements for their substrates (e.g., they may need oligomeric cell wall material) or for the topological presentation of their substrates, which may not be satisfied in the currently used model reactions.

3. Localization of PBPs

For the PBPs that have been studied in some detail, the active site seems to be oriented towards the outer surface of the plasma membrane. The carboxypeptidase activity of *B. subtilis* protoplasts could be inhibited by 6-APA immobilized on sepharose (STORM et al. 1974). Furthermore, polypeptide fragments still capable of radioactive penicillin binding could be released from protoplasts (STORM et al. 1974; WAXMAN and STROMINGER 1978) or membranes of several bacteria by treatment with trypsin. In *B. subtilis*, the hydrophilic, penicillin-binding peptides contained the amino terminal residues of the proteins (obviously including the active site of the protein).

Treatment of either the purified carboxypeptidase (PBP 5, mol. wt. 50,000) or protoplasts of *B. subtilis* with papain or trypsin released a similar set of water-soluble, penicillin-binding peptides (mol. wt. 47,000, 35,000, and 15,000–18,000) plus a hydrophobic polypeptide with a length of 20–30 amino acid residues (WAXMAN and STROMINGER 1979b; COYETTE et al. 1978). It seems that the latter serve to anchor the PBP in the lipid region of the membrane. In fact, purified PBP 5 of *B. ther-*

mophilus could be resorbed into lipid vesicles without loss of activity, indicating that the protein has reattached to the lipid membrane in the native (outward-looking) orientation (WAXMAN and STROMINGER 1979a).

4. Labeling of PBPs in Live, Growing Bacteria

The recent introduction of high specific radioactivity tritiated benzylpenicillin (ROSEGAY 1981), ^{3}H-labeled *N*-alkyl ampicillin (SCHMIDT et al. 1981) and ^{125}I-labeled β-lactam derivatives (SCHWARZ et al. 1981), all with specific radioactivities in the range of 30 Ci per mmole and higher, allowed further increase in the sensitivity and speed of detection of PBPs. The synthesis of high specific radioactivity ^{3}H-penicillin (ROSEGAY 1981), developed in a cooperative effort between the Rockefeller University Microbiology Laboratory and colleagues at the Merck Institute for Therapeutic Research, has allowed us to examine PBPs in live, growing bacteria. The general importance of such in vivo studies is multifold: titration of PBPs in membrane preparations does not take into account the existence of a permeability barrier that might be present in the cell. This makes the interpretation of correlations between the antibiotic "affinities" versus antimicrobial effectiveness difficult (see later). The preparation of membranes may cause selective inactivation or may alter in some other way the properties of some PBPs; the experience with model enzymes shows that the nature of the microenvironment has major influence, not only on the kinetic parameters but even on the catalytic nature of enzyme activities. An example of such differences between the results of in vivo and in vitro labeling (GUTMANN et al. 1980) is shown in Table 2. The reasons for the major shifts in the distribution of bound penicillin (see e.g., PBPs 2a/b and 4, labeled in vivo versus in vitro) are not yet known.

Labeling of PBPs in live cells should also allow studies on the biosynthesis and physiology of these interesting membrane proteins. An illustration of the results of such studies is shown in Fig. 7. Growing group A streptococci were briefly ex-

Table 2. Some properties of the PBPs of group A streptococci – comparison of the results in vivo and in vitro labeling techniques. (GUTMANN and TOMASZ 1981)

PBP	MolWt	Amount of penicillin bound [a] (%)			Initial half-life of deacylation (min)	
		In vivo	In crude lysate	In vitro	In vivo	In vitro
1	95,000	11.8	11.4	4.3	93	84
2a/b [b]	82,000 81,000	74.0	72.3	49.3	127	148
3	70,000	8.5	10.0	3.9	ND [c]	81
4	50,000	0.7	0.8	37.0	16	20
5	47,000	5.0	5.5	5.5	16	24

[a] Determined after exposure to a saturating concentration of [^{3}H] penicillin (0.5 μg/ml) for 10 min

[b] Not resolved in most experiments

[c] ND, not determined

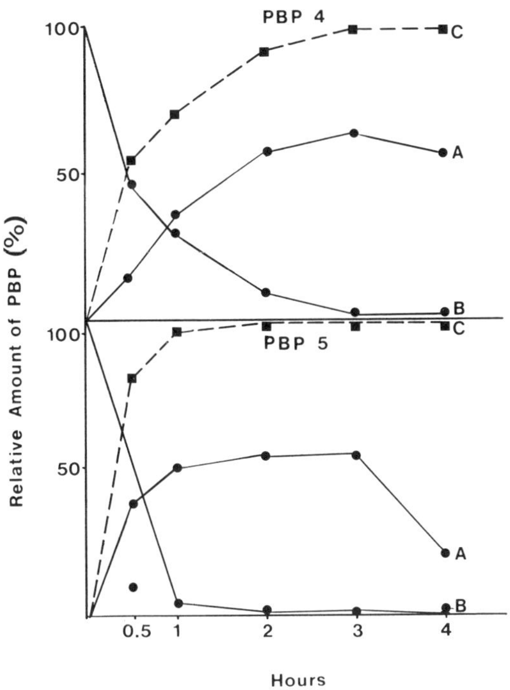

Fig. 7. In vivo acylation and deacylation of PBPs in group A streptococci. A 30-ml exponential-phase culture (about 5×10^7 CFU/ml) was incubated with 10 μg chloramphenicol (CAP) per milliliter to stop biosynthesis of proteins. The culture was divided into two 15-ml portions (cultures A and B). Culture A received 0.5 μg of nonradioactive penicillin per ml, and culture B received 0.5 μg of (^{3}H)penicillin per ml. Both cultures were incubated at 37 °C for 10 min and then chilled to 4 °C. The bacteria were harvested by centrifugation at $12{,}000 \times g$ for 5 min and washed twice with cold THB in the presence of 10 μg of CAP per milliliter. Finally, the cells were suspended in about 15 ml of prewarmed THB containing 10 μg CAP/ml. The suspension volumes of cultures A and B were adjusted to give cell suspensions which had identical light-scattering values. Each culture was then incubated at 37 °C for 4 h, and at different times 1-ml samples were removed to assay for the PBPs. Samples from culture B [which had been exposed to (^{3}H)penicillin] were centrifuged immediately and processed. Samples from culture A (which had been exposed to nonradioactive penicillin) were incubated with (^{3}H)penicillin for 10 min and then processed for the assay of PBPs. Culture B was used to evaluate the degree of deacylation of PBPs, whereas culture A was used to determine the PBPs available for reacylation by (^{3}H) penicillin.
The relative intensities of the PBP bands on fluorograms were quantitated by densitometry. The intensity of each PBP band from the zero-time sample in culture B was defined as 100%, and all results for cultures A and B were expressed as percent changes relative to the corresponding 100% values. The third curve (*curve C*) on the graph shows the percentage of individual PBPs that became deacylated at particular sampling times. These values were calculated by subtracting the band intensity of a PBP at a particular sampling time from the corresponding zero-time value and expressing the difference as a percentage of the zero-time value. Thus, curve C simply shows the relative amounts of the PBPs expected to be present in the deacylated form. If all such PBPs were available for another round of reaction with (^{3}H)penicillin, then we would expect the values on curve A (experimentally determined) to coincide with the values on curve C. The discrepancy between the two curves expresses quantitatively the loss of each PBP. (GUTMANN and TOMASZ 1981)

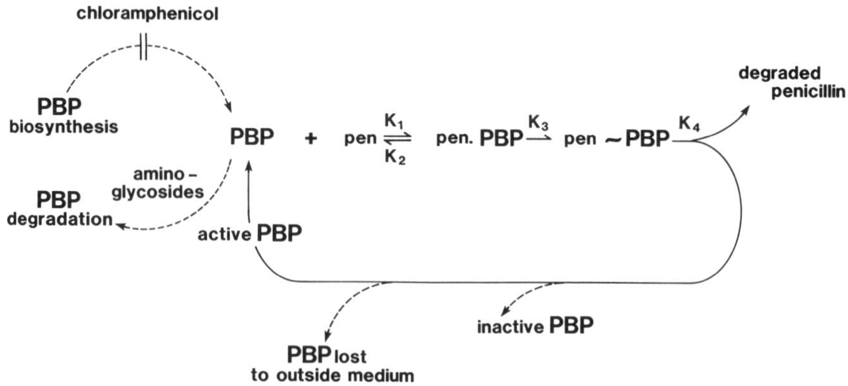

Fig. 8. Interaction of penicillin with bacterial PBPs in growing bacteria. *Dashed lines* indicate processes observable by in vivo labeling of the PBPs of live, growing bacteria

posed to saturating concentrations of ^{3}H penicillin. After removal of the unbound reagent, the bacteria were incubated in full growth medium and the rate of release of radioactivity from the different PBPs was determined (curve *B* in Fig. 7). In a parallel experiment (aimed at determining the rates of reacylation), the cells first received nonradioactive penicillin (to block all PBPs) and then the rate of recovery of PBPs was determined by pulses of ^{3}H penicillin during incubation in growth medium containing chloramphenicol (to prevent synthesis of new PBP molecules) (curve *A* in Fig. 7). These types of experiments have revealed some interesting differences between the in vitro and in vivo reactions. In essence, an incomplete recovery of some of the PBPs was noted after a "round" of reaction with penicillin. This loss of activity could be partially accounted for by two processes: (1) inactivation, and (2) release of a fraction of the penicilloyl-PBP complexes into the medium (GUTMANN et al. 1980). Another interesting process discovered in such in vivo experiments was the rapid and extensive proteolytic degradation of PBPs upon preincubation of the streptococci with bactericidal aminoglycosides (GUTMANN and TOMASZ 1981). Some of these processes, approachable by the technique of in vivo labeling, are depicted in Fig. 8.

5. Selective Affinity of PBPs for Various β-Lactams

One of the major discoveries of the PBP technology was the finding that individual PBPs of a bacterium may have widely different selective affinities for structurally different β-lactam antibiotics (SPRATT 1975). The selective affinity of PBPs for various β-lactams is usually determined by competition assays in which membrane preparations (or live bacteria) are allowed to briefly preincubate with various concentrations of the nonradioactive β-lactam, followed by back-titration of the "available" PBPs by exposure to saturating concentrations of radioactive penicillin. The fluorograms are then quantitated by densitometry. An illustration of the method is shown in Fig. 9.

The selective affinities of various β-lactams for individual PBPs are usually expressed in terms of the concentration of the drug needed to cause 50% inhibition

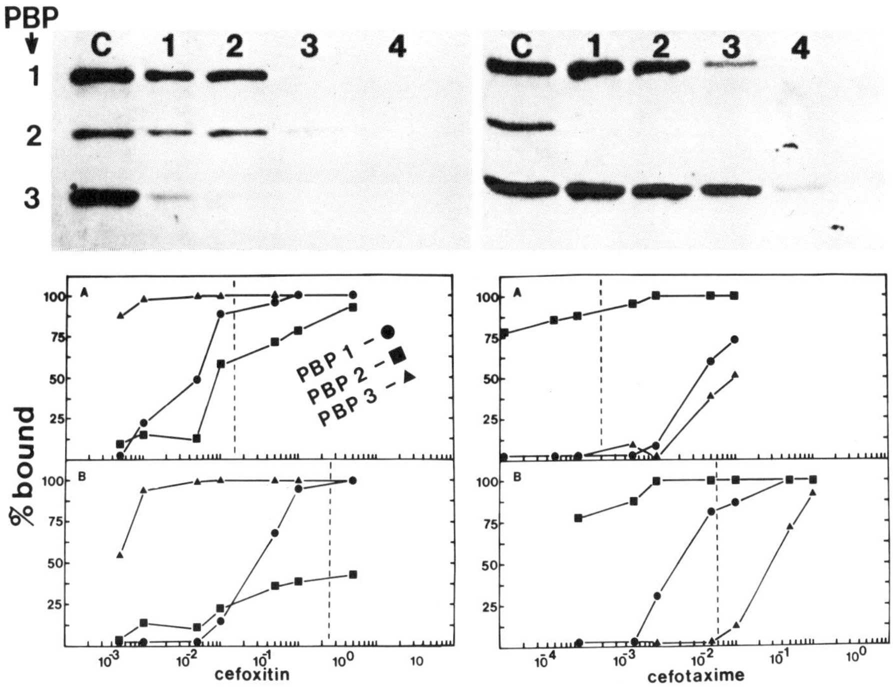

Fig. 9. Selective affinities of β-lactam antibiotics for the PBPs of *N. gonorrhoeae*. Upper portion shows the gel fluorographs from competition assays in which increasing concentrations of cefoxitin (*left*) and cefotaxime (*right*) were incubated with gonococcal membranes. Residual PBPs were then determined by addition of (^{3}H)penicillin. *C* represents a control with received saturating (^{3}H)penicillin only. Lanes 1–4 received 5 ng, 50 ng, 500 ng, and 50 μg/ml respectively. These experiments were performed with the resistant transformant TR3 (corresponds to B titration curves in lower portion). The *lower portion* of the figure shows plots from densitometric tracings of a similar experiment in which live cells of gonococci were exposed to the antibiotics. Exponentially growing cells of strain FA 19 and its isogenic resistant transformant TR3 were exposed to increasing concentrations (μg/ml) of cefotaxime or cefoxitin, for 15 min. Residual PBPs were measured by addition of (^{3}H)penicillin for 15 min. After electrophoresis and fluorography, the amount of (^{3}H)penicillin bound was determined by densitometry. The values were then converted, using a (^{3}H)penicillin-treated reference, into the percentage of unlabeled competing antibiotic bound. Sets A are FA 19 titrations and sets B are transformant TR3 titrations. *Vertical dashed line* represents MIC. (DOUGHERTY et al. 1981).

of the subsequent binding of radioactive penicillin. Extensive tabulations of such I_{50} or ID_{50} values for various β-lactams vis-à-vis individual PBPs may be found in several current publications (SPRATT 1979; GEORGOPAPADAKOU and LIU 1980; NOGUCHI et al. 1979; CURTIS et al. 1979a, b).

6. Selective Morphological Effects

The ability of various β-lactams to cause a variety of morphological changes in bacteria, often in a concentration-dependent manner, has been known for some time (GARDNER 1940; DUGUID 1946; ROLINSON et al. 1977; GREENWOOD and O'GRADY 1973). For instance, benzylpenicillin at low concentrations was shown to induce the formation of filaments in *E. coli*, while higher concentrations caused a halt in growth, followed by rapid lysis. Certain cephalosporins were shown to cause primarily filament formation even within a broader range of drug concentrations (LORIAN and ATKINSON 1976) and the amidino penicillins (mecillinam) and some of the more recently isolated penems and carbapenems caused the conversion of gram-negative bacilli to osmotically stable, round forms (LUND and TYBRING 1972; MELCHIOR et al. 1973; SPRATT et al. 1977c; PRIOR and WARNER 1974). In 1975 Spratt established the strikingly specific correlation between these morphological effects and the inhibition of specific PBPs, by demonstrating that selective inactivation of PBPs (by an appropriate β-lactam) would result in specific morphological changes: stop in longitudinal growth and lysis could be associated with inhibition of PBPs 1b (plus 1a); round cell morphology with inhibition of PBP 2; and filamentation with inhibition of PBP 3 (SPRATT 1975). Several members of *Enterobacteriaceae* were shown to possess PBPs of similar morphological specificity (although they may have had somewhat different molecular sizes from the comparable PBPs of *E. coli*) GEORGOPAPADAKOU and LIU 1980; NOGUCHI et al. 1979; CURTIS et al. 1979a, b; SPRATT 1977a; LORIAN et al. 1979).

Filament formation during β-lactam treatment was also observed in the gram-positive *Clostridium perfringens* (WILLIAMSON and WARD 1981) and in a strain of *Streptococcus bovis* (LORIAN and ATKINSON 1978); cells of several streptococci were shown to elongate and form bulges at the incipient septa, during treatment with *low* concentrations of penicillin (DRING and HURST 1969; WILLIAMSON et al. 1980a); an anaerobic oral fusiform bacterium was described as responding to mecillinam treatment in an anomalous manner, i.e., by filamentous growth (ONOE et al. 1981).

The specificity of these effects was confirmed by the isolation of bacterial mutants defective in PBPs. Conditional mutants of *E. coli* extensively defective in PBP 1b, or double mutants defective in PBP 1b and thermosensitive in PBP 1a, underwent rapid lysis upon shifting to the nonpermissive temperature (MATSUHASHI et al. 1977, 1978). Mutants defective in PBPs 2 or 3 grew as either round or filamentous forms, respectively (SPRATT 1975). Mutants lacking PBPs 4, 5, and 6, individually or as double mutants, showed no morphological effect and grew normally (SPRATT 1977a; MATSUHASHI et al. 1979).

It seems, therefore, that individual PBPs perform distinct physiological functions. PBPs 1a and 1b seem to perform some function for the structural integrity of the cells; the function of PBP 2 seems essential for the maintenance of bacillary shape; PBP 3 is needed for cell division. No clear physiological function, either in terms of morphology or need for bacterial survival (at least in test tube cultures), could be assigned to PBPs 4, 5, and 6, although mutants defective in PBP 5 showed increased sensitivity to penicillin (TAMAKI et al. 1978) and lowered PBP 4 was detected in *E. coli* mutants tolerant to the lytic action of cephaloridine, which also showed substantially lowered endopeptidase (and hydrolytic transglycosylase) activities (KITANO et al. 1980).

The selectivity of morphological effects is seldom complete (the apparent exception being mecillinam which only reacts with PBP 2) so that for the establishment of the specific PBP target responsible for a morphological effect, it is important to examine the bacteria at different antibiotic doses.

Because of the selective affinity of mecillinam for PBP 2 and certain cephalosporins for PBPs 1 and 3, and because of the accompanying specific morphological effects, these β-lactams have been extensively used as diagnostic tools to establish tentative functional similarities between PBPs of different bacterial species. This has been quite successful within the group of Enterobacteriaceae. It is quite likely that at least some of the large variations observed in the MIC values of certain β-lactams against various groups of bacteria (see Table 1) reflect differences in the structure of antibiotic recognition sites of PBPs.

Titration of selective affinities with the PBPs of *E. coli* has also been used to classify β-lactams of different chemical structure, and some correlations between structure and selective PBP affinities have begun to emerge. It is clear from Fig. 10 that the parent compounds (penicillanic acid or cephalosporanic acid and their 6- or 7-amino derivatives) have relatively poor binding capacities. However, upon modification of the basic structures, a striking and selective increase in PBP affinities may be observed. Replacement of the H substituent at position C7 in cephalosporins with the $-OCH_3$ group of cephamycins greatly increases binding to PBPs 5, 6 (and 4). Strong binding to carboxypeptidases by cephamycins (as compared to cephalosporins) has also been reported in other bacteria (YOCUM et al. 1980b). It is also worth noting that the cephamycin-PBP 5 complexes in *E. coli* exhibit a much slower deacylation than the comparable complexes with benzylpenicillin (OHYA et al. 1978).

Beta lactam	Structure	Binding to PBP-s of E. coli						
		1a	1b	2	3	4	5	6
Penicillanic acid	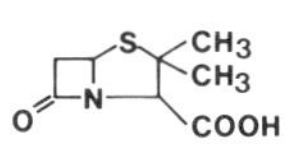	170	400	200	>500	>500	>500	>500
6-amino penicillanic acid	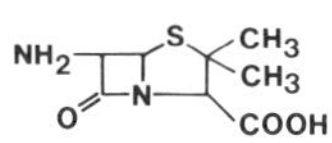	12	>50	3	>50	>50	>50	>50
Cephalosporanic acid	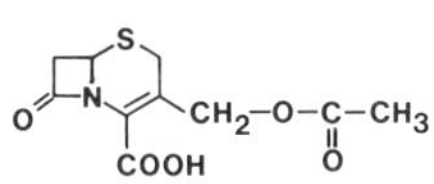	270	500	300	>500	>500	>500	>500
7-amino cephalosporanic acid	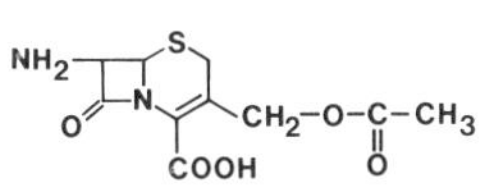	30	500	58	>500	>500	>500	>500

Fig. 10a

Fig. 10a–e. Selective binding of β-lactams to PBPs of *E. coli*. The *numbers* represent the concentrations of the antibiotics (μg/ml) needed to cause a 50% inhibition of penicillin binding to the corresponding PBP, in competition experiments using membrane preparations from *E. coli* and preincubation with the competing β-lactam followed by incubation with saturating concentration of radioactive benzylpenicillin. The data were compiled from CURTIS et al. 1979a, b; CURTIS and ROSS 1980; OHYA et al. 1978; SPRATT 1977b; SPRATT 1980; SPRATT et al. 1977; SYKES et al. 1981a; NOGUCHI et al. 1979

Beta lactam	Structure (Selective binding to PBPs 1a/b and 3)	Binding to PBS-s of E. coli						
		1a	1b	2	3	4	5	6
Cephalothin	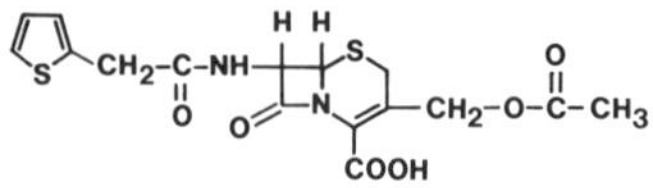	<0.25	16	37	1	60	125	130
Cephaloridine	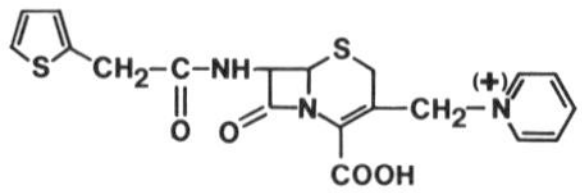	0.25	2.5	50	8	17	250	250
Cephsulodine	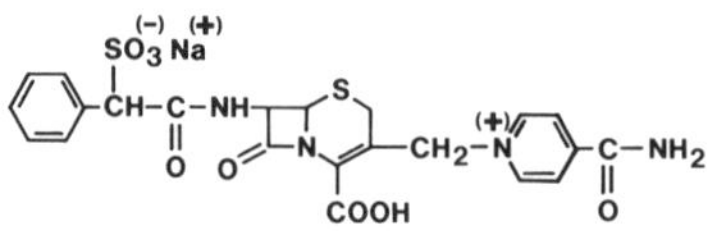	0.47	3.7	250	250	250	250	250
Cefotaxime(syn)	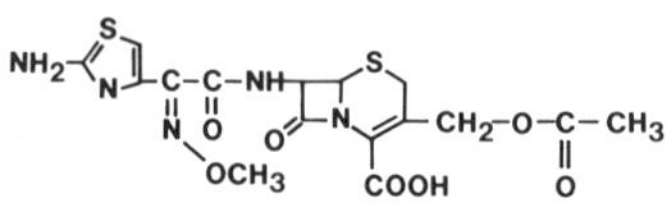	0.05	0.7	5	0.05	30	50	50
Cefotaxime(anti)	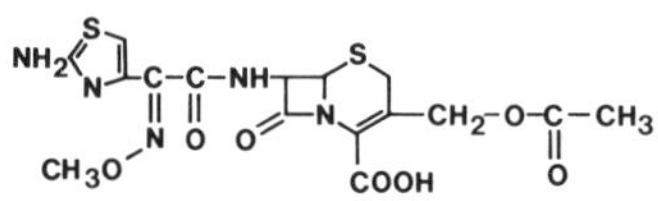			inactive				

Fig. 10b

Beta lactam	Structure (Selective binding to PBP 2	Binding to PBP-s of E. coli						
		1a	1b	2	3	4	5	6
Mecillinam	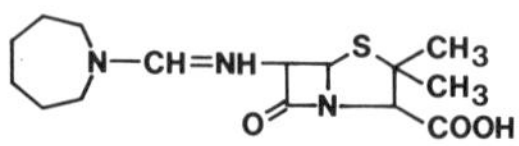	>250	>250	0.25	>250	>250	>250	>250
Thienamycin	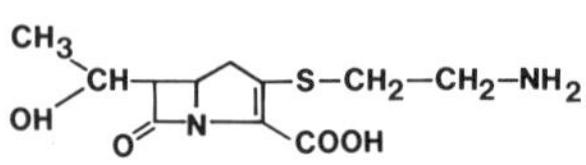	1.1	0.06	31	0.15 5.5	1	3.8	
Clavulanic acid	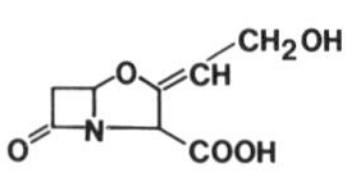	52	4.1	310	11	21	15	
Synthetic penem	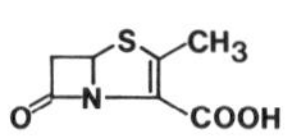	(+)	++	(+)	-	-	-	

Fig. 10c

The same $-OCH_3$ substitution appears to lower binding to PBP 2 of *E. coli* (OHYA et al. 1978). It seems that thienamycin and other synthetic penems have high affinity for PBP 2, while piperacillin, mezlocillin, and monobactams are highly selective for PBP 3. Figure 10 illustrates some of these results.

Beta lactam	Structure (Selective binding to PBP 3)	Binding to PBPs of E. coli 1a	1b	2	3	4	5	6
Cephalexin	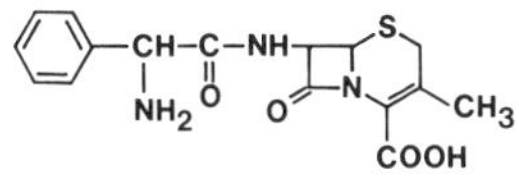	4	240	250	8	30	250	250
Piperacillin	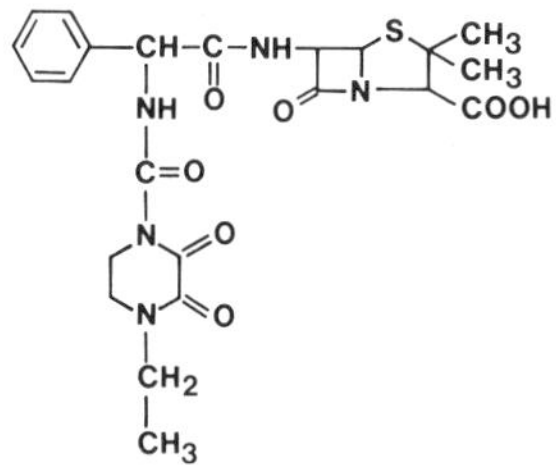	4.5		0.5	0.2	>10	>10	>10
Mezlocillin	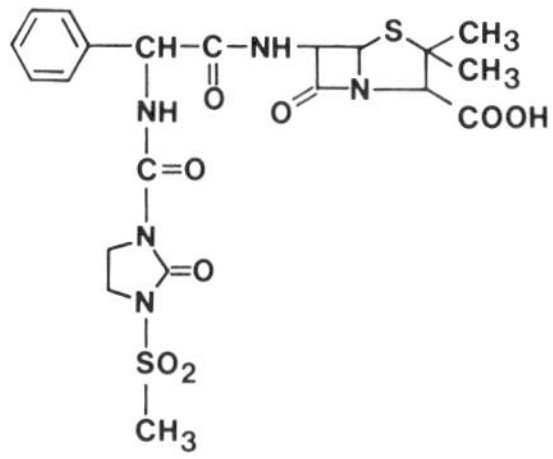	1.5	8	0.9	0.025	>25	>25	>25
Benzylpenicillin (R=H)	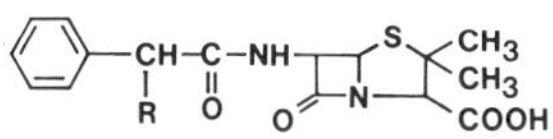	0.5	3	0.8	0.9	1.0	24	19
(Ampicillin)($R=NH_2$)		1.4	(3.9)	(0.7)	(0.9)	(2.0)	(140)	(9)
Azthreonam	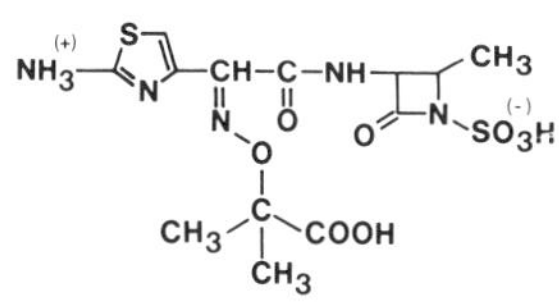	10	100	100	0.1	100	100	

Fig. 10d

Beta lactam	Structure (Selective binding to PBPs 4, 5, 6)	Binding to PBPs of E. coli 1a	1b	2	3	4	5	6
R-45656	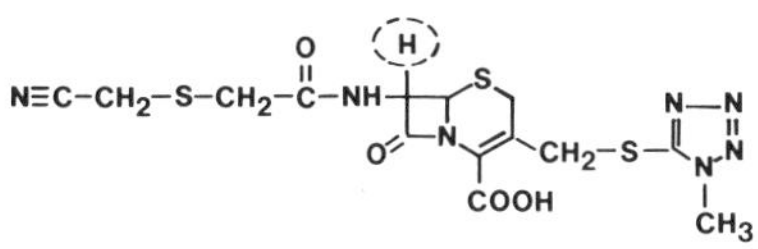	0.2	0.1	7	0.7	4	>125	>125
CS-1170(cefmetazole)	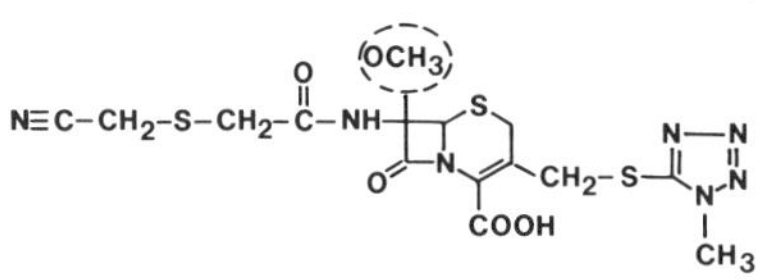	0.4	0.4	>125	0.7	0.2	0.6	1.0
Cefoxitin	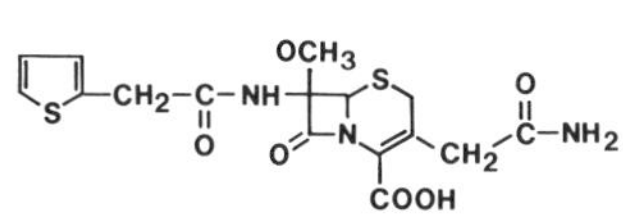	0.1	3.9	>250	5.8	7.0	0.6	0.9

Fig. 10e

It is not clear whether these striking changes in PBP affinities reflect the specificities of secondary, tertiary, etc. recognition sites on these proteins. Alternatively, they may be related to differences in the microenvironments of various PBPs within the plasma membrane which may influence access to the active site of PBPs. It should also be remembered that in most of the published work on selective PBP affinities, the possibility of a very high deacylation rate (giving false negative results) has not been routinely tested.

VI. Penicillin-Sensitive Enzymes in Cell Wall Synthesis

The picture emerging from the studies briefly surveyed in the previous sections is that the biochemical targets of β-lactam antibiotics are a group of proteins (PBPs) anchored in the bacterial plasma membrane. At least some of these proteins can catalyze carboxypeptidase (endopeptidase) and transpeptidase reactions with a variety of model substrates, i.e., the same types of reactions that were originally proposed in 1965 as the likely biochemical targets of penicillin action. However, selective inactivation of individual PBPs leads to strikingly unique morphological consequences, implying that these penicillin-sensitive proteins perform a whole range of distinct physiological functions. Furthermore, the biochemical equivalents of these functions are clearly more complex than the reactions demonstrated with the model peptide substrates.

Recent studies with wall-membrane complexes (TYNECKA and WARD 1975; WARD 1974; TAKU and FAN 1976; SCHRADER and FAN 1974), reverting L-forms (ELLIOTT et al. 1975) and whole bacterial systems (MIRELMAN et al. 1972, 1976; VAN HEIJENOORT et al. 1978; TIPPER and WRIGHT 1979), have revealed a considerable variety in the ways activities of the transpeptidase and carboxypeptidase enzymes are utilized in cell wall synthesis. A relatively newly developed experimental system for such studies involved bacteria made permeable by treatment with organic solvents and fed bactoprenol-linked disaccharide-peptide or UDP-linked precursors (TAKU and FAN 1976; SCHRADER and FAN 1974; MIRELMAN and NUCHAMOVITZ 1979). Formation of polymeric material (insolubility in trichloroacetic acid) or attachment of the precursor to the preformed cell wall (insolubility in hot SDS) may be assayed separately. In other experiments, bacteria were incubated either in specially limited medium (allowing wall synthesis but no cytoplasmic syntheses) (SHOCKMAN et al. 1958) or full growth medium, and the incorporation of radioactive precursors (glucosamine, glycine, diaminopimelic acid or lysine) into cell wall material was assayed, after appropriate fractionation procedures that solubilized all but the cell wall murein.

Studies with these methods have produced evidence indicating that several bacterial systems *(E. coli, B. megaterium, P. aeruginosa, Bacillus licheniformis, Micrococcus luteus)* are capable of forming poorly crosslinked oligomers of cell wall material, apparently by a penicillin-insensitive transglycosylase reaction (VAN HEIJENOORT et al. 1978); WESTON et al. 1977). In reverting protoplasts of autolysin defective bacteria, the extension of long strands of what appears to be oligomeric murein material has been observed by electron microscopy (ELLIOTT et al. 1975). In some of these systems, evidence has been produced indicating that those oligomers can be "chased" into mature cell wall material (FUCHS-CLEVELAND and GILVARG 1976; MIRELMAN and NUCHAMOVITZ 1979). These results have been interpreted to indicate that the bactoprenol-pyrophosphate-linked disaccharide-pentapeptide units may first undergo polymerization via transglycosylation to oligomeric intermediates (reaction 1 in Fig. 11) and it is these, rather than the monomers, that serve as the direct precursors for attachment to the preexisting cell wall material (MIRELMAN 1981). Although the general validity of these observations is not fully established and not yet generally accepted (ROGERS 1981), the results and their interpretation offer plausible, physiologically distinct functions for the multiple transpeptidase and carboxypeptidase activities that have been described in several bacteria.

The oligomers may have been exposed to some degree of intramolecular transpeptidation, as judged by the presence of a limited number of crosslinks, the formation of which is insensitive to penicillin. However, the attachment of these TCA-insoluble (and SDS-soluble) oligomers to preexisting cell wall material occurs by a penicillin-sensitive transpeptidation ("anchoring") (reaction 2 in Fig. 11) (MIRELMAN 1981). A very few, even a single such transpeptide linkage appears to be sufficient to establish insolubility in hot SDS, which has been used as the operational test for the incorporation reaction. It is assumed that the attached oligomeric chains undergo further transpeptidation during a maturation process (newly incorporated cell wall was found to have less than the average degree of crosslinking) (reaction 4 in Fig. 11). This latter process appears to be less sensitive to penicillin than the anchoring reaction. Another reaction that must follow is the establishment of glycosidic linkages between the precursor material and the reducing end of a glycan chain in the preexisting cell wall (reaction 3 in Fig. 11).

Another type of attachment may also be observed in *S. aureus* and various other bacteria in which incorporation of cell wall precursors into the preexisting wall (i.e., hot SDS-insoluble material) continues (with a slow rate) in the presence of penicillin (MIRELMAN et al. 1972). This seems to represent a situation in which the attachment of precursor material (monomers or, possibly, oligomers) occurs via the penicillin-insensitive transglycosylase reaction (reaction 5). The presence of uncrosslinked disaccharide-pentapeptides in the newly synthesized portion of the cell wall has been demonstrated (TIPPER and STROMINGER 1965). Since in *Staphylococcus* over 90% of the cell wall peptides are crosslinked, this attachment reaction must eventually be followed by a penicillin sensitive transpeptidation (reactions 6, 7).

In most of the transpeptidase-catalyzed anchoring reactions studied so far, the carboxy terminal D-alanine carbonyl groups in the oligomeric precursors serve as "donors," and free primary amino groups on the peptide side chains of the preexisting wall provide the "acceptors." In a third version of the cell wall incorporation reaction described in *Gaffkya homari* (HAMMES and KANDLER 1976), the inverse situation has been observed: pentapeptide side-chains in the preexisting cell wall are donors and the precursor material is made up primarily of disaccharide-tetrapeptide units from which the terminal D-alanine residues have been removed by a prior carboxypeptidase reaction. In this organism, the anchoring transpeptidation reaction is catalyzed by a penicillin-resistant enzyme (reaction 9). Nevertheless, the *whole* process of cell wall synthesis is penicillin sensitive due to the antibiotic sen-

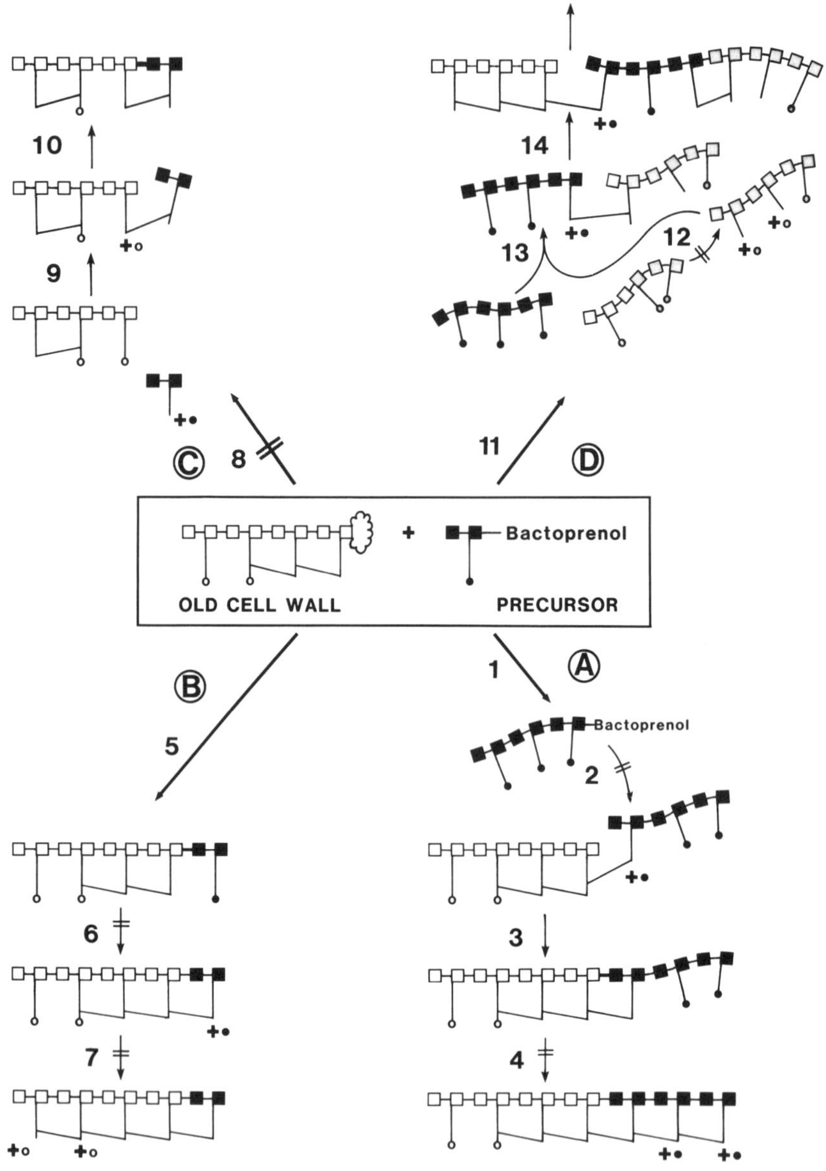

Fig. 11. Terminal reactions in cell wall biosynthesis. The figure illustrates in a schematic fashion four different types of reaction sequences observed and/or postulated to occur during the incorporation of the bactoprenol-linked disaccharide pentapeptide cell wall precursor subunits into the preexisting (old) cell wall (see schematic structures within the rectangle at the center of the figure). The squares represent the *N*-acetyl-glucosamine and *N*-acetyl muramic acid residues, respectively in the glycan chain of old (*empty squares*) or newly made (*black squares*) cell wall material. The *circles* at the end of the stem peptides represent the carboxy terminal D-alanine units in the old (*empty*) or new (*black*) cell wall subunits. In scheme *A*, the precursor disaccharide peptide is first polymerized by a penicillin insensitive transglycosylase (*1*) and these product oligomers are "anchored" on an available R3 amino-group of the old cell wall, by a penicillin sensitive transpeptidase (*2*). Formation of gly-

sitivity of the carboxypeptidase preparing the tetrapeptide units (reaction 8) which appear to be highly preferred precursors for the cell wall synthetic reaction in this bacterium (HAMMES and KANDLER 1976).

Analysis of cell wall synthesis in a thermosensitive filament-forming mutant of *E. coli* has led to a further interesting proposition concerning the possibly distinct functioning of the transpeptidase–carboxypeptidase system (MIRELMAN et al. 1977). It was found that shifting to the nonpermissive temperature (or treatment with cephalosporins) caused a halt in septation, inhibition of carboxypeptidase activity, and continued longitudinal cell wall synthesis with increased transpeptidation. Shift down (or removal of the inhibitor) reinitiated cell division and increased carboxypeptidase activity. As an interpretation of those findings, it was suggested that the relatively high carboxypeptidase activity in normally dividing cells converts many of the side chains of a portion of the newly made cell wall oligomers to tetrapeptides (reaction 12), thus preventing them from taking part in the normal anchoring reaction as donors. On the other hand, these modified oligomers may now serve as acceptors in transpeptidation reactions with other newly made, but unchanged (pentapeptide containing) oligomers (reaction 13). This link-up of newly made donors with newly made acceptors would represent the beginning of septum formation which, in a sense, would represent a combination of the *G. homari*-type and the more conventional anchoring reaction.

In bacterial cell walls, with limited degree of average cross-linking (e.g., the wall of *E. coli*), the unlinked side-chain peptides are mostly tetrapeptides (and some tripeptides) indicating, most probably, carboxypeptidase activity. (Alternatively, tetrapeptide side chains could have been generated by an endopeptidase reaction.) The possible role of such an activity (e.g., reaction 7) in regulating the degree of crosslinkage has long been recognized (TIPPER and STROMINGER 1968).

This brief survey indicates that, of the three types of enzyme activities (transglycosylase, transpeptidase, and carboxypeptidase) involved with cell wall synthesis, each appears to catalyze a number of reactions of sufficiently different nature to indicate that there might exist several transglycosylases, transpeptidases, and carboxypeptidases in a single bacterial cell. In the case of transglycosylase, these would correspond to reactions 3, 5, or 10 in Fig. 11. Distinct transpeptidases may catalyze the anchoring reaction of cell wall elongation (reaction 2), the transpeptidation occurring during the maturation of cell wall (reaction 4) and the polymerization in septal wall synthesis (reaction 13).

Similarly, distinct carboxypeptidase activities may be involved with the formation of nascent acceptor-type oligomers (reaction 12 or 8) and with the removal of

---

cosidic bonds (*3*) and possible D,D carboxypeptidase action (*4*) are also illustrated. In scheme *B*, the attachment of newly made subunits to old cell wall occurs by a penicillin insensitive transglycosylation (*5*) followed by transpeptidase (*6*) and D,D carboxypeptidase (*7*) activities. Scheme *C* illustrates the reaction sequence on *Gaffyka homari*, with the old cell wall providing the carbonyl donors and the penicillin sensitive reaction catalyzed by a D,D carboxypeptidase (*8*), while the "anchoring" transpeptidase (*9*) is penicillin insensitive. Scheme *D* illustrates the hypothetical septal cell wall synthesis. Ligation (*13*) of newly made (*11*) cell wall oligomers with (*black*) and without (*grey*) the terminal D-alanine residues [the latter having been produced by D,D carboxypeptidase action (*12*)] is eventually followed by attachment to the preexisting longitudinal cell wall by transpeptidation (*14*). For details, see text

terminal D-alanine residues from already anchored cell wall oligomers (reaction 7 possibly, as a means of controlling the degree of crosslinking).

The existence of multiple, functionally different transpeptidases is consistent with the observation that formation of chemically different crosslinks (occurring in bacteria with type AII peptidoglycan) have different penicillin sensitivities (Mirelman and Bracha 1974). Additional, conceivably distinct enzyme activities might be responsible for the cell wall thickening observed in the absence of the normally equatorial wall synthesis in gram-positive cocci during inhibition of protein biosynthesis (Shockman et al. 1958).

These findings and models then require the existence of more than one transpeptidase and carboxypeptidase in a single bacterium. Evidence for the existence of multiple forms of these enzymes has already been indicated in work on the purification of penicillin-sensitive enzymes (Blumberg and Strominger 1974).

1. Penicillin-Sensitive Enzymes as PBPs

The introduction of PBP technology to the analysis of penicillin-sensitive proteins provided a tremendous stimulus and resolution to biochemical studies on bacterial cell wall synthesis. One of the major benefits of the PBP method was that it provided a rapid technique for the identification of mutants lacking specific PBPs. Examination of the physiological properties, β-lactam sensitivities and murein-related enzyme activities in such mutants has led to the identification of PBPs 5 and 6 (responsible for over 80% of the penicillin bound by *E. coli* membranes) with the major D,D-carboxypeptidase (carboxypeptidase 1A, determined by the *dac* B locus) while PBP 4 seems to be identical to the carboxypeptidase 1B – endopeptidase (*dac* C locus) of *E. coli* (Spratt and Strominger 1976; Tamura et al. 1976).

E. coli mutants defective in carboxypeptidase activity (*dac* A mutants defective in PBP 5, and *dac* B mutants defective in PBP 4 as well as double mutants of these) have been isolated and were found to be physiologically normal (Spratt 1977a; Matsuhashi et al. 1979), as far as ability to grow was concerned, and this was originally interpreted to mean that these PBPs perform no function essential for the survival of the cells, thus negating the hypothesized physiological and biosynthetic roles of these enzymes (see above).

However, a closer examination revealed: (a) that PBP 5–defective mutants have an increased sensitivity to penicillin (Tamaki et al. 1978); (b) that it is not unusual in enzyme-defective mutants that the phenotype related to the activity is only revealed in deeply defective mutants, and even in double mutants of *E. coli* defective both in PBPs 4 and 5 a residual (5%–10%) carboxypeptidase activity is still detectable, possibly representing the activity of PBP 6, which may be sufficient to perform the physiologically important functions of these enzymes (Amanuma and Strominger 1980). This is also consistent with the finding that the cell walls of PBP 4, 5 double mutants have a normal degree of crosslinking (Sharpe et al. 1974) and show only a temporary increase (over that seen in wild type cells) in the concentration of pentapeptides in newly made cell wall material. However, mutants defective both in PBPs 4 and 5 do not form filaments, and thus the postulated regulatory role of carboxypeptidases in septation must belong to some other PBP, possibly PBP 3 (Botta and Park 1981).

The problems encountered with the definitive identification of enzyme activities in PBPs 1, 2, and 3 did not allow similarly detailed biochemical investigations. However, it has been proposed, for instance, that PBP 1b of *E. coli* may be the main "anchoring" transpeptidase; PBP 3 may be involved, either as a second transpeptidase or as a distinct carboxypeptidase, in the formation of septal walls; and PBP 4 might be a secondary transpeptidase catalyzing transpeptidation during cell wall maturation (DEPEDRO et al. 1980).

D. Physiological Consequences of β-Lactam Inhibition

The investigations on biochemical targets of penicillin, briefly surveyed in the previous section, produced a much more complex picture than was envisioned in 1965 when the penicillin sensitivity of the transpeptidation reaction was discovered. Bacteria appear to contain a number of different transpeptidases and carboxypeptidases and a number of different penicillin-sensitive proteins with distinct physiological roles. Must all of these proteins be inhibited in order to bring about the antibacterial effects of penicillin? This question was further complicated by the finding that different β-lactams have highly selective affinities for one or another PBP and yet, each of these β-lactams could interfere with bacterial growth. Is there more than one mechanism for the inhibition of a bacterial cell, depending on which β-lactams are used? Are the functions of some of the PBPs dispensable, while others with more essential physiological roles are the only relevant antibacterial targets of penicillin? Experiments with the *E. coli* mutants lacking PBPs 4 and 5, without an apparent effect on bacterial survival, have lent some credence to this latter idea. The testing of various approaches to sort out the physiologically important PBPs ("killing targets") from among all the detectable binding proteins has become one of the major activities of the field. This section will illustrate some of the approaches used.

I. Search for the Killing Targets

If the multiple PBPs of bacteria include one or more so-called killing targets for penicillins, while others perform only less vital physiological functions (e.g., PBPs 4, 5, and 6 of *E. coli*) then it should be possible to identify the former by comparing the degree of inhibition of PBPs and the degree of inhibition of the corresponding bacterium, as a function of the antibiotic concentration. The principle of this argument is that PBPs that are saturated either *below* or far *above* the MIC concentration would not qualify as killing targets. Several PBPs have been eliminated on these grounds. The cases include *E. coli* mutants lacking over 90% of their PBPs 5 and/or 4 (SPRATT 1977a; MATSUHASHI et al. 1979), staphylococci defective in PBP 4 (WYKE et al. 1981), and the PBP 5 of *B. subtilis* that may be inhibited to over 90% by 6-aminopenicillanic acid (6-APA) (BLUMBERG and STROMINGER 1971) or PBP 3 of pneumococci which is 90% saturated by one-tenth of the MIC-concentrations of cefoxitin (WILLIAMSON et al. 1980a). All these conditions allow apparently normal growth of the bacteria. Conversely, the inhibition of saturation of PBP 5 in *B. megaterium* required almost 10^4-fold higher concentrations of cephalosoporins than the growth inhibitory concentration; for this reason, it was not considered a physiologically important target (REYNOLDS et al. 1978).

If certain PBPs were indeed the killing targets of β-lactam antibiotics, one might expect some numerical correlation between the degree of saturation of these binding proteins and the MIC value for the same β-lactam. Indeed, such correlations have been claimed to exist between the concentration of β-lactams needed to cause half saturation (ID_{50}) of the *E. coli* PBP 1 b and the MIC value; log/log plots of these values fell on a nearly straight line (NOZAKI et al. 1979).

In *E. coli* and other *Enterobacteriaceae* in which certain classes of β-lactams have special affinities for either PBPs 1 or 2 or 3, an additional resolution for this type of experiment was available. Inhibitors of PBPs 1, 2, and 3 in *E. coli* all cause inhibition of bacterial growth and killing and eventual lysis, in addition to including the distinct morphological alterations described in the previous section. It was shown that the MIC for such β-lactams is closest to the concentrations of these drugs needed to half-saturate the most sensitive PBP (CURTIS et al. 1979a, b; SPRATT 1980). As an illustration, the I_{50} values of cephaloridine (MIC = 2 μg/ml) for PBPs 2 through 6 were all higher than 8 μg/ml; for 1 b it was 2.5 and for 1 a, 0.25. In the case of mecillinam (MIC = 0.05 μg/ml), I_{50} for all but PBP 2 (< 0.25 μg/ml) were higher than 250 μg/ml. The I_{50} of cephalexin (MIC = 8 μg/ml) for PBP 3 was 8 μg/ml while for the rest of the PBPs it was higher than 30 μg/ml, except for 1 a, where it was 4 μg/ml (CURTIS et al. 1979b). Similarly, conditional mutants defective in PBPs 1 a plus 1 b or in PBP 3 not only exhibited expected selective morphological effects but also died (SUZUKI et al. 1978).

On the basis of these findings, Spratt suggested the *E. coli* may have three killing targets (SPRATT 1980) corresponding to PBP 1 b, 2, and 3 and, depending on the nature of the β-lactam, bacteria may be killed by three different mechanisms.

The notion that there might be more than one mechanism by which β-lactams can inhibit and kill *E. coli* is supported by the different phenomena accompanying these inhibitions: cells inhibited by drugs selective for PBP 1 b cause rapid cellular lysis, apparently due to the triggering of cell wall hydrolyzing enzymes (KITANO and TOMASZ 1979b). PBP 2 inhibitors first cause a conversion of cultures from the rod to the round morphology by continued growth and cell divisions. Subsequently, such cells stop dividing, then enlarge and eventually lyse, in a process(es) that has been claimed to also involve cyclic AMP (AONO et al. 1979). The lysis in cultures inhibited by β-lactams selective for PBP 3 is a delayed phenomenon following substantial growth in the filamentous state.

The existence of several distinct mechanisms for the inhibition of bacteria by β-lactam antibiotics is also implied by the observed synergistic effects between pairs of structurally different β-lactams [e.g., mecillinam plus penicillin (GRUNBERG et al. 1976)] and by the fact that intrinsic resistance to certain β-lactams is not accompanied by cross-resistance to others [e.g., resistance to oxacillin in pneumococci (ZIGHELBOIM and TOMASZ 1979); to cloxacillin in *B. subtilis* (BUCHANAN and STROMINGER 1976); to mecillinam in *E. coli* (MATSUHASHI et al. 1974)].

While evidence for a variety of different growth inhibitory processes is clearly available, the notion that these differences can be completely explained on the basis of the selective inhibitions of the three PBPs is less convincing. *E. coli* mutants lacking PBP 2 can go on growing with a round cell morphology (SPRATT 1977c). Similarly, analysis of PBP 3-defective mutants could separate the morphological effect (inhibition of septation) related to the defective PBPs, from the lethal effect that may be related to some other, minor PBPs that have not yet been characterized (HIROTA 1981).

The suggestion that inhibition of PBP 3 is in itself sufficient to cause a halt in bacterial growth has been reexamined by a careful continuous observation of cells growing on the surface of agar in the presence of cefotaxime, a cephalosporin with high selective affinity for PBP 3 at the concentration used. It was found that bacteria would continue to grow in a filamentous form for at least 5 cell generations and, upon transfer to drug-free medium, such bacteria gave rise to normal, dividing cells along the entire length of the filaments (GALE et al. 1981). The eventual lysis of *E. coli* filaments formed during treatment with PBP 3-specific cephalosporins may be due to the gradual binding of the antibiotic to PBP 1b. This was actually observed during the treatment of *E. coli* cultures with a radioactively labeled cephalosporin (LY 146142): the culture growing in the filamentous form started lysing only after longer incubation periods when radioactive labeling of PBP 1 also became evident (CHASE and REYNOLDS 1980b).

These findings suggest that inhibition of PBP3 alone may not be a lethal event in *E. coli*. Similarly, inhibition of PBP 2 alone does not seem to be lethal either, since mutants lacking PBP 2 can apparently go on to grow with a round cell morphology, and it is not clear what additional event causes the growth inhibition and death of mecillinam-treated *E. coli*.

II. Labeling of PBPs in Live Bacteria

One problem with the above approaches is that the comparisons made were between ID_{50} values measured in vitro, in membrane preparations, while the MIC concentration refers to the effect of the antibiotic on live cells and it is known that the latter is often a function of other variables as well (e.g., drug penetration, β-lactamases, etc.). A different approach, in which PBPs of live, growing bacteria are labeled, avoids this problem. In order to reconstruct the condition of the MIC assay it is important that the bacteria are treated with the radioactive β-lactam under conditions which permit exponential growth. With ^{14}C-labeled penicillin, this introduces a technical problem in that the membranes labeled in vivo have to be subsequently isolated and concentrated in order to have sufficient amount of radioactive label without too high concentrations of protein. This *can* be achieved, however. Reynolds titrated growing cultures of *B. megaterium* with radioactive penicillin and found that at or close to the concentration of penicillin just sufficient to inhibit the formation of colonies on agar, the only PBP showing labeling was PBP 1 (REYNOLDS et al. 1978).

However, in another variant of the in vivo approach, a radioactive cephalosporin (LY 121998) was shown to saturate PBP 1 at concentrations *below* that of the MIC (CHASE and REYNOLDS 1980b).

Another approach used by these workers compared the known in vitro half-lives of β-lactam–PBP complexes with the time needed to resume incorporation of precursors into the cell wall, either in wall-membrane preparations (CHASE and REYNOLDS 1980 a) or in *B. megaterium* made permeable by toluene treatment (REYNOLDS and CHASE 1981). In the in vitro system, the time of resumption of wall synthesis (requiring transpeptidation) showed good correlation with the 60 min half-life of PBP 1–penicillin complex. The half-life of the rest of PBP–β-lactam complexes is much longer (4 h). On the other hand, resumption of wall synthesis, in the more permeabilized in vivo system, occurred too fast (2–3 min) to be explicable by the recovery of a substantial fraction of PBP 1.

III. In Vivo Labeling of PBPs in Pneumococci

The availability of high specific radioactivity ^{3}H-penicillin (ROSEGAY 1981), has allowed the performance of in vivo PBP labeling experiments in a simplified and faster form that does not require concentration of the labeled PBPs prior to application to the SDS-gels (WILLIAMSON et al. 1980 a). Portions (1 ml) of exponentially growing pneumococcal cultures were pretreated for 10 min with various concentrations of 18 different β-lactam antibiotics [ranging in MIC value from 6 ng to 114 μg per ml (cephalosporin C)]. Next, a single saturating concentration of ^{3}H-penicillin was added and 10 min later all cultures were processed for the PBP assay. Quantitative scoring of the fluorograms provided a large body of information confirming the observations first made in *E. coli*, namely that structurally different β-lactams have a wide variety of selective affinities for one or the other of the five resolvable PBPs of pneumococci. When the 50% saturation values were plotted against the corresponding MIC values for each PBP and for each β-lactam in a log/log plot, a straight line relationship was obtained with only one of the five PBPs, namely PBP 2b, and only with respect to 12 of the 18 antibiotics tested (Fig. 12). This finding suggested that PBP 2b may be an important β-lactam target in pneumococci.

It should be noted, however, that the actual drug concentrations at the 50% saturation were at least 2-fold higher than the MIC values. If a correlation existed between the MIC value and the half-saturation value of PBP 2b, one would expect that exposure of the bacterium to the different β-lactams, each at the corresponding MIC concentration, should result in 50% inhibition of PBP 2b. However, this was not the case. When the degrees of saturation of PBP 2b were examined upon exposure to the MIC-equivalents of the 18 β-lactams, an enormous spread of saturation values, ranging from 8% to over 90%, was found (WILLIAMSON et al. 1980 a).

The possible cause of the failure to demonstrate a fully convincing correlation between the degree of PBP saturation and the MIC value may have to do with the differents shapes of saturation curves. In addition, the failure to reproduce the correlation calls attention to another factor often overlooked in these types of experiments – the dimension of the MIC value is not drug concentration but drug dose, i.e., concentration multiplied by time of exposure. Bacterial cultures that have received the MIC-equivalent concentrations of β-lactams are known to continue their exponential growth for a considerable length of time, which may be as long as 2–3 cell generations. The length of this residual growth is independent of cell concentration and is inversely related to the concentration of the antibiotic.

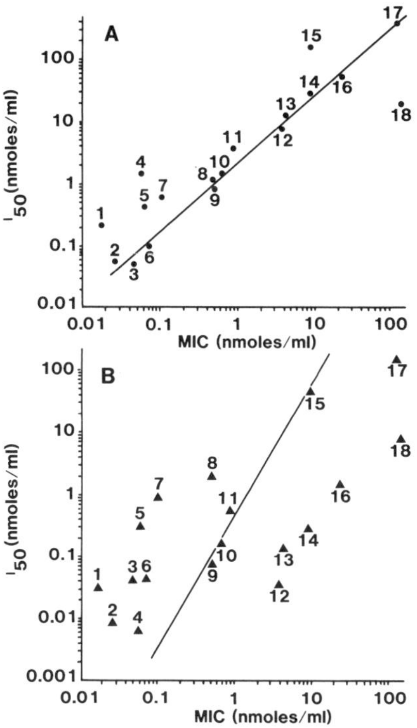

Fig. 12. Correlation between MICs of the antibiotics tested and their affinities (I_{50}) values for (*A*) PBP 2b and (*B*) PBP 3. Numbers represent the following antibiotics: benzylpenicillin (*1*), cefotaxime (*2*), piperacillin (*3*), cephaloridine (*4*), nafcillin (*5*), ampicillin (*6*). dicloxacillin (*7*), methicillin (*8*), cephalothin (*9*), oxacillin (*10*), sulbenicillin (*11*), cefoxitin (*12*), cefadroxil (*13*), cephalexin (*14*), mecillinam (*15*), cefsulodin (*16*), 6-APA (*17*), cephalosporin C (*18*). (WILLIAMSON et al. 1980a)

The precise reasons why bacteria can continue to grow in the presence of drug concentrations that will, eventually, cause growth inhibition are not well understood. In vivo labeling experiments with pneumococci indicate that at least two factors contribute to this: the surprisingly slow kinetics of saturation of PBPs and the production of new PBP molecules through biosynthesis. An added complication may arise from the suggestion that very low concentrations of β-lactams may selectively inhibit the synthesis (availability?) of PBPs in some bacteria (HAMILTON and LAWRENCE 1975; WHITE et al. 1979).

IV. Dynamic Experiments with the Labeling of PBPs in Growing Pneumococci

In an attempt to evaluate the contribution of the antibiotic exposure time to PBP labeling and the related antibacterial effects, a series of experiments was performed in which growing cultures of pneumococci were exposed to different concentrations of ^{3}H-penicillin for various lengths of time in order to examine the degrees and rates of PBP labeling during the entire course of drug exposure, including times

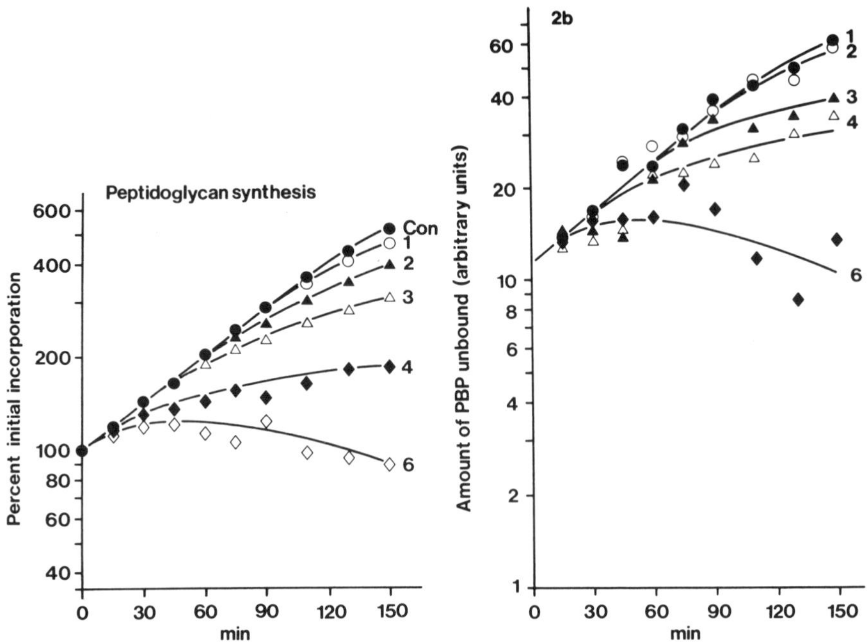

Fig. 13. Correlation between the rate of peptidoglycan synthesis and the cellular concentration of "free" PBP 2b in pneumococci. Cultures of a *lyt*$^-$ mutant of pneumococcus received different concentrations of (^{3}H)penicillin at zero time and the rates of cell wall biosynthesis and the fraction of the various PBPs left "free" (i.e., unbound) of the antibiotic, were assayed at frequent intervals. Shown is the parallel behavior between the amounts of available (unbound) PBP 2b and the rates of lysine incorporation into the cell wall. (WILLIAMSON and TOMASZ 1982)

sufficiently long to bring culture growth to a halt. During the course of this experiment, the following measurements were made: growth (turbidity), rates of peptidoglycan and protein synthesis, and the degree of saturation of PBPs.

Several observations relevant to our discussion were made. Upon addition of the radioactive penicillin to the cultures at various multiples of the MIC, the cultures continued to grow for various periods, the lengths of which were inversely related to the concentration of the antibiotic. The rates of cell wall synthesis (measured as the incorporation of lysine into a hot SDS-insoluble residue) and protein synthesis increased, closely paralleling the increase in cell mass during this residual growth. As the culture growth slowed down and came to a halt, so did the rate increase in cell wall synthesis. Only at high antibiotic concentration (16 × MIC), when residual growth was limited, did the rate of cell wall synthesis actually undergo a rapid and gradual decline to values below those of the pre-inhibition rates (Fig. 13).

Individual PBPs became labeled with penicillin, each with a different characteristic rate, depending upon the drug concentration. Interestingly, there was proportionality between the rate of cell wall synthesis and the amounts of PBP 2b available (i.e., *not* bound by penicillin). This proportionality has remained valid for all penicillin doses and all rates of cell wall synthesis. This observation suggests that the cellular concentration of PBP 2b may limit the rate of attachment of cell wall precursors.

Another interesting observation was made when the degrees of saturation of PBPs were determined *at* the times when the turbidity increase of the culture showed the first observable signs of the onset of growth inhibition. These times varied inversely with the drug concentration: it corresponded to 150, 120, 90, 72, and 45 min of residual growth in cultures treated with 1×, 2×, 3×, 4×, and 6× the MIC concentrations of ^{3}H-penicillin, respectively. It was found that after cultures had received such minimal growth inhibitory doses (MID) of penicillin, each PBP showed a different but characteristic degree of saturation which was thus related to antibiotic dose (rather than concentration alone).

One may consider these as minimal degrees of saturation of the five PBPs at which bacterial cell wall synthesis and cellular growth will start to slow down. Thus, in this proposition, the functioning of *each* PBP, rather than a few select killing targets, may be needed for normal growth. The lack of correlation between degrees of PBP saturation noted upon the exposure of the bacteria to longer than the minimal inhibitory doses (MID) may be due to the fact that the slowdown in cell wall synthesis rapidly initiates various indirect secondary effects in the bacteria (e.g., deregulation of autolysins, changes in plasma membrane permeability) and the rates and degrees of further inhibition of cellular growth will depend upon these processes rather than on the inhibited cell wall synthesis.

V. PBP Alterations in Intrinsically β-Lactam-Resistant Bacteria

Alterations in the PBPs of several intrinsically β-lactam-resistant bacteria have been described (Buchanan and Strominger 1976; Zighelboim and Tomasz 1980; Hartman and Tomasz 1980; Dougherty et al. 1980; Reynolds et al. 1978; Brown and Reynolds 1980). In some of these cases, it was shown by genetic transformation or by the isolation of revertants that the penicillin resistance was actually accompanied by and was, presumably, causally related to the PBP alteration (Buchanan and Strominger 1976; Zighelboim and Tomasz 1980). Since these bacteria were apparently "forced" to modify their PBPs in order to retain the ability to grow in the presence of the antibiotic, the determination of PBP changes could be used to identify the physiologically important binding proteins. In penicillin-resistant laboratory isolates of *B. megaterium*, the altered protein was PBP 1 (Reynolds et al. 1978). In *B. subtilis* mutants exhibiting gradually elevated levels of cloxacillin resistance, the altered protein was PBP 2 (Buchanan and Strominger 1976).

VI. Several Physiologically Important PBPs in Pneumococci

The multiply drug-resistant clinical isolates of South African strains of pneumococci also show greatly elevated (as high as 1,000-fold) penicillin resistance and altered PBP patterns (Zighelboim and Tomasz 1980). It was possible to transfer penicillin resistance to isogenic background by several consecutive rounds of genet-

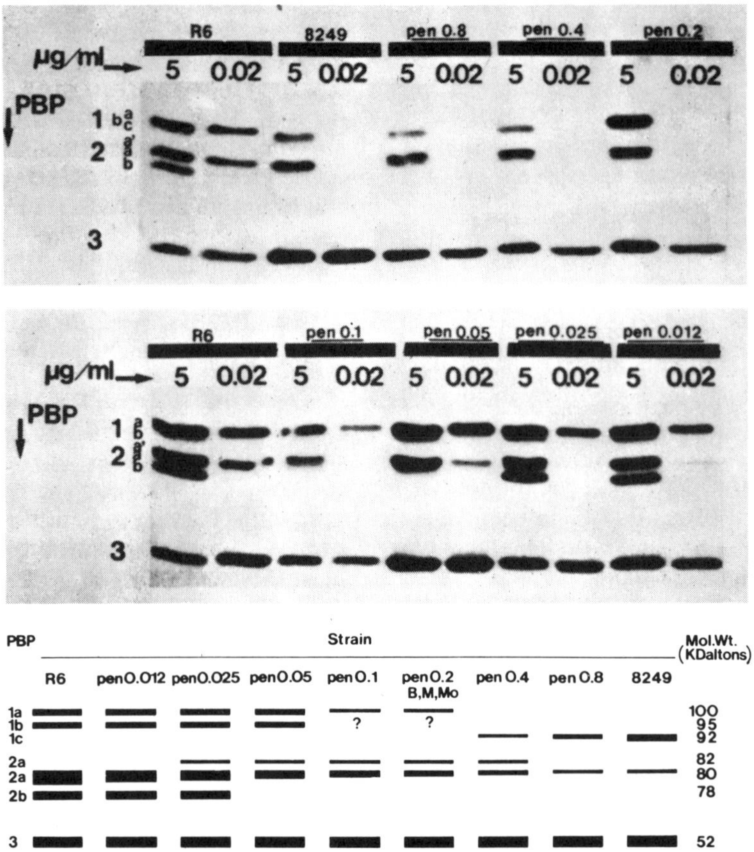

Fig. 14. Altered PBPs in the intrinsically penicillin-resistant (South African) strains of pneumococci.
PBPs of the penicillin-sensitive laboratory strain R6, a penicillin-resistant (South African) strain 8 249 and a series of penicillin-resistant transformants (obtained by transforming the R6 strain with DNA from strain 8 249) were visualized by in vivo labeling with (^{3}H)penicillin (at concentrations 5 and 0.02 μg/ml) and fluorography (*upper part* of figure). *Pen 0.012, pen 0.025, pen 0.05* etc. refer to the various classes of transformants and the numbers indicate the highest concentration of penicillin that still allowed normal growth of the bacteria in an MIC-type assay.
The *lower part* of the figure is a schematic respresentation of the PBPs of a series of isogenic transformants. The *thickness of bars* indicates intensity of the bands in the fluorograms. The penicillin-sensitive recipient strain (R6) and the DNA donor penicillin-resistant strain (8 249) are included as controls. Strains M, Mo, and B are independent clinical isolates from the Oklahoma Children's Hospital. (ZIGHELBOIM and TOMASZ 1980; WILLIAMSON et al. 1981).

ic transformation, which produced a series of strains differing from one another in distinct levels of penicillin resistance. Determination of the PBP patterns in these transformants allowed the identification of a gradual and stepwise shift in the PBP pattern from that characteristic of the recipient (penicillin-sensitive) bacteria to the pattern of the DNA donor (resistant) bacteria (Fig. 14).

These findings indicate that the acquisition of resistance to gradually increasing penicillin concentrations forces the bacteria to modify at least four of the five PBPs. The alterations involved change in penicillin affinity and disappearance of a particular PBP, as well as production of PBPs with new electrophoretic mobility. These changes appeared to represent a unique biochemical strategy, since intrinsically penicillin-resistant pneumococci isolated from a completely different source (Oklahoma Children's Hospital) showed specific PBP alterations comparable to those observed in the South African derivatives with the same MIC value (HAKENBECK et al. 1980). These findings were interpreted as indicating that at least four of the five pneumococcal PBPs perform physiologically indispensable functions and are therefore lethal targets of penicillin action in this bacterium.

The observations with the pneumococcal resistant mutants (ZIGHELBOIM and TOMASZ 1980) and the results of PBP labeling experiments using the MIC concentrations of various β-lactams (WILLIAMSON et al. 1980a) illustrate the complexity of the correlation between the degree of penicillin binding to PBPs and the degree of inhibition of cell wall synthesis or cellular growth. Some recent experiments further document this. A comparison of the titration profiles of the PBPs of *S. faecalis* strains differing greatly in penicillin MICs showed no detectable difference between the penicillin affinities of the PBPs (ELIOPOULOS et al. 1981). Similarly, the substantial variation in the penicillin MIC value of some *S. faecalis* strains with growth temperature was not accompanied by changes in the PBP affinities for the antibiotic (FONTANA et al. 1980). A striking example of the lack of correlation between MIC value and PBP affinity for the drug was provided by studies with the methicillin-resistant *S. aureus* (HARTMAN and TOMASZ 1980). It was possible to show (both by in vivo labeling and in membrane preparations) that the dramatic increase in methicillin resistance (from a MIC value of 0.4–3,200 μg/ml) was accompanied by an almost quantitative parallel decrease in the methicillin affinities of PBPs 1, 2, and 3. It is known that the MIC values of these mutants depend on the pH value of the cultures, in that resistance is virtually lost (i.e., not expressed) in cultures grown at low pH (5.2–5.5). When the PBP "affinities" of such low pH cultures of genetically methicillin-resistant, but phenotypically methicillin-sensitive, staphylococci were examined, the surprising observation was made that the PBPs retained their low antibiotic affinities. In other words, bacterial growth (and cell wall synthesis) was inhibited and the cells lost viability during exposure to low concentrations of methicillin, which only caused insignificant (1%–5%), binding to the PBPs, i.e., the great majority of those proteins remained available for their normal functioning.

These experiments brought into focus another difficulty inherent in comparing the degrees or rates of inhibition of PBPs with those of inhibition of cell wall synthesis or bacterial growth. It is not clear what fraction of an essential PBP is needed in an available form to allow a given rate of cell wall synthesis and it is even less clear what degree of inhibition of cell wall synthesis is required to cause interference with cellular growth. The observations described here suggest that quantitatively minor inhibitions may cause drastic antibacterial effects, and that growth conditions and secondary factors (both in the bacterium and in its environment) that do not react directly with the antibiotic molecule can have a decisive influence over whether or not a given degree of PBP inhibition will be translated into interference with growth.

E. Variations in the Physiological Effects of Penicillins

I. The Single Target – Unbalanced Growth Model

The complex and sometimes conflicting results of the experiments described in the previous section underline the importance of taking a different approach to understanding the mode of action of penicillin in which the starting point and object of the investigation is the physiology of the penicillin-treated cell.

More or less parallel with the many biochemically oriented early studies on the mode of action of penicillin, a large body of microbiological observations on the aberrant morphology, loss of viability and lysis of penicillin-treated bacteria has accumulated in the literature since the early 1940s. Although penicillin itself was discovered due to its lytic action on staphylococci, it was also recognized quite early that such lytic (and bactericidal) effects depended on growth conditions. Simultaneous treatment of cultures with a bacteriostatic sulfa drug would prevent penicillin-induced lysis, and starvation of nutritional auxotrophs would protect against the bactericidal effect of penicillin (Davis 1948; Hobby et al. 1942).

It was also observed long ago that, in some strains of bacteria, the irreversible (i.e., killing and lytic) versus reversible (i.e., growth inhibitory) effects of penicillin varied as independent functions of the drug concentration. In other words, it was found that raising the drug concentration above a threshold level higher than the MIC, could actually inhibit drug-induced killing and lysis (Eagle and Musselman 1948; Demerec 1945).

In an early attempt to combine biochemical and microbiological findings into a single coherent model for the mode of action of penicillin, the requirement for growth in the killing and lytic effect was combined with the already established inhibition of murein transpeptidase in a model to explain the mechanism of antibacterial effects of penicillin. The essential points of this model, until recently quite popular are as follows: (1) In the presence of penicillin, incorporation of precursors into the bacterial cell wall continues (via a transglycosylase-type reaction) but (2) the crosslinking of the incorporated disaccharide-peptides required for the mechanical stability of the wall is prevented by the virtually irreversible inhibition of the transpeptidase, creating (3) mechanically weak spots in the newly made portion of the wall. These (4) would subsequently rupture under the mechanical/osmotic pressure of the continuously increasing cytoplasmic mass, leading to cell lysis, thus explaining the well-known requirement for "active growth" in the lytic action of penicillin. (5) The aberrant morphology of penicillin-treated cells would then represent an expression of ill-defined structural defects exhibited by the bacteria prior to lysis.

Within the context of this model, the frequently quoted statement that penicillin kills bacteria by inhibiting the murein transpeptidase was indeed a reasonable one.

However, recent findings indicate that the mechanism of penicillin-induced antibacterial effects are much more complex than was depicted by this unbalanced growth model. As to points (1) and (2), it seems that in most bacteria the incorporation of precursor units into the preexisting wall is catalyzed by a transpeptidase which is sensitive to penicillin. Thus, in such bacteria the mechanism for creating "weak spots" does not exist. Concerning points (3) and (4), recent findings indicate that lysis is an enzyme-catalyzed process and the requirement for active growth probably has to do with the control of these hydrolases rather than with the osmotic turgor of cells (TOMASZ 1979a). As to point (5), the morphological effects of penicillin treatment represent the specific symptoms of the inhibition of a number of specific penicillin-sensitive proteins, rather than the loss of structural integrity.

II. From Inhibited Enzyme to Inhibited Target Cell

On a more general ground, one may argue that even when the nature of the drug-sensitive reaction is well understood (and this is certainly not the case with β-lactams), the question of how and why specific interference with a metabolic reaction leads to inhibition of cellular growth or division is far from obvious (TOMASZ et al. 1979). Neither is it self-evident why even a complete and irreversible inhibition of an essential enzyme should cause irreversible inactivation of the whole cell, since during the test for bacterial survival (i.e., after removal of the excess drug), cells might be expected to resynthesize new molecules of the inhibited enzyme (unless, of course, protein synthesis is also inhibited). The pathway from inhibited target enzyme to inhibited (non-growing or non-dividing) bacterium varies tremendously in "length" and complexity, and the actual mechanism gearing the whole cell to a halt may be remote from the site of inhibition. For instance, in a stringently controlled *(Rel+)* bacterium, removal of the essential aminoacid does not cause inhibition of growth by the cell's running out of an essential building block. Instead, the drop in the internal concentration of the aminoacid activates a complex regulatory circuit involving guanosine tetraphosphate, a multifunctional effector, the accumulation of which causes the inhibition of several key synthetic enzymes in RNA, lipid and cell wall syntheses (NIERLICH 1978). Similar variation exists in the mechanism of action of irreversible antimicrobial agents. Polymyxin and complement may kill bacteria by direct damage to the plasma membrane (KOIKE and MATSUO 1969; MULLER-EBERHARD 1975). In contrast, interference with DNA synthesis may trigger a complex indirect killing mechanism. For instance, thymidine starvation may cause loss of viability by triggering the lytic cycle of defective lysogenic prophage. In bacteria "cured" of prophage, the lethality of thymidine starvation depends on the *rec A* gene. The dramatically reduced lethality of thymidine starvation in *rec* A^- mutants seems to be related to the low levels of protein X (the *rec A* gene product). In the *rec* A^+ cells, inhibition of DNA synthesis stimulates production of protein X (a protein known to be involved with complex membrane functions) and it has been suggested that the phenomenon of "thymineless death" is actually caused by a change in the energized state of the plasma membrane induced by protein X (INOUYE 1971). Thus, whether or not thymidine starvation causes irreversible loss of viability would depend entirely on secondary processes, coupled to the primary interference with DNA synthesis.

These examples are described in order to help set the stage for a more detailed discussion of the extraordinarily complex antimicrobial mechanisms of β-lactams.

III. Inhibition of Growth, Loss of Viability, Lysis

At least two types of factors seem to contribute to this complexity. First, as was discussed in previous sections of this review, β-lactam antibiotics can inhibit not

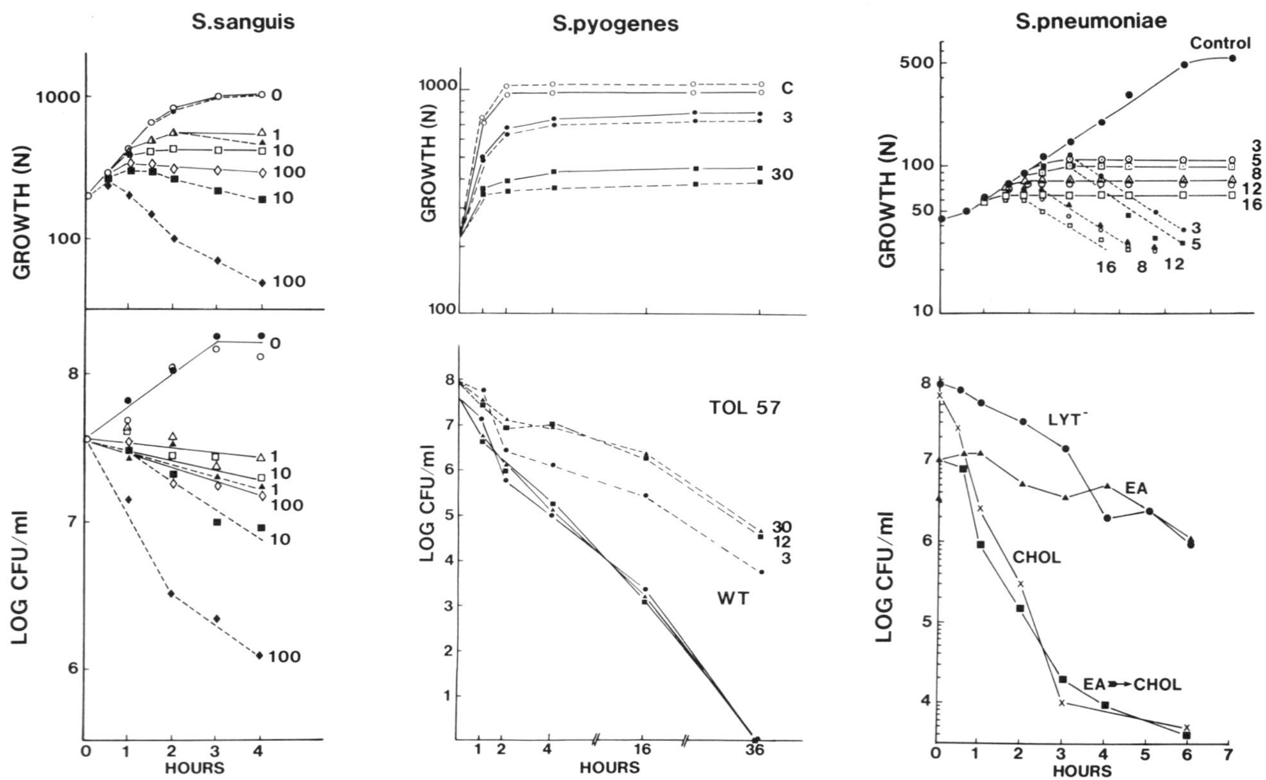

Fig. 15. Different physiological responses to penicillin treatment in three strains of streptococci. Growth, lysis, and viable titer of the cultures were measured during exposure of cultures to various concentrations of benzylpenicillin, expressed as multiples of the minimal inhibitory concentration (MIC) values *(see numbers next to the curves)*. In the experiment with the penicillin tolerant *S. sanguis*, *dashed lines* represent cultures which also received 1.5 Unit/ml of C phage associated lysin added to the growth medium with or without penicillin. In the experiment with *S. pyogenes* the response of wild type (*wt*) cells and that of a penicillin-tolerant mutant (*tol* 27) are shown. The cultures of *S. pneumoniae* were grown either in choline (*CHOL*)-containing (*dashed lines*) or in ethanolamine (*EA*)-containing medium (*solid lines*). These bacteria exhibit phenotypic tolerance to penicillin when grown in the EA-containing medium. The lower panel also shows the rate of loss of viability during penicillin treatment of a *lyt*⁻ mutant of pneumococcus as well as in a culture in which phenotypic tolerance was abolished by the readdition of choline to the medium of EA-grown pneumococci (EA→*CHOL*). (HORNE and TOMASZ 1980; GUTMANN and TOMASZ 1982; TOMASZ 1974)

one but a whole number of functionally different targets (penicillin binding proteins, PBPs) in bacteria and the nature and/or number of targets inhibited may depend on both the chemical sturcture of the β-lactam and the species of the bacterium as well.

A second factor contributing to the complexity of the mechanism is only now beginning to be recognized. It seems that β-lactam antibiotics can cause at least three major mechanistically different types of antibacterial effects: inhibition of growth, loss of viability, and lysis, and that the type of response could vary with the bacterial species, with the β-lactam structure, and with the environmental conditions as well. As an illustration, Fig. 15 shows the three different responses to penicillin treatment by three streptococci which all have comparable (low) MIC values to penicillin (0.006–0.01 μg/ml) (HORNE and TOMASZ 1977). It can be seen that the antibiotic inhibits the growth of all three bacterial species, but only in pneumococci does cell lysis and killing of the bacteria occur. In the group A streptococci, growth inhibition and rapid loss of viability occur without lysis, while in *Streptococcus sanguis*, the primary response is inhibition of growth accompanied by only very slow loss of viability and no lysis. Biochemical experiments have shown that in each of the three strains, penicillin causes rapid inhibition of the incorporation of cell wall precursors. Thus, the primary biochemical effects appeared to be similar. Yet these cells differed greatly in their ultimate response to penicillin. The lower panels of Fig. 15 show that the penicillin response of each of these bacteria may be altered either by modification of the growth medium or by the introduction of secondary mutations. Thus, the addition of lysozyme to the medium of *S. sanguis* converted the response of these cells to a cidal and lytic effect (HORNE and TOMASZ 1980). Mutants of group A streptococci exhibiting a slower rate of loss in viability could be isolated (GUTMANN and TOMASZ 1982) and a variety of genetic and physiological manipulations [e.g., replacing the choline component of the growth medium with ethanolamine (TOMASZ 1968), lowering the pH of the medium, adding trypsin (LOPEZ et al. 1976) or the lipid-teichoic acid Forssman antigen (HOLTJE and TOMASZ 1975a)] would convert the lytic response of pneumococci to a response similar to that of *S. sanguis*. The term "penicillin tolerance" was coined to describe this primarily bacteriostatic response to penicillin (TOMASZ et al. 1970).

IV. The PBPs of Penicillin-Tolerant Bacteria

In a close analogy with the diverse and mechanistically different morphological effects of β-lactams in gram-negative bacilli, there seems to exist a spectrum of antibacterial effects as well. Furthermore, the nature of these effects can be modulated by environmental factors. The possibility that the nature of antibacterial effects may be determined by differences in the nature of the inhibited PBPs was examined in lysis-prone and tolerant mutants of pneumococci (WILLIAMSON et al. 1980c) and *E. coli* (KITANO and TOMASZ 1979a), but with negative results. It was found that the PBPs of pneumococci with the lytic response to penicillin showed the same penicillin titration profiles as the bacteria in which the lytic response was suppressed either by physiological manipulations (e.g., growth at low pH or in the presence of chloramphenicol) or by the introduction of lyt^- mutations. Identical

PBP patterns were also observed in tolerant versus kill-sensitive group A streptococci and in an *E. coli* mutant that showed slow lysis and slow loss of viability at one growth temperature, and the typical fast lysis and killing at another (KITANO and TOMASZ 1979a).

Thus, in sharp contrast with the situation in the intrinsically penicillin-resistant bacteria, in tolerance the bacteria appeared to have a normal complement of normally accessible PBPs.

V. Penicillin-Induced Death, Without Lysis (Group A Streptococci)

Penicillin-treated group A streptococci are unable to resume cell division after removal of the drug from the medium, despite the fact that the antibiotic-treated cells show no sign of the usual sort of structural damage seen in other bacteria (HORNE and TOMASZ 1977). One possible mechanism for such a phenomenon would be an irreversible inhibition of vital PBPs, provided that protein synthesis would also be inhibited [and thus preventing production of new PBPs (TOMASZ et al. 1979)]. This possibility was tested, with negative results (GUTMANN et al. 1980). The turnover rate of PBPs was determined in group A streptococci that were exposed to ^{3}H-penicillin while growing. It was found that even after exposure to antibiotic doses that caused irreversible inactivation ("death") of 99.9% of the cells, almost 80% of the PBPs had continued to catalyze cycles of acylation and deacylation by the radioactive antibiotic (and thus, presumably, these proteins were also capable of catalyzing their physiological reactions in cell wall biosynthesis). These data suggest that the irreversibility of penicillin action in this bacterium cannot be explained by some uniqueness in the interaction between PBPs and the antibiotic molecule. In support of this conclusion was the observation that the PBP patterns of the kill-sensitive wild-type streptococci and of the tolerant mutants isolated from them were indistinguishable (GUTMANN and TOMASZ 1982). However, several alternative mechanisms remain plausible, such as membrane damage by the induction of a phospholipase (due to some indirect perturbation of the plasma membrane during inhibition of wall synthesis), or the production of a limited number of irreparable "nicks" in the cell wall through the action of a murein hydrolase that, for some reason, would not cause extensive degradation of murein (TOMASZ 1979b).

VI. Reversible Growth-Inhibitory Effect of Penicillin

In order to appreciate the full range of possible biological effects of penicillin, one should remember that in appropriately supplemented (osmotically protective) media, penicillin can induce the formation of spheroplasts or L-forms in several species of bacteria and these wall defective forms have been known to continue synthesis of both cytoplasmic and cell surface components (LEDERBERG and ST CLAIR 1958; DIENES and WEINBERGER 1951).

A particularly interesting and illuminating set of experiments has been reported on the effect of penicillin in *Streptococcus mutans* cells and protoplasts (prepared by an enzymatic method) from the same bacteria (MYCHAJLONKA et al. 1980; SHOCKMAN and LAMPEN 1962). *S. mutans*, like *S. sanguis*, is a penicillin-tolerant bacterium: even high doses (100 × MIC) of the antibiotic do not cause lysis (and only cause a relatively limited decline in viability). An analysis of polymer syntheses in this bacterium revealed that cell wall, protein and RNA syntheses were all about equally sensitive to inhibition by penicillin and, after a timely removal of the antibiotic, polymer syntheses (and growth of the inhibited cultures) would resume.

Inhibition of protein synthesis (and, presumably, other polymer syntheses as well) does eventually occur even in lysis-prone bacteria. However, as the authors of the study have suggested, the *rapid* inhibition of protein synthesis upon the addition of penicillin may be unique to these bacteria and it may provide a mechanism for tolerance, i.e., resistance against penicillin-induced lysis (even if lytic enzymes were present), since non-growing bacterial cells are resistant to the lytic and cidal action of cell wall inhibitors. The biochemical basis of the phenotypic tolerance of non-growing bacteria is not well understood. (Some recent studies describing a possible mechanism for non-growing *E. coli* are described later in this review).

Another interesting idea that emerged from these studies was the possibility that the type of physiological response to penicillin treatment (i.e., inhibition of growth; killing or lysis) may also depend upon at which stage of the cell cycle the target bacterium was at the time of the penicillin-induced inhibition of cell wall synthesis, since the activity of autolytic enzymes (i.e., the agents required for cell lysis) undergoes substantial fluctuation during the cell cycle (ROSENTHAL et al. 1975; SHOCKMAN et al. 1974). Studies with synchronized bacterial cultures should make it possible to test some aspects of this proposition. This type of mechanism may explain why, even in lysis-prone cultures, a varying proportion of the bacteria may survive prolonged exposure to penicillin. Most interestingly, conversion of penicillin-inhibited bacteria to protoplasts resulted in the release of penicillin inhibition, and the protoplasts continued to make biopolymers with a reasonable rate even in the presence of a high concentration of penicillin corresponding to 100 times the MIC for intact bacteria. These phenomena were not due to the presence of osmotic stabilizer. Since the protoplasts are apparently capable of producing soluble murein material as well, it seems that the growth-inhibitory effects of penicillin in the intact cells must be somehow mediated by the final stages in the assembly of insoluble cell wall or, to use the authors' metaphor, these terminal stages in cell wall replication must be able to "talk back" to cytoplasmic syntheses, possibly through some effector molecule (ISHIGURO and RAMEY 1976) or via the plasma membrane (ROSENTHAL et al. 1975; SHOCKMAN et al. 1981).

Another interesting system, which illuminates the same problem is an L-form of *P. mirabilis* which can continue to multiply (in the form of pleiomorphic cells) in the presence of several hundred micrograms of penicillin, a concentration highly inhibitory for the intact *Proteus* cells. These L-forms even produce cell walls of normal chemical composition, except for a relatively minor decrease in the degree of crosslinking (from 23%–12%) and a drop in the number of muramic acid 6-O-acetyl groups (MARTIN and GMEINER 1979; GMEINER and KROLL 1981).

These systems promise much valuable information about mechanisms by which cell wall synthesis and cytoplasmic syntheses are coordinated.

VII. Penicillin Tolerance in Bacteria with Suppressed Murein Hydrolase Activity

Since tolerant and lysis-prone pneumococci were shown to have identical PBP patterns, the mechanism of the bactericidal and lytic effects of penicillin must involve factors other than the primary targets of penicillin action. In 1970, during the biochemical analysis of penicillin-tolerant pneumococci, one major factor associated with these irreversible effects was identified as the pneumococcal murein hydrolase, an *N*-acetylmuramic acid–L-alanine amidase (TOMASZ et al. 1970). Pneumococci in which the activity of this enzyme was suppressed, (either by mutation or by some physiological manipulation), had the same MIC value and showed the same kinetics of growth inhibition as the lysis-prone wild-type bacteria, except that the rate of loss of viability was slower and the eventual culture lysis, measured by optical techniques, did not occur in the lysis-negative cells.

That the tolerant (i.e., primarily bacteriostatic) response of lysis-defective pneumococci is related to the suppression of the activity of the pneumococcal murein hydrolase has since been corroborated by several additional lines of evidence. Penicillin tolerance and a defective autolytic system were found to co-transform during genetic transformation in which DNA from lysis-defective mutants was used and the property of lysis-defect was positively selected for (JIANG and TOMASZ 1981).

Further proof for the key role of murein hydrolase in the lytic (and killing) effects of penicillin was provided by physiological experiments in which the addition of specific inhibitors of the enzyme to the growth medium could protect wild-type pneumococci against the lytic effects of penicillin. Such agents are high concentrations of the autolysin-inhibitor Forssman antigen (HOLTJE and TOMASZ 1975b), trypsin (the amidase is sensitive to proteolysis) (LOPEZ et al. 1976), and antibodies prepared against purified autolysin (GARCIA et al. 1982).

An additional intriguing observation was made regarding the autolysin-defective mutants. It was possible to coat live cells of the mutant bacteria with purified wild type enzyme. Such bacteria, upon transfer to growth medium, would continue to grow with normal generation times. However, upon addition of penicillin, these autolysin-coated cells behaved like "phenocopies" of wild-type pneumococci, i.e., they underwent normal lysis (TOMASZ and WAKS 1975a). Another striking similarity between this system and wild-type pneumococci was that lysis could be prevented by pretreating the "phenocopy" cells with inhibitors of protein or RNA synthesis prior to the addition of penicillin (TOMASZ and WAKS 1975b). Identical results were obtained when excess autolysin was present in the medium throughout the experiments.

A close comparison of the kinetics of penicillin inhibition in this latter system with that of wild-type pneumococci has revealed that, in both systems, the *time of onset* of lysis was the same inverse function of penicillin concentration, while the eventual *rate of culture lysis* was primarily the function of the concentration of purified autolysin added to the growth medium. This suggested that the first phase of penicillin exposure somehow weakens the control of endogenous enzyme (and/or sensitizes the bacterial surface to exogenous enzyme) while the rate-limiting factor in the second phase may be the cell-wall-degrading activity of the murein hydrolase (TOMASZ and WAKS 1975b).

Table 3. Penicillin tolerance in murein hydrolase-defective bacterial mutants

Strain	Resistance to lytic agents	Murein hydrolase implicated	Probable cause of antibiotic tolerance	Reference
S. pneumoniae				
$LYT^{-}TOL^{+}$	All cell wall inhibitors, detergents, bacteriophage Dp-l.	Amidase (0.1–0.5%)	Low level of hydrolase	Tomasz et al. (1970)
$LYT^{+}TOL^{+}$	β-lactams, D-cycloserine; lysed by vancomycine, lysed be detergents	Normal level of amidase	Block in "trigger pathway"(?)	Williamson and Tomasz (1980)
E. coli C-80				
$LYT^{-}TOL^{+}$	β-Lactams	Transglycosylase and endopeptidase	Low level of hydrolases	Kitano and Tomasz (1979)
x2452 LYT^{+}ts TOL^{+}	β-Lactams	Normal level of autolysins	Ts block in "trigger pathway"(?)	
B. licheniformis				
$LYT^{-}TOL^{+}$	All cell wall inhibitors	Amidase, glucosaminidase	Low level of hydrolases	Fein and Rogers (1976)
B. subtilis				
$LYT^{-}TOL^{+}$	All cell wall inhibitors(?)	Amidase(?)	Low level of hydrolase	Ayusawa et al. (1975)
S. faecalis				
$LYT^{-}TOL^{+}$	All cell wall inhibitors	Muramidase	Low level of hydrolase	Shungu et al. (1979)

The penicillin tolerance of lysis-defective bacterial mutants was subsequently confirmed in several other bacterial species (Table 3). It should be noted that none of these mutants showed defective growth, and tolerance was associated with the loss of a variety of catalytically different murein hydrolases (Forsberg and Rogers 1971; Ayusawa et al. 1975; Shungu et al. 1979; Kitano and Tomasz 1979a; Fein and Rogers 1976; Chatterjee et al. 1976).

More recently, the phenomenon of penicillin tolerance was detected among clinical isolates of several pathogenic species (Sabath et al. 1977; Best et al. 1974; Mayhall et al. 1976; De Leys and Juni 1977; Kim et al. 1979; Storch and Krogstad 1981; Liu et al. 1981;Savitch et al. 1978; Allen and Sprunt 1978). In most cases, antibiotic tolerance was defined as relative resistance to the bactericidal effect of penicillin after overnight treatment with the antibiotics (i.e., high MBC values relative to the MIC; MBC/MIC > 32). Only in some of these has there been some evidence presented for a defective murein hydrolase activity. Because of the complexity of the irreversible effects of penicillin, the phenomenon of tolerance may involve a variety of different "defects" which may or may not be directly related to low autolytic activity.

VIII. Penicillin-Induced Lysis and Death in E. coli

Analysis of the penicillin response of *E. coli* has revealed several new features that may be of significance in some other bacteria as well. Treatment with β-lactams has been shown to induce cell wall degradation in *E. coli* (Schwarz et al. 1969; Schwarz and Weidel 1965). However, a comparison of the specific activities of a number of structurally different β-lactams (compared to one another on the basis of common biological activity – MIC units) as "triggers" of cell wall degradation showed that β-lactams with high affinity for PBP 1 b had higher activity than antibiotics with selective affinities for PBP 3 or PBP 2 (Kitano and Tomasz 1979b; Reynolds and Chase 1981). Rates of killing by the same β-lactams showed parallel differences.

Unlike the pneumococcus, which has one murein hydrolase activity only, *E. coli* is known to have several hydrolytic enzymes capable of splitting covalent bonds in murein material (see Fig. 1). Penicillin-induced wall hydrolysis appears to involve the hydrolytic transglycosylase (this activity has nothing to do with the "transglycosylase" responsible for the catalysis of formation of β-1,4 glycosidic linkages in the murein) and/or the endopeptidase (Kitano et al. 1980). This conclusion is based on the nature of enzymatic defects in *E. coli* mutants selected for tolerance (survival) during exposure to varying doses of cephaloridine (Kitano and Tomasz 1979b). In several classes of such mutants, a 25%–30% decrease in the hydrolytic transglycosylase and a superimposed decrease in endopeptidase activity was noted. In contrast to the situation in lysis-defective pneumococci, the activity of *E. coli N*-acetylmuramic acid L-alanine amidase did not change. Another interesting, and contrasting, property of these *E. coli* mutants, relative to the pneumococcal *lyt*$^-$ mutants, was the quantitative nature of tolerance in the *E. coli* cells. The double hydrolytic defect was characteristic of the more extensively tolerant mutants (i.e., mutants that were capable of surviving larger doses of cephaloridine

Table 4. Decreased murein hydrolase activities in β-lactam tolerant mutants of *E. coli* K12. (KITANO et al. 1980)

Mutant	Doubling time (min)	MIC (µg/ml) (Cephaloridine)	Tolerance ratio[a] (Cephaloridine)	Relative activities of Trans-glycosylase[b]	Relative activities of Endo-peptidase	Relative activities of Amidase[c]
C-31	69	1.95	8	33.3	110	123
C-54	90	3.90	8	31.5	84.2	113
C-61	84	7.80	12	47.0	44.3	116
C-80	69	3.90	16	34.2	44.6	114
C-254	66	3.90	16	34.8	39.1	103
C-263	79	3.90	8	29.4	123	101
Parent	55	1.95	(1)	100	100	100

[a] Minimal lysis permissive concentration/MIC
[b] Murein transglycosylase
[c] *N*-acetyl muramic acid L-alanine amidase

treatment) (KITANO et al. 1980). Some properties of these mutants are shown in Table 4.

Figure 16 further illustrates the drug (and PBP) specificity of tolerance in the *E. coli* mutants. It may be seen that treatment of the tolerant mutants with β-lactams that are selective inhibitors of PBPs 2 and 3 evoked the characteristic morphological alteration from the bacteria although lysis in PBP 1 b inhibitors did not occur. This finding suggests that the characteristic *rapid* lysis and death of β-lactam-treated *E. coli* is due to triggering of the unregulated activities of the transglycosylase (and endopeptidase) through some consequence of the inhibition of PPB 1 b. It is not clear what *degree* of inhibition of this binding protein is needed to bring about an irreversible triggering of the hydrolases. Apparently, as little as 25% saturation in PBP 1 b is sufficient to initiate cell killing (REYNOLDS and CHASE 1981). Preliminary studies in our laboratory indicate that this quantitative relationship between PBP inhibition and degree of triggering may depend upon environmental factors.

IX. How and Why Does Penicillin Cause Cell Wall Degradation?

The observations briefly summarized above do not provide an answer to the question of why penicillin treatment causes enzymatic degradation of cell walls. An explicitly described model providing predictions which could be tested was outlined in 1964 by Weidel and Pelzer; this model will herein be referred to as the "enzymic unbalance" model (WEIDEL and PELZER 1964). In short, it was proposed that the ubiquitous bacterial murein hydrolases may perform an essential physiological function in cell wall replication, by acting in concert with synthetic enzymes for which they provide points of insertion of new cell wall building blocks into the

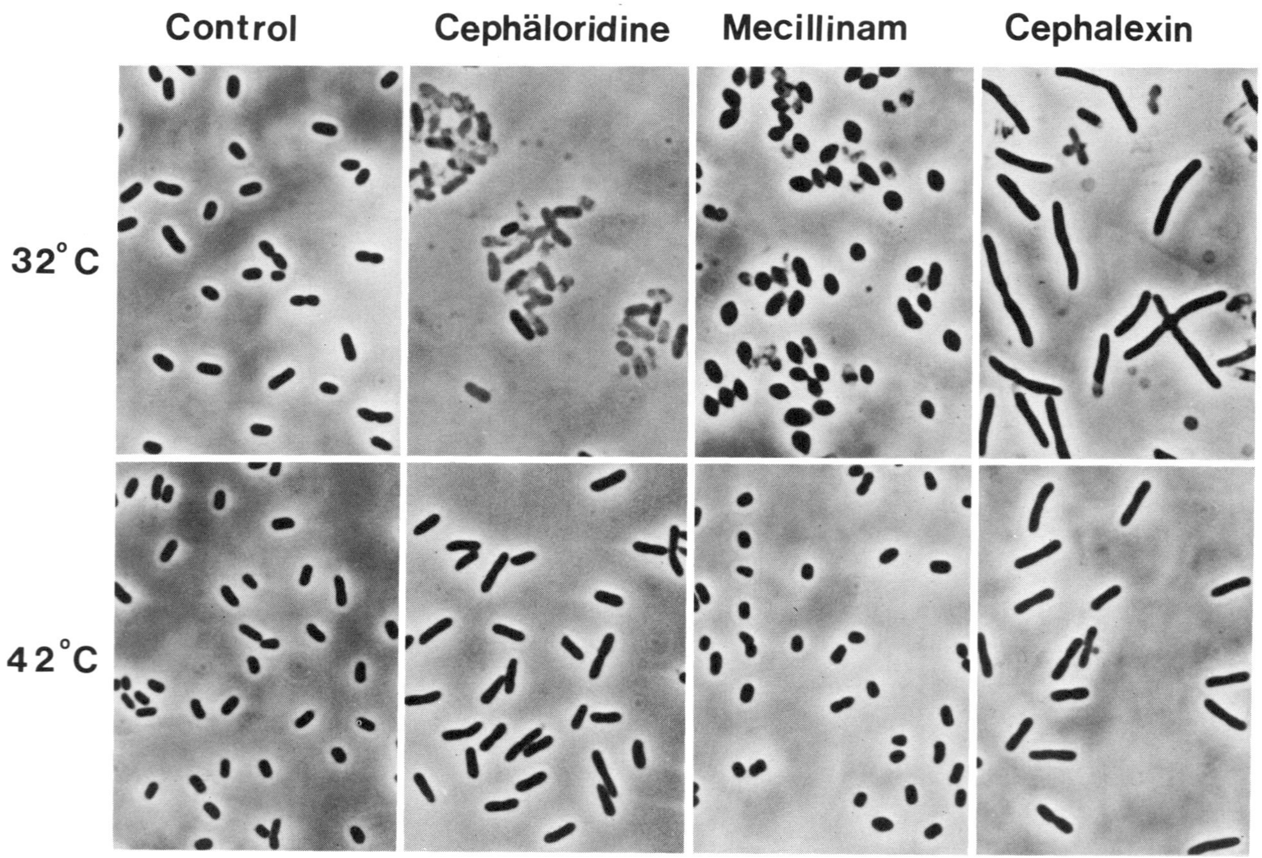

Fig. 16. Selective inhibition of the lytic effect of β-lactams in a temperature-sensitive tolerant strain of *E. coli*. Cells grown at 32 °C and 42 °C were exposed to 4 times the MICs of various β-lactam antibiotics for 3 h. (KITANO and TOMASZ 1979a)

preexisting cell wall. This model fully explained the phenomenon of lysis in bacteria inhibited in their cell wall synthesis. Implicit in this model was the expectation that hydrolase-defective mutants should be able to survive penicillin treatment. Indeed, the penicillin tolerance of lysis-defective pneumococci was first interpreted as an experimental proof of this model (TOMASZ et al. 1970).

However, gradually more and more difficulties were encountered with this interpretation. (1) The type of catalytic activity (amidase) implicated in lysis of pneumococci was not easy to accommodate into the model. (2) If hydrolases were essential for growth, one would expect to find some growth defect in the lysis-defective cells. However, close examination of lysis-defective pneumococci showed no indication of abnormalities that would affect replication of the bacteria. None of the lysis-defective (tolerant) mutants isolated in pneumococci and other bacterial species were found to be conditional mutants. (3) Yet, the mutationally lowered autolytic activity was clearly implicated in penicillin-induced lysis, since the lysis-defective bacteria were tolerant to penicillin. Thus, one is forced to conclude that penicillin-induced lysis is catalyzed by enzymes which are not essential for the growth of bacteria. (4) Finally, recent observations on the mode of cell wall synthesis in many bacterial species depict a completely different picture about the nature of cell wall growing points than what was envisioned originally. It seems that breaks in the glycan backbone of preexisting cell wall are not essential for either the polymerization or the attachment of new wall building blocks (see Sect. E).

Thus, why and how inhibition of cell wall synthesis initiates cell wall degradation has remained an enigma. If cell lysis is not an obvious, automatic consequence of the inhibition of cell wall synthesis, then there is a need for a new term, a word to express the notion that the abnormal destructive activity of murein hydrolases is actually "provoked" or "initiated" by inhibitors of cell wall synthesis. For the lack of a better word, we proposed the term "triggering" for this purpose (TOMASZ and WAKS 1975b; TOMASZ 1981), without implying any detailed mechanism.

X. Possible Causes of Penicillin-Induced Cell Wall Degradation in E. coli

We examined three simple alternative possibilities for the explanation of the rapid degradation of cell wall material observed during exposure of *E. coli* to β-lactam antibiotics. First, radioactively labeled cell walls isolated from control and from penicillin-treated bacteria were compared with respect to their susceptibilities to degradation by crude autolytic extracts from *E. coli*. Next, we tested the possibility that β-lactams somehow stimulate the *activity* of autolysins or increase the cellular concentration of these enzymes. All these experiments yielded negative results (KITANO and TOMASZ 1979b).

When thinking about the mechanism by which penicillin treatment triggers cell wall degradation, one should remember that continuous and substantial enzymatic degradation of cell wall material is known to occur in several bacterial species during normal growth, i.e., without any deleterious effect on the physiology of the cells. Studies with gonococci indicate that upon the addition of penicillin, these bacteria either continue or actually slow down their normal cell wall turnover, which seems to be primarily catalyzed by an *N*-acetylmuramic acid-L-alanine amidase type autolysin. On the other hand, the addition of penicillin seems to "trigger" another type of cell wall hydrolytic activity (transglycosylase?) that is only a minor contributor to the normal turnover of murein material (GOODELL et al. 1978; SINHA and ROSENTHAL 1981). These observations provide further support for the notion that penicillin treatment induces some regulatory defect in the control of autolytic enzymes.

XI. Penicillin-Induced Lysis and Natural Inhibitors of Autolysis

The discovery by Joachim Höltje in 1975 that the pneumococcal Forssman antigen is a powerful and specific inhibitor of the pneumococcal autolytic enzyme (HÖLTJE and TOMASZ 1975a) has turned our attention to the metabolism of this lipid-teichoic acid in penicillin-treated cells. It was found that high concentrations of Forssman antigen added to the growth media could induce phenotypic tolerance, i.e., prevent penicillin-induced lysis of pneumococci without interfering with the penicillin-induced growth-inhibition (HÖLTJE and TOMASZ 1975b). In addition, penicillin treatment was shown to cause the release of a substantial fraction of Forssman antigen into the growth medium of both lysis-defective and lysis-prone bacteria (TOMASZ and WAKS 1975b). Similar phenomena were subsequently observed with the polyglycerophosphate-type lipoteichoic acids and with certain autolysin-inhibitory phospholipids in several other bacterial species (CLEVELAND et al. 1975; CARSON et al. 1979; HINKS et al. 1978).

On the basis of these findings, an alternative hypothesis was proposed to explain how inhibition of cell wall synthesis may provoke autolytic cell wall degradation (TOMASZ and WAKS 1975b; TOMASZ and HÖLTJE 1977). The "triggering" model attempts to put a number of experimental findings into a plausible but hypothetical scheme. These observations are: (1) the tolerance of autolysin-defective bacterial mutants against the lytic (and bactericidal) effect of penicillin; (2) the fact that the autolytic activities involved in lysis appear to be non-essential for bacterial growth; (3) the tendency of autolysis-defective mutants to grow in chains; (4) the existence of natural autolysin inhibitors; (5) their release from bacteria during penicillin treatment; (6) the induction (triggering) of autolytic cell wall degradation after brief treatment of bacteria with penicillins.

In essence, this model proposes that in pneumococci, and perhaps in other bacteria as well, the murein hydrolases involved in the degradation of cell walls are not essential enzymes involved with cell wall replication but, rather, these enzymes are inhibited in the growing bacteria by natural inhibitors such as lipoteichoic acids. The physiological role of such enzymes may be in the catalysis of cell separation at the end of cell division (lysis-defective mutants tend to form chains). Penicillin treatment is assumed to initiate a chain of events that eventually results in the release of the negative control of these hydrolases either by dissociation of the hypothetical enzyme-inhibitor complexes, or by inactivation (deacylation?) of the inhibitor. Loss of the inhibitors to the medium may be part of this decontrolling ("triggering") process.

The same kinds of processes may be involved in the control of autolytic enzymes irrespective of what the specific physiological role of these enzymes will eventually turn out to be. H. J. Rogers (ROGERS 1965) has made the original proposal that autolytic enzymes may perform a variety of as yet ill-defined roles as "plasticizers" in the expansion of cell wall material. Clearly, for both the proper as well as for the abnormal functioning of such enzymes, one would have to assume the existence of some kind of control mechanism.

It is tempting to speculate that the physiologically relevant activity of these hydrolases (e.g., catalysis of daughter cell separation) is also triggered at the end of the cell cycle by a transient, genetically programmed halt in cell wall synthesis by a mechanism similar to the one triggered by penicillin treatment, except that the physiological activity would be localized, transient, and properly timed (TOMASZ and HÖLTJE 1977). One may then consider penicillin induced lysis as a premature triggering of some terminal events in bacterial cell division (cell separation).

It should be pointed out that experiments with synchronized cultures of pneumococci have not yet been performed to test this proposition. On the other hand, hydrolase activity extractable from cells seems to decrease (rather than increase) at the time of cell separation in both *S. faecalis* (HINKS et al. 1978) and *E. coli* (HAKENBECK and MESSER 1977).

XII. Attempts to Define the Events Responsible for the Triggering of Autolytic Activity in Pneumococci

The main question emerging from the above discussion is this: what specific evidence, if any, exists concerning the biochemical nature of events that are postulated to bring about the triggering of murein hydrolase activity in penicillin treated bacteria? In an attempt to answer this question, Russell Williamson has isolated a novel type of tolerant mutant of pneumococci, which had normal levels of autolytic activity and yet could not be triggered to lyse (and died only slowly) during penicillin treatment. The rationale for selecting such mutants was as follows: if there indeed existed events *between* the inhibited PBPs and the triggering of autolytic activity, mutants defective in such intermediate events preceding the onset of uncontrolled autolysin activity would be obviously masked in autolysin defective mutants. Therefore, we tried to isolate mutants that are tolerant to penicillin *despite* the fact that they contained a normal level of autolytic activity. Such mutants were indeed isolated (WILLIAMSON and TOMASZ 1980). These $lyt^{+}tol^{+}$ mutants, in contrast to the familiar $lyt^{-}tol^{+}$ mutants, had a normal level of autolytic activity, and could be lysed by detergents and in the stationary phase of growth. However, they were resistant to the lytic effects of substantial doses of penicillin (20 × MIC for 6–10 h at 32 °C), while they had virtually the same MIC value as the parental cells. An unexpected property of these mutants was that they could still be lysed by vancomycin and bacitracin, while they showed cross-tolerance to D-cycloserine. These novel types of mutants are reminiscent of the thermosensitive penicillin-tolerant mutants of *E. coli* which also had high (normal) levels of autolytic activity even at the higher temperature at which the lytic (and cidal) effects of penicillin were suppressed (KITANO and TOMASZ 1979a).

The existence of $tol^{+} lyt^{+}$ mutants is consistent with a postulated inhibitory or trigger pathway connecting the penicillin-inhibited targets with the uncontrolled murein hydrolase activity. The fact that tolerance in these bacteria was drug-specific suggests that there might be more than one such pathway in pneumococci, indicating the complexity of the regulatory circuitry of murein hydrolases.

It should be emphasized that nothing is known about the biochemical nature of this postulated pathway – it is not known whether the "signals" generated in the inhibited bacterium are low molecular weight or soluble compounds (e.g., UDP-linked cell wall precursors or cell wall oligomers); some local structural alteration in the newly made cell wall (e.g., hypo-crosslinking); or some aspect of the plasma membrane structure (TOMASZ 1979b).

F. Environmental Factors That Modulate the Antibacterial Effects of Penicillin

As one starts modifying the growth conditions of the bacteria during penicillin treatment, a great variety of effects may be observed, which illustrates how profound an influence the environment of the target bacterium can have upon the outcome of encounter between the antibiotic and the cell. In most cases, the mechanism of the phenomena is not well understood, although some of them may be mediated by the penicillin-induced secretion of cell surface components into the growth medium (see below). Most of the modifying effects have to do with influencing the killing or lytic effects of penicillin, although drastic changes in the β-lactam MIC values with pH of the medium (HARTMAN and TOMASZ 1980) and with temperature of growth (FONTANA et al. 1980) were also noted. Some of these effects will be briefly illustrated by a few examples, mostly from observations made in our laboratory.

I. Protection Against the Lytic (and Cidal) Effects by Alteration of the pH of the Medium

Cultures of pneumococci, *B. subtilis*, *S. faecalis*, *E. coli* or staphylococci each have a characteristic pH range that is optimal for the lytic effects of penicillin. Below (or above) this pH range, the bacteria acquire a kind of phenotypic tolerance to cell wall synthesis inhibitors, including penicillin (LOPEZ et al. 1976). As a mechanism for this effect, lowering of autolytic activity or the production of more rigid plasma membrane have been considered. Cultures of group B streptococci develop such a pH-related phenotypic tolerance spontaneously at around the middle of the logarithmic phase of growth (HORNE and TOMASZ 1981b). The relative acidity of the natural environment of this bacterium in the female urogenital tract may contribute to the difficulties encountered in the attempts at prophylactic use of penicillin (FRANCIOSI et al. 1973).

II. The Effect of Exogenous Murein Hydrolases on Penicillin-Treated Tolerant Bacteria

Figure 16 demonstrates that addition of heterologous lysozymes (from human urine or from the C-phage) causes rapid killing and lysis of the penicillin tolerant *S. sanguis*, provided that the bacteria have also been treated with penicillin or other cell wall inhibitors. Enzyme added to the medium of growing cells has no effect, and penicillin alone only inhibits growth. The two together, however, convert the tolerant response of *S. sanguis* to a lytic response. It is interesting that different β-lactams have different specific activities (expressed on the basis of the corresponding MIC units) in sensitizing the cells to the enzymes (HORNE and TOMASZ 1980).

III. Synergistic Bactericidal Action of Penicillin and Human Polymorphonuclear White Blood Cells (PMN)

Treatment of group B streptococci with a variety of β-lactams, each at sub-MIC (or MIC) concentration, was found to cause a substantial stimulation of the bactericidal effect of PMN on the antibiotic-treated bacteria. The effect required the presence of specific antibody and thus, presumably, involved a stimulated phagocytosis (HORNE and TOMASZ 1981 a).

A variety of synergistic effects between β-lactams and enzymes, and immune factors has been described in the pioneering studies of Warren and his colleagues, and numerous current investigations have demonstrated synergistic as well as antagonistic effects between β-lactams and various components of the immune system (ROOT et al. 1981; FRIEDMAN and WARREN 1974; FRIEDMAN and WARREN 1976, EFRATI et al. 1976; TRAUB and SHERRIS 1970; ZAK and KRADOLFER 1979; VOSBECK et al. 1979; WAKS and TOMASZ 1978; HAKENBECK et al. 1978).

IV. Inhibition of Penicillin-Induced Lysis by Extracellular Lipids and Lipoteichoic Acids

Addition of high concentrations of the Forssman antigen to the growth medium of lysis-prone pneumococci causes these bacteria to grow in chains and protects the cells against penicillin-induced lysis (HÖLTJE and TOMASZ 1975 a). Both of these phenomena are characteristic of cells with suppressed autolytic systems, and since the Forssman antigen is a powerful inhibitor of the pneumococcal autolysin, it has been suggested that the mechanism of the phenomenon involves the inhibition of autolysin molecules at the cell surface. Similar phenotypic tolerance was induced by the addition of the autolysin-inhibitory cardiolipin to the medium of penicillin-treated *S. faecalis* (CLEVELAND et al. 1976). Overproduction and secretion of lipoteichoic acids was observed and proposed as the mechanism of tolerance in some strains of *S. aureus* (BEST et al. 1974).

V. Penicillin-Induced Release of Cell Surface Components into the Medium

During studies on the mode of action of penicillin on tolerant pneumococci, it was observed that the antibiotic treatment caused a rapid and substantial release of several pneumococcal surface components into the surrounding medium. The components released include the Forssman antigen (HORNE et al. 1977), nascent wall teichoic acid and murein material (HORNE and TOMASZ 1979), lipids, and membrane proteins. The release was specifically induced only by cell wall inhibitors; it required active metabolism and was reversible by the timely addition of penicillinase.

Penicillin-induced release of surface components was subsequently also demonstrated in *S. sanguis* (HORNE and TOMASZ 1979), gonococci (GOODELL et al. 1978) and group A and B streptococci (HAKENBECK et al. 1978). In the latter, the materials released included the type B capsule (HORNE and TOMASZ 1981 a). This penicillin-induced secretion process was probably related to the release of lipid and cell wall material demonstrated earlier, in several bacteria (ELLIOTT et al. 1975; MIRELMAN et al. 1972; JOSEPH and SHOCKMAN 1975). The reason for bringing up this phenomenon in this section of the review is that the secretion of biologically active surface components is likely to be involved with the sensitization phenomena described above. The removal of inhibitory or antiphagocytic structures from the surface of the target cells may be responsible for the hypersensitivity of penicillin-treated bacteria to extracellular enzymes and phagocytic cells.

The penicillin-induced release of bacterial components with powerful biological activities [e.g., teichoic acid inducers of the complement alternative pathway (WINKELSTEIN and TOMASZ 1978), endotoxins, immune adjuvant cell wall fragments, chemotactic stimulants, etc.] into the vascular system of an invaded host may play a role in the modulation of immune response mounted against the invading bacterium, and the same phenomenon may also be involved with inflammatory tissue damage.

VI. Phenotypic Tolerance in Nongrowing Cells

It has long been known that nongrowing bacteria are inert to the killing and lytic effects of penicillin. This seems to be generally true for all bacteria. The ability of nongrowing cells to survive penicillin treatment is the basis of auxotrophic mutant selection (LEDERBERG and ZINDER 1948) and is also thought to be responsible for the antagonistic effects of bacteriostatic agents on the chemotherapeutic effectiveness of penicillin (LEPPER and DOWLING 1951). It has been suspected that this phenomenon may involve the bacterial autolytic system, but no conclusive evidence has been found (PRESTIDGE and PARDEE 1957). A more recent study with amino acid-starved *E. coli* suggests that the resistance of such bacteria to penicillin-induced lysis reflects a defect in the autolytic system that develops rapidly upon the removal of required amino acid. It was found that such nongrowing cells were difficult to "trigger" into cell wall degradation by physico-chemical treatments (e.g., chaotropic agents, EDTA, organic solvents, etc.) which would cause the rapid and extensive autolysis of cell walls in the growing cells (GOODELL and TOMASZ 1980).

A closer examination indicated that the defective component was the cell wall, and not the autolytic enzyme. It was found that the most recently made cell wall, i.e., the murein synthesized during amino acid starvation, became less susceptible to crude, homologous autolytic extract isolated from the normal bacteria. It was suggested that a structural alteration in the murein, possibly involving hypercrosslinking, may be responsible for this effect.

A large number of additional observations in the literature describes effective antimicrobial activity of β-lactams against bacteria in a complex environment at concentrations of the antibiotic below the MIC values measured in vitro. For instance, nocardicin (KUNUGITA et al. 1981) and some cephamycins (YAMADA et al. 1981) were reported to produce better PD50 (protective dose) values than would have been predicted on the basis of their in vitro inhibitory power against the same bacteria. Gram-negative bacteria treated with subinhibitory doses of mecillinam were shown to have increased serum sensitivity (TRAUB and SHERRIS 1979; TAYLOR et al. 1981). Staphylococci, pretreated with subinhibitory concentrations of penicillin, were found to become sensitive to extracellular killing by PMN (ROOT et al. 1981; FRIEDMAN and WARREN 1974; EFRATI et al. 1976).

Some recent observations indicate that adherence to certain types of surfaces increases the survival of bacteria during treatment with penicillin (GWYNN et al. 1981). Other studies suggest that penicillin treatment can selectively (i.e., without killing the bacteria) interfere with the adherence of group A streptococci to ephithelial surfaces (VOSBECK et al. 1979; OFEK et al. 1975; ALKAN and BEACHEY 1978; BEACHEY and OFEK 1976; OFEK et al. 1979). Similarly, the effective attachment of the penicillin-tolerant *S. sanguis* to traumatized rabbit heart values was inhibited by in vitro pretreatment of the bacteria with penicillin doses that caused release of about 85% of the acylated lipoteichoic acids but no loss of viability (NEUHAUS et al. 1980). One can imagine that these surface alterations may lead to either synergistic or antagonistic interactions with the immune system. An example of the latter would be the loss of surface components that are receptors for components of the immune system. The penicillin-induced loss of teichoic acid complexes capable of triggering the alternative pathway of complement has been reported (WINKELSTEIN and TOMASZ 1978). Such complexes released into the vascular system may adhere to host epithelial surfaces, or in the kidneys, and this may initiate a misdirected attack of complement leading to tissue damage.

The findings listed were selected to document the breadth of variability in the antibacterial effects of penicillin, and the myriad of factors that can modulate the antibacterial effectiveness of β-lactam antibiotics in vivo in an infected host. A more complete catalogue of such findings may be found in one of several recent reviews (BEACHEY et al. 1981; VOSBECK et al. 1979).

To what extent these cooperative effects actually occur during penicillin chemotherapy is not clear. Several of these phenomena occur during exposure of the bacteria to sub-MIC concentrations of penicillin, at which only some of the bacterial PBPs, classified as physiologically "dispensable targets," would be expected to be labeled by penicillin. Thus, in the complex environment of an invaded host, such PBPs may, by definition, become lethal targets of β-lactam action. A relatively minor perturbation of the cell surface, reparable during growth in vitro, may become a fatal vulnerability for the bacteria in vivo.

G. Conclusion

The mode of action of penicillin, as defined at the beginning of this review, is composed of a number of recognizable stages, only *some* of which involve a direct chemical interaction between bacterial surface components and the β-lactam molecules. In most cases, the journey of the antibiotic molecules would begin with the crossing of surface boundaries and end at the outer surface of the bacterial plasma membrane. By this time, the antibiotic molecule will have interacted with several bacterial components; it will have had to pass a number of chemically and physically diverse barriers, some in the immediate microenvironment of the bacterium (e.g., a phagosomal membrane or extracellular polysaccharide), others on the bacterium itself (e.g., outer membrane lipids and lipopolysaccharides; porins; and the murein and nonmurein components of the cell wall). The antibiotic molecule may encounter β-lactamases – in the periplasmic space. Clearly, the success of arriving fast, in an active form and at sufficient concentrations, to the ultimate biochemical targets in the plasma membrane will depend on the chemical structure of the particular β-lactam, which will affect, favorably or unfavorably, the interactions of the drug molecule with the various bacterial components encountered during the journey through the cell surface. The final and most important group of these components are the PBPs, and the "choice" of PBP, the rate of its acylation, and the stability of the complex will all be partly dependent on the chemistry of the antibiotic molecule. In our current view, it is up to this point that the chemical structure of the antibiotic will *directly* influence the inhibitory activity of the molecules.

This, however, does not mean that the type and degree of the antimicrobial effect (MIC, MBC etc.) is *fully* determined by the reaction with the PBP molecules, since the end of the physical journey of the β-lactam at the PBPs just signals the beginning of the process of antibacterial activity, i.e., the interference with bacterial metabolism which, in turn, may lead to the development of a variety of physiological defects and which may culminate in a halt of cellular growth, irreversible loss of viability or physical disintegration (dissolution) of the cell. While it is virtually certain that the antibacterial effects of β-lactams are, in the long run, ultimately all the consequences of the inhibition of the biochemical function(s) of the PBPs, it is becoming increasingly clear that the degree of inhibition of PBPs need not directly translate into the MIC or MBC value. Whether or not a certain degree of inhibition of one or more PBPs will lead to a reversible or irreversible inhibition of the whole cell will also depend to a great extent on bacterial factors that do not directly react with the penicillin molecule. Furthermore, environmental factors, such as pH, nutrients, the presence or absence of immune factors, etc. may exert a critical influence on the eventual fate of the penicillin-treated bacterium. The generally acknowledged predictive value of the in vitro MIC values for the performance of the antibiotic in vivo need not mean that the *mechanisms* of in vitro and in vivo antibacterial effects are also the same.

The notion that the physiological effects of penicillin may be only indirectly related to the inhibition of the primary biochemical targets of this drug was originally made explicit in 1975 and 1977, in an explanation of the mechanism of the irreversible antibacterial effects of penicillin as these related to the phenomenon of antibiotic tolerance in pneumococci (TOMASZ and WAKS 1975b; TOMASZ and HÖLTJE

1977). It was suggested that, contrary to the common notion, penicillin may be a bacteriostatic agent in the sense that the *primary effect* of penicillin may be inhibition of growth. However, this may only be observed in the tolerant cells, since in most wild-type bacteria the inhibited cells go on to lose viability and lyse, due to secondary effects (such as deregulation of autolytic enzymes) that are triggered by the inhibition of cell wall synthesis.

Although this model was proposed primarily to explain the irreversible effects of penicillin, it was also pointed out that the question of how interference with cell wall synthesis should cause inhibition of growth, as happens in tolerant bacteria, is not a trivial one either. It was suggested that, similarly to the coordinate regulation of protein and RNA syntheses, inhibition of cell wall synthesis may lead to inhibition of other polymer syntheses via some change in the cellular concentration of some effector compound, such as a guanosine-tetraphosphate. Some of the anomalous results obtained in attempts to correlate PBP labeling with the MIC values (see Sect. D) suggest that, indeed, "indirect" mechanisms proposed for the killing and lytic effects may also be valid for the reversible (growth inhibitory) effects of penicillins.

Mode of action type studies with β-lactam antibiotics should continue to provide numerous potential benefits for the academically oriented scientist. As one is trying to follow the path of the penicillin molecule to its cellular targets, or when one tries to reconstruct the mechanism by which inhibition of penicillin sensitive enzymes may lead to the actual antimicrobial effects (e.g., inhibition of protein synthesis or deregulation of cell wall hydrolysing enzymes), one finds the problem of the mode of action of penicillin entangled with numerous aspects of bacterial surface biology. This happens to be one of the least understood areas of microbiology, and one of the major scientific benefits of studies on the mode of action of β-lactams is in the amount of basic knowledge such efforts have the potential of generating on a variety of general problems. These problems include, for example, the structure and regulation of porin function; the mechanism by which the murein sacculus, a vast network of glycopeptide polymers covering the entire cell surface, is enlarged by the addition of new subunits that have to be transported to the precise sites of wall growth zones; the structure and topographic distribution of membrane-bound enzymes that catalyze these processes; the coordination of cell wall and cell membrane synthesis with chromosome replication within the process of cell division, etc. Luria has called attention to our rather scant knowledge concerning such "macro-regulatory phenomena" (LURIA 1970).

The other thesis of this review is that current studies on the mode of action of β-lactam antibiotics also have the potential of providing important leads for the pharmaceutical chemist interested in the development of antibiotics of improved performance.

The quantitative expression of a drug's ultimate performance as an antimicrobial agent is represented by the minimal growth inhibitory, or minimal bactericidal concentration (MIC or MBC), values or by the minimal protective dose (PD_{50}). These simple numbers, which allow the comparison of various drugs with one another, have been used by the pharmaceutical industry for the evaluation of β-lactam structure-activity relationships. While this approach has been a fruitful one as proven by the development of a number of β-lactams of improved characteristics, it is also clear that the understanding of the relationship between β-lactam structure and antibacterial activity will require the breaking down of the MIC values to their component terms. The MIC value represents the sum-total of contributions from each level of interaction between the drug molecule and the bacterium, such as coefficients characterizing the access of drug-sensitive targets, terms expressing the stability of the antibiotic to β-lactamases or other side reactions, and kinetic constants (relating the interaction between drug sensitive enzymes and the inhibitor). In addition, the MBC may also include a number of largely unknown parameters that express the individual contributions of secondary factors (e.g., autolysin activity, the cell divisional stage of the target cell), since both the MBC and the MIC values of β-lactams can vary considerably with the growth conditions in several bacteria. Some of this is illustrated by the data in Table 1. For instance, the very large variations in the penicillin MIC values against various strains of *E. coli* and *Pseudomonas* are related to rate-limiting drug access and/or β-lactamase production. In contrast, the very high cephalosporin MIC of *S. faecalis* is most likely determined by the low affinity of those antibiotics for some critical PBPs. The fluctuations in the in vitro β-lactam MIC values for *Legionella* most likely reflect the relative sensitivity of the drugs to cephalosporinases (PASCULLE et al. 1981). The very poor activity of the monobactam SQ 26776 against most gram-positive strains may reflect some basic structural difference between the PBPs of gram-negative and those gram-positive bacteria. In the methicillin-resistant *S. aureus* or in the penicillin-resistant pneumococci and gonococci, the elevated MIC values appear to be related to altered PBPs. The high MBC values in *S. sanguis* or in some of the tolerant staphylococci correlate with the low autolytic activity in these bacteria.

The unexpectedly low PD_{50} values (i.e., lower than predicted from their in vitro MICs) observed with nocardicin (KUNUGITA et al. 1981) or some cephamycin derivatives (YAMADA et al. 1981) demonstrate that factors that come into play only in the in vivo environment of the bacteria may definitively alter (in these cases, improve) the antibacterial effectiveness of a β-lactam antibiotic.

A full understanding of the contributions of all these factors to the antibacterial effectiveness of a drug would be tantamount to a complete characterization of its mode of action, and this has not yet been achieved for any of the β-lactam antibiotics. Nevertheless, specific assays capable of characterizing the various levels of interaction of a β-lactam with its target cell are now available. Permeability coefficients; stability to β-lactamases; affinity to PBPs; capacity to interfere with murein biosynthesis or with model transpeptidation; specific activity for "triggering" autolysis, causing specific morphological change or sensitizing to the antibacterial effects of immune factors; interference with bacterial adherence, etc., can all be measured. Individual β-lactams differ from one another in these assays. Obviously, the use of all these criteria in the screening of new β-lactam antibiotics would be an impossibly burdensome task and this should, ideally, be a cooperative effort for the academic scientists and pharmaceutical chemists – an investment that would surely pay off, in the longer run.

Nevertheless, a good case could be made for a more immediate utilization of modern knowledge gained from mode-of-action studies in the development of new antibiotics. Some of the new information about mode of action of penicillins could already be converted to highly specific assays that could be sharply targeted on certain types of bacteria or bacteria in specific kinds of environments. The isolation of such truly novel β-lactam antibiotics as thienamycin, nocardicin or the monobactams would not have been possible without the use of new types of hypersensitive strains [e.g., deep rough mutants and/or *E. coli* deficient in PBP 1 b (1)] in the screening process. From titration of the selective affinities of a large number of β-lactams for the individual PBPs of various bacteria, some correlations between chemical structure and PBP affinity have begun to emerge; this should permit better interpretation of the traditional structure-activity relationships. Semisynthetic derivatives of monobactams appear to be particularly promising in this respect. Isolation of several PBPs and success with the crystallization of some penicillin-sensitive carboxypeptidases should also generate much useful information with potential use in drug design. The dramatically lowered penicillin or methicillin affinities of the PBPs in intrinsically resistant clinical isolates of staphylococci, streptococci, and gonococci raise the possibility of screening for structurally new β-lactams modified to give increased affinities for these mutationally altered PBPs (and possibly provide lower MIC values against the resistant bacteria). Enough information is available about the regulation of bacterial autolytic enzymes and their role in the irreversible effects of penicillins to use some of this knowledge for the selection of β-lactams with superior "killing" power. Similarly, new knowledge available on the mechanism of transport of β-lactams across cellular membranes or on the regulation of porin function, or information concerning the role of bacterial adherence in certain infections, should all be exploitable by those interested in rational drug design. Indeed, it seems that we have entered an era in which there is no end to the possibilities of translating specific mechanistic knowledge into practical pharmaceutical chemistry.

Three major practical conclusions may be drawn from the foregoing discussion:

(1) It seems that in thinking about the mode of action of penicillin it is more realistic to widen one's focus from inhibited bacterial enzymes to an entire inhibitory pathway of multiple steps and factors that connect the penicillin sensitive bacterial enzymes to the inhibited bacterial cell. Still, additional factors come into play and modulate the mode of antibiotic action as the target bacterium is moved from the in vitro culture tube to the complex environment of the infected host. It is quite possible that studies on this latter aspect of penicillin action would soon lead to the analysis of the mechanism of bacterial disease, thus further enlarging the context and importance of mode-of-action studies.

(2) Given the tremendous number of structurally different β-lactams available (Williams 1981) and the great bacterium-to-bacterium variation in the mode of antibacterial action of these compounds, one might make a good case for developing β-lactam antibiotics in the direction of highly selective narrow-spectrum and antibacterial agents. General arguments in favor of such "selective" limited warfare against bacterial pathogens may be found in the literature.

(3) The multiple factors – some in the target cells, others in their environment – that seem to affect, directly and indirectly, the final outcome as well as every stage of encounter between β-lactams and bacteria raise the possibility of a variety of properly targeted secondary drugs that might be used in synergistic combination with β-lactams. One such example is provided by the success with the lactamase

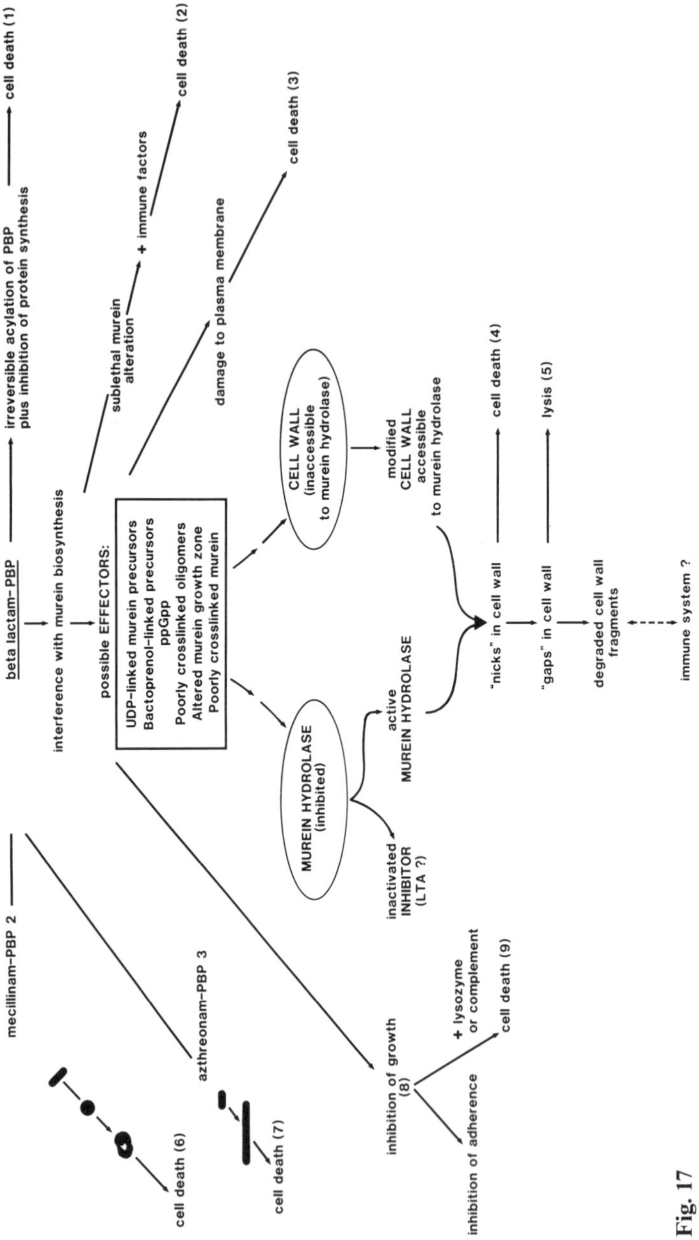
beta lactam–PBP
irreversible acylation of PBP
plus inhibition of protein synthesis
cell death (1)
interference with murein biosynthesis
sublethal murein
alteration
+ immune factors
cell death (2)
damage to plasma membrane
cell death (3)
possible EFFECTORS:
UDP-linked murein precursors
Bactoprenol-linked precursors
ppGpp
Poorly crosslinked oligomers
Altered murein growth zone
Poorly crosslinked murein
CELL WALL
(inaccessible
to murein hydrolase)
modified
CELL WALL
accessible
to murein hydrolase
MUREIN HYDROLASE
(inhibited)
active
MUREIN HYDROLASE
inactivated
INHIBITOR
(LTA ?)
"nicks" in cell wall
cell death (4)
"gaps" in cell wall
lysis (5)
degraded cell wall
fragments
immune system ?
mecillinam–PBP 2
cell death (6)
azthreonam–PBP 3
cell death (7)
inhibition of growth
(8)
+ lysozyme
or complement
cell death (9)
inhibition of adherence

Fig. 17

inhibitor – β-lactam combinations. However, other functionally cooperative "partner" drugs could also be sought. These could include, for instance, inhibitors capable of suppressing the production of extracellular capsule (COSTERTON 1979), or outer membrane lipopolysaccharides, agents that could destabilize the bacterial autolytic enzyme (and thus stimulate the irreversible outcome of penicillin inhibition), etc.

Optimal performance in passing the cellular boundaries, resistance to β-lactamases, and reactivity with the appropriate PBP, etc., may impose difficult and opposing structural requirements. The general and obvious advantage of the partner-drug approach would be that in an ideal case it might exempt the β-lactam structure from at least some of these demands, so that the chemistry of the β-lactam could be mainly targeted on the PBPs.

Figure 17 is a graphic summary of some of the observed and/or postulated mechanisms by which inhibition of PBPs may lead to the antibacterial effects of β-lactam antibiotics.

Fig. 17. Variation in the antibacterial effects of β-lactam antibiotics. In *E. coli*, selective inhibition of PBPs 2 and 3 may lead to distinct mechanisms of cell death at the end of the unique morphological changes induced in the bacteria (see *6* and *7*). In the same bacterium, inhibition of PBP 1 b (plus 1 a?) appears to cause death and lysis by upsetting the regulation of murein hydrolase(s). Some or all of these physiological consequences of PBP inhibition may be mediated by possible effectors, i.e., compounds accumulating in the β-lactam treated bacteria and/or an altered (hypo-crosslinked?) murein synthesized by the antibiotic treated cells. Penicillin treatment that only causes reversible inhibition of growth in a test tube culture may sensitize bacteria to the bactericidal action of exogenous lysozyme or complement (*9*). The same – sublethal – effect of penicillin may effectively interfere with bacterial adhesion.
The scheme is intended to illustrate the proposition that β-lactam antibiotics may bring about the inhibition of a bacterial cell by a number of different mechanisms that may vary with the particular β-lactam, with the bacterial species and with factors in the bacterium's environment. All the inhibitory effects are assumed to be consequences of the inhibition of the physiological function(s) of one or more PBP. The figure illustrates a variety of conceivable pathways leading to inhibition of growth (as observed in some penicillin-tolerant bacteria – *pathway 8*), cell death (*1–4*), and lysis (*5*). Observations suggesting these mechanisms have been discussed in the text. Mechanisms 1, 3, or 4 have been considered for the lethality of group A streptococci (nonlytic death). It is also conceivable that a variation in the *degree* of structural damage to the murein layer by the triggered activity of murein hydrolases may be the basis of the various, more or less severe, physiological consequences of β-lactam action, such as "sensitization" of the cells to hostile agents (e.g., immune factors) or interference with the normal ability to adhere to surfaces. A more extensive "nicking" of the murein may cause irreversible damage to reproductive capacity (*4*). Extensive hydrolysis of bonds in the murein should cause exposure (and rupture) of the plasma membrane and degradation of cell wall.
According to this view, any factor, genetic, physiological or environmental, that can interrupt the chain of secondary events towards irreversibility, could cause β-lactam tolerance, which may have a variety of different mechanisms, some related to the level of murein hydrolase activity, others involving changed control of hydrolases, etc. Bacterial mutants with β-lactam tolerance related to a "hardier" plasma membrane structure, may also exist

References

Albers-Schonberg G, Aricson BH, Hensens OD, Hirschfield J, Hogsteen K, Kaczka EA, Rhodes RE, Kahan JS, Kahan FM, Ratcliffe RW, Walton E, Ruswinkle LJ, Morin RB, Christensen GB (1978) Structure and absolute configuration of thienamycin. J Am Chem Soc 100:6491–6499

Alkan ML, Beachey EH (1978) Excretion of lipoteichoic acid by group A streptococci: influence of penicillin on excretion and loss of ability to adhere to human oral mucosal cells. J Clin Invest 61:671–677

Allen BL, Sprunt K (1978) Discrepancy between minimum inhibitory and minimum bactericidal concentrations of penicillin for group A and group B β-hemolytic streptococci. J Pediatrics 93:69–71

Amanuma H, Strominger JL (1980) Purification and properties of penicillin-binding protein 5 and 6 from *Escherichia coli* membranes. J Biol Chem 255:11173–11180

Ambler RP (1980) The structure of β-lactamases. Philos Trans R Soc Lond B 321–331

Aono R, Yamasaki M, Tamura G (1979) High and selective resistance to mecillinam in adenylate cyclase-deficient or cyclic adenosine 3′,5′ monophosphate receptor protein deficient mutants of *Escherichia coli.* J Bacteriol 137:839–845

Araki Y, Shimada A, Ito E (1966) Effect of penicillin on cell wall mucopeptide synthesis in a *Escherichia coli* particulate system. Biochem Biophys Res Commun 23:518–525

Ayusawa D, Yoneda Y, Yamane K, Maruo B (1975) Pleiotropic phenomena in autolytic enzyme(s) content, flagellation, and simultaneous hyperproduction of extracellular α-amylase and protease in a *Bacillus subtilis* mutant. J Bacteriol 124:459–469

Beachey EH, Ofek I (1976) Epithelial cell binding of group A streptococci by lipoteichoic acid on fimbriae denuded of M protein. J Exp Med 143:759–771

Beachey EH, Eisenstein BI, Ofek I (1981) Sublethal concentrations of antibiotics and bacterial adhesion. Ciba Found Symp 80:288–305

Best GK, Best NH, Koval AV (1974) Evidence for participation of autolyins in bactericidal action of oxacillin on *Staphylococcus aureus.* Antimicrob Agents Chemother 6:825–830

Blumberg PM, Strominger JL (1971) Inactivation of D-alanine carboxypeptidase by penicillins and cephalosporins is not lethal in *Bacillus subtilis.* Proc Natl Acad Sci USA 68:2814–2817

Blumberg PM, Strominger JL (1974) Interaction of penicillin with the bacterial cell: penicillin binding proteins and penicillin-sensitive enzymes. Bacteriol Rev 38:291–315

Blumberg PM, Yocum RR, Willoughby E, Strominger JL (1974) Binding of ^{14}C penicillin G to the membrane bound and purified D-alanine carboxypeptidases from *Bacillus stereorothermophilus* and *Bacillus subtilis* and its release. J Biol Chem 249:6828–6835

Botta GA, Park JT (1981) Evidence for involvement of penicillinbinding protein 3 in murein synthesis during septation but not during cell elongation. J Bacteriol 145:333–340

Brown DFJ, Reynolds PE (1980) Intrinsic resistance to β-lactam antibiotics in *Staphylococcus aureus.* FEBS Lett 122:275–278

Brown KN, Percival A (1978) Penetration of antimicrobials into tissue culture cells and leukocytes. Scand J Inf Dis Suppl 14:251–260

Buchanan CE, Strominger JL (1976) Altered penicillin-binding components in penicillin-resistant mutants of *Bacillus subtilis.* Proc Natl Acad Sci USA 73:1816–1820

Buchanan CE, Hsia J, Strominger JL (1977) Antibody to the D-alanine carboxypeptidase of *Bacillus subtilis* does not cross react with other penicillin-binding proteins. J Bacteriol 131:1008–1010

Carson D, Pieringer RA, Daneo-Moore L (1979) Effect of growth rate on lipid and lipoteichoic acid composition in *Streptococcus faecium.* Biochem Biophys Acta 575:225–233

Chase HA, Reynolds PE (1980a) In: FEMS symp microbial envelopes, abstr 92, Saimaranta, Finland

Chase HA, Reynolds PE (1980b) The interaction of β-lactam antibiotics with penicillin-binding proteins studies in vivo. Soc Gen Microbiol 7:78

Chase HA, Shephard ST, Reynolds PE (1977) Studies on the penicillinbinding components of *Bacillus megaterium.* FEBS Lett 76:199–206

Chase HA, Fuller C, Reynolds PE (1981) The role of penicillin-binding proteins in the action of cephalosporins against *Escherichia coli* and *Salmonella typhimurium*. Eur J Biochem 117:301–310

Chatterjee AN, Wong W, Young FE, Gilpin RW (1976) Isolation and characterization of a mutant of *Staphylococcus aureus* deficient in autolytic activity. J Bacteriol 125:961–967

Cleveland RF, Holtje J-V, Wicken AJ, Tomasz A, Daneo-Moore L, Shockman GD (1975) Inhibition of bacterial wall lysins by lipoteichoic acids and related compounds. Biochem Biophys Res Commun 67:1128–1135

Cleveland RF, Wicken AJ, Daneo-Moore L, Shockman GD (1976) Inhibition of wall autolysis in *Streptococcus faecalis* by lipoteichoic acids and lipids. J Bacteriol 126:192–197

Cooper PD (1956) Site of action of radiopenicillin. Bact Rev 20:28–48

Costerton JW (1979) *Pseudomonas aeruginosa* in nature and disease. In: Sabath LD (ed) *Pseudomonas aeruginosa*. H. Huber, Bern, pp 15–24

Coyette J, Ghuysen JM, Fontana R (1978) Solubilization and isolation of the membrane-bound D,D-carboxypeptidase of *Streptococcus faecalis* ATCC 9790: properties of the purified enzyme. Eur J Biochem 88:297–305

Curtis NAC, Ross GW (1980) Factors influencing the interaction of β-lactam antibiotics with bacteria: penetration, resistance to β-lactamases, affinity for β-lactam binding protein targets. In: Gregory GI (ed) Recent advances in the chemistry of beta lactam antibiotics. The Royal Society Chemistry, London, pp 203–216

Curtis NAC, Orr D, Ross GW, Boulton MG (1979a) Competition of β-lactam antibiotics for the penicillin-binding proteins of *Pseudomonas aeruginosa*, *Enterobacter cloacae*, *Klebsiella aerogenes*, *Proteus rettgeri*, and *Escherichia coli*: comparison with antibacterial activity and effects upon bacterial morphology. Antimicrob Agents Chemother 16:325–328

Curtis NAC, Orr D, Ross GW, Boulton MG (1979b) Affinities of penicillins and cephalosporins for the penicillin-binding proteins of *Escherichia coli* K-12 and their antibacterial activity. Antimicrob Agents Chemother 16:533–539

Curtis SJ, Strominger JL (1978) Effects of sulfhydryl reagents on the binding and release of penicillin G by D-alanine carboxypeptidase IA of *Escherichia coli*. J Biol Chem 253:2584–2588

Davis BD (1948) Isolation of biochemically deficient mutants of bacteria by penicillin. J Am Chem Soc 70:4267

DeLeys RJ, Juni E (1977) Unusual effects of penicillin G and chloroamphenicol on the growth of *Moraxella osloensis*. Antimicrob Agents Chemother 12:573–576

Demerec M (1945) Production of straphylococcus strains resistant to various concentrations of penicillin. Proc Natl Acad Sci USA 31:16–24

DePedro MA, Schwartz U, Nishimura Y, Hirota Y (1980) On the biological role of penicillin-binding proteins 4 and 5. FEMS Microbiol Lett 9:219–221

Dideberg O, Frere J-M, Ghuysen J-M (1979) Crystallographic data for the D,D-carboxypeptidase-endopeptidase of low penicillin sensitivity excreted by *Streptomyces albus* G. J Mol Biol 129:677–679

Dienes L, Weinberger HJ (1951) The L forms of bacteria. Bacteriol Rev 15:245–288

Dougherty TJ, Koller AE, Tomasz A (1980) Penicillin-binding proteins of penicillin-susceptible and intrinsically resistant *Neisseria gonorrhoeae*. Antimicrob Agents Chemother 18:730–737

Dougherty TJ, Koller AE, Tomasz A (1981) Competition of β-lactam antibiotics for the penicillin-binding proteins of *Neisseria gonorrhoeae*. Antimicrob Agents Chemother 20:109–114

Dring GJ, Hurst A (1969) Observations on the action of benzylpenicillin on a strain of *Streptococcus lactis*. J Gen Microbiol 55:185–194

Duguid JP (1946) The sensitivity of bacteria to the action of penicillin. Edinburgh Med J 53:401–412

Dusart J, Reynolds PE, Ghuysen J-M (1981) Penicillin binding proteins and model transpeptidase activity of the plasma membranes of *Streptomyces* strains R61 and *rimosus*. FEMS Microbiol Lett 12:299–303

Eagle H, Musselman AD (1948) The rate of bactericidal action of penicillin in vitro as a function of its concentration and its paradoxically reduced activity at high concentrations against certain organisms. J Exp Med 88:99–131

Efrati C, Sacks T, Ne'eman N, Lahav M, Ginsburg I (1976) The effect of leucoyte hydrolases on bacteria. VIII. The combined effect of leukocyte extracts, lysozyme, enzyme "cocktails," and penicillin on the lysis of *Staphylococcus aureus* and group A streptococci in vitro. Inflammation 1:371–407

Eliopoulos GM, Wennersten C, Moellering RC Jr (1981) Abstr 502: Resistance to β-lactam antibiotics in *Streptococcus faecium*. 21 Intersci conf antimicrob agents and chemotherapy, American Society for Microbiology

Elliott TSJ, Ward JB, Rogers HJ (1975) Formation of cell wall polymers by reverting protoplasts of *Bacillus licheniformis*. J Bacteriol 124:623–632

Fein JE, Rogers HJ (1976) Autolytic enzyme-deficient mutants of *Bacillus subtilis* 168. J Bacteriol 127:1427–1442

Fischer J, Belasco JG, Charnas RL, Koshla S, Knowles JR (1980) β-Lactamase inactivation by mechanism-based reagents. Philos Trans R Soc Lond B 289:309–319

Flynn EH (1972) Cephalosporins and penicillins: chemistry and biology. Academic, New York

Fontana R, Canejan P, Satta G, Coyette J (1980) Identification of the lethal target of benzylpenicillin in *Streptococcus faecalis* by in vivo penicillin binding studies. Nature 287:70–72

Forsberg C, Rogers HJ (1971) Autolytic enzymes in growth of bacteria. Nature 229:272–273

Franciosi RA, Knostman JD, Zimmerman RA (1973) Group B streptococcal neonatal and infant infections. J Pediatrics 82:707–718

Frere J-M, Ghuysen J-M, Degelaen J, Loffet A, Perkins HR (1975a) Fragmentation of benzylpenicillin after interaction with the exocellular D,D-carboxypeptidase-transpeptidases of *Streptomyces* R61 and R39. Nature 258:168–170

Frere J-M, Ghuysen J-M, Perkins HR (1975b) Interaction between the exocellular D,D-carboxypeptidase-transpeptidase from *Streptomyces* R61, substrate and β-lactam antibiotics: a choice of models. Eur J Biochem 57:353–359

Friedman H, Warren GH (1974) Enhanced susceptibility of penicillin-resistant staphylococci to phagocytosis after in vitro incubation with low doses of nafcillin. Proc Soc Exp Biol Med 146:707–711

Friedman H, Warren GH (1976) Antibody-mediated bacteriolysis: enhanced killing of cyclocillin treated bacteria. Proc Soc Exp Biol Med 153:301–304

Fuchs-Cleveland E, Gilvarg C (1976) Oligomeric intermediate in peptidoglycan biosynthesis in *Bacillus megaterium*. Proc Natl Acad Sci USA 73:4200–4204

Gale EF, Cundliffe E, Reynolds PE, Richman MH, Waring MJ (1981) The molecular basis of antibiotic action. Wiley, London

Garcia E, Rojo JM, Garcia P, Ronda C, Lopez R, Tomasz A (1982) Preparation of antiserum against the pneumococcal autolysin-inhibition of autolysin activity and some autolytic processes by the antibody. FEMS Microbiol Lett 14:133–136

Gardner AD (1940) Morphological effects of penicillin on bacteria. Nature 146:837–838

Gensmantel NP, McLellan D, Morris JJ, Page MT, Proctor P, Randahand GS (1980) Mechanisms in the reactions of some β-lactam antibiotics and their derivatives. In: Gregory GI (ed) Recent advances in the chemistry of beta lactam antibiotics. The Royal Society of Chemistry, London, pp 227–239

Georgopapadakou NH, Liu FY (1980) Penicillin-binding proteins in bacteria. Antimicrob Agents Chemother 18:148–157

Ghuysen J-M (1968) Use of bacteriolytic enzymes in determination of wall structure and their role in cell metabolism. Bacteriol Rev 32:425–464

Ghuysen J-M (1976) The bacterial D,D-carboxypeptidase-transpeptidase enzyme system: a new insight into the mode of action of penicillin. In: Brown WE (ed) ER Squibb lectures on chemistry and microbial products. University of Tokyo Press, Tokyo, pp 1–164

Ghuysen J-M (1977) The concept of the penicillin target from 1965 until today. J Gen Microbiol 101:13–33

Ghuysen J-M, Frere JM, Leyh-Bouille M, Perkins HR, Nieto M (1980) The active centres in penicillin-sensitive enzymes. Philos Trans R Soc Lond B 289:119–135
Ghuysen J-M, Frere J-M, Leyh-Bouille M, Dideberg O (1981) The D-alanyl-D-ala peptidases; mechanism of action of penicillins and δ^3-cephalosporins. In: Salton MRJ, Shockman GD (eds) β-Lactam antibiotics. Academic, New York, pp 127–152
Ghuysen J-M, Leyh-Bouille M, Frere J-M, Dusart J, Marquet A, Perkins HR, Nieto M (1974) The penicillin receptor in Streptomyces. Ann NY Acad Sci 235:236–266
Gmeiner J, Kroll H-P (1981) Murein biosynthesis and *O*-acetylation of *N*-acetyl muramic acid during the cell-division cycle of *Proteus mirabilis*. Eur J Biochem 117:171–177
Goodell EW, Tomasz A (1980) Alteration of *Escherichia coli* murein during amino acid starvation. J Bacteriol 144:1009–1016
Goodell EW, Fazio M, Tomasz A (1978) Effect of benzylpenicillin on the synthesis and structure of the cell envelope of *Neisseria gonorrhoeae*. Antimicrob Agents Chemother 13:514–526
Govan JRW (1975) Mucoid strains of *Pseudomonas aeruginosa:* the influence of culture medium on the stability of mucus production. J Med Microbiol 8:513–522
Greenwood D, O'Grady F (1973) The two sites of penicillin action in *Escherichia coli*. J Infect Dis 128:791–794
Grunberg E, Cleeland R, Beskid G, DeLorenzo WF (1976) In vivo synergy between 6β-amidinopenicillamic acid derivatives and other antibiotics. Antimicrob Agents Chemother 9:589–594
Gutmann L, Tomasz A (1981) Degradation of the penicillin-binding proteins in aminoglycoside-treated group A streptococci. EMS Microbiol Lett 10:323–326
Gutmann L, Tomasz A (1982) Penicillin-resistant and penicillin-tolerant mutants in group A streptococci. Antimicrob Agents Chemother 22:128–136
Gutmann L, Williamson R, Tomasz A (1980) Physiological properties of penicillin-binding proteins in group A streptococci. Antimicrob Agents Chemother 19:872–880
Gwynn MN, Webb LT, Rolinson GN (1981) Regrowth of *Pseudomonas aeruginosa* and other bacteria after the bactericidal action of carbenicillin and other β-lactam antibiotics. J Inf Dis 144:263–269
Hakenbeck R, Messer W (1977) Oscillations in the synthesis of cell wall components in synchronized cultures of *Escherichia coli*. J Bacteriol 129:1239–1244
Hakenbeck R, Waks S, Tomasz A (1978) Characterization of cell wall polymers secreted into the growth medium of lysis-defective pneumococci during treatment with penicillin and other inhibitors of cell wall synthesis. Antimicrob Agents Chemother 13:302–311
Hakenbeck R, Tarpay M, Tomasz A (1980) Multiple changes of penicillin-binding proteins in penicillin-resistant clinical isolates of *Streptococcus pneumoniae*. Antimicrobiol Agents Chemother 17:364–371
Hamilton TE, Lawrence PE (1975) The formation of functional penicillin-binding proteins. J Biol Chem 250:6578–6585
Hammarstrom S, Strominger JL (1975) Degradation of penicillin G to phenylacetyl-glycine by D-alanine carboxypeptidase from *Bacillus stearothermophilus*. Proc Natl Acad Sci USA 72:3463–3467
Hammes WP, Kandler D (1976) Biosynthesis of peptidoglycan in *Gaffkya homari:* the incorporation of peptidoglycan into the cell wall and the direction of transpeptidation. Eur J Biochem 70:97–106
Hammes WP, Winter J, Kandler O (1979) The sensitivity of the pseudomurein containing genus *Methanobacterium* to inhibitors of murein synthesis. Arch Microbiol 123:275–279
Hancock REW, Nikaido H (1978) Outer membranes of gram-negative bacteria. XIX. Isolation from *Pseudomonas aeruginosa* PAO1 and use in reconstitution and definition of the permeability barrier. J Bacteriol 136:381–390
Hartman BJ, Tomasz A (1980) Altered penicillin-binding proteins in methicillin-resistant strains of *Staphylococcus aureus*. Antimicrob Agents Chemother 19:726–735
Hinks RP, Daneo-Moore L, Shockman GD (1978) Cellular autolytic activity in synchronized populations of *Streptococcus faecium*. J Bacteriol 133:822–829
Hirota et al., quoted in Waxman DJ, Strominger JL (1981) In: Morin RB, Gorman M (eds) Beta lactam antibiotics – chemistry and biology. Academic, New York

Hobby GL, Meyer K, Chaffee M (1942) Observation on the mechanism of penicillin. Proc Soc Exp Biol Med 50:281–285

Höltje J-V, Tomasz A (1975a) Lipoteichoic acid, a specific inhibitor of autolysin activity in pneumococcus. Proc Natl Acad Sci USA 72:1690–1694

Höltje J-V, Tomasz A (1975b) Biological effects of lipoteichoic acids. J Bacteriol 124:1023–1027

Hoover JRE, Dunn GL (1979) The β-lactam antibiotics. In: Wolff ME (ed) Burger's medicinal chemistry, 4th edn, pt 3. Wiley, New York, pp 83–172

Horne D, Tomasz A (1977) Tolerant response of *Streptococcus sanguis* to β-lactams and other cell wall inhibitors. Antimicrob Agents Chemother 11:888–896

Horne D, Tomasz A (1979) Release of lipoteichoid acid from *Streptococcus sanguis:* stimulation of release during penicillin treatment. J Bacteriol 137:1180–1184

Horne D, Tomasz A (1980) Lethal effect of a heterologous murein hydrolase on penicillin-treated *Streptococcus sanguis*. Antimicrob Agents Chemother 17:235–246

Horne D, Tomasz A (1981a) Hypersusceptibility of penicillin-treated group B streptococci to bactericidal activity of human polymorphonuclear leukocytes. Antimicrob Agents Chemother 19:745–753

Horne D, Tomasz A (1981b) pH-dependent penicillin tolerance of group B streptococci. Antimicrob Agents Chemother 20:128–135

Horne D, Hakenbeck R, Tomasz A (1977) Secretion of lipids induced by inhibition of peptidoglycan synthesis in streptococci. J Bacteriol 132:704–717

Imada A, Kitano K, Kintaka K, Muroi M, Asai M (1981) Sulfazecin and isosulfazecin, novel β-lactam antibiotics of bacterial origin. Nature 289–590–591

Inouye H (1971) Pleiotropic effect of the *recA* gene of *Escherichia coli;* uncoupling of cell division from deoxyribonucleic acid replication. J Bacteriol 106:539–542

Ishiguro EE, Ramey WD (1976) Stringent control of peptidoglycan biosynthesis in *Escherichia coli* K-12. J Bacteriol 127:1119–1126

Ishino F, Mitsui K, Tamaki S, Matsuhashi M (1980) Dual enzyme activities of cell wall peptidoglycan synthesis, peptidoglycan transglycosylase, and penicillin-sensitive transpeptidase in purified preparations of *Escherichia coli* penicillin-binding protein 1A. Biochem Biophys Res Commun 97:287–293

Izaki K, Matsuhashi M, Strominger JL (1966) Glycopeptide transpeptidase and D-alanine carboxypeptidase: penicillin-sensitive enzymatic reactions. Proc Natl Acad Sci 55:656–663

Izaki K, Matsuhashi M, Strominger JL (1968) Biosynthesis of the peptidoglycan transpeptidase and D-alanine carboxypeptidase; penicillin-sensitive enzymatic reaction in strains of *Escherichia coli.* J Biol Chem 243:3180–3192

Jiang R, Tomasz A (1981) Abstract 505: genetic transformation of defective autolysis and penicillin tolerance in *S. pneumoniae*. 21st Intersci conf antimicrob agents and chemotherapy, American Society for Microbiology

Joseph R, Shockman GD (1975) Synthesis and excretion of glycerol teichoic acid during growth of two streptococcal species. Infect Immun 12:333–338

Kandler O, Schleifer KH, Dandl R (1968) Differentiation of *Streptococcus faecalis* Andrewes and Horder and *Streptococcus faecium* Orla-Jensen based on the amino acid composition of their murein. J Bacteriol 96:1935–1939

Kim KS, Yoshimori RN, Imagawa DT, Anthony BF (1979) Importance of medium in demonstrating penicillin tolerance in group B streptococci. Antimicrobiol Agents Chemother 16:214–216

Kitano K, Tomasz A (1979a) *Escherichia coli* mutants tolerant to β-lactam antibiotics. J Bacteriol 140:955–963

Kitano K, Tomasz A (1979b) Triggering of autolytic cell wall degradation in *Escherichia coli* by β-lactam antibiotics. Antimicrob Agents Chemother 16:838–848

Kitano K, Williamson R, Tomasz A (1980) Murein hydrolase defect in the β-lactam tolerant mutants of *Escherichia coli.* FEMS Microbiol Lett 7:133–136

Knox J, DeLucia M, Murthy N, Kelly J, Moews P, Frere J-M, Ghuysen J-M (1979) Crystallographic data for a penicillin receptor: exocellular D,D-carboxypeptidase-transpeptidase from *Streptomyces* R61. J Mol Biol 127:217–224

Koike M, Iida K, Matsuo IK (1969) Electron microscopic studies on the mode of action of polymyxin. J Bacteriol 97:448–452
Konig H, Kandler O (1978) The amino acid sequence of the peptide moiety of the pseudomurein from *Methanobacterium thermoautotrophicum*. Arch Microbiol 121:271–275
Kozarich JW, Strominger JL (1978) A membrane enzyme from *Staphylococcus aureus* which catalyzes transpeptidase, carboxypeptidase, and penicillinase activities. J Biol Chem 253:1272–1278
Kunugita K, Tamaki S, Matsuhashi M (1981) Nocardicin A, general aspects and mechanism of action. In: Salton M, Shockman GD (eds) β-Lactam antibiotics. Academic, New York, pp 185–197
Lawrence PJ, Strominger JL (1970) Biosynthesis of the peptidoglycan of bacterial cell walls. J Biol Chem 245:3653–3659
Lederberg J (1956) Bacterial protoplasts induced by penicillin. Proc Natl Acad Sci USA 42:574–577
Lederberg J (1957) Mechanism of action of penicillin. J Bacteriol 73:144
Lederberg J, St Clair J (1958) Protoplasts and L-type growth of *Escherichia coli*. J Bacteriol 75:143–160
Lederberg J, Zinder N (1948) Concentration of biochemical mutants of bacteria with penicillin. J Am Chem Soc 70:4267–4268
Lepper MH, Dowlinger HF (1951) Treatment of pneumococcal meningitis with penicillin compared with penicillin plus aureomycin. Arch Intern Med 88:489–494
Linnett PE, Strominger JL (1974a) Amidation and cross-linking of the enzymatically synthesized peptidoglycan of *Bacillus stearothermophilus*. J Biol Chem 249:2489–2496
Linnett PE, Strominger JL (1974b) Biosynthesis and cross-linking of the γ-glutamyl glycine containing peptidoglycan of vegetative cells of *Sporosarcina ureae*. J Biol Chem 249:2497–2506
Liu H, Zighelboim S, Tomasz A (1981) Abstr 506: penicillin tolerance in multiply drug-resistant natural isolates of *Streptococcus pneumoniae*. 21st Intersci conf antimicrob agents and chemotherapy, American Society for Microbiol
Lopez R, Ronda-Lain C, Tapia A, Waks SB, Tomasz A (1976) Suppression of the lytic and bactericidal effects of cell-wall inhibitory antibiotics. Antimicrob Agents Chemother 10:697–706
Lorian V, Atkinson B (1976) Effects of subinhibitory concentrations of antibiotics on cross walls of cocci. Antimicrob Agents Chemother 9:1043–1055
Lorian V, Atkinson B (1978) Effect of serum on gram-positive cocci grown in the presence of penicillin. J Infect Dis 138:865–871
Lorian V, Atkinson B, Amaral L (1979) Effects of subminimum inhibitory concentrations of antibiotics on *Pseudomonas aeruginosa:* the MIC/MAC ratio. In: Sabath LD (ed) Pseudomonas aeruginosa, Huber, Berne, pp 193–205
Lund F, Tybring L (1972) 6-Amidinopenicillanic acids – a new group of antibiotics. Nature 236:135–137
Luria S (1970) Phage, colicins, and macroregulatory phenomena. Science 168:1166–1170
Martin HH (1964) Composition of the mucopolymer in cell walls of the unstable and stable L-forms of *Proteus mirabilis*. J Gen Microbiol 36:641–650
Martin HH, Gmeiner J (1979) Modification of peptidoglycan structure by penicillin action in cell walls of *Proteus mirabilis*. Eur J Biochem 95:487–495
Matsuhashi M, Kamiryo T, Blumberg PM, Linett P, Willoughby E, Strominger JL (1974) Mechanism of action and development of resistance to a new amidinopenicillin. J Bacteriol 117:578–587
Matsuhashi M, Takagaki Y, Maruyama IN, Tamaki S, Nishimura Y, Suzuki H, Ogino U, Hirota Y (1977) Mutants of *Escherichia coli* lacking in highly penicillin-sensitive D-alanine carboxypeptidase activity. Proc Natl Acad Sci USA 74:2976–2979
Matsuhashi M, Maruyama IN, Takgaki Y, Tamaki S, Nishimura Y, Hirota Y (1978) Isolation of a mutant of *Escherichia coli* lacking penicillinase-sensitive D-alanine carboxypeptidase 1A. Proc Natl Acad Sci USA 75:2631–2635
Matsuhashi M, Tamaki S, Curtis SJ, Strominger JL (1979) Mutational evidence for identity of penicillin-binding protein 5 in *Escherichia coli* with the major D-alanine carboxypeptidase 1A activity. J Bacteriol 137:644–647

Mayhall CG, Medoff G, Marr JJ (1976) Variation in the susceptibility of strains of *Staphylococcus aureus* to oxacillin, cephalothin, and gentamicin. Antimicrob Agents Chemother 10:707–712

Melchior NH, Blom J, Tybring L, Birch-Anderson A (1973) Light and electron microscopy of the early response of *Escherichia coli* to a 6β-amidinopenicillamic acid (FL 1060). Acta Pathologica Microbiol Scand Sect B 81:393–407

Mirelman D (1981) Assembly of wall peptidoglycan polymers. In: Salton M, Shockman GD (eds) β-Lactam antibiotics. Academic, New York, pp 67–86

Mirelman D, Bracha R (1974) Effect of penicillin on the in vivo formation of the D-alanyl-L-alanine peptide cross-linkage in cell walls of *Micrococcus luteus*. Antimicrob Agents Chemother 5:663–666

Mirelman D, Nuchamovitz Y (1979) Biosynthesis of peptidoglycan in *Pseudomonas aeruginosa:* mode of action of β-lactam antibiotics. Eur J Biochem 94:541–549

Mirelman D, Bracha R, Sharon N (1972) Role of the penicillin-sensitive transpeptidation reaction in attachment of newly synthesized peptidoglycan to cell walls of *Micrococcus luteus*. Proc Natl Acad Sci USA 69:3355–3359

Mirelman D, Yashouv-Gan Y, Schwarz U (1976) Peptidoglycan biosynthesis in a thermosensitive division mutant of *Escherichia coli.* Biochem 15:1781–1790

Mirelman D, Yashouv-Gen Y, Schwarz U (1977) Regulation of murein biosynthesis and septum formation in filamentous cells of *Escherichia coli* PAT 84. J Bacteriol 129:1593–1600

Muller-Eberhard HJ (1975) Complement. Ann Rev Biochem 44:697–724

Mychajlonka M, McDowell TD, Shockman GD (1980) Inhibition of peptidoglycan, ribonucleic acid, and protein synthesis in tolerant strains of *Streptococcus mutans*. Antimicrob Agents Chemother 17:572–582

Nakae T (1976) Outer membrane of *Salmonella:* Isolation of protein complex that produces transmembrane channels. J Biol Chem 251:2176–2178

Nakae T, Nikaido H (1975) Outer membrane as a diffusion barrier in *Salmonella typhimurium.* J Biol Chem 250:7359–7365

Nakagawa J, Matsuhashi M (1980) Fragmentation of penicillin binding protein 1 Bs of Escherichia coli by proteolytic enzymes: A preliminary study on the location of the penicillin-binding site on the bifunctional peptidoglycan synthetase enzyme. Agric Biol Chem 44:3041–3044

Nayler JHC (1973) Advances in penicillin research. In: Harper NJ, Simmonds AB (eds) Advances in drug research, vol 7. Academic, New York, pp 1–105

Neuhaus E, Lowy F, Chang D, Horne D, Tomasz A, Steigbigel N (1980) Penicillin (P) tolerant (T) *S. viridans:* effect of P on host bacterial interaction. Abstr 20th Intersci Conf Antimicrob Agents Chemother, American Society for Microbiology

Nierlich D (1978) Regulation of bacterial growth, RNA, and protein synthesis. Ann Rev Microbiol 32:393–407

Nikaido H (1976) Outer membrane of *Salmonella typhimurium:* transmembrane diffusion of some hydrophobic substances. Biochem Biophys Acta 433:118–132

Nikaido H (1979) Permeability of the outer membrane of bacteria. Angew Chem Int Ed Engl 18:337–350

Nikaido H (1981) Outer membrane permeability of bacteria: resistance and accessibility of targets. In: Salton M, Shockman GD (eds) β-Lactam antibiotics. Academic, New York, pp 249–260

Nikaido H, Nakae T (1979) The outer membrane of gram-negative bacteria. Adv Microb Physiol 20:163–250

Nishimura Y, Takeda Y, Nishimura A, Suzuki H, Inouye M, Hirota Y (1977) Synthetic Col-El plasmids carrying genes for cell division in *Escherichia coli.* Plasmid 1:67–77

Nishino T, Kozarich JW, Strominger JL (1977) Kinetic evidence for an acyl-enzyme intermediate in D-alanine carboxypeptidases of *Bacillus subtilis* and *Bacillus stearothermophilus*. J Biol Chem 252:2934–2939

Nixdorff K, Fitzer H, Gmeiner J, Martin HH (1977) Reconstitution of model membranes from phospholipid and outer membrane proteins of *Proteus mirabilis;* role of proteins in the formation of hydrophilic pores and protection of membranes against detergents. Eur J Biochem 81:63–69

Noguchi H, Matsuhashi M, Matsuhashi S (1979) Comparative studies of penicillin-binding proteins in *Pseudomonas aeruginosa* and *Escherichia coli*. Eur J Biochem 100:41–49

Nozaki Y, Imada A, Yoneda M (1979) SCE-963, a new potent cephalosporin with high affinity for penicillin-binding proteins 1 and 3 of *Escherichia coli*. Antimicrob Agents Chemother 15:20–27

Ofek I, Beachey EH, Eisenstein BI, Alkan ML, Sharon N (1979) Suppression of bacterial adherence by subminimal inhibitory concentrations of β-lactam and aminoglycoside antibiotics. Rev Inf Dis 1:832–837

Ofek I, Beachey EH, Jefferson W, Campbell GL (1975) Cell membrane-binding properties of group A streptococcal lipoteichoic acid. J Exp Med 141:990–1003

Ohya S, Yamazaki M, Sugawara S, Tamaki S, Matsuhashi M (1978) New cephamycin antibiotic, CS-1170: binding affinity to penicillin-binding proteins and inhibition of peptidoglycan cross-linking reactions in *Escherichia coli*. Antimicrob Agents Chemother 14:780–785

Onoe T, Umemoto T, Sagawa H, Suginaka H (1981) Filament formation of *Fusobacterium nucleatum* cells induced by mecillinam. Antimicrob Agents Chemother 19:487–489

Park JT (1952) Uridine-5′-pyrophosphate derivatives. J Biol Chem 194:897–904

Park JT, Johnson MJ (1949) Accumulation of labile phosphate in *Staphylococcus aureus* grown in the presence of penicillin. J Biol Chem 179:585–592

Park JT, Strominger JL (1957) Mode of action of penicillin: biochemical basis for the mechanism of action of penicillin and for its selective toxicity. Science 125:99–101

Pasculle AW, Dowling JN, Weyand RS, Sniffen JM, Cordes LG, Gorman GM, Feeley JC (1981) Susceptibility of Pittsburgh pneumonia agent *(Legionella micdadei)* and other newly recognized members of the genus *Legionella* to nineteen antimicrobial agents. Antimicrob Agents Chemother 20:793–799

Pellon G, Bondet C, Michel G (1976) Peptidoglycans synthesized by a membrane preparation of *Micrococcus luteus*. J Bacteriol 125:509–517

Prestidge LS, Pardee AB (1957) Induction of bacterial lysis by penicillin. J Bacteriol 74:48–59

Prior RB, Warner JF (1974) Morphological alteration of *Pseudomonas aeruginosa* by ticarcillin: a scanning electron microscope study. Antimicrob Agents Chemother 6:853–855

Rasmussen JR, Strominger JL (1978) Utilization of a depsipeptide substrate for trapping acyl-enzyme intermediates of penicillin-sensitive D-alanine carboxypeptidases. Proc Natl Acad Sci USA 75:84–88

Reynolds P, Chase H (1981) β-Lactam-binding proteins: identification as lethal targets and probes of β-lactam accessibility. In: Salton MRJ, Shockman GD (eds) β-Lactam antibiotics. Academic, New York, pp 153–168

Reynolds PE, Shepherd ST, Chase HA (1978) Identification of the binding protein which may be the target of penicillin action in *Bacillus megaterium*. Nature 271:568–570

Richmond M (1981) β-Lactamases and bacterial resistance to β-lactam antibiotics. In: Salton MRJ, Shockman GD (eds) β-Lactam antibiotics. Academic press, New York, pp 261–273

Rolinson GN, Macdonald AC, Wilson DA (1977) Bactericidal action of β-lactam antibiotics on *E. coli* with particular reference to ampicillin and amoxycillin. J Antimicrob Chemother 3:541–553

Rogers HJ (1965) The outer layers of bacteria: the biosynthesis of structure, 15th Symposium Soc Gen Microbiol, pp 186–219

Rogers HJ (1981) Some unsolved problems concerned with the assembly of the walls of gram-positive organisms. In: Salton MRJ, Shockman GD (eds) β-Lactam antibiotics. Academic, New York, pp 87–100

Root RK, Isturiz R, Molavi A, Metcalf JA, Malech HL (1981) Interactions between antibiotics and human neutrophils in the killing of staphylococci: studies with normal and cytochalasin B-treated cells. J Clin Invest 67:247–259

Rosegay A (1981) High specific activity (Phenyl-^{3}H) benzylpenicillin *N*-ethylpiperidine salt. J Labelled Compounds and Radiopharm 18:1337–1340

Rosenthal RS, Jungkind D, Daneo-Moore L, Shockman GD (1975) Evidence for the synthesis of soluble peptidoglycan fragments by protoplasts of *Streptococcus faecalis*. J Bacteriol 124:398–409

Sabath LD, Wheeler N, Laverdiere M, Blazeric C, Wilkinson B (1977) A new type of penicillin resistance of *Staphylococcus aureus*. Lancet 1:443–447
Salton MRJ (1964) The bacterial cell wall. Elsevier, Amsterdam
Savitch CB, Barry AL, Hoeprich PD (1978) Infective endocarditis caused by *Streptococcus bovis* resistant to the lethal effect of penicillin. Arch Intern Med 138:931–934
Schleifer KH, Kandler O (1972) Peptidoglycan types of bacterial cell walls and their taxonomic implications. Bact Rev 36:407–477
Schrader WP, Fan DP (1974) Synthesis of cross-linked peptidoglycan attached to previously formed cell wall by toluene-treated cells of *Bacillus megaterium*. J Biol Chem 249:4815–4818
Schmidt LS, Botta G, Park JT (1981) Effects of furazlocillin, a β-lactam antibiotic which binds selectively to penicillin-binding protein 3 on *Escherichia coli* mutants deficient in other penicillin-binding proteins. J Bacteriol 145:632–637
Schwarz U, Ashus A, Frank H (1969) Autolytic enzymes and cell division of *Escherichia coli*. J Mol Biol 41:419–429
Schwarz U, Seeger K, Wengenmayer F, Strecker H (1981) Penicillin-binding proteins of *Escherichia coli* identified with a ^{125}I-derivative of ampicillin. FEMS Microbiol Lett 10:107–108
Schwarz U, Weidel W (1965) Zum Wirkungsmechanismus von Penicillin. A Naturforsch 206:147–157
Sharpe A, Blumberg PM, Strominger JL (1974) D-Alanine carboxypeptidase and cell wall cross-linking in *Bacillus subtilis*. J Bacteriol 117:926–927
Shockman GD, Lampen JO (1962) Inhibition by antibiotics of the growth of bacterial and yeast protoplasts. J Bacteriol 84:508–512
Shockman GD, Kolb JJ, Toennies G (1958) Relations between bacterial cell wall synthesis, growth phase, and autolysis. J Biol Chem 230:961–977
Shockman GD, Daneo-Moore L, Higgins ML (1974) Problems of cell wall and membrane growth, enlargement, and division. Ann NY Acad Sci 235:161–197
Shockman GD, Daneo-Moore L, McDowell TD, Wong W (1981) Function and structure of the cell wall – its importance in the life and death of bacteria. In: Salton MRJ, Shockman GD (eds) β-Lactam antibiotics. Academic press, New York, pp 31–65
Shungu DL, Cornett JB, Shockman GD (1979) Morphological and physiological study of autolytic-defective *Streptococcus faecium* strains. J Bacteriol 138:598–608
Sinha RK, Rosenthal RS (1981) Effect of penicillin G on release of peptidoglycan fragments by *Neisseria gonorrhoeae:* characterization of extracellular products. Antimicrob Agents Chemother 20:98–103
Smith J, Hamilton-Miller JMT, Knox R (1969) Bacterial resistance to penicillins and cephalosporins. J Pharm Pharmac 21:337–358
Spratt BG (1975) Distinct penicillin-binding proteins involved in the division, elongation, and shape of *Escherichia coli* K12. Proc Natl Acad Sci USA 72:2999–3003
Spratt BG (1977a) Temperature-sensitive cell division mutants of *Escherichia coli* with thermolabile penicillin-binding proteins. J Bacteriol 131:293–305
Spratt BG (1977b) Properties of the penicillin-binding proteins of *Escherichia coli* K-12. Eur J Biochem 72:341–352
Spratt BG (1977c) The mechanism of action of mecillinam. J Antimicrob Chemother 3 (Suppl B):13–19
Spratt BG (1979) In: Mitsuhashi S (ed) Microbial drug resistance, vol 2, pp 349–360. Japan Scientific Societies Press, Tokyo
Spratt BG (1980) Biochemical and genetical approaches to the mechanism of action of penicillin. Philos Trans R Soc Lond B 289:273–283
Spratt BG, Strominger JL (1971) Identification of the major penicillin-binding proteins of *Escherichia coli* as D-alanine carboxypeptidase 1A. J Bacteriol 127:660–663
Spratt B, Strominger J (1976) Identification of the major penicillin-binding proteins of *Escherichia coli* as D-alanine carboxypeptidase 1A. J Bacteriol 127:660–663
Spratt BG, Jobanputra V, Zimmerman W (1977) Binding of thienamycin and clavulanic acid to the penicillin-binding proteins of *Escherichia coli* K-12. Antimicrob Agents Chemother 12:406–409

Steber J, Schleifer KH (1975) *Halococcus morrhuae:* a sulfated heteropolysaccharide as the structural component of the bacterial cell wall. Arch Microbiol 105:173–177

Storch GA, Krogstad DJ (1981) Abstr 503: Autolysin and cell wall as determinants of the entercoccal response to penicillin. 21 st Intersci conf antimicrob agents and chemotherapy, American Society of Microbiology

Storm DR, Blumberg PM, Strominger JL (1974) Inhibition of the *Bacillus subtilis* membrane-bound D-alanine carboxypeptidase by 6-aminopenicillinic acid covalently coupled to sepharose. J Bacteriol 117:783–785

Strominger JL (1970) Penicillin-sensitive enzymatic reactions in bacterial cell wall synthesis. Harvey Lect 64:171–213

Strominger JL, Willoughby E, Kamiryo T, Blumberg PM, Yocum RR (1974) Penicillin-sensitive enzymes and penicillin-binding components in bacterial cells. Ann NY Acad Sci 235:210–224

Suzuki H, Nishimura Y, Hirota Y (1978) On the process of cellular division in *Escherichia coli;* a series of mutants of *E. coli* altered in the penicillin-binding proteins. Proc Natl Acad Sci 75:664–668

Suzuki H, Van Heijenoort J, Tamura T, Mizoguchi J, Hirota Y, Van Heijenoort J (1981) In vitro peptidoglycan polymerization catalysed by penicillin binding protein 1b of *Escherichia coli* K-12. FEBS Let 110:245–249

Sykes RB, Bonner DP, Bush K, Georgopapadakou NH (1981a) Azthreonam (SQ 26,776), a synthetic monobactam specifically active against aerobic gram-negative bacteria. Antimicrob Agents Chemother 21:85–92

Sykes RB, Cimarusti CM, Bonner DP, Bush K, Floyd DM, Georgopapadakou NH, Koster WH, Liu WC, Parker WL, Principe PA, Rathnum ML, Slusarchyk WA, Trejo WH, Wells JS (1981b) Monocyclic β-lactam antibiotics produced by bacteria. Nature 291:489–491

Taku A, Fan DP (1976) Identification of an isolated protein essential for peptidoglycan synthesis as the *N*-acetylglucosaminyltransferase. J Biol Chem 251:6154–6156

Tamaki S, Nakajawa J, Maruyama IN, Matsuhashi M (1978) Supersensitivity to β-lactam antibiotics in Escherichia coli caused by a D-alanine carboxypeptidase IA mutation. Agric Biol Chem 42:2147–2150

Tamura T, Imae Y, Strominger JL (1976) Purification to homogeneity and properties of two D-alanine carboxypeptidases 1 from *Escherichia coli.* J Biol Chem 251:414–423

Tamura T, Suzuki M, Nishimura Y, Mizoguchi J, Hirota Y (1980) On the process of cellular division in *Escherichia coli:* isolation and characterization of penicillin binding proteins 1a, 1b, and 3. Proc Natl Acad Sci USA 77:4499–4503

Taylor PW, Gaunt H, Unger F (1981) Effect of subinhibitory concentration of mecillinam on the serum susceptibility of *Escherichia coli* strains. Antimicrob Agents Chemother 19:786–788

Thorpe SJ, Perkins HR (1979) Deoxycholate enhancement of an intermediate of peptidoglycan synthesis in *Micrococcus luteus.* FEBS Lett 105:151–154

Tipper JD, Berman MF (1969) Structures of the cell wall peptidoglycans of *Staphylococcus epidermidis* Texas 26 and *Staphylococcus aureus* Copenhagen. I. chain length and average sequence of crossbridge peptides. Biochem 8:2183–2192

Tipper DJ, Strominger JL (1965) Mechanism of action of penicillins: a proposal based on their structural similarity to acyl-D-alanyl-D-alanine. Proc Natl Acad Sci USA 54:1133–1141

Tipper D, Strominger JL (1968) Biosynthesis of the peptidoglycan of bacterial cell walls. XII. Inhibition of cross-linking by penicillins and cephalosporins: studies in *Staphylococcus aureus* in vivo. J Biol Chem 243:3169–3179

Tipper DJ, Wright A (1979) The structure and biosynthesis of bacterial cell walls. In: Gonsalus LC (ed) The bacteria, vol 7. Academic, New York, pp 291–426

Tomasz A (1968) Biological consequences of the replacement of choline by ethanolamine in the cell wall of pneumococcus: chain formation, loss of transformability and loss of autolysis. Proc Natl Acad Sci USA 59:86–93

Tomasz A (1974) The role of autolysins in cell death. Ann NY Acad Sci 235:439–448

Tomasz A (1979a) The mechanism of the irreversible antimicrobial effects of penicillins: how the β-lactam antibiotics kill and lyse bacteria. Ann Rev Microbiol 33:113–137

Tomasz A (1979b) From penicillin-binding proteins to the lysis and death of bacteria: a 1979 view. Rev Infect Dis 1:434–467

Tomasz A (1981) Penicillin tolerance and the control of murein hydrolases. In: Salton MRJ, Shockman GD (eds) β-Lactam antibiotics. Academic, New York, pp 227–247

Tomasz A, Höltje J-V (1977) Murein hydrolases and the lytic and killing action of penicillin. In: Schlessinger JD (ed) Microbiology 1977. American Society Microbiology, Washington, pp 209–215

Tomasz A, Waks S (1975a) Enzyme replacement in a bacterium: phenotypic correction by the experimental introduction of the wild-type enzyme into a live enzyme-defective mutant pneumococcus. Biochem Biophys Res Commun 65:1311–1319

Tomasz A, Waks S (1975b) Mechanism of action of penicillin; triggering of the pneumococcal autolytic enzyme by inhibitors of cell wall synthesis. Proc Natl Acad Sci USA 72:4162–4166

Tomasz A, Albino A, Zanati E (1970) Multiple antibiotic resistance in a bacterium with suppressed autolytic system. Nature 227:138–140

Tomasz A, Kitano K, Lopez R, DeFreitas C (1979) Variations in the mechanism of antibacterial effects of β-lactams. In: Kalman T (ed) Drug action and design: mechanism-based enzyme inhibitors. Elsevier North Holland, Amsterdam, pp 197–221

Traub WH, Sherris JC (1970) Studies on the interaction between serum bactericidal activity and antibiotics in vitro. Chemother 15:70

Tynecka A, Ward JB (1975) Peptidoglycan synthesis in *Bacillus licheniformis:* the inhibition of cross-linking by benzylpenicillin and cephaloridine in vivo accompanied by the formation of soluble peptidoglycan. Biochem J 146:253–267

Umbreit JN, Strominger JL (1973) D-Alanine carboxypeptidase from *Bacillus subtilis* membranes. II. Interaction with penicillins and cephalosporins. J Biol Chem 248:6767–6771

Van Heijenoort Y, Derrien M, Van Heijenoort J (1978) Polymerization by transglycosylation in the biosynthesis of the peptidoglycan of *Escherichia coli* K12 and its inhibition by antibiotics. FEBS Lett 89:141–144

Veale DR, Finch H, Smith H, Wilt K (1976) Penetration of penicillin into human phagocytes containing *Neisseria gonorrhoeae:* intracellular survival and growth at optimum concentrations of antibiotic. J Gen Microbiol 95:353–363

Vosbeck K, Handschin H, Menge E-B, Zak O (1979) Effects of subminimal inhibitory concentrations of antibiotics on adhesiveness of *Escherichia coli* in vitro. Rev Infect Dis 1:845–851

Waks S, Tomasz A (1978) Secretion of cell wall polymers into the growth medium of lysis-defect pneumococci during treatment with penicillin and other inhibitors of cell wall synthesis. Antimicrob Agents Chemother 13:293–301

Ward JB (1974) The synthesis of peptidoglycan in an autolysin-deficient mutant of *Bacillus licheniformis* NCTC 6346 and the effect of β-lactam antibiotics, bacitracin, and vancomycin. Biochem J 141:227–241

Ward JB, Perkins HP (1974) Peptidoglycan biosynthesis by preparations from *Bacillus licheniformis:* cross-linking of newly synthesized chains to preformed cell wall. Biochem J 139:781–784

Waxman DJ, Strominger JL (1978) Abstract: active water-soluble fragments of bacterial D-alanine carboxypeptidases. Fed Proc 37:1393

Waxman DJ, Strominger JL (1979a) Cleavage of a *COOH*-terminal hydrophobic region from D-alanine carboxypeptidase, a penicillin-sensitive bacterial membrane enzyme. J Biol Chem 254:4863–4875

Waxman DJ, Strominger JL (1979b) Abstr 54, Cold spring harbor conf on memb biogenesis. Structure of the *COOH*-terminal hydrophobic region of a penicillin-sensitive bacterial D-alanine carboxypeptidase

Waxman DJ, Strominger JL (1980) Sequence of active site peptides from the penicillin-sensitive D-alanine carboxypeptidase of *Bacillus subtilis:* mechanism of penicillin action and sequence homology to β-lactamases. J Biol Chem 255:3964–3976

Weidel W, Pelzer H (1964) Bag-shaped macromolecules – a new outlook on bacterial cell walls. Adv Enzymol 26:193–232

Weston A, Ward JB, Perkins HR (1977) Biosynthesis of peptidoglycan in wall plus membrane preparations from *Micrococcus luteus:* direction of chain extension, length of chains, and effect of penicillin on cross-linking. J Gen Microbiol 99:171–181

White JS, Astill M, Lawrence PJ (1979) Effect of cephapirin on formation of D-alanine carboxypeptidase on growing *Bacillus subtilis* cells. Antimicrob Agents Chemother 13:204–208

Wickus GG, Strominger JL (1972a) Penicillin-sensitive transpeptidation during peptidoglycan biosynthesis in cell-free preparations from *Bacillus megatherium:* I. Incorporation of free diaminopimelic acid into peptidoglycan. J Biol Chem 247:5297–5306

Wickus GG, Strominger JL (1972b) Penicillin-sensitive transpeptidation during peptidoglycan biosynthesis in cell-free preparations from *Bacillus megatherium:* II. Effect of penicillins and cephalosporins on bacterial growth and in vitro transpeptidation. J Biol Chem 247:5307–5311

Williams JD (1981) The needs for new antibiotics for infection in man. In: Ninet L, Bost PE, Bouanchaud DH, Florent J (eds) The future of antibiotherapy and antibiotic research. Academic Press, pp 117–126

Williamson R, Tomasz A (1980) Antibiotic-tolerant mutants of *Streptococcus pneumoniae* that are not deficient in autolytic activity. J Bacteriol 144:105–113

Williamson R, Tomasz A (1982) Interactions of ^{3}H-benzylpenicillin with growing pneumococci, abstr A-11. Annual Meeting American Society of Microbiology 1982

Williamson R, Ward BJ (1981) Deficiency of autolytic activity in *Bacillus subtilis* and *Streptococcus pneumoniae* is associated with decreased permeability of the wall. J Gen Microbiol 125:325–334

Williamson R, Calderwood S, Tomasz A, Moellering RC Jr (1980a) Studies on the intrinsic resistance to β-lactams in group D streptococci, abstr 20th intersc conf antimicrob agents Chemotherap, American Society of Microbiology

Williamson R, Hakenbeck R, Tomasz A (1980b) In vivo interaction of β-lactam antibiotics with the penicillin-binding proteins of *Streptococcus pneumoniae.* Antimicrob Agents Chemother 18:629–637

Williamson R, Hakenbeck R, Tomasz A (1980c) The penicillin-binding proteins of *Streptococcus pneumoniae* grown under lysis-permissive and lysis-protective (tolerant) conditions. FEMS Microbiol Lett 7:127–131

Williamson R, Zighelboim S, Tomasz A (1981) Penicillin-binding proteins of penicillin-resistant and penicillin-tolerant *Streptococcus pneumoniae.* In: Salton MRJ, Shockman GD (eds) β-Lactam antibiotics. Academic, New York, pp 215–225

Winkelstein JR, Tomasz A (1978) Activation of the alternate complement pathway by pneumococcal cell wall teichoic acid. J Immunol 120:174–178

Wise EM, Park JT (1965) Penicillin: its basic site of action as an inhibitor of a peptide cross-linking reaction in cell wall mucopeptide synthesis. Proc Natl Acad Sci USA 54:75–81

Woese CR, Magrum LJ, Fox GE (1978) Archaebacteria. J Mol Evol 11:245–252

Woodward RB (1980) Penems and related substances. Phil Trans R Soc Lond B 289:239–250

Wyke A, Ward BJ, Hayes MV, Curtis NAC (1981) A role in vivo for penicillin-binding protein 4 of *Staphylococcus aureus.* Eur J Biochem 119:389–393

Yamada Y, Goi H, Watanabe T, Tsurucka T, Miyauchi K, Yoshida T, Hoshiko S, Kazano Y, Inouye S, Niida T, Matsuhashi M (1981) Abstr 53: Studies on the bactericidal mechanism of a new cephamycin, MT-141. 21st Intersci Conf Antimicrob Agents and Chemother, American Society for Microbiology

Yocum RR, Waxman DJ, Rasmussen JR, Strominger JL (1979) Mechanism of penicillin action: penicillin and substrate bind covalently to the same active site serine in two bacterial D-alanine carboxypeptidases. Proc Natl Acad Sci USA 76:2730–2734

Yocum RR, Rasmussen JR, Strominger JL (1980a) The mechanism of action of penicillin: penicillin acylates the active site of *Bacillus stearothermophilus* D-alanine carboxypeptidase. J Biol Chem 255:3977–3986

Yocum RR, Waxman DJ, Strominger JL (1980b) The interaction of penicillin with its receptors in bacterial membranes. Trends Biochem Sci 5:97–101

Zak O, Kradolfer F (1979) Effects of subminimal inhibitory concentrations of antibiotics in experimental infections. Rev Infect Dis 1:862–879

Zighelboim S, Tomasz A (1979) Stepwise acquisition of resistance to oxacillin in Streptococcus. In: Schlessinger D (ed) Microbiology 1979. American Society of Microbiology, pp 290–292

Zighelboim S, Tomasz A (1980) Penicillin-binding proteins of multiply antibiotic-resistant South African strains of *Streptococcus pneumoniae*. Antimicrob Agents Chemother 17:434–442

Zimmermann W, Rosselet A (1977) Function of the outer membrane of *Escherichia coli* as a permeability barrier to β-lactam antibiotics. Antimicrob Agents Chemother 12:368–372

CHAPTER 3

Strain Improvement and Preservation of β-Lactam-Producing Microorganisms

R. P. ELANDER

A. Introduction

The initial discovery of FLEMING's contaminating *Penicillium* fungus and its remarkable antibacterial properties now date back more than 50 years. Although the Oxford group proposed in 1943 that penicillin contained a fused β-lactam ring, its structure was not generally accepted until it was confirmed by x-ray crystallographic studies of HODGKIN and LOW in 1945 (CROWFOOT et al. 1949; ABRAHAM 1978). The reactivity of the β-lactam ring is undoubtedly one of the major factors for its intrinsic antibacterial activity.

Exploitation of the second major class of β-lactam substances from fungi began with the discovery of the cephalosporin-producing organism, *Acremonium chrysogenum* by BROTZU in Sardinia some 30 years ago and the chemical isolation of cephalosporin C as a contaminant in a crude preparation of penicillin N by NEWTON and ABRAHAM (1955). Cephalosporin C was found to be resistant to acid and to enzymatic hydrolysis and was shown to be more active than the natural penicillins against gram-negative bacteria. These characteristics attracted the attention of clinicians because of the increasing incidence of bacterial resistance to penicillins (ABRAHAM 1979). A major impetus for the commercial exploitation of cephalosporin C was the discovery of a practical method for chemically splitting cephalosporin C to 7-aminocephalosporanic acid (7-ACA) by MORIN et al. (1962). This stimulated the development of the semisynthetic cephalosporins which was analogous historically to the rapid progress in chemotherapy induced by the discovery of 6-aminopenicillanic acid nucleus (6-APA) and its semisynthetic derivatives. Similarly, the rapid start in the development of superior semisynthetic cephalosporins over the last decade parallels the history of the semisynthetic penicillins over the past two decades.

During the past 10 years, a number of new β-lactam stuctures have been discovered in the filamentous bacteria *Streptomyces* and *Nocardia*, and in genera of gram-negative bacteria, including *Pseudomonas*, *Chromobacterium*, *Gluconobacteria*, *Acetobacter* and *Agrobacterium*. The β-lactamase-resistant cephamycins were reported in the United States by the Eli Lilly company (HIGGENS and KASTNER 1971; NAGARAJAN et al. 1971) and Merck and Company (STAPLEY et al. 1972), and in Japan (HASEGAWA et al. 1975; FUKASE et al. 1976).

The discovery of the monocyclic nocardicins in strains of *Nocardia* by scientists at the Fujisawa Pharmaceutical Co., Ltd. opened new avenues of biosynthesis and also total chemical synthesis of certain nocardicin antibiotics (AOKI et al. 1976; KAMIYA 1977).

A new chapter in the history of β-lactam antibiotics was opened with the discovery of the species of *Streptomyces* which produce novel β-lactam structures. These β-lactam molecules react with enzymes responsible for the degradation of penicillins and cephalosporins and have been termed β-lactamase inhibitors.

Clavulanic acid, isolated from strains of *Streptomyces clavuligerus*, has no substituent at C-6 of the β-lactam ring and is fused with an oxazolidine ring (BROWN et al. 1976). Also, a novel related antifungal β-lactam antibiotic has recently been reported by KRONE et al. (1981). The antibiotic is structurally related to clavulanic acid (hydroxyethylclavam) and is produced by *Streptomyces antibioticus* subsp. *antibioticus*. The olivanic acid compounds produced by *Streptomyces olivaceus* represent another interesting group of β-lactamase inhibitors (BROWN et al. 1977) and PS-5, another β-lactamase inhibitor, has recently been described in Japan (OKAMURA et al. 1978). One of the newer and more exciting β-lactams is thienamycin isolated from *Streptomyces cattleya*. It has a β-lactam ring with a side-chain that contains no nitrogen and is fused to a five-membered ring containing a double bond without sulfur or oxygen (KAHAN et al. 1979). The thienamycin complex of antibiotics represents one of the most potent natural antibacterial substances known to man.

The carpetimycins represent new carbapenem antibiotics produced by *Streptomyces* sp. KC-6043 reported by scientists from the Kowa Company, Ltd. (NAKAYAMA et al. 1980). They are related to the thienamycins, olivanic acid derivatives, and PS-5 antibiotics. Carpetimycins A and B have strong activity against both gram-positive and gram-negative bacteria and are also active against β-lactamase-producing strains.

Other new carbapenem antibiotics reported are C-1939 S_2 and H_2 (IMADA et al. 1980). They are produced by a new subspecies of *Streptomyces griseus*, subsp. *cryophilus*, isolated from Swedish soil at 4 °C. The activity was discovered by a sensitive and selective screen developed at Takeda Chemical Industries, Ltd. using a penicillin-supersensitive strain of *Pseudomonas aeruginosa* and activity against a battery of penicillinase and cephalosporinase enzymes.

The most recently discovered β-lactam antibiotics are produced by acidophilic pseudomonads. The antibiotics are monocyclic β-lactams containing a rare sulfamate group and a side-chain on C-3 of the azetidine ring composed of D-alanine and D-glutamic acid. A methoxy group is attached to C-3 which is probably responsible for the resistance of the molecule to β-lactamase degradation. Due to the unusual nature of the sulfonic acid residue attached to the nitrogen of the β-lactam ring, the antibiotics have been termed sulfazecins by the Takeda scientists (IMADA et al. 1981). A related molecule to sulfazecin has been very recently discovered by Squibb researchers. The antibiotics termed monobactams are produced by strains of gram-negative bacteria including species of the following genera: *Chromobacterium*, *Gluconobacter*, *Acetobacter*, and *Agrobacterium* (SYKES et al. 1981).

Total chemical synthesis of penicillin, cephalosporin and several of the newer carbapenem and monocyclic lactams have been reported but their yields are extremely poor and presently cannot compete with microbial biosynthesis (SHEEHAN and HENERY-LOGAN 1959; WOODWARD et al. 1966; KAMIYA 1977). Thus, all known β-lactam compounds are natural products of microbial or plant origin and their industrial production thus far depends on large-scale fermentation technology.

The increased pace of discovery of novel β-lactams during the last 10 years has been due largely to the development of new highly selective screens and to more sensitive methods of antibiotic screening. The improved methodology includes the use of highly sensitive test bacteria mutagenized to be supersensitive to a variety of the newer β-lactam antibiotics (AOKI et al. 1976; HOSODA et al. 1977; KITANO et al. 1975, 1977). Some of the hypersensitive mutants have been mutated for chromosomal β-lactamase deletions and have been reported to have genetic lesions leading to changes in their outer and inner membrane proteins (TAMAKI et al. 1978). Of the inner membrane proteins, the most likely to be involved in increased β-lactam antibiotic sensitivity are the penicillin-binding proteins (PBPs). There are at least nine inner-bound membrane proteins thus far reported to bind radioactive penicillin G (SPRATT 1977).

Another major factor contributing to the increased discovery of novel β-lactam antibiotics was the development and implementation of sophisticated β-lactamase enzyme inhibition screens. The strategy of the β-lactamase inhibition has been recently reviewed by COLE (1979). The β-lactamase inhibition screen was important in the discovery of the clavulanic acids, olivanic acids, and PS-5 and related metabolites. Other important factors contributing to increased β-lactam discovery were the rapid development of improved preparative and analytical high-pressure liquid chromatography equipment and improved high resolution nuclear magnetic resonance (NMR) and mass spectroscopic methodology.

This chapter will describe strain improvement, biology, and fermentation behavior of the important β-lactam-producing organisms. More comprehensive reviews are available including fermentation technology and screening methodology involved in the fermentation development and discovery of β-lactam substances (ELANDER and AOKI 1982; CASSIDY 1981). Other areas covered in this chapter include general methodologies and strategies used for strain improvement in the organisms producing nocardicin antibiotics. A brief review of essential strain maintenance and long-term preservation of microbial cultures is also included.

B. Distribution of β-Lactam Antibiotics and Related Metabolites in Nature

The occurrence of microbial and plant metabolites containing the β-lactam ring is widespread in nature. The β-lactam ring has been found in steroidal alkaloids of certain higher plants. A summary of the distribution of microorganisms known to elaborate β-lactam antibiotics is shown in Fig. 1.

Penicillin was originally discovered to be a byproduct of Fleming's now famous laboratory contaminant which was classified taxonomically as *Penicillium notatum* (FLEMING 1929). Later, penicillin was found to be produced by a variety of penicillia (SANDERS 1949) including strains of *Penicillium chrysogenum* (RAPER et al. 1944; Table 1). During the ensuing few years, a number of diverse fungi other than penicillia were reported to synthesize a variety of β-lactam metabolites (Table 2). These include eukaryotic species of *Aspergillus* (DULANEY 1947), *Malbranchea* (RODE et al. 1947), *Cephalosporium* (BURTON and ABRAHAM 1951; ROBERTS 1952), *Emericellopsis* (GROSKLAGS and SWIFT 1957; ELANDER et al. 1961), *Paecilomyces*

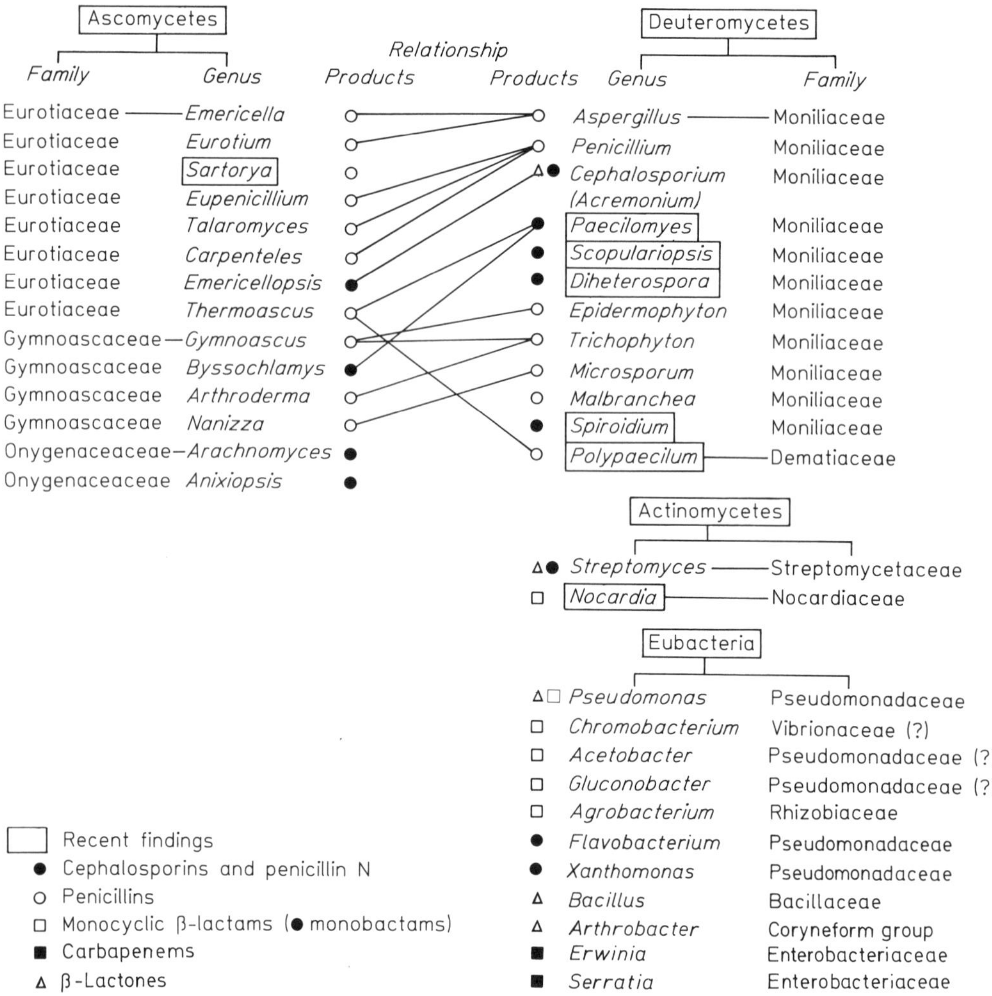

Fig. 1. Distribution of β-lactam-producing microorganisms

(Fleischman and Pisano 1961), *Epidermophyton* (Uri et al. 1963), *Trichophyton* (Uri et al. 1963; Elander et al. 1969), *Anixiopsis* (Kitano et al. 1975, 1977), *Diheterospora* (Higgens et al. 1974), *Scopulariopsis* (Higgens et al. 1974), and *Spiroidium* (Kitano et al. 1975, 1977). Prokaryotic microorganisms classified as *Streptomyces* (Miller et al. 1962; Nagarajan et al. 1971) and *Nocardia* (Aoki et al. 1976; Aoki and Okuhara 1980) also produce a variety of β-lactam molecules.

The discovery of monocyclic β-lactam cell-wall-active antibiotics from *Nocardia uniformis* was significant in that the activity was detected using a β-lactam supersensitive mutant of *Escherichia coli* (Aoki et al. 1976). The nocardicin complex is known to consist of seven different components with nocardicin A being the most active (Fig. 2).

Table 1. Penicillin antibiotics produced by *Penicillium chrysogenum*

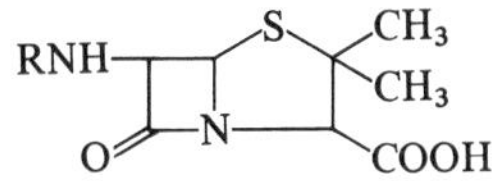

R-Side-chain	Common name	Reference
H	Penicin, Penicillin nucleus, 6-APA (6-Aminopenicillanic acid)	Kato (1953), Batchelor et al. (1959)
$HO_2C{-}CH(NH_2)(CH_2)_3{-}CO{-}$ (L-α-Aminoadipic acid)	Isopenicillin N	Flynn et al. (1962), Cole and Batchelor (1963)
$CH_3CH_2CH{=}CHCH_2CO{-}$ (β-γ-Hexanoic acid)	Penicillin F (2-Pentenylpenicillin)	Florey et al. (1949)
$CH_3(CH_2)_4{-}CO{-}$ (Caproic acid)	Penicillin dihydro F (Amylpenicillin)	Florey et al. (1949)
$CH_3(CH_2)_6{-}CO{-}$ (Octanoic acid)	Penicillin K (Heptylpenicillin)	Florey et al. (1949)
$C_6H_5{-}CH_2{-}CO$ (Phenylacetic acid)	Penicillin G (Benzylpenicillin)	Moyer and Coghill (1946)
$p{-}OH{-}C_6H_5{-}CH_2{-}CO{-}$ (*p*-Hydroxyphenylacetic acid)	Penicillin X	Raper and Fennel (1946)
$C_6H_5{-}O{-}CH_2{-}CO{-}$ (Phenoxyacetic acid)	Penicillin V (Phenoxymethylpenicillin)	Behrens (1949)

Two compounds containing a four-membered β-lactam ring have been reported in the ground-cover plant *Pachysandra terminalis* (Kikuchi and Uyeo 1967). These compounds do not possess antibacterial activity and are steroidal alkaloids. β-Lactam compounds have also been reported in the eubacteria. The wildfire-toxin of *Pseudomonas tabaci* has been reported to be a β-lactam compound (Stewart 1971). Another related β-lactam metabolite from *Pseudomonas* has also been identified (Taylor et al. 1972). Newer monocyclic monobactam antibiotics produced by a variety of gram-negative bacteria have been reported recently (Imada et al. 1981; Sykes et al. 1981).

Before 1971, descriptions of cephalosporin-producing strains were very limited, i.e., one strain of the asexual *Cephalosporium* (Newton and Abraham 1955) and a few species of its sexual form, *Emericellopsis (Acremonium)* (Elander et al. 1961). Recently, cephalosporin-producing microorganisms have been found to be widely distributed in nature. These include the molds *Anixiopsis* (Kitano et al. 1975, 1977), *Arachnomyces* (Kitano et al. 1975, 1977), *Diheterospora* (Higgens et al. 1974), *Paecilomyces* (Higgens et al. 1974; Kitano et al. 1974; Pisano and Vellozi 1974), *Scopulariopsis* (Higgens et al. 1974), and *Spiroidium* (Kitano et al. 1975, 1977), and several species of *Streptomyces* (Nagarajan et al. 1971; Stapley et al. 1972; Higgens et al. 1974; Hasegawa et al. 1975). The successive findings of new cephalosporin-producing fungi at the Takeda Laboratories was due to the advancement of the analytical methods developed for the isolation of β-lactam antibiotics and the use of a specific mutant of *Pseudomonas*, highly sensitive to ce-

Table 2. β-Lactam antibiotics produced by fungi

R Side-chain		Common name	Organism	Reference
A. Penicillins		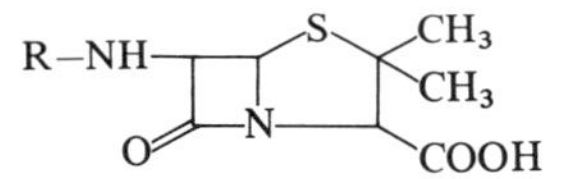		
H		Penicillin nucleus, 6-APA (6-aminopenicillanic acid)		Cole and Robinson (1961)
HO_2C—$CH(NH_2)(CH_2)_3$—CO— (D—α—aminoadipic acid)		Penicillin N, synnematin B, cephalosporin N	All strains that produce cephalosporin	Abraham et al. (1954), Newton and Abraham (1955), Olson et al. (1953), Crawford et al. (1952)
$HO_2CCH(NH_2)CH_2SCH_2CO$—		RIT—2214	*A. chrysogenum* (*lys*$^-$) ATCC 20389	Troonen et al. (1976)
B. Cephalosporins		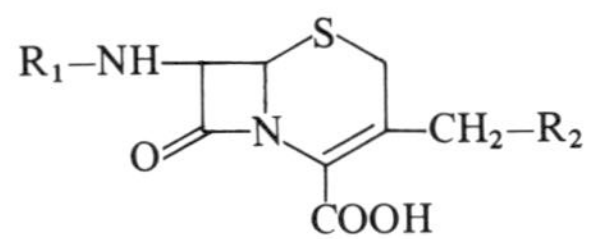		
R_1	R_2			
HO_2C—$CH(NH_2)(CH_2)_3$—CO— (D—α—aminoadipic acid)	—$OCOCH_3$	Cephalosporin C	*C. acremonium* (also classified as *A. chrysogenum*)	Newton and Abraham (1955)
			Emericellopsis glabra	Elander et al. (1961)
			C. polyaleurum	Tubaki (1973)
			Arachnomyces minimus	Kitano et al. (1975, 1977)
			Anixiopsis peruviana	Kitano et al. (1975, 1977)
			Spiroidium fuscum	Kitano et al. (1975, 1977)
			Paecilomyces persicinus	Pisano and Vellozzi (1974)
			Paecilomyces carneus	Higgens et al. (1974)
HO_2C—$CH(NH_2)(CH_2)_3$—CO—	—OH	Deacetylcephalosporin C	*C. acremonium* and mutants	Jeffery et al. (1961)
				Queener and Capone (1974)
				Kanzaki et al. (1974)
				Liersch et al. (1976)
				Fujisawa et al. (1975)
			C. polyaleurum	Kanzaki and Fujisawa (1976)
			Arachnomyces minimum	Kitano et al. (1975)
			Anixiopsis peruviana	Kitano et al. (1975)
			Spiroidium fascum	Kitano et al. (1975)
			P. persicinus	Pisano and Vellozzi (1974)
			P. carneus	Higgens et al. (1974)

$HO_2C—CH(NH_2)(CH_2)_3—CO—$	—H	Deacetoxycephalosporin C	*C. acremonium* and mutants	KANZAKI et al. (1974) QUEENER and CAPONE (1974) LIERSCH et al. (1976)
			C. polyaleurum	KANZAKI and FUJISAWA (1976)
			C. chrysogenum[a]	HIGGENS et al. (1974)
			Cephalosporium sp.	HIGGENS et al. (1974)
			Emericellopsis sp.	ELANDER et al. (1961) HIGGENS et al. (1974)
			Diheterospora chlamydosporia	HIGGENS et al. (1974)
			Scopulariopsis sp.	HIGGENS et al. (1974)
			Arachnomyces minimus	KITANO et al. (1975, 1977)
			Anixiopsis peruviana	KITANO et al. (1975, 1977)
			Spiroidium fuscum	KITANO et al. (1975, 1977)
			P. persicinus	PISANO and VELLOZZI (1974)
			P. carneus	HIGGENS et al. (1974)
$HO_2C—CH(NH_2)(CH_2)_3—CO—$	$—SCH_3$	F—1	*C. acremonium* mutant	KANZAKI et al. (1974
$HO_2C—CH(NH_2)(CH_2)_3—CO—$	$—S_2O_3H$	F—2	*C. acremonium* mutant	KANZAKI and FUJISAWA (1976)
$HO_2C—CH(NH_2)(CH_2)_3—CO—$	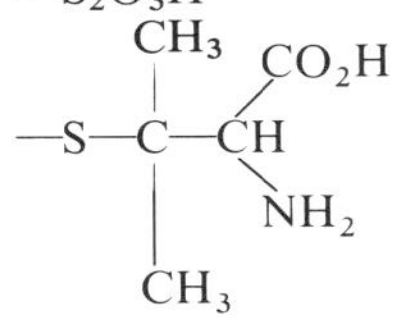	C43—219	*C. acremonium* mutant	KITANO et al. (1975)
$HO_2C—CH(CH_2)_3—CO—$ (with $NH—COCH_3$ on CH)	—H	*N*-acetyldeacetoxycephalosporin C	*C. acremonium* mutant	TRAXLER et al. (1975)
$HO_2C—(CH_2)_3—CO—$	—H	C—1778a	*C. chrysogenum*	KITANO et al. (1975)
$HO_2C—(CH_2)_3—CO—$	—OH	C—1778b	*C. chrysogenum*	KITANO et al. (1975)
$HO_2C—(CH_2)_3—CO—$	$—OCOCH_3$	C—1778c	*C. chrysogenum*	KITANO et al. (1975)
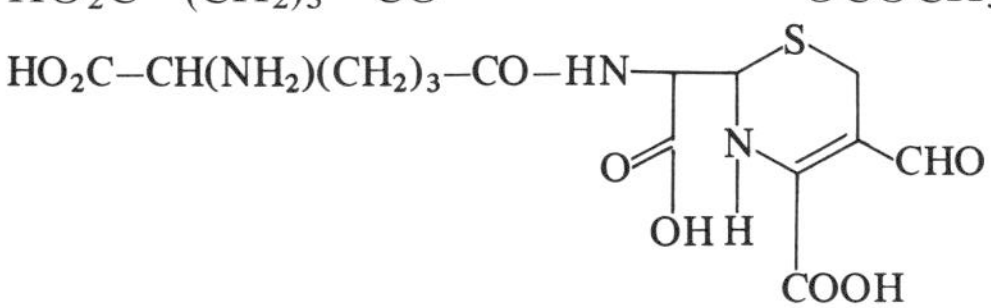		C—2	*C. acremonium* mutant	FUJISAWA and KANZAKI (1975)

[a] Most strains which produce deacetoxycephalosporin C also produce cephalosporin C and deacetylcephalosporin C

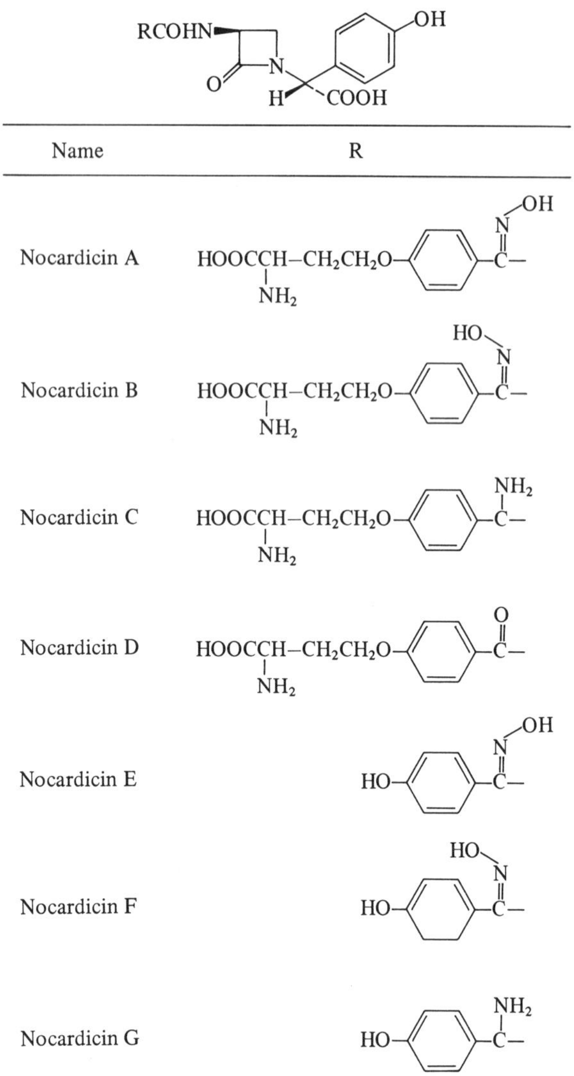

Fig. 2. Structures of nocardicin antibiotics

phalosporins, with which KITANO et al. (1975, 1976, 1977) succeeded in detecting trace amounts. Other sensitive screening procedures have been detailed by AOKI et al. (1977) and OMURA et al. (1979).

Cephalosporins and various metabolites related to the biosynthesis of β-lactam antibiotics in cephalosporin-producing strains are summarized in Table 2. HIGGENS et al. (1974) reported that the majority of the deacetoxycephalosporin C–producing strains accumulate cephalosporin C and deacetylcephalosporin C. Indeed, in almost every strain, the production of cephalosporin C is accompanied by that of deacetylcephalosporin C and deacetoxycephalosporin C. From these facts, it may be generalized that those strains which produce one of the three cephalosporin compounds concomitantly produce two other cephalosporin antibiotics.

The mechanism of synthesis of deacetylcephalosporin C and deacetoxycephalosporin C in microorganisms has been determined with mutants of *A. chrysogenum*. In the case of the latter, deacetoxycephalosporin C is synthesized de novo by some of the cephalosporin C–negative mutants (FUJISAWA et al. 1973, 1975). In contrast, deacetylcephalosporin C may be accumulated through enzymic or chemical hydrolysis of cephalosporin C in other deacetylcephalosporin C–producing microorganisms, since acetylhydrolase has been demonstrated in the culture broth of an *A. chrysogenum* mutant (FUJISAWA et al. 1973, 1975; KANZAKI et al. 1974; LIERSCH et al. 1976) and in *Streptomyces* species (BRANNON et al. 1972). A trace quantity of deacetylcephalosporin C in the fermentation broths of *A. chrysogenum* was reported to be formed by chemical hydrolysis (HUBER et al. 1968).

Compound F-1 (Table 2) was detected in culture broths of potent cephalosporin C-producing strains (KANZAKI et al. 1974). It may be produced through a chemical or biochemical reaction between cephalosporin C and methanethiol which could originate from added methionine by the action of a methionine-degrading enzyme.

A mutant of *A. chrysogenum*, No. 1011, produced a cephem compound F-2 (Table 2) in a culture broth (KANZAKI and FUJISAWA 1976). The compound F-2 was determined to be a Bunte salt, in which the *O*-acetyl group of cephalosporin C was replaced by thiosulfate nonbiologically (DEMAIN et al. 1963). Therefore, compound F-2 may be produced from thiosulfate which is formed from methionine added to the medium and cephalosporin C.

An *A. chrysogenum* mutant, No. C-43-219, accumulated a small amount of a new cephem compound, C-43-219 (KITANO et al. 1975). The compound was identified as 7-(D-5-amino-5-carboxyvaleramido)-3-(1,1-dimethyl-2-amino-2-carboxyethylthiomethyl)-3-cephem-4-carboxylic acid, which may be formed from cephalosporin C and penicillamine (Table 2).

It is known that deacetoxycephalosporin C is formed through de novo synthesis in the mutants of *A. chrysogenum* defective in cephalosporin C or deacetylcephalosporin C productivity (KANZAKI et al. 1974). Details are not known about the biosynthesis of deacetoxycephalosporin C in other microorganisms.

The discovery of cephalosporins in streptomycetes was an epoch-making event in the following aspects. One was the fact that prokaryotes also produced cephalosporins and that such organisms are widely distributed in nature. The other was the demonstration of the occurrence of a new family of cephem compounds, 7-methoxy-cephem derivatives. The new cephalosporins were noteworthy for the fact that introduction of the methoxyl group to the cephem nucleus increased activity against gram-negative bacteria, especially against *Proteus* species which produce β-lactamase (MILLER et al. 1972).

A deacetoxycephalosporin C–producing mutant of *A. chrysogenum* CP71, blocked in the synthesis of cephalosporin C, was found to accumulate a new cephem compound (TRAXLER et al. 1975). The new compound was identified as *N*-acetyl-deacetoxycephalosporin C (Table 2). The titers of this compound in the three independently obtained deacetoxycephalosporin C–producing mutants varied from 0.05 to 0.2 mg/ml.

KITANO et al. (1975) isolated and identified a family of cephem compounds containing a glutaryl group instead of the α-aminoadipyl residue (Table 2). These compounds were accumulated in a trace amount in culture broths of *A. chrysogenum*. Hydrophilic β-lactam compounds have been found to involve only the α-aminoadipyl group or its *N*-acetyl derivative as a side chain. The discovery of this family of cephalosporins is important, but the mechanism of its biosynthetic pathway remains to be determined.

A new hydrolysis product (C-2) was found to be accumulated in the culture broths of *A. chrysogenum* mutants Nos. 20, 29, 26, and 40, which were defective in acetyl CoA: deacetylcephalosporin C acetyltransferase and, therefore, could not accumulate cephalosporin C, but could accumulate deacetylcephalosporin C (FUJISAWA and KANZAKI 1975). The compound C-2 was isolated from the culture filtrate of the deacetylcephalosporin C–producing mutant No. 40 and identified as D-5-amino-5-carboxyvaleramido (5-formyl-4-carboxy-2*H*, 3*H*, 6*H*-tetrahydro-1,3-thiazinylglycine) by its chemical and physical properties (Table 2). It was postulated that compound C-2 was formed through hydrolysis of the β-lactam ring of 7-(5-amino-5-carboxyvaleramido)-3-formyl-3-cephem-4-carboxylic acid, which may be synthesized by oxidation of deacetylcephalosporin C.

Penicillins fall into two major types: hydrophobic and hydrophilic molecules. From the standpoint of antibiotic production, there are interesting differences between strains producing them. Organisms which produce a hydrophilic penicillin, penicillin N, never produce a significant amount of hydrophobic penicillins and fail to respond to the addition of side-chain percursors. A hydrophilic penicillin, isopenicillin N, possessing the L-α-aminoadipyl group at C-6 as the side-chain, is sometimes observed in culture broths of hydrophobic penicillin producers. However, not only is the amount very small but also the major portion is contained within the mycelium. Furthermore, biochemical approaches suggest it to be an intermediate of the synthesis of a hydrophobic penicillin. Thus, it is considered not to be a final product. To date, isopenicillin N has not been detected in the broths of cultures producing penicillin N.

Microorganisms which produce penicillin N are very similar to those producing cephalosporins. Fungi and streptomycetes which produce cephalosporins always produce penicillin N, but not all penicillin N–producing strains produce cephalosporins. In fact, only a few penicillin N–producing strains synthesize cephalosporins. Interestingly, this relationship also holds true for mutants of *Cephalosporium* species (LEMKE and NASH 1972; KANZAKI and FUJISAWA 1976).

Cephalosporin-producing organisms produce 6-aminopenicillanic acid and penicillin N as the only penam compounds. When *A. chrysogenum* was cultivated in a complex medium, 6-aminopenicillanic acid was produced (LEMKE and NASH 1972), but it was not detected in cultures propagated on a synthetic medium (SMITH et al. 1967). The function of 6-aminopenicillanic acid in the metabolism of β-lactam antibiotics in cephalosporin-producing organisms remains to be determined, although it is believed to be a shunt metabolite.

The so-called "tripeptide theory" where a common precursor of β-lactam antibiotics is a tripeptide, α-aminoadipylcysteinylvaline, has been supported by most β-lactam antibiotic investigators. The tripeptide was first isolated from mycelia of *P. chrysogenum* by ARNSTEIN and MORRIS (1960). LODER and ABRAHAM (1971) later isolated three peptides, P3, P2, and P1 from the mycelium of *A. chrysogenum*. The peptides P3, P2, and P1 were found to contain α-aminoadipic acid, cysteine, valine. P2 and P1 are tetrapeptides containing glycine; P2 contains valine and P1 α-hydroxyvaline.

Independent of this work, KANZAKI et al. (1974) obtained several kinds of antibiotic-negative mutants of *A. chrysogenum*. They observed mutants which accumulated two peptides extracellularly among both penicillin N – and cephalosporin C–negative strains. The peptides, S-1 and S-2, were determined to be the dimer of δ-(L-α-aminoadipyl)-L-cysteinyl-D-valine and the disulfide of δ-(L-α-aminoadipyl)-L-cysteinyl-D-valine and methanethiol, respectively. Methanethiol may be derived from methionine added to the culture medium. The amounts of S-1 and S-2 were approximately 500 and 50 µg/ml, respectively. The thiol compounds are responsible for severe odor problems in less efficient production strains of *A. chrysogenum*. Sulfate-efficient strains with decreased dependence on methionine result in fewer pollution problems in large-scale cephalosporin C production (ELANDER 1975).

Several natural microbial β-lactam compounds containing novel ring systems were known prior to 1975. These substances were not inhibitors of microbial cell-wall synthesis and, thus, bore little relationship to the classic penicillins or cephalosporins. An example of this type of compound is X-372A (Table 3). It was reported by SCANNELL et al. (1975) to be an antimetabolite. The modest antimicrobial activity of this streptomycete compound was evident in a synthetic medium and its inherent weak activity could be reversed by the addition of glutamate to the medium.

Another novel monocyclic β-lactam called FR-1923 was reported in broths of *Nocardia uniformis* subsp. *tsuyamanensis* by AOKI et al. (1976). The substance is known as nocardicin A (Table 3) and was the major component in a series of related metabolites. The compound has only slight in vitro activity against *Pseudomonas aeruginosa* but has marked in vivo activity in mice infected with a carbenicillin-resistant strain of *Pseudomonas aeruginosa*. AOKI et al. (1977) suggested that the enhanced in vivo activity may be the result of the antibiotic's ability to alter the bacterial cell in such a way as to render it more susceptible to phagocytosis. This effect was also suggested by enhanced activity when organisms were incubated in the presence of nocardicin A and white blood cells.

Clavulanic acid is a member of an interesting group of novel β-lactam metabolites produced by a strain of *S. clavuligerus* (ATTC 15380) which also produces penicillin N and a number of cephalosporins (BROWN et al. 1976). The compound was detected by a screen designed to select activities which inhibit the destruction of penicillin antibiotics by a variety of bacterial penicillinases, i.e., β-lactamase inhibitors. Clavulanic acid (Table 3) and three related structures have been described (COLE et al. 1976). Despite extensive investigation, clavulanic acid or its related metabolites were not found in sensitive classic antibacterial assays (GORMAN and HUBER 1977). The structure of clavulanic acid (Table 3) is unique because it is composed of a fused oxazolidine ring and the nonacylamido-substituted azetidinone. Also, the stereochemistry of the two asymmetric centers in clavulanic acid is the same as in the penicillins. The present marketing strategy for β-lactamase inhibitors is a combination of clavulanic acid with a second, more potent β-lactam antibiotic.

In 1976, the Beecham Group Ltd. reported a compound (MM-4550, Table 3) produced by a strain of *S. olivaceus*, which had the property of inhibiting the hydrolysis of penicillins and cephalosporins by β-lactamases (BROWN et al. 1976). The

Table 3. Representative β-lactam antibiotics produced in bacteria and actinomycetes

Compound	Structure	Organism	Reference
Cephamycin C	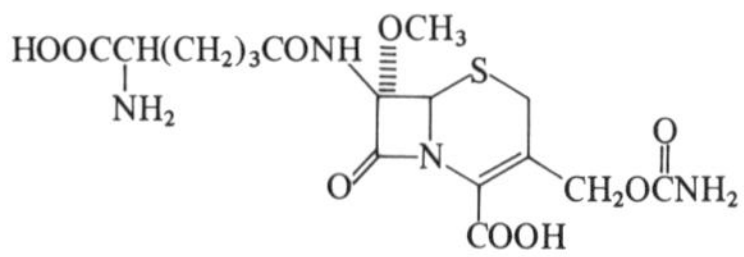	*S. clavuligerus*	NAGARAJAN et al. (1971) HIGGENS and KASTNER (1971)
Wildfire Toxin (Tabtoxin)	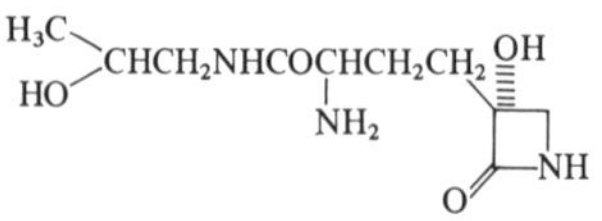	*Pseudomonas tabaci*	STEWART (1971)
X–372A	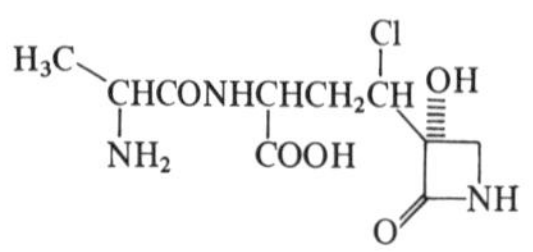	*Streptomyces* sp. 372A	SCANNELL et al. (1975)
Clavulanic acid	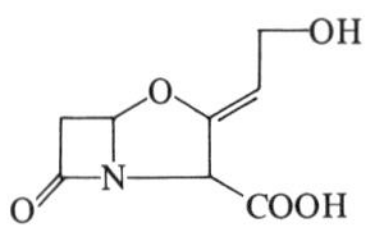	*S. clavuligerus*	BROWN et al. (1976) READING and COLE (1977)
Nocardicin A	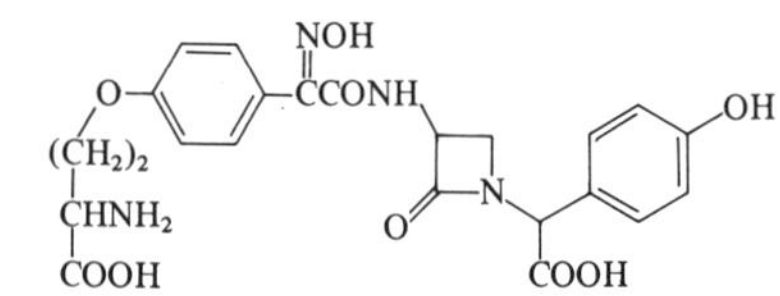	*Nocardia uniformis*	AOKI et al. (1976)
Thienamycin	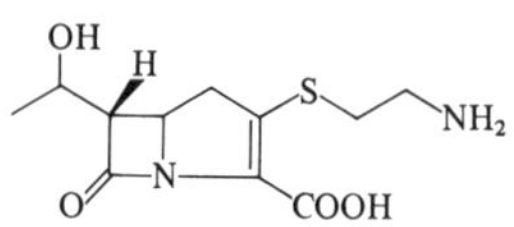	*S. cattleya*	KAHAN et al. (1979)
Carpetimycins	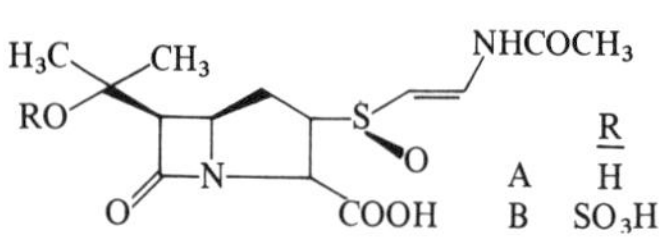	*Streptomyces* sp. KC–6643	NAKAYAMA et al. (1980)
C–19393 S_2 and H_2	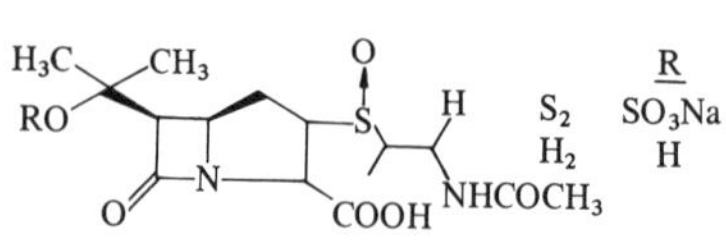	*Streptomyces griseus* subsp. *cryophilus*	IMADA et al. (1980)
Sulfazecin	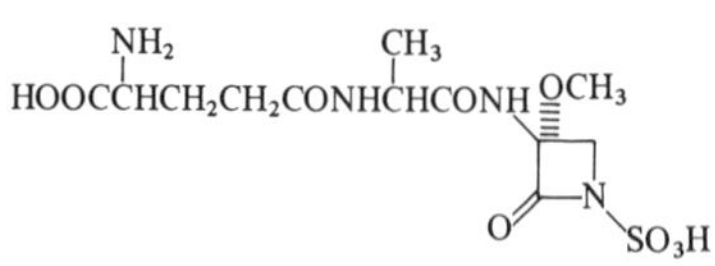	*Pseudomonas acidophila*	IMADA et al. (1981)
Hydroxyethyl-clavam	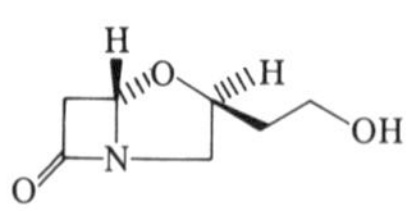	*Streptomyces antibioticus* subsp. *antibioticus*	KRONE et al. (1981)

three compounds have been designated MM-4550, MM-13902, and MM-17880 (Table 3). All three of these compounds were able to protect penicillins and cephalosporins against destruction by β-lactamases with MM-13902 being the most potent inhibitor.

Another new β-lactamase inhibitor antibiotic was reported by OKAMURA et al. (1978, 1979a, b). The producer organism has been classified as *Streptomyces cremeus* subsp. *auratilis* (ATTC 31358) and was shown to have good inhibitory activity against a variety of gram-positive and gram-negative bacteria. The substance also inhibited a variety of β-lactamase enzymes. The new molecule has been called PS-5 and, structurally, is a new β-lactam having a 1-carbapenem structure (see Fig. 9) as in thienamycin.

An exciting recent β-lactam antibiotic from the Merck Institute termed thienamycin was reported by KAHAN et al. (1976, 1979). The antibiotic is highly unstable chemically and is extremely active against a broad spectrum of microorganisms including *Pseudomonas*. It is produced by a new strain of *Streptomyces* classified as *S. cattleya* (NRRL-8057). The *trans*-stereochemistry of the β-lactam appears to be unique as all biologically active penicillins and cephalosporins previously known have the *cis*-configuration at these two carbon atoms. This unique stereochemistry may contribute to the β-lactamase stability of thienamycin (GORMAN and HUBER 1977).

Thienamycins are also produced by strains of *Streptomyces fulvoviridis* and *Streptomyces flavogriseus* (NRRL-8139-40). Chemically, the thienamycins are extremely complex in that they contain three asymmetric centers and, thus, each structure represents eight possible compounds. *N*-acetylthienamycin and *n*-acetylepithienamycins are known which possess varying low antibacterial activities against strains of *Pseudomonas*. On the basis of the reported literature, microorganisms capable of synthesizing the thienamycin ring system can form a variety of substituents on the β-lactam ring, thereby increasing the probability of discovering many new thienamycin- and olivanic acid–related antibiotics.

C. Strain Improvement Programs in Commercially Important β-Lactam Fermentation Organisms

Mutation and genetic recombination have played important roles in the fermentation development of penicillin and cephalosporin antibiotics. The low productivity of the original strains of *P. chrysogenum* and *C. acremonium* (now classified as *A. chrysogenum*) and inherent advantages of both the natural and semisynthetic penicillin and cephalosporin antibiotics over others led to an exploitation of the genetic potential of beneficial mutations to generate superproductive commercial strains of these β-lactam-producing fungi. Mutation has proved to be important in other areas of antibiotic research also: a) It has resulted in the development of genetically blocked mutants which have been useful in the elucidation of biosynthetic pathways for β-lactam antibiotics. b) It has led to the discovery of a number of new β-lactam primordial peptides and closed-ring β-lactam derivatives which have not been discovered to date in fermentation broths of wild-type isolates. c) The feeding of fraudulent precursor analogs to mutants blocked in side-chain precursors has resulted in the synthesis of new β-lactam molecules. This mutasynthetic approach may result in a variety of novel molecules with superior antibiotic properties.

Classic mutation and selection techniques, important in the development of highly productive mutants in the absence of fundamental knowledge, have now been largely replaced by more rational (directed) selection techniques grounded on more scientific bases. The application of directed selection, coupled with programs using recombinational genetics, the new techniques of protoplast fusion, and the potentials of recombinant DNA, should provide rationales for the development of new tailor-made recombinant strains elaborating β-lactam antibiotics.

I. Mutation and Enhanced Penicillin Formation in P. chrysogenum

Large programs concerned with the induction, selection, and utilization of superior penicillin-producing variants of *P. chrysogenum* have now been proceeding for over 30 years. From the screening of hundreds of thousands of strains, a series of superior penicillin-producing mutants has been developed from strain Wisconsin Q-176, and distant relatives are now used throughout the world for the manufacture of penicillin (see Fig. 3 and Table 4; BACKUS and STAUFFER 1955; ELANDER 1976, 1979).

During the period of intensive screening work, attention was focused on strain characteristics which correlated with high yield. The Wisconsin group showed a correlation between increased productivity and reduced sporulation and growth (ELANDER et al. 1976; QUEENER et al. 1975). In the Wisconsin series, the greatest change was observed in the early ancestry. Between the NRRL-1951 and Q-176 strains, growth and sporulation fell by 60%, with a concomitant titer increase of sixfold. Later, an additional threefold increase in antibiotic titer was associated with only an additional 10% reduction in mycelial vigor. These changes may represent a correlated response due to linkage of loci determining growth with those influencing penicillin titer. Screening can also be utilized to isolate strains with improved growth and sporulation characteristics. The latter was most important for long-term preservation and for providing vigorous vegetative development in tank fermentations (ELANDER et al. 1973). The correlation of strain vigor, decreased sporulation, and weak vegetative development may reflect conflicting physiologi-

Table 4. Improvement in penicillin G by Panlabs' strains of *P. chrysogenum*. (SWARTZ 1979; COONEY 1979)

Strain	Penicillin G (mg/ml)	Conversion yield (g pen G/g glucose)
P-2	9.0	0.05
P-7	17.4	0.10
P-11	21.6	0.12
P-13	27.0	0.09
P-15	29.4	0.12

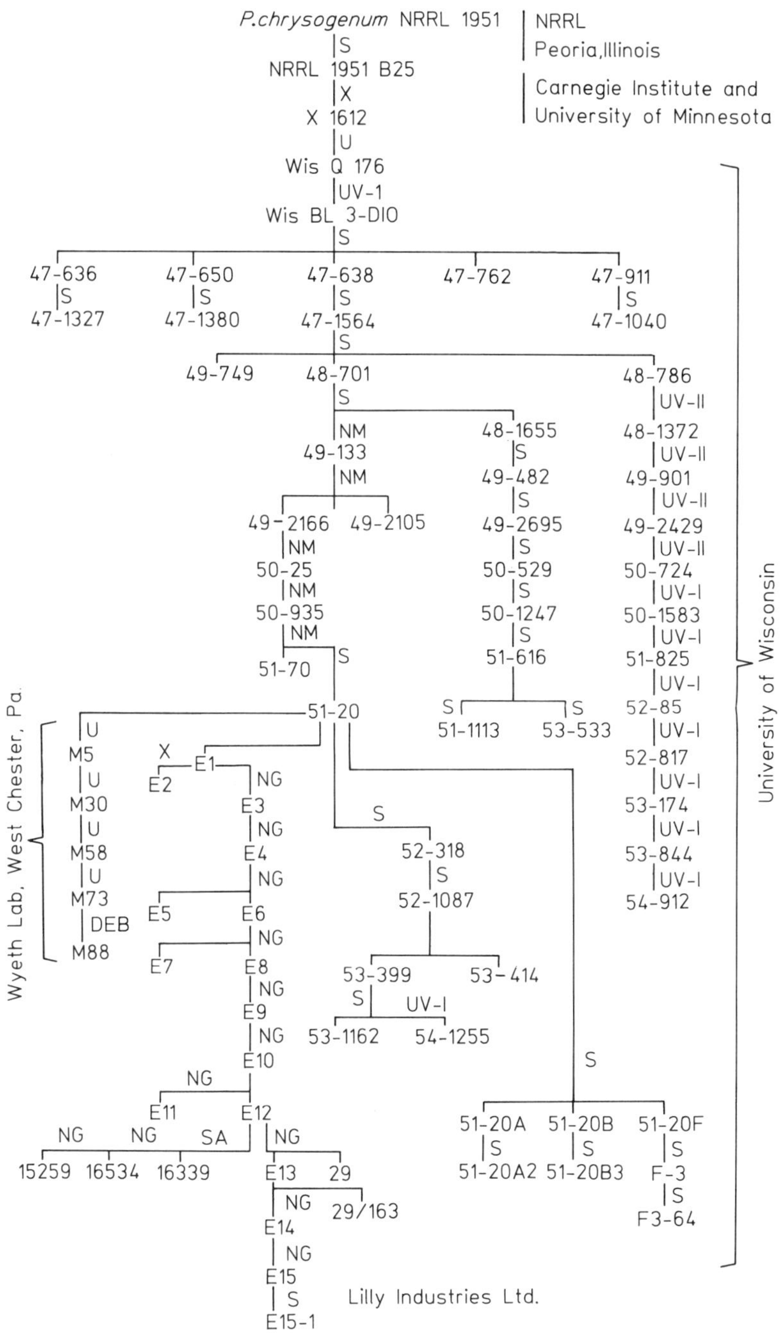

Fig. 3. The development of some industrial strain lineages of *P. chrysogenum* (ELANDER 1967)

cal or metabolic balances of pleiotropic effects of high-yield-determining genes. However, it is not possible to assess the basis of genetic and environmental interactions as related to improved yield because of the lack of relevant information. There are correlations which include strain tolerance to phenylacetic acid (FUSKA and WELWARDOVA 1969), ability to accumulate intracellular sulfate (SEGEL and JOHNSON 1961), ability to assimilate carbohydrate and precursor (PAN et al. 1972), sensitivity to iron (PAN et al. 1975), penicillin acylase activity (ERICKSON and DEAN 1966), levels of acetohydroxyacid synthetase (GOULDEN and CHATTAWAY 1969), and acyltransferase activity (PREUSS and JOHNSON 1967).

II. Mutagenesis and Yield Improvement in the Cephalosporin C Organism, Acremonium chrysogenum

A strain improvement program was initiated in the 1950s to improve the low levels of cephalosporin C in BROTZU's strain of *A. chrysogenum*. Mutagenesis of the Brotzu isolate resulted in the selection of a mutant, M-8650, which was the progenitor strain for many industrial programs (ELANDER et al. 1976). The synthesis of cephalosporin C in laboratory fermentations by a series of improved UV variants is shown in Figure 4. An improved mutant (CW-19) developed at Eli Lilly and Co. produced threefold more antibiotic than the Brotzu culture. When CW-19 was fermented under more favorable conditions, the culture synthesized 15 times more antibiotic than the progenitor strain. The CW-19 variant also had a significantly improved cephalosporin C to penicillin N ratio (ELANDER 1975). The CW-19 mu-

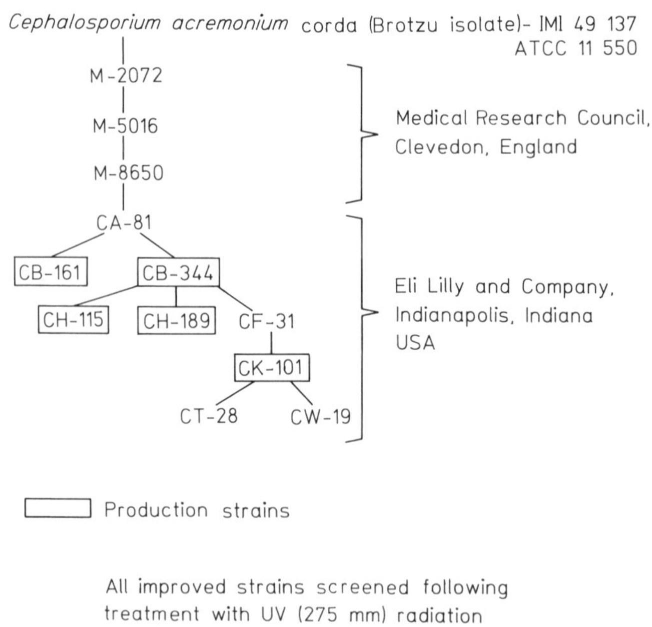

Fig. 4. The lineage of early improved commercial strains of *A. chrysogenum* (ELANDER et al. 1976)

tant has been used for a number of biosynthetic studies (DREW and DEMAIN 1977; KONOMI et al. 1979). Biometric considerations of the data using normal populations of UV survivor strains showed an 11–1 advantage for "normal" clones versus "abnormal" clones in searching for mutants producing 20% higher antibiotic titers. The probability statements were calculated for many survivor populations on a statistical basis (BROWN and ELANDER 1966). The improved UV variants differed markedly from the progenitor strains in cultural and biochemical properties. Untreated populations of the improved variants showed a progressive reduction in colony diameter, decreased vegetative development and decreased sporulation vigor, features which were also characteristic of the improved penicillin variants (ELANDER 1976). FASANI et al. (1974) reported that dimethylsulfate- and phenethyl alcohol–treated populations yielded higher producing cephalosporin C variants. The highest antibiotic producers were obtained by phenethyl alcohol treatment. Strains of *A. chrysogenum* or *Cephalosporium polyaleurum* resistant to polyene antibiotics produced 10 g cephalosporin C/liter (Takeda Pharmaceutical Co., Japanese Patent JA-110723, 16 January 1975). In another patent, polyploid clones were reported to be potent cephalosporin C producers. The higher ploidy clones were induced by exposure to camphor followed by selection of large cells (Takeda Pharmaceutical Co., Japanese Patent JS-109680, 16 January 1975).

Submerged cultures of *A. chrysogenum* form arthrospores, and the differentiation coincides with the maximal rate of cephalosporin C synthesis. In the improved variants, arthrospore formation was proportional to the increased antibiotic formation (NASH and HUBER 1971). Methionine supplementation enchanced the onset of differentiation, and the requirement for methionine was increased for higher yielding mutants (NASH and HUBER 1971). Methionine and sulfate metabolism is important with respect to cephalosporin C synthesis, and the metabolism of methionine, through its oxo and hydroxy analogs, is to stimulate cellular differentiation.

Cysteine is the immediate donor of sulfur to cephalosporin C but the amino acid is not stimulatory for cephalosporin C synthesis in media containing sulfate (DENNEN and CARVER 1969). Methionine stimulates antibiotic synthesis, but the stimulation is not due to sulfur donation but to an unresolved role in antibiotic regulation. NÜESCH et al. (1973) and DREW et al. (1976) have obtained mutants with blocks between sulfate and cysteine, cystathionine, and homocysteine. These mutants still require methionine with respect to cephalosporin C stimulation. An interesting Ciba *slp* mutant, blocked in the sulfate reduction pathway prior to sulfide formation, was able to assimilate more exogenous methionine and synthesized four times more antibiotic than its sulfide-proficient parent (NÜESCH et al. 1973). Revertant strains of the mutant assimilated less methionine and synthesized low levels of cephalosporin C. DREW and DEMAIN (1977) showed a similar result with the 274-1 mutant. NÜESCH and co-workers have proposed that higher levels of cephalosporin C obtained with non-sulfate-utilizing mutants were due to their inability to synthesize cysteine, an amino acid which acts as a repressor of methionine permease (NÜESCH et al. 1973).

In a study with improved mutants at Eli Lilly and Co., QUEENER et al. (1975) reported that the specific activity of glutamate dehydrogenase was derepressed whereas two mutants in a low-yielding series had repressed levels of glutamate dehydrogenase. The altered regulation pattern for this enzyme may have removed a nitrogen limitation for cephalosporin C synthesis. An inverse relationship appeared to exist between vegetative development and enhanced cephalosporin C synthesis.

Mutants of *A. chrysogenum*, altered in sulfur metabolism and in their potential to synthesize cephalosporin C from sulfate, have been derived (NISS and NASH 1973; TREICHLER et al. 1978, 1979). One of the mutants (M8650-I), corresponded to the *cys*-3 mutant of *Neurospora crassa* in which the locus exerts coordinate control over the synthesis of sulfate permease as well as arylsulfatase. Mutant M8650-I was improved in sulfate transport and repressed for arylsulfatase, and it utilized sulfate as effectively as methionine in providing sulfur for cephalosporin C. In this connection, the parent strain, M8650, is considered to be a derepressed mutant of arylsulfatase synthesis. The sulfatase repression in M8650-*sp*-I may be related to the accumulation of sulfide which regulates sulfatase synthesis, since sulfide is believed to be a corepressor of sulfatase in fungi. Mutants of *A. chrysogenum* are increasingly derepressed for arylsulfatase and concomitantly exhibit increased potentials for synthesis of antibiotics from methionine (DENNEN and CARVER 1969).

Another mutant, IS-5, with enhanced potential to use sulfate for cephalosporin C production, produced two times more antibiotic than its parent, with sulfate (KOMATSU et al. 1975). Cephalosporin C production by this mutant was sensitive to methionine, in contrast to its parent. In addition to the mutant IS-5, several other mutants with an increased potential to produce higher levels of cephalosporin C from sulfate were methionine sensitive. Therefore, the increase in productivity from sulfate and in methionine sensitivity may be metabolically related and caused by the same mutational event.

KOMATSU and KODAIRA (1977) reported enzymatic studies on sulfate-efficient strains of *A. chrysogenum*. In sulfate-starved cells, norleucine showed an inhibitory effect on cephalosporin C and penicillin N formation in the presence of inorganic S sources and L-cysteine. However, antibiotic production was stimulated by methionine in the parental strain. High cysteine pools were formed in the sulfate-efficient strains. One of the cysteine biosynthetic enzymes, L-serine sulfhydrylase, was elevated twofold in the mutant, thereby rendering the improved mutant with a high pool of cysteine, an important biosynthetic intermediate of cephalosporin C.

Two excellent reviews have been published by TREICHLER et al. (1978, 1979) describing the use of mutant strains of *A. chrysogenum* blocked in important steps in sulfur metabolism. Mutants blocked in methionine synthase and cystathionine γ-lyase and/or requiring *O*-acetyl-L-homoserine and resistant to methylselenide ($OAH^-/MeSe^R$) provided additional credence that L-cystathionine mediates induction of L-cysteine incorporation into cephalosporins (TREICHLER et al. 1979).

III. Rational Screening or Selection for Improved Mutants or Mutants Producing Modified β-Lactam Antibiotics

In efforts to improve the efficiency of large-scale strain improvement programs, rational screening and selection procedures have been reported to be more efficient than random blind screening for the isolation of improved variants. Many of the techniques involve the use of prescreening on agar of mutagenized cells prior to laboratory fermentation studies. More importantly, the techniques are based on known or probable biochemical mechanisms and, therefore, remove much of the empiricism commonly associated with random screening.

1. Mutants Screened Directly on Agar Plates

Direct demonstration of antibiotic production by a colony growing on solidified fermentation medium can be observed by overlaying of a sensitive organism after colonial development of either *Penicillium* or *Acremonium*. The colony-plate method had advantages in that it can eliminate many of the poorly producing isolates, thereby increasing the probability of discovering superior mutants in laboratory programs. The application of the colony-plate procedure has meaning only if plate performance is correlated with submerged fermentation performance. The program has been useful in isolating superior cephalosporin producers by researchers at the University of Wisconsin (ELANDER et al. 1961) and has recently been advocated by TRILLI et al. (1978). The Wisconsin workers sprayed plates containing mature fungal colonies from mutagenized spores with suspensions of *Alcaligenes faecalis*. Strains having a greater inhibition zone diameter compared to colony diameter (potency index) were examined in flask fermentations. With this procedure, approximately 60% of the isolates were discarded prior to the flask evaluation stage. Using the above technique, the Wisconsin workers obtained a strain showing a fivefold improvement over a 4-year period in a small-scale program. TRILLI et al. (1978) grew colonies of *Acremonium chrysogenum* originating from mutagenized spores on small discs of agar medium. After 5 days of growth, the antibiotic contents of the discs were assayed with a sensitive assay organism. By varying the concentration of nitrogen in the agar, these workers were able to control the quantities of antibiotic produced. The relation of agar disc inhibition zone diameter to log shake-flask titer was linear with short incubation times, but shifted toward a higher order upon more prolonged incubation periods. Interestingly, their results suggest that the shake-flask performance test underestimated the improvement in strain productivity. BALL and MCGONAGLE (1978) adopted the potency index method of ELANDER et al. (1961) to improve the penicillin yields of industrial strains at Glaxo Ltd. In this technique, colonies on agar are surrounded by a bacterial suspension and following further incubation, zones of lysis appear around the colony. The zone size was reduced by the incorporation of penicillinase into the agar. A variety of techniques which increase the sensitivity of bioassay screening on solid media have been described by DULANEY and DULANEY (1967).

2. Selection of Mutants for Resistance to Toxic Antibiotic Precursors or Analogs of Precursors

Analogs of end products may act as false feedback effectors, thereby inhibiting growth of the producer organism. The side-chain precursor of penicillin G, phenylacetic acid, is a highly toxic agent to strains of *Penicillium chrysogenum*. FUSKA and WELWARDOVA (1969) reported that a high percentage of a population of strains resistant to high concentrations of phenylacetic acid were superior penicillin producers. Amino acid analogs are often used for the selection of deregulated mutants which overproduce the corresponding amino acid. The isolation of deregulated mutants of *P. chrysogenum* and *A. chrysogenum* has been limited to some extent by the lack of toxicity of available amino acid analogs (MASUREKAR and DEMAIN 1974; FRIEDRICH and DEMAIN 1977a, b). Native resistance of most fungi to commonly used analogs is well documented (LEMKE 1969; LEMKE and BRANNON 1972). Since penicillins and cephalosporins are derived from α-aminoadipic acid, cysteine, and valine, it was suggested that deregulation of these amino acid pathways might lead to the selection of superior strains (DREW and DEMAIN 1977; DEMAIN and MASUREKAR 1974; ELANDER and CHANG 1979). Recently, MEHTA and NASH (1979) showed that the relationship between the carbon source in test media markedly influenced the toxicity of a number of amino acid analogues in a high-producing strain of *A. chrysogenum*.

GODFREY (1973) reported that analog-resistant mutants of the cephalosporin-producing actinomycete, *Streptomyces lipmanii*, showed increased cephamycin production. Trifluoroleucine and 2-amino-ethyl-L-cysteine were particularly effective. NÜESCH et al. (1973) reported that strains of *A. chryosgenum* resistant to selemomethionine experience impaired methionine uptake and were poor producers of cephalosporin. They used the methionine analogs, DL-methionine-DL-sulfoxide, DL-norleucine, and DL-ethionine in studies on the effects of methionine, sulfate, and sulfur metabolism on cephalosporin synthesis.

3. Selection of Mutants Resistant to Metallic Ions

Ions of heavy metals such as mercuric ions (Hg^{2+}), cupric ions (Cu^{2+}) and related organometallic ions are known to complex with β-lactam antibiotics and with their thio precursors. One can theorize that mutants which become resistant to these metallic ions may do so by overproducing β-lactam compounds which complex with the metal ions as a means of detoxifying these metallic substances, or the metals may interact with β-lactam biosynthetic enzymes containing –SH groups (CHANG and ELANDER 1979).

GODFREY (1973) reported the use of phenylmercuric acetate resistance in attempts to isolate high-yielding strains of the cephamycin-producing organism *S. lipmanii*. He found decreased production with phenylmercuric acetate-resistant mutants. NISS and NASH (1973) reported on the use of a strain of *A. chrysogenum* resistant to potassium chromate, a compound known to impair sulfate uptake. A mutant designated as M8650-*chr* showed severe impairment for the synthesis of cephalosporin C from sulfate. However, the chromate resistance mutation did not alter the capability of the resistant mutant to synthesize cephalosporin C from methionine. MARZLUF (1970) working with *N. crassa*, reported that chromate-resistant mutants were defective in sulfate transport. LEMKE (1969) reported the effects of a variety of toxic substances on the growth of *A. chrysogenum*. CHANG and ELANDER (1979) reported that several strains of *A. chrysogenum* resistant to mercuric chloride and phenylmercuric acetate were better cephalosporin producers in shake-flask fermentation.

4. Isolation of Specific Morphological Mutants of A. chrysogenum

Cells of *A. chrysogenum* are morphologically heterogeneous in submerged culture. The maximal rate of cephalosporin synthesis during the fermentation is normally associated with the differentiation of hyphal filaments to swollen, septate fragments or arthrospores, which in turn develop into yeastlike cells in the final stage of the fermentation. The arthrospore and yeast-phase cells are the cell types which are most actively engaged in antibiotic synthesis (NASH and HUBER 1971). CHANG and ELANDER (1979) isolated three kinds of morphological mutants of *A. chrysogenum* and evaluated each type for its capacity to synthesize cephalosporins in shake-flask fermentations.

a) Proficient Producers of Arthrospores

These mutants were obtained by microscopically examining treated colonies for arthrospore formation. NASH and HUBER (1971) reported that submerged cultures of *A. chrysogenum* differentiate into small swollen fragments termed arthrospores and the differentiation coincides generally with the maximal rate of cephalosporin C synthesis. In their improved variants, arthrospore formation was proportional to increased antibiotic formation. Methionine supplementation enhanced the onset of differentiation and the requirements for methionine were increased for high-yielding mutants.

b) Mutants Forming Small Compact Colonies on Chemically Defined Medium

Improved mutants of *A. chrysogenum* have been correlated with progressive reduction in colony diameter and vegetative development (ELANDER et al. 1976).

c) Conditional Thin Colonies

This class of morphological mutants grows poorly on a sulfate-limiting medium, but grows to full thickness on a sulfate-sufficient medium, presumably because of its greater demand for sulfate. A similar type of morphological mutant has been isolated by OKANISHI and GREGORY (1970) in *Candida tropicalis* which produced methionine-rich protein for potential utility as single-cell protein. In contrast to the *A. chrysogenum* mutants which formed thinner colonies on a sulfate-limiting medium, the *Candida* mutants formed smaller colonies on an identical medium.

Mutants forming colonies which rapidly differentiated into arthrospores were more proficient in generating cephalosporins. Colonies which were more efficient on a sulfate-limiting medium were capable of generating more cephalosporin C on sulfate-containing media (ELANDER and CHANG 1979).

5. Use of Auxotrophic Strains or Revertants of Auxotrophic Strains

TREICHLER et al. (1979) reported that methionine-requiring mutants of *A. chrysogenum* produced five times more cephalosporin C on media supplemented with 4 g methionine/liter compared to the parental strain on the addition of methionine (2 g/liter) which was optimal for maximal cephalosporin C synthesis. However, the high concentration of methionine required undoubtedly resulted in high fermentation costs.

Table 5. Comparison of random screening versus directed screening/selection procedure in strains of *Penicillium chrysogenum* and *Acremonium chrysogenum*. (Adapted from CHANG and ELANDER 1979)

Type	Treated	Organisms examined	Screening procedure	No. tested	No. retained	% Retained[a]
Random screening	UV, NG[b]	*P. chrysogenum* and *C. acremonium*	None	860	7	0.81
Directed screening/selection	UV, NG	*P. chrysogenum* and *C. acremonium*	1. Colony-plate	438	6	1.36
			2. Auxotrophs	35	2	5.71
			3. Haploidization-inducing agents	503	8	1.59
			4. Mitotic inhibitors	225	3	1.33
			5. Mercury	162	2	1.23
			6. Amino acid analogs	567	8	1.41
			7. Sulfur analogs	452	22	3.98
		C. acremonium (only)	1. Methionine analogs	605	22	3.64
			2. Increased sensitivity to methionine			
			A. Growth	247	4	1.62
			B. β-Lactam synthesis	52	2	3.85

[a] Superior on both primary and secondary screening tests
[b] NG, nitrosoguanidine

Modification of the structure of a feedback-sensitive enzyme through auxotrophic mutation followed by replacement with a second, reversion, mutation is a common procedure employed industrially for the selection of strains with altered regulatory control mechanisms (DULANEY and DULANEY 1967).

Table 5 shows a comparison of random empirical screening procedures against a variety of directed rational screening/selection techniques in a large strain improvement program with penicillin and cephalosporin producers at Bristol-Myers and Co. The data clearly demonstrate the superiority of rational screening/selection procedures as expressed by the numbers of isolates retained for preservation and tertiary examination prior to small-tank evaluations. Such data are probably representative of those obtained in current industrial laboratories involved in rational screening/selection for improved mutants.

6. Mutational Biosynthesis and New Biosynthetic β-Lactams

Mutation of microorganisms producing secondary metabolites has resulted in the selection of biochemical or blocked mutants capable of producing new modified metabolites either directly or in response to addition of some precursor analog. The modified metabolites usually possess the basic structural features of the parent compound, but either lack certain functional groups or contain ones which often convey differing biological activities. The biosynthetic approach using mutants and biosynthetic analogs has been useful in the generation of new aminoglycoside antibiotics.

To date, there has been only a single report of a new biosynthetic analog produced by mutants of β-lactam-producing fungi in response to the feeding of biosynthetic precursor analogs. TROONEN et al. (1976) reported on a lysine auxotroph of *Acremonium chrysogenum* ATCC 20389 producing cephalosporin C and penicillin N only, in media supplemented with DL-α-aminoadipic acid. The mutant was found to incorporate a fraudulent side-chain analogue, L-S-carboxymethylcysteine, to generate a new biosynthetic penicillin. The new penicillin (RIT-2214) was identified as 6-(D)-{[2-amino-2-carboxy) ethylthio]-acetamido}-penicillanic acid (Table 2). However, no corresponding modified 7-aminocephalosporanic acid derivative was reported. LEMKE and NASH (1972) reported lysine-requiring strains of *A. chrysogenum* which were unable to synthesize either penicillin N or cephalosporin C. The mutants grew in a minimal medium supplemented with lysine but not with α-aminoadipate. The presence of exogenous DL-α-aminoadipic acid was sufficient for both growth and the production of penicillin N and cephalosporin C (NASH et al. 1974).

Incorporation of side-chain precursors appears to be nonspecific for strains of *P. chrysogenum* and has generated a variety of biosynthetic penicillins. However, in *A. chrysogenum*, only the L-S-carboxymethyl-cysteine analog has been reported to be incorporated into a new penicillin N analog. It was proposed that L-S-carboxymethyl-cysteine or a derivative may interfere with an enzyme involved in an oxidative process essential for the synthesis of cephalosporin C (TROONEN et al. 1976). However, the lack of production of a cephalosporin with the new side chain is more probably due to the narrow substrate specificity of the ring-expansion enzyme (KOHSAKA and DEMAIN 1976).

Two mutant strains of the Merck patented strain of *S. cattleya* NRRL 8507, were reported to produce the *N*-acetyl and deshydroxycarbapenems related to thienamycin (ROSI et al. 1981). One of the mutants, SWRI-M459, produced an *N*-acetyl carbapenem corresponding to *N*-acetylthienamycin. The second mutant, S-WRI-M5301, produced a deshydroxy analog thienamycin corresponding to NS-5 (deshydroxythienamycin). The Sterling–Winthrop report is the first report of the use of mutant strains to produce thienamycin analogs. The mutants may also prove to be important in the eventual elucidation of the biosynthetic pathway for the thienamycin class of β-lactam antibiotics and, possibly, the determination of the pathways for related carbapenem antibiotics.

D. Actinomycetes Producing New β-Lactam Antibiotics

I. Cephamycins (7-Methoxycephalosporins)

The observation that a *Streptomyces* species was capable of producing penicillin N indicated the possibility of the production of β-lactam antibiotics by microorganisms belonging to the *Actinomycetales* (MILLER et al. 1962; HIGGENS et al. 1974). In 1971, the screening for new antibiotic substances at the Lilly Research

Table 6. Natural 7-methoxy cephem compounds

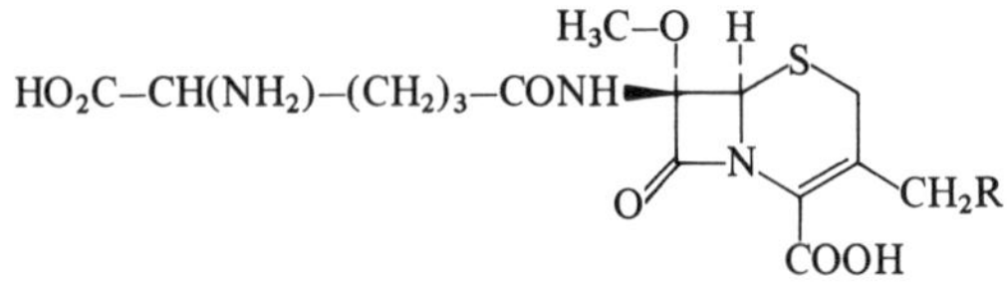

Compound	R	Reference
Cephamycin C (A–16886 B)	$-OCONH_2$	NAGARAJAN et al. (1971) STAPLEY et al. (1972)
A–16886 A	$-OCOCH_3$	NAGARAJAN et al. (1971)
Cephamycin A	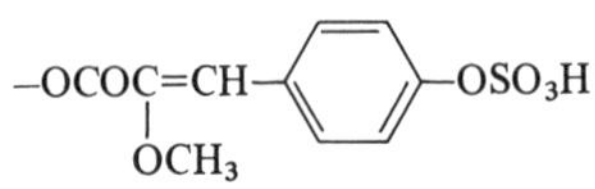	STAPLEY et al. (1972)
Cephamycin B	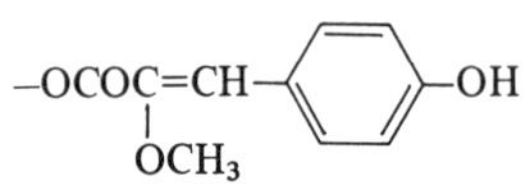	STAPLEY et al. (1972)
C–2801 X	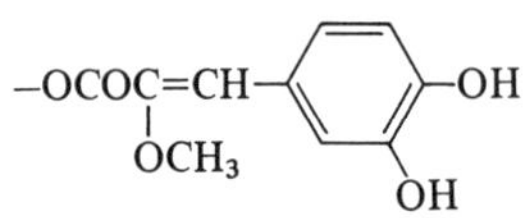	Jap. Patent 50–53594
SF–1623	$-S-SO_3H$	Jap. Patent 50–82291
WS–3442D	–H	Jap. Patent 49–26488

Laboratories resulted in the discovery of three new β-lactam antibiotics produced by two species of *Streptomyces* (HIGGENS et al. 1974). *Streptomyces lipmanii* produced AO16884, 7-(5-amino-5-carboxyvaleramido)-7-methoxycephalosporanic acid. A new species *S. clavuligerus* (HIGGENS and KASTNER 1971) yielded two β-lactam antibiotics, A-16886 A and A-16886 B, 7-(5-amino-5-carboxyvaleramido)-3-carbamoyloxymethyl-3-cephem-4-carboxylic acid, and 7-(5-amino-5-carboxy-valeramido)-7-methoxy-3-carbamoyloxymethyl-3-cephem-4- carboxylic acid (Table 6). Simultaneously, scientists at the Merck Research Laboratories reported a new family of 7-methoxycephem antibiotics (STAPLEY et al. 1972) which they called cephamycins, from several species of *Streptomyces*. Cephamycins A and B were first discovered in the fermentation broths of *S. griseus*. Cephamycin C, which was later found to be identical to A-16886 B, was produced by a new species, *Streptomyces lactamdurans*, now classified as *Nocardia lactamdurans*. Strains of *Streptomyces* producing cephamycins were collected from various soil samples; most of them produced both cephamycins A and B. Only a single strain produced cephamycin C among 27 cephamycin producers belonging to eight species.

In 1975, another member of cephamycin group, C-2801 X was found to be produced by two new species, *Streptomyces heteromorphus* and *Streptomyces panayensis* by HASEGAWA et al. (Japanese Patent 50-53594). C-2801 X is closely related to cephamycin B in its chemical structure, but has an additional hydroxy function at the aromatic moiety of cephamycin B. Researchers at the Fujisawa Pharmaceutical Co. reported the production of 7-methoxycephem antibiotics from a new species, *Streptomyces wadayaensis* (Japanese Patent 49-26488). A strain of *Streptomyces chartreusis* has been found also to produce an antibiotic of the cephamycin group (Japanese Patent 50-82291).

1. Cephamycin Fermentations

The fermentation of 7-methoxycephalosporin antibiotics by *S. lipmanii* and *S. clavuligerus* has been described (NAGARAJAN 1972).

For the production of cephamycins A and B (STAPLEY et al. 1972) a seed culture of *S. griseus* NRRL 3851 was developed in a medium having the following composition: beef extract, 3.0 g; N-Z amine, 10 g; NaCl, 5.0 g; and distilled water, 1,000 ml. Development of media used for the fermentation is shown in Table 7. The production of cephamycins A and B in media A, B, and C was 9 μg/ml, 13 μg/ml, and 50 μg/ml, respectively. The screening of superior natural variants resulted in the production of cephamycins A and B at a concentration of 130–170 μg/ml in medium C. The inoculum for *N. lactamdurans* NRRL 3802 for the production of cephamycin C was developed in a medium composed as follows: peptone (Aradmine), 10 g; dextrose, 10 g; $MgSO_4 \cdot 7H_2)$, 0.05 g; phosphate buffer, 2.0 ml (KH_2PO_4, 91.0 g; Na_2HPO_4, 95.0 g; water, 1,000 ml; pH 7.0; and distilled water, 1,000 ml; the pH was adjusted to 6.5. The maximum activity, obtained after 5 days of incubation in medium E, was 20 μg/ml. The strain propagated in medium F yielded a potency of 50 μg/ml. Medium F with dextrose omitted (medium G) resulted in potency increase to 110 μg/ml. The transfer of cultures through multiple stages of seed development in the seed medium resulted in a reduction of titer. This was corrected by the use of medium G in all stages of inoculum development, where multiple seed build-up was required in large-scale fermentation.

In the production of SF-1623 at the Meiji Research Laboratories (Japanese Patent 50-82291), a seed culture of *S. chartreusis* SF-1623 was developed in a medium (500 ml) which consisted of: sucrose, 10 g; soy bean meal, 30 g; water, 1 liter (pH adjusted to 7.0) at 28 °C for 24 h. The contents of inoculum culture were transferred to second-stage seed culture (20 liters) in a stainless-steel fermentor and incubated for 20 h. The seed was used to inoculate a fermentation medium (200 liters) having the following composition: glycerol, 1.5%; dextrin, 1.5%; soy bean meal, 2.0%; $CaCO_3$, 0.15%; sodium thiosulfate, 0.05% (pH 7.0). The fermentation was carried out at 28 °C. At 24 and 28 h, a sterile solution of sodium thiosulfate was added at concentrations of 0.15% and 0.2%, respectively. After 72 h, a potency of 80 μg/ml was obtained.

For the production of C-2801 X, a seed culture of *S. heteromorphus* was developed in a medium composed of: glucose, 2%; soluble starch, 3%; corn-steep liquor, 1%; soy bean meal, 1%; peptone, 0.5%; $CaCO_3$, 0.5% (pH 7.0, 500 ml in 2-liter flasks) at 20 °C for 40 h. The biomass was used to inoculate 30 liters of a

Table 7. Fermentation media used for the production of cephamycins

Component	Amount
Medium A (pH 7.0)	
N – Z amine	2.5 g
Beef extract	1.0 g
NaCl	5.0 g
Soybean meal	10.0 g
Distiller's solubles	2.0 g
Corn-steep liquor (wet)	5.0 g
Dextrose	20.0 g
K_2HPO_4	2.0 g
$CaCO_3$	10.0 g
Distilled water	1,000 ml
Medium B (pH 7.2)	
Dextrose	10.0 g
L-Asparagine	1.0 g
K_2HPO_4	0.1 g
$MgSO_4$, $7H_2O$	0.5 g
Yeast extract	0.5 g
Trace element mix	10 ml
Distilled water	1,000 ml

Component	Amount
Medium C (pH 7.0)	
Corn-steep liquor (wet)	40.0 g
Dextrose	20.0 g
NaCl	2.5 g
$MgSO_4$, $7H_2O$	0.5 g
Polyglycol 2000	0.25% (v/v)
Distilled water	1,000 ml
Medium D (pH 7.1)	
L-Proline	15.0 g
Glycerol	20.0 g
Sucrose	2.5 g
Na-glutamate	1.5 g
NaCl	5.0 g
K_2HPO_4	2.0 g
$CaCl_2$	0.4 g
$MnCl_2$, $4H_2O$	0.1 g
$FeCl_3$, $6H_2O$	0.1 g
$ZnCl_2$	0.05 g
$MgSO_4$, $7H_2O$	1.0 g
Distilled water	1,000 ml

Component	Amount
Medium E (pH 7.0)	
Soybean meal	30.0 g
Distiller's solubles	7.5 g
Dextrose	20.0 g
NaCl	2.5 g
$CaCO_3$	10.0 g
Distilled water	1,000 ml
Medium F (pH 7.0)	
Amber BYF 300 yeast	10.0 g
Distiller's solubles	20.0 g
Dextrose	10.0 g
Distilled water	1,000 ml
Medium G (pH 7.0)	
Amber BYF 300 yeast	10.0 g
Distiller's solubles	20.0 g
Distilled water	1,000 ml

seed medium in a 50-liter stainless-steel fermentor. The second-stage seed culture was carried out at 28 °C with agitation at 280 rpm and an airflow of 1 vol/vol per minute for 25 h. The growth (10 liters) was transferred to a fermentor containing a medium which consisted of: sucrose, 3%; cotton seed meal (Proflo), 2%; corn-steep liquor, 1%; $FeSO_4$, 0.05%; K_2HPO_4, 0.05%; NaCl, 0.3%; $CaCO_3$, 0.5% (pH 7.0, 100 liters medium in 200-liter fermentor). The fermentation was carried out at 28 °C with an agitation rate of 200 rpm and an airflow rate of 1 vol/vol per minute for 66 h until a maximal potency was obtained. In the case of *S. panayensis*, the same procedure was employed. The peak activity was obtained at 54–66 h.

In the production of WS 3442 D (Japanese Patent 49-26488), a medium composed of: glycerin, 3%; soy bean meal, 2%, gluten meal, 1%; cotton seed meal, 1%, D,L-methionine, 0.2%, was used for the first- and second-stage seeds and also in the fermentation stage.

2. Improvement in Strains of Nocardia lactamdurans

Two methods of genetic recombination have been employed for strain improvement in a cephamycin-producing strain of *N. lactamdurans*, formerly classified as *Streptomyces lactamdurans* by scientists at Merck (Wesseling and Lago 1981). In the first method, protoplast fusion of two diverged mutant lines yielded a recombinant strain which produced 12% more cephamycin C than the parental strains. The improvement obtained was near that expected for the sum of the two mutations. The Merck workers also reported the intergeneric recombination between another cephamycin organism, *S. griseus*, and *N. lactamdurans*. Biochemical mutants of the above two strains producing cephamycins were mated and a recombinant was isolated which produced 8% more cephamycin C than the wild type *N. lactamdurans* grandparent.

II. Nocardicins

The excellent antibacterial activity and the low toxicity of β-lactam antibiotics derived from penicillin and cephalosporin nuclei has prompted researchers, especially in pharmaceutical companies, to undertake screening programs directed toward the discovery of new β-lactam antibiotics. In the Fujisawa Pharmaceutical Company, a screening program using β-lactam-supersensitive mutants (Aoki et al. 1977) has resulted in detection of novel β-lactams in the fermentation broths of an actinomycete (Aoki et al. 1976). The antibiotics, called nocardicins, proved to be monocyclic β-lactam compounds. The culture producing nocardicins was isolated from a soil sample collected at Tsuyama City, Okayama Prefecture, Japan. Taxonomic studies on the strain showed that it belonged to the genus *Nocardia* and that it closely resembles *N. uniformis*, although some minor differences were observed between the characteristics of the strain and the described properties of *N. uniformis*. The strain has been designated *N. uniformis* subsp. *tsuyamanensis* and has been deposited in the American Type Culture Collection, Rockville, Maryland as ATCC 21806.

Another culture producing nocardicin A has been isolated from a soil sample collected in Tokyo, Japan (Iguchi et al., unpublished work). The isolate was characterized by its growth on media in high pH range (pH 9.5–10.0) and its inability to grow in neutral pH range (pH 6.5–7.0). Taxonomic studies have shown that the strain resembles *Streptomyces flavovirens*, *Streptomyces atroolivaceus*, *S. fluvoviridis*, and *S. flavogriseus* in its properties except for its alkalophilic character. Close examination showed, however, that the strain was distinct from any of them in several morphological and/or physiological characteristics and it has been designated *Streptomyces alcalophilus* sp. nov.

1. Strain Improvement

Two major problems were encountered during the initial stages of strain improvement with *N. uniformis* subsp. *tsuyamanensis*. First, their organism was found to be sensitive to β-lactam antibiotics including nocardicin A, which was the product of the strain itself. When 2 mg/ml nocardicin was added at various times to the culture of a descendant of the wild isolate, strain no. 1923, its growth was completely inhibited (Fig. 5). The cells were fragmented and lysed when observed microscopically. A strain improvement program was initiated for the selection of mutants which were able to form colonies on agar plates containing varying concentrations of nocardicin A. Mutagenic treatment with NTG or UV radiation was employed and mutants resistant to nocardicin A in varying degrees were obtained (Fig. 6).

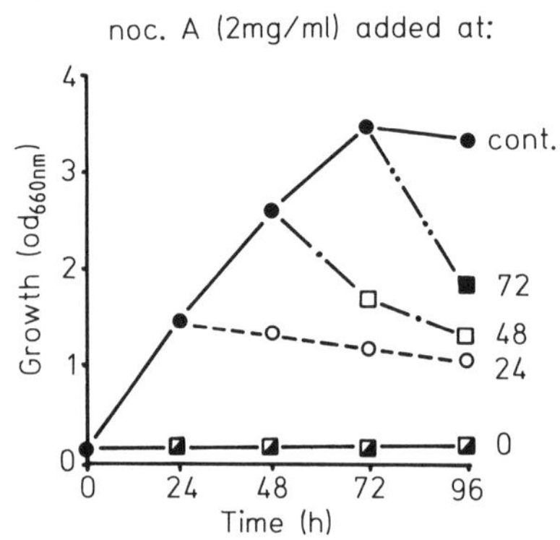

Fig. 5. The effect of exogenous nocardicin A on the growth of *N. uniformis* strain 1923

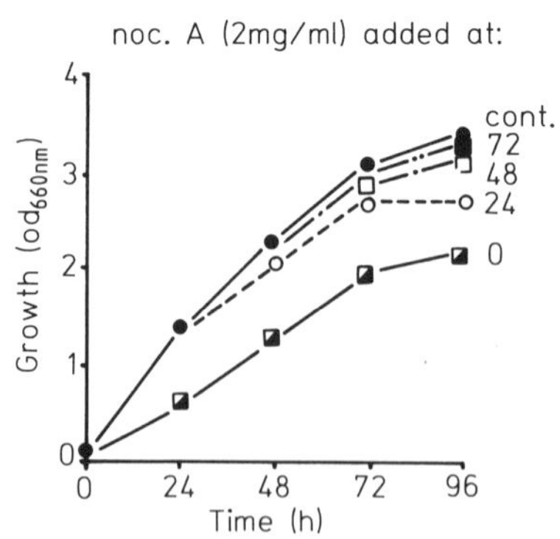

Fig. 6. The effect of exogenous nocardicin A on the growth of *N. uniformis* mutant strain No. 7649

Another problem encountered was β-lactamase production by the producing organism, which destroyed nocardicin A as well as other β-lactam antibiotics upon formation (Table 8). The β-lactamase was secreted into the culture medium. Among nocardicin A–resistant mutants, strains with decreased β-lactamase activity were frequently observed (Fig. 7). Thus, the next step in strain improvement ef-

Table 8. Degradation of various β-lactam antibiotics by an enzyme from *N. uniformis* subsp. *tsuyamanensis* no. 926. (H. Aoki 1980, personal communication)

Substrate	Relative rate of degradation (%)
Penicillin G	100
Ampicillin	116
Carbenicillin	23
6-APA	6
Dicloxacillin	0
Cephalosporin C	7
Cephaloridine	52
Cephalothin	18
Cephalexin	2
Cefazolin	12
7-ACA	2
Nocardicin A	0.5

Reaction conditions:
Concentration of substrate: 5 μmol/ml,
pH 7.0 (0.1 M phosphate buffer), 37 °C, 2 h

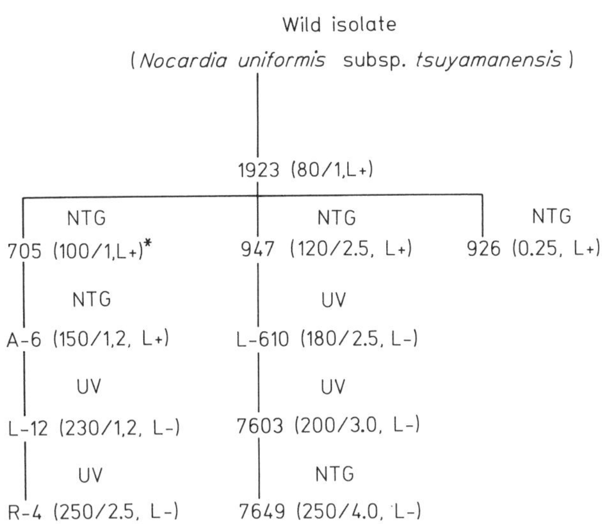

* The figures in parentheses are production in units/ml, resistance to nocardicin A in mg/ml, and presence (L+) or absence (L−) of β-lactamase

Fig. 7. The lineage of nocardicin A-producing strains

Table 9. Enrichment of strains with improved productivity following selection of nocardicin A-resistant mutants. (H. AOKI 1980, personal communication)

	Frequency of occurrence (%)		
	Productivity (% of parent's potency)		
	<50	50–130	>130
Isolates from normal agar plate	2.6	96.7	0.7
Isolates from agar plates containing 2.5 mg/ml nocardicin A	17.3	78.5	4.2

forts was to screen β-lactamase-negative mutants from among the nocardicin A-resistant strains. A simple method was devised for the detection of β-lactamase production. Mutagen-treated spore populations were plated on an agar medium. Soft agar, containing a dilution of a culture of *Staphylococcus aureus* 209P and penicillin G (10 μg/ml), was overlayed and the plates were incubated at 37 °C for 18 h. A growth zone of *Staphylococcus* cells appeared around the colonies which produced β-lactamase, which decomposed penicillin G. β-Lactamase-negative mutants were screened as colonies which did not show a detectable growth zone around them. Stable isolates were chosen from the β-lactamase-negative mutants. Once the productivity of β-lactamase was lost, the resulting sensitivity of the nocardicin-producer to nocardicin A proved to be a practical technique for the selection of superior mutants. The frequency of appearance of variants superior to the parent in nocardicin A productivity was higher when the mutagen-tested spores were plated and colonies were selected on a medium containing nocardicin A at a concentration which inhibited growth of the parent strain (Table 9).

2. Nocardicin A Fermentation

The nocardicin fermentation followed a general pattern in that a spore suspension prepared on agar slants with a medium listed in Table 10 was used to inoculate seed flasks (Japanese Patent 52-64494). The seed culture was transferred to fermentation flasks or stainless steel fermentors containing media also shown in Table 10. Fermentations with strain R-4 in medium I resulted in the production of nocardicin A at a concentration of 110 μg/ml. Close examination of the chemical structure of nocardicin A suggested the possible involvement of several amino acids, including tyrosine, glycine, serine, and homoserine as precursors of the antibiotic. Both D- and L-tyrosine, and several substances related to tyrosine metabolism, were examined for their effect on nocardicin production. They showed a marked stimulatory effect on nocardicin production (Japanese Patent 52-64494; HOSODA et al. 1977; Table 11). The addition of glycine, alanine, serine, homoserine, and related substances showed stimulatory effects when added with tyrosine to the medium, although they had no effect when added alone (Table 12). Evaluation of various formulas resulted in the selection of media II and III. The titer in these me-

Table 10. Media used for the production of nocardicin A. (H. AOKI 1980, personal communication)

Component	Amount	Component	Amount
Seed medium		Medium II	
Sucrose	20.0 g	Soluble starch	10.0 g
Cotton seed meal	20.0 g	Glucose	5.0 g
Dried yeast	10.0 g	Yeast extract	2.0 g
KH_2PO_4	2.18 g	Peptone	10.0 g
$Na_2HPO_4 \cdot 12H_2O$	1.43 g	Ca-pantothenate	0.2 g
Water	1,000 ml	KH_2PO_4	18.0 g
pH 6.0		$Na_2HPO_4 \cdot 12H_2O$	12.0 g
		$MgSO_4 \cdot 7H_2O$	5.0 g
Medium I		Water	1,000 ml
Soluble starch	20.0 g	pH 6.0	
Yeast extract	4.0 g		
K_2HPO_4	3.5 g	Medium III	
$Na_2HPO_4 \cdot 12H_2O$	1.5 g	Starch	10.0 g
$MgSO_4 \cdot 7H_2O$	1.0 g	Cotton seed meal	20.0 g
Water	1,000 ml	Dried yeast	20.0 g
pH 6.0		KH_2PO_4	21.8 g
		$Na_2HPO_4 \cdot 12H_2O$	14.3 g
		$MgSO_4 \cdot 7H_2O$	5.0 g
		Water	1,000 ml
		pH 6.0	

Table 11. The effect of tyrosine and related substances on production of nocardicin A. (H. AOKI 1980, personal communication)

Compound [a]	Amount (μg/ml)	Nocardicin A (μg/ml)
L-Tyrosine	200	310
	300	310
D-Tyrosine	200	365
	300	410
p-Hydroxyphenyl-pyruvic acid	200	180
	300	200
p-Hydroxyphenyl-glycolic acid	100	170
	200	220
p-Hydroxyphenyl-glyoxalic acid	100	345
	200	340
L-*p*-Hydroxyphenyl-glycine	200	330
	300	440
Shikimic acid	200	200
	300	260
Control	–	110

[a] Test samples were added to medium I. After 144 h of fermentation at 30 °C, the potency of nocardicin A in fermentation broth was measured

Table 12. The effect of the addition of amino acids on the production of nocardicin A. (H. AOKI 1980, personal communication)

Compound[a]	Nocardicin A titer (μg/ml)	
	Medium I	Medium I + L-Tyr. (300 μg/ml)
Glycine	170	525
L-Alanine	170	470
L-Serine	155	490
L-Homoserine	160	440
D,L-α-Aminobutyric acid	180	525
L-α,β-Diaminopropionic acid	180	455
Control	160	310

[a] Test compound was added at the concentration of 600 μg/ml in medium I

Table 13. The effect of the addition of tyrosine and glycine on the production of nocardicin A. (H. AOKI 1980, personal communication)

L-Tyrosine (μg/ml)	Glycine (μg/ml)	Nocardicin A titer (μg/ml)
0	0	540
0	1,000	550
0	2,000	530
1,000	0	900
1,000	1,000	950
1,000	2,000	1,000
2,000	0	930
2,000	1,000	1,000
2,000	2,000	1,200
3,000	0	950
3,000	1,000	1,000
3,000	2,000	1,100

L-Tyrosine and glycine were added to medium III

dia were 400 and 500 μg/ml, respectively. The combination of tyrosine and glycine in medium III resulted in an increased production of nocardicin A (Table 13).

During the investigation of the chemical structure of nocardicin A, hydrogenation of the antibiotic was carried out to yield reduced nocardicin A (HASHIMOTO et al. 1976). The structure of this compound has been established (Table 3) and the compound was designated nocardicin C. Nocardicin C showed extremely low antibacterial activity even against β-lactam-supersensitive mutants used for detection of nocardicin A (AOKI et al. 1977). Mutants were developed from *Pseudomonas aeruginosa* NCTC 10490, selected in vitro for their high sensitivity to nocardicin C which was prepared chemically. By the use of one of these mutants, Ps-III, two antibacterial spots were observed on thin-layer chromatography of crude nocardicin A crystals. The compound that was active only on Ps-III was separated, isolated, and designated nocardicin B (KURITA et al. 1976). Later, nocardicin B was found to be an anti-isomer of nocardicin A at the oxime function (HASHIMOTO et al. 1976). Using the sensitive mutant, Ps-III, a search was carried out for minor components which might be present in the fermentation broths of a strain of *N. uniformis* subsp. *tsuyamanensis* improved for nocardicin A production. A bioautogram of a thin-layer chromatogram of the concentrated filtrate revealed seven spots having Ps-III activity including those of nocardicin A and B. Each of the five new compounds were isolated and their structures have been established (HOSODA et al. 1977). Nocardicin C and D have been identified as the amino and keto derivatives of nocardicin A. Nocardicin E and F are also steroisomers of each other at the oxime function, E having syn- and F having anti-configuration. Nocardicin G has been found to be an amino derivative of nocardicin E (Fig. 2). The production of nocardicin C and D is low (0.19 mg/liter and 10 mg/liter, respectively) and nocardicin E and F are produced in slightly higher concentrations (0.55 mg/liter, 3.33 mg/liter, respectively), although a precise determination of the production was not made. Some mutants of a nocardicin A–producing strain showed high production of nocardicin G (ELANDER and AOKI, 1982).

III. Clavulanic Acid

The clavulanic acid–producing strain *Streptomyces clavuligerus* ATTC 27064 was reported to produce several β-lactam compounds, including cephamycin C, deacetoxycephalosporin C, and penicillin N (READING and COLE 1977). The organism was grown on an agar medium having the following composition: yeast extract, 10 g; glucose, 10 g; Oxoid agar No. 3, 20 g; water, 1,000 ml (pH 6.8) at 26 °C. It was used to inoculate a seed-stage medium which consisted of: Oxoid malt extract, 10 g; Oxoid bacteriological peptone, 10 g; glycerol, 20 g; tap water, 1,000 ml; pH was adjusted to 7.0 with a sodium hydroxide solution. The flasks were incubated for 3 days at 26 °C. The fermentation stage consisted of flasks containing DAS medium having the following composition: dextrin, 20 g; Araksoy 50 soybean flour, 10 g; Scotasol dried distillers solubles, 1 g; $FeSO_4 \cdot 7H_2O$, 0.1 g; distilled water, 1,000 ml (pH 7.0). The seed and fermentation flasks (500 ml) contained 100 ml medium and were incubated at 26 °C on a rotary shaker operating with 2-inch throw and agitation rate of 240 rpm. Fermentations in large-scale fermentors were also carried out using the DAS medium with antifoam added before sterilization. Growth from an agar slant in a Roux bottle (10 days at 26 °C) was scraped into 100 ml 0.05% Triton X-100 aqueous solution and used to inoculate 50 liters of medium in a stainless-steel fermentor (90 liters, baffled). The seed fermentor was agitated by a disc turbine impeller at 240 rpm, and aerated at 50 liters/min at 26 °C. After 72 h, the seed culture was used to provide 5% vegetative inoculum into 150 liters of DAS medium contained in a 300-liter baffled fermentor. The fermentor was agitated at 210 rpm and aerated at 150 liters/min at 26 °C for 4 days, by which time the clavulanic acid titer ranged from 150 to 200 μg/ml.

IV. Hydroxyethylclavam

Hydroxyethylclavam, a novel antifungal β-lactam antibiotic, was isolated from *Streptomyces antibioticus* subsp. *antibioticus*. It is structurally related to clavulanic acid and it shows good activity against gram-positive and gram-negative bacteria on defined medium and has a broad spectrum against fungi. The antibacterial activity can be antagonized by methionine, homocysteine, and cystathionine. The antibiotic is stable to β-lactamases and has no β-lactamase inhibitory effect. Its structure is shown in Table 3 (KRONE et al. 1981).

V. Thienamycin

Thienamycin (Table 3) is produced in the fermentation broth of *Streptomyces cattleya* as a component of a complex of β-lactam antibiotics, including penicillin N, cephamycin C, and *N*-acetylthienamycin (KAHAN et al. 1976, 1979; STAPLEY et al. 1977). A 250-ml baffled flask containing 50 ml seed medium was inoculated with a lyophilized culture, slant or frozen vial of *S. cattleya* NRRL 8057 and incubated at 28 °C for 24 h on a rotary shaker at 160 rpm. The seed medium consisted of: yeast autolysate, 10 g; glucose, 10 g; KH_2PO_4, 182 mg; Na_2HPO_4, 190 mg; $MgSO_4 \cdot 7H_20$, 50 mg; distilled water, 1,000 ml (pH 6.5). The seed culture was used to inoculate, at a ratio of 1:50, five 2-liter baffled flasks containing 500 ml seed medium. After 24 h of incubation, the growth was added at a ratio of 1:500 to 467 liters of medium in a 756-liter stainless-steel fermentor. This tank was operated for 24 h at 28 °C with an agitation of 130 rpm and an airflow rate of 0.3 m^3/min. After 24 h, 453 liters of the growth was transferred to a 5,670-liter fermentor containing 4,082 liters of production medium. The medium had the following composition: cerelose, 25 g; corn-steep liquor, 15 g; distiller's solubles, 10 g; cotton seed meal, 5 g; $CoCl_2 \cdot 6H_2O$, 10 mg; tap water, 1,000 ml. After adjustment of pH to 7.3, $CaCO_3$ (3 g/liter) and Polyglycol 2,000 (2.5 ml/liter) were added. The tank was operated at 24 °C with an agitation rate of 70 rpm and an airflow rate of 1.54 m^3/min. The peak thienamycin levels were 1–4 μg/ml with the original strain of *S. cattleya.*

VI. Olivanic Acids

The olivanic acid family is produced by *S. olivaceus* ATCC 21379 (BUTTERWORTH et al. 1979). The culture was grown in a glucose-yeast extract agar medium for 7 days at 28 °C. Seed and production fermentations were carried out in 500-ml flasks containing 100 ml media and incubated at 28 °C on a rotary shaker at 240 rpm, with a 50-mm throw. The seed stage was incubated for 48 h and the final fermentation was incubated for 48–72 h. Pilot-scale fermentations were carried out in baffled stirred tanks containing 50 liters of medium and inoculated with 2.5 liters of seed biomass. The fermentations were carried out with an aeration rate of 1.0 vol/vol per minute. β-Lactamase-inhibitor activity was observed in media A and C (Table 14). The results indicated that a relatively low nitrogen content and a high C:N ratio were required. Evaluation of medium components resulted in the selection of media consisting of 1% soy bean flour and 2% glucose. Addition of trace amounts of cobalt chloride (0.05–1.0 mg/liter) stimulated the production of olivanic acid complex remarkably. The addition of calcium carbonate (0.02%) and sodium sulfate (0.05%) to the medium also resulted in some increase in the production titer. In fermentations with the optimum medium, the olivanic acid complex

Table 14. Media used for the production of olivanic acids. (H. Aoki 1980, personal communication)

Component	Amount	Component	Amount
Medium A		Medium C	
Glucose	25.0 g	Glucose	20.0 g
Soybean flour	40.0 g	$NaNO_3$	4.0 g
Distiller's solubles	5.0 g	Malt extract	20.0 g
NaCl	2.5 g	Water	1,000 ml
Water	1,000 ml	pH 7.3	
pH 7.5		Medium D	
Medium B		Glucose	10.0 g
Glucose	20.0 g	Egg albumin	0.5 g
Yeast extract (paste)	4.0 g	K_2HPO_4	0.5 g
Malt extract (paste)	10.0 g	$MgSO_4 \cdot 7H_2O$	0.2 g
Water	1,000 ml	$Fe_2(SO_4)_3$	0.05 g
pH 7.3		Water	1,000 ml
		pH 7.3	

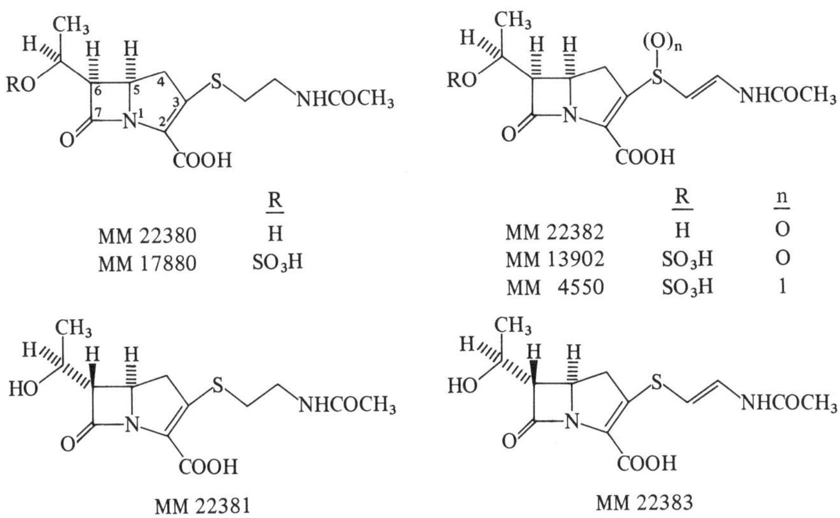

Fig. 8. Structures of new olivanic acids produced in fermentation

reached a maximum titer at approximately 40 h. Several new olivanic acid components have been recently reported by Box et al. (1979) and they appear to be isomers of previously reported structures (Fig. 8).

VII. PS-5 and Related Carbapenems

An antibiotic of the desthia-carbapenem family, PS-5, was reported to be produced in fermentation broths of *Streptomyces cremeus* subsp. *auratilis* ATCC 31358 and

Table 15. Media used for the production of PS-5

Component	Content
Seed medium	
Beef extract (Difco)	0.3%
Bacto-tryptone (Difco)	0.5%
Defatted soybean meal	0.5%
Glucose	0.1%
Soluble starch	2.4%
Yeast extract	0.5%
$CaCO_3$	0.4%
pH 7.5	
Production medium (ML – 19M2)	
Glycerol	4.0%
Peptone	0.5%
Glucose	0.2%
Potato starch	0.2%
Defatted soybean meal	2.5%
Dry yeast	0.5%
NaCl	0.5%
$CaCO_3$	0.2%
pH 6.4	

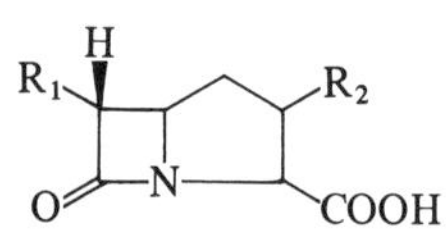

	R_1	R_2
Thienamycin	$-CH(OH)CH_3$	$-S-CH_2-CH_2-NH_2$
PS–4	$-CH(OH)CH_3$	$-S-CH=CH-NH-COCH_3$
PS–5	$-CH_2-CH_3$	$-S-CH_2-CH_2-NH-COCH_3$
PS–6	$-CH(CH_3)CH_3$	$-S-CH_2-CH_2-NH-COCH_3$
PS–7	$-CH_2-CH_3$	$-S-CH=CH-NH-COCH_3$

Fig. 9. Structures of new PS-5 antibiotics in fermentation broths of *Streptomyces cremeus* subsp. *auratilis* (Japanese Patent 54-154598)

Streptomyces fluvoviridis (OKAMURA et al. 1979a, b). These organisms were isolated from soil samples treated in repeated moistening–drying cycles for 1–2 months (OKAMURA et al. 1979b).

For the production of PS-5 by *S. cremeus* subsp. *auratilis*, growth from the seed culture incubated in 500-ml flasks for 48 h on a rotary shaker was used to inoculate 15 liters of seed medium in a 30-liter jar fermentor. The fermentor was operated at 28 °C with an agitation rate of 200 rpm and an airflow rate of 0.5 vol/vol per minute for 24 h. One liter of the culture was transferred to 100 liters of production medium (Table 15) in a 200-liter fermentor. The fermentor was operated at 28 °C with agitation at 200 rpm and an airflow of 0.5 vol/vol per minute for 72 h. PS-5 production was stimulated by the addition of vitamin B_{12} to the fermentation medium. Recently, several new PS-5 derivatives have been reported in fermentation broths of *S. cremeus* subsp. *auratilis* (Fig. 9).

VIII. C-19393 S_2 and H_2

Two new carbapenem antibiotics, C-19393 S_2 and H_2, were recently isolated by scientists at Takeda Chemical Industries Ltd. (IMADA et al. 1980). The producing organism has been classified as *Streptomyces griseus* subsp. *cryophilus* and was isolated from a soil sample collected in Sweden. The organism is related toxomically to *S. griseus* in its gross cultural characteristics and spore chain morphology. It differs from the described species of *S. griseus* listed in Bergey's Manual, 8th Edition, by its inability to use D-mannitol and to grow at 37 °C, the optimal growth temperature for *S. griseus*. The Takeda C-19393 strain had the remarkable capability of growing at 4 °C, a property not shared by 13 other strains of *S. griseus* including the type strain ISP 5236. On the basis of its capacity to grow at 4 °C, the Takeda workers named the C-19393 strain *S. griseus* subsp. *cryophilus* (IFO 13886). The growth temperature range for the C-19393 strain is 4°–36 °C and the optimal temperature range for sporulation is 21°–24 °C. The organism is propagated on "T" agar medium, which is a concoction of tomato paste, oatmeal, and an edible beef extract. Sporulation is abundant at 7 days of incubation at 24 °C (IMADA et al. 1980). The seed medium used by Takeda for the C-19393 fermentation contained, in grams/liter: glucose, 20; soluble starch, 30; soy bean flour, 10; corn-steep liquor, 10; polypeptone, 5; NaCl, 3; and $CaCO_3$, 5. The fermentation medium had the following composition, in grams/liter: glucose, 30; soluble starch, 30; soy bean meal, 15; cotton seed meal, 15; K_2HOP_4, 0.25; $CoCl_2$, 0.002; and Actol antifoam (Takeda Chemical Ind.), 0.5. The pH of both the seed and fermentation media was adjusted to pH 7.0 with 2 N NaOH prior to sterilization.

The addition of $CoCl_2$ stimulated the production of the C-19393 antibiotics and the $CoCl_2$ could be replaced by the addition of vitamin B_{12}. The optimal concentration of $CoCl_2$ was between 0.3 and 20 μg/ml. The following protocol was used for pilot-scale fermentations in 2,000-liter stainless-steel fermentors. Spores from slants propagated on "T" agar for 7 days were added to 500 ml seed medium in a 2-liter Sakaguchi flask which was shaken at 28 °C for 48 h on a reciprocating shaker. The seed culture was then transferred into 30 liters of seed medium contained in a 50-liter fermentor and agitated (280 rpm) and sparged (30 liters/min) for 48 h at 28 °C. The fermentation stage was carried out in a 2,000-liter stainless-steel fermentor containing 1,200 liters of fermentation medium. The fermentation was carried out for 5 days at 30 °C with an aeration rate of 840 liters/min and an agitation rate of 180 rpm.

The assay procedure for determining the concentration of the stable C-19393 antibiotics employed mutants of *Escherichia coli* lacking chromosomal β-lactamase and penicillin-binding protein 1 B. The β-lactamase inhibitor activity using *Klebsiella pneumoniae* has been described by BROWN et al. (1976).

Structurally, the antibiotics produced by the C-19393 are two new species of carbapenems designated S_2 and H_2. The structures are shown in Table 3. The C-19393 strain also elaborates in active fermentation a variety of other β-lactam antibiotics including penicillin N, epithienamycins, and olivanic acid derivatives (HOSODA et al. 1977). The S_2 and H_2 compounds possess a broad antimicrobial spectrum, are resistant to a variety of β-lactamase enzyme and are relatively stable in aqueous solution. The H_2 component is more stable than cephalosporin C in aqueous solution. The C-19393 S_2 and H_2 antibiotics also have synergistic effects with other β-lactam antibiotics including ampicillin and cefotiam against β-lactamase-producing strains of bacteria (IMADA et al. 1980).

IX. Carpetimycins

Carpetimycins A and B are two recent carbapenem antibiotics related to thienamycin, olivanic acid derivatives, and the PS-5 class of antibiotics. The chemical determination of the two compounds indicated a new class of carbapenem antibiotics, which are shown in Table 3. They possess *cis*-oriented β-lactam protons similar to those present in the penams and cephams and they are characterized by an α-hydroxypropyl group on the β-lactam ring and a sulfoxide function having an *R*-configuration. They are also stable entities in aqueous solution. The carpetimycins were discovered by scientists at the Kowa Company Ltd. (Japan) and are produced in the culture filtrates of *Streptomyces* sp. KC-6643 (NAKAYAMA et al. 1980).

The strain was cultured in an Erlenmeyer flask which contained 100 ml of a medium composed of starch, 3.6%; soy bean meal, 2.2%; cotton seed oil, 1.5%; $Na_2HPO_4 \cdot 12H_2O$, 0.62%; KH_2PO_4, 0, 0.1%; $MgSO_4 \cdot 7H_2O$, 0.05%; $FeSO_4 \cdot 7H_2O$, 0.001%; $CoCl_2 \cdot 6H_2O$, 0,0005%, on a rotary shaker at 29 °C for 72 h. Five-hundred milliliters of the culture broth was inoculated into 100 liters of the same medium in a 200-liter fermentor. The fermentation was carried out at 29 °C under an aeration rate of 100 liters/min, an agitation rate of 240 rpm, and a back pressure of 0.5 kg/cm^2.

E. Unicellular Bacteria Producing Sulfazecins and Related Structures

Scientists at the Takeda Chemical Industries have recently reported on the isolation of new species of *Pseudomonas* producing two novel monocyclic β-lactam antibiotics named sulfazecin and isosulfazecin (IMADA et al. 1981). The two *Pseudomonas* strains producing the novel monocyclic structures were isolated from soil suspensions on agar plates acidified to pH 4.5. All species of *Pseudomonas* heretofore described by DOUDOROFF and PALLERONI (1974) fail to grow at pH 4.0. The acidophilic pseudomonads selected at Takeda were categorized into taxonomic groups producing either sulfazecin or its isomer and were selected for their capability to synthesize β-lactam antibiotics using both selective and sensitive screening procedures. The procedures involved mutant strains of *P. aeruginosa*, PsC^{ss}, supersensitive to cephalothin (KITANO et al. 1976) and a strain of *E. coli* PG8 lacking chromosomal β-lactamase and the penicillin-binding protein PBP1B. The active broths of the pseudomonads elaborating the sulfazecins also induced the formation of spheroplasts and were slightly inactivated by β-lactamases.

The chemical structure of the antibiotic sulfazecin produced by the strain *Pseudomonas acidophila* G-6302 was determined to be 3 (*R*)-3- -D-glutamyl-D-alanylamino-3-methoxyazetin-2-one-1-sulphonic acid and was thus named because the sulphonic acid residue was structurally unique in its direct link to the nitrogen atom of the azetidin-2-one. Another structural feature of the molecule is the presence of a methoxyl group attached to the azetidine ring which is responsible for the β-lactamase resistance and a dipeptide side-chain composed of glutamic acid and alanine (Table 3). An optical isomer of sulfazecin was isolated from a related strain, *Pseudomonas mesoacidophila* strain SB-72310.

The Takeda workers reported that the 1-sulpho-2-oxaazetidinine moiety was essential for its antibacterial activity and its presence differentiated sulfazecin and its isomer from all known β-lactam antibiotics, including the monocyclic Fujisawa β-lactam nocardicin. They also emphasized that the unique sulphamate group ($-N \cdot SO_3H$) was rarely found in nature and the only naturally occurring natural products containing the sulphamate structure are heparin and its related *N*-sulphonated glycones.

The active fermentations of both strains producing sulfazecins were carried out in a 2,000-liter fermentor for 72 h at 28 °C. The fermentor contained a medium of the following composition: glycerol (3%); glucose (0.1%); sodium thiosulfate (0.1%); peptone (0.5%); meat extract (0.5%); NaCl (0.5%); and contained a total volume of 1,200 liters. The antibiotics were purified using activated charcoal, anion exchange resin, and Sephadex followed by crystallization as free acid from aqueous methanol.

The *Pseudomonas* strains producing the sulfazecins are polar-flagellated gram-negative rods, strictly aerobic, oxidase negative, and poly-β-hydroxybutyric acid accumulating, with no nutritional requirements. Arginine dihydrolase was found in strain SB-72310, but not in strain G-6302. The G–C content of the DNA was 64 mol% in strain G-6302 and 70 mol% in strain SB-72310. The two strains are also unique in their pH dependence for growth. Growth was poor at a pH of > 8.3 and > 8.9, respectively.

F. Maintenance and Long-Term Preservation of Strains of Penicillium chrysogenum and Acremonium chrysogenum

The preservation and long-term storage of fungal cultures with capability for producing constant high yields of desirable metabolites in large-scale production fermentations is of prime importance for a successful commercial fermentation process. Ideally, preservation procedures must provide conditions in which mutant strains are preserved for a long period of time free from phenotypic change with respect to high production capability of a particular metabolic product. During recent years the storage of fungi in the liquid or gas phase of liquid nitrogen appears to be the best currently available procedure (DAILY and HIGGENS 1973; PERLMAN and KIKUCHI 1977; WELLMAN and STEWART 1973; ELANDER 1978).

In my laboratories, the preferred procedure for preparing a fungal culture for the fermentation process consists of propagating a cell mass, either conidia, arthrospores, or vegetative mycelium, from a master source and dispensing a constant amount with or without substituting another menstruum for extracellular fluid, into a number of vials. The vials as a group are frozen either rapidly (in the lyophilization process) or at a sustained rate (under liquid nitrogen refrigeration). When inoculum is to be used, it is thawed rapidly in a water bath and propagated through as few stages as possible. Philosophically, we assume that the high-yielding fungal mutant is genetically mixed and inheritantly unstable. We have developed procedures which infuse a minimal stress on the culture during storage, or during any propagation step in the inoculum development process. We rely on plate counts for viability determinations and population patterns and laboratory productivity tests as judgement criteria for successful preservation. Herein is described the evolution of our experimental procedures and experimental data supporting our contention that liquid nitrogen preservation, when practical, is the currently best available preservation procedure for high productivity mutants of fungi producing penicillin and cephalosporin antibiotics.

Judgment criteria used for successful long-term preservation should cover the following parameters: percent recovery (viable units) after 6 months and 1 or more years of storage following initial preservation; uniformity in colony population pattern before and after preservation; and more importantly, stability of high antibiotic productivity in laboratory, pilot, and production-scale fermentations.

I. Studies with P. chrysogenum

A comparison of conidial viabilities of four Bristol production strains of *P. chrysogenum* following lyophilization, storage at −20 °C, or preservation in the vapor phase of liquid nitrogen (−167 °C) is presented in Table 16. The highest percent viabilities were indicated for storage under liquid nitrogen, where 100% viability was recorded. This increase is due to the probable breaking up of spore clumps upon exposure to the ultracold liquid nitrogen temperatures. Storage of conidia at liquid nitrogen temperatures also resulted in the least amount of change in colony population pattern following liquid nitrogen storage. Also, productivities in fermentation trials were maximal for liquid nitrogen preservation.

Storage of spores at −20 °C resulted in loss of 30% after storage for a 6-month period. The greatest change in colony population pattern was also observed when conidia of *P. chrysogenum* were stored at −20 °C. The numbers of variant-type colonies for two strains ranged from 9.4%–11.8%, respectively. Variant-type colonies types generally yield inferior penicillin productivity and this was depicted in actual fermentation trials. Fermentation productivity was decreased by 10% over that recorded for liquid nitrogen.

Table 16. Comparison of conidial viability following lyophilization, storage at −20 °C and liquid nitrogen storage (−167 °C) of *P. chrysogenum*

Strain	Storage condition	CFU[a] (× 10^6/ml)		% Via-bility	Change in colony popula-tion pattern (% variant type)	Relative pro-ductivity
		Before stg.[b]	After stg.			
3130-1L	Lyophilization	22	20	90.9	1.2	97.4
3168-1L	Lyophilization	13	14	77.7	3.8	96.8
4114-FS	Storage at − 20 °C	16	12.4	77.5	9.4	92.4
4130-FS	Storage at − 20 °C	28	20	71.4	11.4	94.5
3130-LN	Storage at −167 °C	24	28	116.6	0.2	104.5
3168-LN	Storage at −167 °C	18	19	105.5	0.09	99.4
4172-LN	Storage at −167 °C	16	15	93.8	1.8	108.9

[a] CFU, colory forming units
[b] stg., storage

Table 17. Survival of strains of *Penicillium chrysogenum*, *Streptomyces* and *Arthrobacter simplex* after prolonged storage (Squibb). (FORTNEY and THOMA 1977)

Process	Organism	Lyoph-ilized	Storage[a]		% Survival
			Temp. (°C)	Years	
Amphotericin	*S. nodosus* 3433	Yes	5, −40	11	0.93
Amphotericin	*S. nodosus* 6093	No	−100 to −200	4	100
Steroid	*A. simplex* 6157	Yes	−100 to −200	8	100
Steroid	*A. simplex* 3062	Yes	5, −40	13	4
Steroid	*A. simplex* 6035	Yes	5, −40	9	3.4
Nystatin	*S. noursei* 3134	Yes	5, −40	13	3
Nystatin	*S. noursei* 6007	No	−100 to −200	4	86.7
Nystatin	*S. noursei* 6007	Yes	−100 to −200	4	85.8
Streptomycin	*S. griseus* 3417	Yes	5, −40	13	2.5
Streptomycin	*S. griseus* 3417	Yes	−100 to −200	5	100
Streptomycin	*S. griseus* 3417	Yes	−100 to −200	5	96.8
Streptomycin	*S. griseus* 6228	Yes	5, −40	8	47.7
Penicillin G	*P. chrysogenum* 6221	No	−100 to −200	3	100

[a] Where 5, −40 is indicated, vials were stored at −40 for last 6 of the years shown; where −100 to −200 is indicated, vials were stored in vapor phase of liquid N_2 where temperature gradient exists

Conidia of a Squibb production culture of *P. chrysogenum* strain 6221 were stored for 3 years in the vapor phase of liquid nitrogen with no loss in conidial viability and minimal loss in production productivity (FORTNEY and THOMA 1977). These workers reported that on studies of 13 organisms used to support five production processes, liquid nitrogen was the best method for preserving production strains (Table 17). They examined various process cultures over a period of 4–8 years and reported cultures were extremely stable in regard to production capability. They routinely prepare several hundred vials per production lot, which meets production needs for several years. The benefits derived from the preparation of

Table 18. Conidial viabilities of *P. chrysogenum* Wis. 54–1255 following storage at +4 °C and −196 °C. (MACDONALD 1972)

Time (months)	Viability at 4 °C relative to:			Viability at −196 °C relative to:		
	Hemo-cytometer count	Initial viability	Viability after storage	Hemo-cytometer count	Initial viability	Viability after storage
0	77.4	100		77.4	100	
0.25	76.5	98.8	100	60.7	78.4	100
4	72.9	94.2	95.3	61.4	79.3	101.1
21	52.4	67.7	68.5	37.7	48.7	62.1
30	14.9	19.3	19.5	60.3	77.9	99.4
36	3.2	4.1	4.0	46.7	60.3	76.9
42	3.1	4.0	4.0	52.3	67.6	86.2

large vial lots were not only to effect economy in the preparation and testing operations but also to be able to study process variables over a period of time with an identical culture source.

MACDONALD (1972) reported that the viability of conidia of *P. chrysogenum* Wis. 54-1255 stored at −196 °C and +4 °C for a period of 3.5 years fell to 68% viability at −196 °C and only 4% viability at +4 °C (Table 18). MACDONALD used entire slopes of slant for this work and this probably resulted in low viabilities compared to conidial suspensions in buffered menstrua with protective agents and no attempts were made to establish controlled conditions for heating or cooling. At the beginning of the experiment where slant cultures were inoculated from the master culture for preservation, 65 colonies were selected from spores obtained from slants before storage, storage at 4 °C for 42 months, and storage at −196 °C for 42 months and tested for penicillin G yield in shake-flask fermentations. Storage at −196 °C for 42 months resulted in penicillin productivity nearly identical to the penicillin productivity from a similar number of conidial isolates not subjected to storage conditions. Colonies originating from conidia stored at +4 °C for 42 months showed that a number of isolates had a loss in productivity.

II. Studies with A. chrysogenum

A comparison of viability of conidia and vegetative cells of various strains of the cephalosporin C fungus, following lyophilization, is shown in Table 19. It is important to note that vegetative cells consisting primarily of swollen hyphal fragments, termed arthrospores, and hyphal cell fragments showed extremely low viability following freezing and desiccation. In these experiments over 98% of the cells were killed following storage for only a 6-month period of lyophilized ampoules at +5 °C. A greater than 99% kill was recorded from ampoules stored for 7 years.

In contrast, conidia of *A. chrysogenum* were considerably more resistant to freezing and desiccation. This was somewhat strain dependent, but viabilities of 35% were recorded for one strain of *A. chrysogenum* following lyophilization and storage at +5 °C for 30 months (Table 19).

Table 19. Comparison of viability following lyophilization of vegetative cells and conidia of *A. chrysogenum*

Strain designation	Cell type	CFU[a] (× 10⁶)		% Viability after treatment	Storage time (mos.)	% Viability after storage	Relative productivity
		Before treatment	After treatment				
2 6-1L	Vegetative	60	0.4	0.7	6	1.1	99.4
					13	0.33	96.4
					84	0.08	86.8
2 29-1L	Vegetative	37	0.6	1.6	16	3.8	92.4
2 29-3L	Vegetative	39	3	7.7	16	4.1	96.3
4 61-1L	Vegetative	84	2.4	2.9	–	–	–
5 6-2L	Conidia	104	50	48	26	21	98.6
1 13-1L	Conidia	6.3	0.4	6.3	1	25	105.8
					55	3.2	101.4
6 62-2L	Conidia	2.1	1.6	76	3	52	93.7
1 70-1L	Conidia	5.1	2.0	39	30	35	95.6
1 74-1L	Conidia	7.2	5.0	69	–	–	–

[a] CFU, colony forming units

Table 20. Comparison of storage of vegetative cells of *A. chrysogenum* at −20 °C and −167 °C

Lot No.	°C Storage temp.	CFU[a] (× 10⁶)		% Viability after freeze	Storage time (mos.)	% Viability after storage	Relative productivity
		Before freeze	After freeze				
2FV	− 20	65	54	83	3	28	92.5
					4	37	38.7
3FV	− 20	46	49	106	8	20	94.4
9FV	− 20	32	19	59	8	62	91.2
14FV	−167	48	46	95	5	154	99.3
15FV	−167	47	38	81	5	138	106.5

Suspending menstruum
Vegetative seed medium + glycerine (5%, V/V) and sucrose (5%, V/V)

[a] CFU, colony forming units

Table 20 shows data for all vegetative cells of strain of *A. chrysogenum* stored at −20 °C and −167 °C (in the vapor phase of liquid nitrogen). It is interesting to note that there was a dramatic increase in the numbers of vegetative cells (arthrospores) following freezing in the vapor phase of liquid nitrogen. An increase of 38% and 54% resulted from two independent liquid nitrogen storage preparations. A similar effect was reported for the alga *Scenedesmus quadricaula* by workers at the Lilly Research Laboratories (DAILY and HIGGENS 1973). They attributed the increase in viability following preservation in liquid nitrogen to cellular fragmentation. Production fermentations were also more uniform using vegetative seed preparations derived from vegetative suspensions stored at −167 °C (Table 20). An occasional drop in productivity was noted for preparations stored at −20 °C. It is, therefore, recommended to store nonsporulating organisms in liquid nitrogen.

References

Abraham EP (1978) Developments in the chemistry and biochemistry of β-lactam antibiotics. In: Hütter R, Leisinger T, Nüesch J, Wehrli W (eds) Antibiotics and other secondary metabolites. Academic Press, New York, pp 141–164

Abraham EP (1979) A glimpse of the early history of cephalosporins. Rev Infect Dis 1:99–105

Abraham EP, Newton GGF, Hale CW (1954) Purification and some properties of cephalosporin N, a new penicillin. Biochem J 58:94–102

Aoki H, Okuhara M (1980) Natural β-lactam antibiotics. Ann Rev Microbiol 34:159–181

Aoki H, Sakai H, Kohsaka M, Konomi T, Hosoda J, Kubochi Y, Iguchi E, Imanaka H (1976) Nocardicin, a new β-lactam antibiotic. I. Discovery, isolation and characterization. J Antibiot 29:492–500

Aoki H, Kunugita K, Hosoda J, Imanaka H (1977) Screening of new and novel β-lactam antibiotics. J Antibiot [Suppl] 30:S-207-2-217

Arnstein HRV, Morris D (1960) The structure of a peptide containing α-aminoadipic acid, cysteine, and valine, present in the mycelium of *Penicillium chrysogenum*. Biochem J 76:357–366

Backus MP, Stauffer JF (1955) The production and selection of a family of strains in *Penicillium chrysogenum*. Mycologia 47:429–463

Ball C, McGonagle MP (1978) Development and evaluation of a potency index screen for detecting mutants of *Penicillium chrysogenum* having increased penicillin yield. J Appl Bacteriol 45:67–74

Batchelor FR, Doyle FP, Nayler THC, Rolinson GN (1959) Synthesis of penicillin = 6-aminopenicillanic acid in penicillin fermentations. Nature 183:257–258

Behrens OK (1949) Biosynthesis of penicillin: In: Clarke HT, Johnson TR, Robinson R (eds) The chemistry of penicillin. Princeton University Press, Princeton, pp 657–679

Box SJ, Hood JD, Sear S (1979) Four further antibiotics related to olivanic acid produced by *Streptomyces olivaceus*. Fermentation, isolation, characterization, and biosynthesis studies. J Antibiot 32:1239–1247

Brannon DR, Fukuda DS, Mabe JA, Huber FM, Whitney JG (1972) Detection of a cephalosporin C acetyl esterase in the carbamate cephalosporin antibiotic producing culture, *Streptomyces clavuligerus*. Antimicrob Agents Chemother 1:237–241

Brown AG, Butterworth D, Cole M, Hanscomb G, Hood JD, Reading C, Rolinson GN (1976) Naturally occuring β-lactamase inhibitors with antibacterial activity. J Antibiot 29:668–669

Brown AG, Corbett DF, Englington AJ, Howarth TT (1977) Structures of olivanic acid derivatives MM4550 and MM13902, two new fused β-lactams isolated from *Streptomyces olivaceus*. J Chem Soc [D] 1977:523–525

Brown WF, Elander RP (1966) Some biometric considerations in an applied antibiotic AB-464 strain development program. Dev Ind Microbiol 7:114–123

Burton HS, Abraham EP (1951) Isolation of antibiotics from a species of *Cephalosporium*: P1, P2, P3, P4, and P5. Biochem J 50:168–174

Butterworth D, Cole M, Hanscomb G, Rolinson GN (1979) Olivanic acids, a family of β-lactam antibiotics with β-lactamase inhibitory properties produced by a *Streptomyces* species. I. Detection, properties, and fermentation studies. J Antibiot 32:287–294

Cassidy PJ (1981) Novel naturally occurring β-lactam antiobitics – a review. Dev Ind Microbiol 22:181–209

Chang LT, Elander RP (1979) Rational selection for improved productivity in strains of *Acremonium chrysogenum* Gams. Dev Ind Microbiol 20:367–379

Cole M (1979) Inhibition of β-lactamases. In: Hamilton-Miller JMT, Smith JT (eds) Beta-Lactamases. Academic Press, New York, pp 205–289

Cole M, Batchelor FR (1963) Aminoadipylpenicillin in penicillin fermentations. Nature 198:383–384

Cole M, Rolinson GN (1961) 6-Aminopenicillanic acid II. Formation of 6-aminopenicillanic acid by *Emericellopsis minima* (Stolk) and related fungi. Proc R Soc Lond [Biol] 154:490–497

Cole M, Howarth TT, Reading C (1976) Ger Offen 2:517, 316

Cooney CL (1979) Conversion yields in penicillin production: theory *vs.* practice. Proc Biochem 14:31–33

Crawford K, Heatley NG, Boyd PF, Hale CW, Kelley BK, Miller GA, Smith N (1952) Antibiotic production by a species of *Cephalosporium.* J Gen Microbiol 6:41–59

Crawfoot D, Bunn CW, Rogers-Low BW, Turner-Jones A (1949) The x-ray crystallographic investigation of the structure of penicillin. In: Clarke HT, Johnson JR, Robinson R (eds) The chemistry of penicillin. Princeton University Press, Princeton, pp 310–366

Daily WA, Higgens CE (1973) Preservation and storage of microorganisms in the gas phase of liquid nitrogen. Cryobiology 10:364–367

Demain AL, Masurekar PS (1974) Lysine inhibition of in vivo homocitrate synthesis in *Penicillium chrysogenum.* J Gen Microbiol 82:143–151

Demain AL, Newkirk JF, Davis GE, Harman RE (1963) Nonbiological conversion of cephalosporin C to a new antibiotic by sodium thiosulfate. Appl Microbiol 11:58–61

Dennen DW, Carver DD (1969) Sulfatase regulation and antibiotic synthesis in *Cephalosporium acremonium.* Can J Microbiol 15:175–181

Doudoroff M, Palleroni NJ (1974) Part 7. Gram-negative aerobic rods and cocci. In: Buchanan RE, Gibbons NE (eds) Bergey's manual of determinative bacteriology, 8th ed. Williams & Wilkens, Baltimore, pp 217–243

Drew SW, Demain AL (1977) Effect of primary metabolites on secondary metabolism. Ann Rev Microbiol 31:343–356

Drew SW, Winstanley DJ, Demain AL (1976) Effect of norleucine on morphological differentiation in *Cephalosporium acremonium.* Appl Microbiol 31:143–145

Dulaney EL (1947) Some aspects of penicillin production by *Aspergillus nidulans.* Mycologia 39:570–582

Dulaney EL, Dulaney DD (1967) Mutant populations of *Streptomyces viridifaciens.* Trans NY Acad Sci 29:782–799

Elander RP (1967) Enhanced penicillin biosynthesis in mutant and recombinant strains of *Penicillium chrysogenum.* In: Stübbe H (ed) Induced mutations and their utilization. Academie-Verlag, Berlin, pp 403–423

Elander RP (1975) Genetic aspects of cephalosporin and cephamycin-producing microorganisms. Dev Ind Microbiol 16:356–374

Elander RP (1976) Mutation to increased product formation in antibiotic producing microorganisms. In: Schlessinger D (ed) Microbiology–1976. American Society of Microbiology, Washington, D.C., pp 517–521

Elander RP (1978) Maintenance and productivity of industrially important fungi (Abstr). XII International Congress of Microbiology, Munich, No. S28.1, p 39

Elander RP (1979) Mutations affecting antibiotic synthesis in fungi producing β-lactam antibiotics. In: Sebek OK, Laskin AI (eds) Genetics of industrial microorganisms. American Society of Microbiology, Washington, D.C., pp 21–35

Elander RP, Aoki H (1982) β-Lactam producing microorganisms – their biology and fermentation behavior. In: Morin RB, Gorman M (eds) Chemistry and biology of β-lactam antibiotics, vol 3. Academic Press, New York, pp 83–153

Elander RP, Chang LT (1979) Microbial culture selection. In: Peppler H, Perlman D (eds) Microbiology technology, 2nd edn, vol 2. Academic Press, New York, pp 243–302

Elander RP, Stauffer JF, Backus MP (1961) Antibiotic production by various species and varities of *Cephalosporium* and *Emericellopsis.* Antimicrob Agents Ann 1:91–102

Elander RP, Gordee RS, Wilgus RM, Gale RM (1969) Synthesis of an antibiotic closely resembling fusidic acid by imperfect and perfect dermatophyte fungi. J Antibiot 22:176–178

Elander RP, Espenshade MA, Pathak SG, Pan CH (1973) The use of parasexual genetics in an industrial strain improvement program with *Penicillium chrysogenum*. In: Vanek Z, Hostalek Z, Cudlin J (eds) Genetics of industrial microorganisms, vol 2. Actinomycetes and fungi. Elsevier, Amsterdam, pp 239–253

Elander RP, Corum CJ, DeValeria H, Wilgus RM (1976) Ultraviolet mutagenesis and cephalosporin synthesis in strains of *Cephalosporium acremonium*. In: Macdonald KD (ed) Second international symposium on the genetics of industrial microorganisms. Academic Press, London, pp 253–271

Erickson RC, Dean LD (1966) Acylation of 6-aminopenicillanic acid by *Penicillium chrysogenum*. Appl Microbiol 14:1047–1048

Fasani M, Marini F, Teatini L (1974) Variability of cephalosporin C production induced by phenethyl alcohol and dimethylsulfate (Astr). Second international symposium on genetics of industrial microorganisms. Academic Press, London, p 31

Fleischman HI, Pisano MA (1961) The production of synnematin B by *Paecilomyces persicinus* in a chemically defined medium. Antimicrob Agents Ann 1:48–53

Fleming A (1929) On the antibacterial action of cultures of a penicillin, with special reference to their use in the isolation of *B. influenzae*. Br J Exp Pathol 10:226–236

Florey HW, Chain EB, Heatley NG, Jennings MA, Sanders AG, Abraham EP, Florey ME (eds) (1949) Antibiotics, vol 2. Oxford University Press, London New York

Flynn EH, McCormick MH, Stamper MC, DeValeria H, Godzeski CW (1962) A new natural penicillin from *Penicillium chrysogenum*. J Am Chem Soc 84:4594–4595

Fortney KF, Thoma RW (1977) Stabilization of culture productivity. Dev Ind Microbiol 18:319–325

Friedrich CG, Demain AL (1977a) Homocitrate synthase as the crucial site of the lysine effect on penicillin biosynthesis. J Antibiot 30:760–761

Friedrich CG, Demain AL (1977b) Effects of lysine analogs on *Penicillium chrysogenum*. Appl Environ Microbiol 34:706–709

Fujisawa Y, Kanzaki T (1975) Occurrence of a new cephalosporoate in a culture broth of a *Cephalosporium acremonium* mutant. J Antibiot 28:372–378

Fujiasawa Y, Shirafuji H, Kida M, Nara K, Yoneda M, Kanzaki T (1973) New findings on cephalosporin C biosynthesis. Nature 246:154–155

Fujiasawa Y, Shirafuji H, Kida M, Nara K, Yoneda M, Kanzaki T (1975) Accumulation of deacetylcephalosporin C by cephalosporin C negative mutants of *Cephalosporium acremonium*. Agric Biol Chem 39:1295–1301

Fukase H, Hasegawa T, Hatano K, Iwasaki H, Yoneda M (1976) C-2801X, A new cephamycin-type antibiotic. J Antibiot 29:113–120

Fuska S, Welwardova F (1969) Selection of productive strains of *Penicillium chrysogenum*. Biologia 24:691–698

Godfrey OW (1973) Isolation of regulatory mutants of the aspartic and pyruvic acid families and their effect on antibiotic production in *Streptomyces lipmanii*. Antimicrob Agents Chemother 4:73–79

Gorman M, Huber F (1977) β-Lactam antibiotics. In: Perlman D (ed) Annual Reports, Fermentation Processes, vol. 1. Academic Press, New York, pp 326–346

Goulden SA, Chattaway FW (1969) End-product control of acetohydroxy acid synthetase by valine in *Penicillium chrysogenum* Q-176 and a high penicillin yielding mutant. J Gen Microbiol 59:111–118

Grosklags JH, Swift ME (1957) The perfect stage of an antibiotic producing *Cephalosporium*. Mycologia 49:305–317

Hasegawa T, Fukase H, Kitano K, Iwasaki H, Yoneda M (1975) Abstract – Annu Meet Agric Chem, Agricultural Soc. Japan, p 80

Hashimoto M, Komori T, Kamiya T (1976) Nocardicin A, a new monocyclic β-lactam antibiotic. J Antibiot 29:890–901

Higgens CE, Kastner RE (1971) *Streptomyces clavuligerus* sp. nov., a β-lactam antibiotic producer. Int J Syst Bacteriol 21:326–331

Higgens EC, Hamill RL, Sands TH, Hoehn MM, Davis NE, Nagarajan R, Boeck LD (1974) The occurrence of deacetoxycephalosporin C in fungi and streptomycetes. J Antibiot 27:298–300

Hosoda J, Konomi T, Tami N, Aoki H, Imanaka H (1977) Isolation of new nocardicins from *Nocardia uniformis* subsp. *tsuyamanensis*. Agric Biol Chem 41:2013–2020

Huber FM, Baltz RH, Caltrider PG (1968) Formation of deacetylcephalosporin C in the cephalosporin C fermentation. Appl Microbiol 16:1011–1014

Imada A, Nozaki Y, Kintaka , Okonogi K, Kitano K, Harada S (1980) C-19393 S_2 and H_2, new carbapenem antibiotics. I. Taxonomy of the producing strain, fermentation, and antibacterial properties. J Antibiot 33:1417–1424

Imada A, Kitano K, Kintaka K, Mursi M, Asai M (1981) Sulfazecin and isosulfazecin, novel β-lactam antibiotics of bacterial origin. Nature 289:590–591

Jeffery JDA, Abraham EP, Newton GGF (1961) Deacetylcephalosporin C. Biochem J 81:591–596

Kahan JS, Kahan FM, Geogelman R, Currie SA, Jackson M, Stapley EO, Miller TW et al. (1976) Thienamycin: a new β-lactam antibiotic. I. Discovery and isolation. Abstract of papers, 16th Intersci Conf Antimicrob Agents Chemother, no. 227. Ann Soc Microbiol, Washington, D.C.

Kahan JS, Kahan FM, Geogleman R, Currie SA, Jackson M, Stapley EO, Miller TW et al. (1979) Thienamycin, a new β-lactam antibiotic. I. Discovery, taxonomy, isolation, and physical properties. J Antibiot 32:1–12

Kamiya T (1977) Studies on the new monocyclic β-lactam antibiotics, Nocardicin A and B. In: Elks J (ed) Recent advances in the chemistry of β-lactam antibiotics (Special Publication No. 28). The Chemical Society, London, pp 281–294

Kanzaki T, Fujisawa Y (1976) Biosynthesis of cephalosporin. Adv Appl Microbiol 20:159–202

Kanzaki T, Fukita T, Shirafuji H, Fujisawa Y, Kitano K (1974) Occurrence of a 3-methylthiomethylcephem derivative in a culture broth of a *Cephalosporium* mutant. J Antibiot 27:361–362

Kato K (1953) Occurrence of penicillin-nucleus in culture broths. J Antibiot Ser A 6:130–136

Kikuchi T, Uyeo S (1967) Pachysandra alkaloids. VIII. Structures of pachyoterminus-A and -B, novel type alkaloids having a β-lactam ring. Chem Pharm Bull 15:549–570

Kitano K, Kintaka K, Suzuki S, Katamoto K, Nara K, Nakao Y (1975) Screening of microorganisms capable of producing β-lactam antibiotics. J Ferment Technol 53:327–338

Kitano K, Kintaka K, Nakao Y (1976) Some characteristics of β-lactam antibiotic-hypersensitive mutant derived from a strain of *Pseudomonas aeruginosa*. J Ferment Technol 54:696–704

Kitano K, Nara K, Nakao Y (1977) Screening of β-lactam antibiotics using a mutant of *Pseudomonas aeruginosa*. J Antibiot [Suppl] 30:S239–S245

Kohsaka M, Demain AL (1976) Conversion of penicillin N to cephalosporin(s) by cell-free extracts of *Cephalosporium acremonium*. Biochem Biophys Res Commun 70:465–473

Komatsu KI, Kodaira R (1977) Sulfur metabolism of a mutant of *Cephalosporium acremonium* with enhanced potential to utilize sulfate for cephalosporin C production. J Antibiot (Tokyo) 30:226–233

Komatsu KI, Mizuno M, Kodaira R (1975) Effect of methionine on cephalosporin C and penicillin N production by a mutant of *Cephalosporium acremonium*. J Antibiot 28:881–888

Konomi T, Herschen S, Baldwin JE, Yoshida M, Hunt NA, Demain AL (1979) Cell-free conversion of δ-(L-α-Aminoadipyl)-L-cysteinyl-D-valine into an antibiotic with the properties of isopenicillin N in *Cephalosporium acremonium*. Biochem J 184:427–430

Krone B, Wanning M, Zähner H, Zeeck A (1981) Hydroxyethylclavam, a new antifungal β-lactam antibiotic (Abstr). 2nd Europ Cong Biotechnol, Eastbourne, England. Soc of Chem Indust, London, p 80

Kurita M, Kazuyoshi J, Komori T, Miyairi M, Aoki H, Kuge S, Kamiya T, Imanaka H (1976) Isolation and characterization of nocardicin B. J Antibiot 29:1243–1245

Lemke PA (1969) A century of compounds and their effect on fungi. Mycopathol Mycol Appl 38:49–59
Lemke PA, Brannon DR (1972) Microbial synthesis of cephalosporin and penicillin compounds. In: Flynn EH (ed) Cephalosporins and penicillins, chemistry, and biology. Academic Press, New York, pp 370–437
Lemke PA, Nash CH (1972) Mutations that affect antibiotic synthesis by *Cephalosporium acremonium*. Can J Microbiol 18:255–259
Liersch M, Nüesch J, Treichler HJ (1976) Final steps in the biosynthesis of cephalosporin C. In: Macdonald KD (ed) Second international symposium on the genetics of industrial microorganisms. Academic Press, New York, pp 179–195
Loder PB, Abraham EP (1971) Isolation and nature of intracellular peptides from a cephalosporin C producing *Cephalosporium* sp. Biochem J 123:471–476
Macdonald KD (1972) Storage of conidia of *Penicillium chrysogenum* in liquid nitrogen. Appl Microbiol 23:990–993
Marsluf GA (1970) Genetic and metabolic controls for sulfate metabolism in *Neurospora crassa:* isolation and study of chromate-resistant and sulfate-transport-negative mutants. J Bacteriol 102:716–721
Masurekar PS, Demain AL (1974) Impaired penicillin production in lysine regulatory mutants of *Penicillium chrysogenum*. Antimicrob Agents Chemother 6:366–368
Mehta RJ, Nash CH (1979) Relationship between carbon source and susceptibility of *Cephalosporium acremonium* to selected amino acid analogues. Can J Microbiol 25:818–821
Miller IM, Stapley EO, Chaiet L (1962) Production of synnematin B by a member of the genus *Streptomyces*. Bacteriol Proc 32
Miller TW, Geogeleman RT, Weston RG, Putter I, Wolf FJ (1972) Cephamycins, a new family of β-lactam antibiotics. Antimicrob Agents Chemother 2:132–135
Morin RB, Jackson BG, Flynn EH, Roeske RW (1962) Chemistry of cephalosporin antibiotics. III. Chemical correlation of penicillin and cephalosporin antibiotics. J Am Chem Soc 84:3400–3401
Morin RB, Jackson BG, Mueller RA, Lavagnino ER, Scanlon WB, Andrews SL (1963) Chemistry of cephalosporin antibiotics. III. Chemical correlation of penicillin and cephalosporin antibiotics. J Am Chem Soc 85:1896–1897
Moyer AJ, Coghill RD (1946) Penicillin VIII. Production of penicillin in surface cultures. J Bacteriol 51:57–78
Nagarajan R (1972) β-Lactam antibiotics from *Streptomyces*. In: Flynn EH (ed) Cephalosporins and penicillins. Academic Press, New York London, pp 636–661
Nagarajan R, Boeck LD, Gorman M, Hamill RL, Higgens CE, Hoehn MM, Stark WM, Whitney JG (1971) β-lactam antibiotics from *Streptomyces*. J Am Chem Soc 93:2308–2310
Nakayama M, Iwasaki A, Kimura S, Mizoguchi T, Tanabe S, Murakami A, Watanabe I, Okuchi M, Itoh H, Saino Y, Kobayashi F, Mori T (1980) Carpetimycins A and B, new β-lactam antibiotics. J Antibiot 33:1388–1390
Nash CH, Huber FM (1971) Antibiotic synthesis and morphological differentiation of *Cephalosporium acremonium*. Appl Microbiol 22:6–10
Nash CH, DeLaHiguera N, Neuss N, Lemke PA (1974) Application of biochemical genetics to the biosynthesis of β-lactam antibiotics. Dev Ind Microbiol 15:114–132
Newton GGF, Abraham EP (1955) Cephalosporin C, a new antibiotic containing sulfur and D-α-aminoadipic acid. Nature 175:548–556
Niss HF, Nash CH (1973) Synthesis of cephalosporin C from sulfate by mutants of *Cephalosporium acremonium*. Antimicrob Agents Chemother 4:474–478
Nüesch J, Treichler HJ, Liersch M (1973) Biosynthesis of cephalosporin C. In: Vanek Z, Hostalek Z, Cudlin J (eds) Genetics of industrial microorganisms, vol 2. Elsevier, Amsterdam, pp 309–334
Okamura K, Hirata S, Okumura V, Fukagawa Y, Shimauchi Y, Kouno K, Ishikura T, Lein J (1978) PS-5, a new β-lactam antibiotic from *Streptomyces*. J Antibiot 31:480–482
Okamura K, Hirata S, Koki A, Hori K, Shibamoto N, Okamura Y, Okabe M et al. (1979a) PS-5, a new β-lactam antibiotic. I. Taxonomy of the producing organism, isolation and physico-chemical properties. J Antibiot 32:262–271

Okamura K, Koki A, Sakamoto M, Kubo K, Mutoh Y, Fukagawa Y, Kouno K et al. (1979b) Microorganisms producing a new β-lactam antibiotic. J Ferment Technol 57:265–272

Okanishi M, Gregory KF (1970) Isolation of mutants of *Candida tropicalis* with increased methionine concentration. Can J Microbiol 16:1139–1143

Olson BH, Jennings JC, Junek AJ (1953) Separation of synnematin into components A and B by paper chromatography. Science 117:76–78

Omura S, Tanaka H, Oiwa R, Nagai T, Koyama Y, Takahashi S (1979) Studies on bacterial cell wall inhibitors VI. Screening method for the specific inhibitors of peptidoglycan synthesis. J Antibiot 32:978–984

Pan CH, Hepler L, Elander RP (1972) Control of pH and carbohydrate addition in the penicillin fermentation. Dev Ind Microbiol 13:103–112

Pan CH, Hepler L, Elander RP (1975) The effect of iron on a high-yielding industrial strain of *Penicillium chrysogenum*. J Ferment Technol 53:854–861

Perlman D, Kikuchi M (1977) Culture maintenance. In: Perlman D (ed) Annual reports, fermentation processes, vol. 1. Academic Press, New York, pp 41–48

Pisano MA, Vellozzi EM (1974) Production of cephalosporin C by *Paecilomyces persicinus* P-10. Antimicrob Agents Chemother 6:447–451

Preuss DL, Johnson MJ (1967) Penicillin acyltransferase in *Penicillium chrysogenum*. J Bacteriol 94:1502–1508

Queener SW, Capone JJ (1974) Deacetoxycephalosporin C accumulation in mutants of *Cephalosporium acremonium*. (Abstr) Genetics of Indust Microorganisms. Academic Press, London, p 33

Queener SW, McDermott JJ, Radue AB (1975) Glutamate dehydrogenase-specific activity and cephalosporin synthesis in the M8650 series of *Cephalosporium acremonium* mutants. Antimicrob Agents Chemother 7:646–651

Raper KB, Fennell DA (1946) The production of penicillin in submerged culture. J Bacteriol 51:761–777

Raper KB, Alexander DF, Coghill RD (1944) Penicillin I. Natural variation and penicillin production in *Penicillium notatum* and allied species. J Bacteriol 48:639–659

Reading E, Cole M (1977) Clavulanic acid: a beta-lactamase inhibiting beta-lactam from *Streptomyces clavuligerus*. Antimicrob Agents Chemother 11:852–857

Roberts JM (1952) Antibiotics produced by species of *Cephalosporium*, with a description of a new species. Mycologia 44:292–306

Rode LJ, Foster JW, Schuhardt VT (1947) Penicillin production by a thermophilic fungus. J Bacteriol 53:565–572

Rosi D, Drozd ML, Kuhrt MF, Terminello L, Came PE, Daum SJ (1981) Mutants of *Streptomyces cattleya* producing N-acetyl and deshydroxy carbapenems related to thienamycin. J Antibiot 34:341–342

Sanders AG (1949) In: Florey HW, Chain EB, Heatley NG, Jennings MA, Sanders AG, Abraham EP, Florey ME (eds) Antibiotics, vol 2. Oxford University Press, London New York, pp 672–685

Scannell JP, Pruess DL, Blount JF, Ax HA, Kellet M, Weiss F, Demmy TC, Williams TH, Stempel A (1975) Antimetabolites produced by microorganisms XIII. (S)-alanyl-3-[α-(S)-chloro-3(S)-hydroxy-2-oxo-3-azetidinymethyl]-(S) alanine, a new β-lactam containing a natural product. J Antibiot 28:1–6

Segel IH, Johnson MJ (1961) Accumulation of intracellular sulfate by *Penicillium chrysogenum*. J Bacteriol 81:91–98

Sheehan JC, Henery-Logan KR (1959) A general synthesis of the penicillins. J Am Chem Soc 81:5838–5839

Smith B, Warren SC, Newton GGF, Abraham EP (1967) Biosynthesis of penicillin N and cephalosporin C. Biochem J 103:877–890

Spratt BG (1977) Properties of the penicillin-binding proteins of *Escherichia coli* K12. Eur J Biochem 72:341–352

Stapley EO, Jackson M, Hernandez S, Zimmerman SB, Currie SA, Mochales S, Mata JM, Woodruff HB, Hendlin D (1972) Cephamycins, a new family of β-lactam antibiotics. I. Production by actinomycetes, including *Streptomyces lactamdurans*, sp. n. Antimicrob Agents Chemother 2:122–131

Stapley EO, Cassidy P, Currie SA, Daoust D, Goegelman R, Hernandez S, Jackson M et al. (1977) Epithienamycins: Biological studies of a new family of β-lactam antibiotics. Abst Intersci Conf Antimicrob Ag Chemother 17th, New York, Paper No. 80, Amer Soc Microbiol, Washington, D.C., 20006

Stewart WW (1971) Isolation and proof of structure of wildfire toxin. Nature 229:174–178

Sykes RB, Cimarusti CM, Bonner DP, Bask K, Floyd DM, Georgopapadakou NH, Koster WH et al. (1981) Monocyclic β-lactam antibiotics produced by bacteria. Nature 291:489–491

Swartz RW (1979) The use of economic analysis of penicillin G manufacturing costs in establishing priorities for fermentation process improvement. Abstr ACS Meeting, 176th, Miami Beach, September 1978

Tamaki S, Nakagawa JI, Marugama IN, Matsuhashi M (1978) Supersensitivity to β-lactam antibiotics in *Escherichia coli* caused by a D-alanine carboxypeptidase 1A mutation. Agric Biol Chem 42:2147–2150

Taylor PA, Schnoes HK, Durbin RD (1972) Characterization of chlorosis inducing toxins from a plant pathogenic *Pseudomonas* sp. Biochim Biophys Acta 286:107–117

Traxler P, Treichler HJ, Nüesch J (1975) Synthesis of N-acetyldeacetoxycephalosphorin C by a mutant of *Cephalosporium acremonium*. J Antibiot 28:605–606

Treichler HJ, Liersch M, Nüesch J (1978) Genetics and biochemistry of cephalosporin biosynthesis. In: Hütter R, Leisinger T, Nüesch J, Wehrli W (eds) Antibiotics and other secondary metabolites. Academic Press, New York, pp 177–199

Treichler HJ, Liersch M, Nüesch J, Dobeli H (1979) Role of sulphur metabolism in cephalosporin C and penicillin biosynthesis. In: Sebek OK, Laskin AI (eds) Genetics of industrial microorganisms. American Society of Microbiology, Washington, D.C., pp 97–104

Trilli A, Michelini V, Mantovani V, Pirt SJ (1978) Development of the agar disc method for the rapid selection of cephalosporin producers with improved yield. Antimicrob Agents Chemother 13:7–13

Troonen H, Roelants P, Boon B (1976) RIT 2214, a new biosynthetic penicillin produced by a mutant of *Cephalosporium acremonium*. J Antibiot 29:1258–1266

Tubaki K (1973) Aquatic sediment as a habitat of *Emericellopsis*, with a description of an undescribed species of *Cephalosporium*. Mycologia 65:938–941

Uri J, Valer G, Bekesi I (1963) Production of 6-aminopenicillanic acid by dermatophytes. Nature 200:896–897

Wellman AM, Stewart GW (1973) Storage of brewing yeasts by liquid nitrogen preservation. Appl Microbiol 26:577–583

Wesseling AC, Lago BD (1981) Strain improvement of cephamycin producers, *Nocardia lactamdurans* and *Streptomyces griseus*. Dev Ind Microbiol 22:641–651

Woodward RB, Heusler K, Gosteli J, Naegele P, Oppolzer W, Ramage R, Ranganathan S, Vorbruggen H (1966) The total synthesis of cephalosporin C. J Am Chem Soc 88:852–853

CHAPTER 4

Genetics of β-Lactam-Producing Fungi

C. BALL

A. Introduction

The genetics of β-lactam-producing fungi are fundamentally interesting and a key feature in the development of industrial microbial genetics. In this review, I will focus mainly on three organisms, *Aspergillus nidulans*, *Penicillium chrysogenum*, and *Cephalosporium acremonium* since these have been the most extensively studied from the genetical point of view. I will adhere to the narrow definition of genetics, namely studies of genetic recombination.

A. nidulans is the "academic" fungus with which it is convenient to carry out fundamental work to provide model examples for work with the other "industrial" fungi. The advantages of *A. nidulans* for fundamental studies include the fact that it has both a sexual and parasexual recombination cycle while *P. chrysogenum* and *C. acremonium* have only parasexual cycles. As a result, *A. nidulans* has been extensively studied genetically and the genetic map is comprehensive particularly when compared with its industrial counterparts. Unfortunately for industry, this situation has been autocatalytic and has tended to refocus the attention of the academic research worker onto *A. nidulans* and away from the other β-lactam-producing fungi.

It is useful to examine the development of industrial microbial genetics including the genetics of β-lactam production in three phases. The first phase was that preceding the First International Symposium on the Genetics of Industrial Microorganisms (GIM 70) in 1970 and largely summarized either at that symposium or in SERMONTI's book (1969). The second phase was the period between 1970 up to the present including the Second and Third International Symposia on the Genetics of Industrial Microorganisms. The third phase, i.e., the future promises to be particularly exciting because genetic engineering techniques involving in vitro recombination of DNA and transformation of protoplasts with hybrid plasmids will have an increasing impact on work with industrial microorganisms and hopefully with β-lactam-producing fungi.

B. Aspergillus nidulans

As stated in the introduction, work with *A. nidulans* serves as a model for studies with other β-lactam-producing fungi. Rather than attempt to cover the whole of *A. nidulans* genetics, I shall cover those aspects that impinge on the genetics of industrial β-lactam production described in later sections. The reader is referred to several reviews for further insight into the classic genetics of *A. nidulans* namely

PONTECORVO et al. (1953), ROPER (1966), and KÄFER (1977). Studies relevant to β-lactams fall into two general areas, namely the mechanics of the parasexual cycle and the genetics of penicillin production.

I. The Parasexual Cycle

The parasexual cycle is characterized by three main stages: (i) heterokaryosis between different parental haploid strains, (ii) nuclear fusion to generate a relatively stable diploid, and (iii) genetic recombination plus chromosome segregation to generate haploid segregants including different types of recombinant. Methods for establishing stages (i) and (ii) are well documented (e.g., SERMONTI 1969) and relatively easy to apply but special methods for dealing with stage (iii) have been developed in order to aid a specific type of genetic analysis to be carried out. Stage (iii) incorporates two types of genetic recombination namely recombination within homologous pairs of chromosomes (mitotic crossing-over and mitotic gene conversion) and exchange of whole chromosomes by nondisjunction (unequal segregation) of whole chromosomes followed by haploidization (reduction to the haploid state). These processes are usually independent events (Fig. 1). Certain chemical and physical agents such as 5-fluorouracil can increase the frequency of mitotic crossing-over and others such as parafluorophenylalanine can increase the frequency of haploidization. It is often desirable to use agents that are not potent mutagens and the term recombinogen is often used to describe such agents. De-

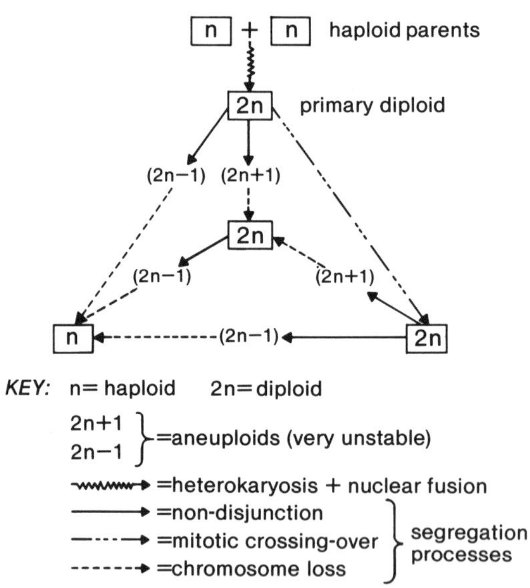

Fig. 1. Some ploidy relationships in the parasexual cycle showing that a primary diploid colony can contain a variety of different segregant genotypes of spontaneous origin. Usually the haploid parents carry different spore color and auxotrophic mutants all of which are recessive. Therefore, the diploid is selected as a prototroph with nonmutant spore color. The latter feature often distinguishes the diploid from heterokaryons which may exhibit the parental mutant spore colors. Segregants can be recognized initially by mutant spore color and later by auxotrophic requirements and spore size

scription of these processes, natural and induced, can be found in the references given earlier and there are more simplified descriptions in BALL (1973b) and MACDONALD and HOLT (1976).

A major use of haploidization in genetic analysis is that all genes on the same chromosome segregate together allowing ready allocation of genes to linkage groups. In contrast, major use of mitotic crossing-over is that ordering of genes on a linkage group is facilitated. Such ordering is also aided by the use of recessive selectable or readily screenable markers such as drug resistance and spore color mutants, respectively.

An important intermediate stage in the haploidization process is the occurrence of aneuploids. These are genetically unbalanced genomes, i.e., containing chromosomes additional to the normal haploid or diploid chromosome complement. They are slower growing than haploids or diploids and readily throw off faster growing haploid or diploid sectors (Fig. 1). They could have significance in industrial strain improvement, i.e., by such means genes that are rate limiting for titer improvement may be duplicated. Studies by KÄFER and UPSHALL (1973) have shown an interesting correlation between morphology of the disomic aneuploids representing one chromosome excess (n + 1) over the normal haploid complement (n) and the particular chromosome duplicated. This has been developed into a method for rapid detection of translocated strains of *A. nidulans* (UPSHALL and KÄFER 1974). Such strains have a tendency to produce disomics for the chromosomes involved in the translocation, which can then be recognized on a morphological basis without the need for extensive genetic analysis. Aneuploids have also been used by UPSHALL et al. (1979) to show that mitotic crossing-over occurs in such strains at high frequency and that cross-overs occur in greatest frequency near the centromere rather than at the extremes of chromosomes arms. This has implications for attempts to produce stable aneuploids by balanced lethals. Such nonallelic lethals would need to be terminal to a chromosome arm to reduce the chance of separation by crossing-over. UPSHALL et al. (1979) have also proposed another interesting method for stabilizing aneuploids. This involved the use of leaky, temperature-sensitive mutants where aneuploids being duplicated for the chromosome carrying the leaky, temperature-sensitive mutant would be faster growing than the haploid at the nonpermissive temperature.

On the subject of duplications, the work of ROPER and co-workers (e.g., see BIRKETT and ROPER 1977) has clearly demonstrated the use of nonreciprocal chromosome translocations in the production of partially duplicated strains which are usually more stable than aneuploids. These duplications can be partly reverted by interstitial loss of chromosomal material, but the frequency of such loss is not very high. Such duplications could be of use in strain improvement of industrial fungi.

II. The Genetics of Penicillin Production

Two groups of workers have studied the genetics of penicillin production in detail. They are MACDONALD and HOLT and co-workers and CATEN and co-workers. In each case the analytical methods were different. MACDONALD and HOLT and co-workers studied penicillin production as a qualitative character mapping to chromosomes not only single genes for titer improvement but also single genes for titer reduction. In contrast, CATEN and co-workers studied penicillin production as a quantitative character and used rigorous statistical techniques.

The work of HOLT and MACDONALD (1968a, b) was the first study of genetic recombination in *A. nidulans* with respect to penicillin production. They showed that recombination between different wild-type isolates could give rise to yield improvement. Later papers described how three specific yield-increasing genes could be allocated to three different chromosomes (DITCHBURN et al. 1976) and how nonproducing mutants could be allocated, following complementation tests, to at least four complementation groups (EDWARDS et al. 1974; HOLT et al. 1976). Most of this work has been extensively reviewed by MACDONALD and HOLT (1976).

The work of CATEN and co-workers started with the studies of MERRICK and CATEN (1975) and MERRICK (1975a, b) using spontaneous genetic variation in different wild-type isolates of *A. nidulans*. By using the biometrical approach i.e., quantifying genetic variability and environmental variability, they were able to assess whether the potential in inbred lines had been exhausted with respect to penicillin titer improvement and to make decisions to outbreed to further improve titer.

Subsequently, SIMPSON and CATEN (1977) carried out analogous studies with genetic variability induced by mutagens. These studies showed that genetic recombination as well as mutation could lead to titer improvement. As part of this study, SIMPSON and CATEN (1979a, b) showed that biometric approaches could be used in the appraisal of relative mutagen efficiency in inducing variability in titer. There had been a scarcity of literature on this subject possibly because of the large task of assessing titer-improving mutations. Use of a low-yielding strain such as *A. nidulans*, in which titer-improving mutations are more frequent, helps to overcome this problem. SIMPSON and CATEN (1979a) were still limited to samples of 100 fermentations in each experiment and their definition of a titer-improving mutation was, therefore, based solely on the statistics of each population of 100 survivors from each treatment. Such a definition is very sensitive to the value of the mean of each population, but SIMPSON and CATEN (1979a) claimed that in their study the means in general did not vary significantly.

Both the quantitative and qualitative approaches to understanding the genetics of penicillin production have significance for yield improvement of industrial microorganisms. The quantitative approach is probably the more appropriate for short-term improvement of high- and low-yielding industrial strains. However, the qualitative approach is less empirical in that it interfaces with knowledge of the penicillin biosynthetic pathway particularly in that nonproducing mutants can represent blocks in such a pathway. It therefore reveals longer term strategies for strain improvement. Furthermore, the qualitative approach enables a very precise determination of the dominance relationships and additivity of genes giving rise to titer improvement.

C. Penicillium chrysogenum

The discovery of diploids in *A. nidulans* by ROPER (1952) rapidly led to their detection in *P. chrysogenum* (PONTECORVO and SERMONTI 1954) and the establishment of the broader elements of the parasexual cycle in this and other fungi (ROPER

Table 1. Possible problems with the asexual and parasexual cycles in A. nonindustrial and B. industrial strains of *P. chrysogenum*. (Based on SERMONTI 1969)

A. Nonindustrial strains (strains closely related to natural isolates and not extensively mutated to produce increases in penicillin yield)
   1. Auxotrophs are obligatory and can sometimes reduce or interact to reduce penicillin titer
   2. A random sample of segregants is not readily obtained (Fig. 1)
   3. Haploid segregants are not exclusively produced (Fig. 1)
   4. Diploids are asexually propagated and unwanted segregation can precede analysis (Fig. 1)

B. Industrial strains (strains extensively mutated to produce increases in penicillin yield)
   1. Features described in A. above
   2. Parental strains can be genetically unstable
   3. Parental strains may sporulate poorly and are slow growing
   4. Variable spore size may prevent use in accurate ploidy classification
   5. A random sample of segregants is never obtained
   6. Parental genotype segregation in "crosses" between strains separated by a large number of mutation steps

1966). The possible use of the parasexual cycle in breeding improved industrial strains was immediately recognized, but there was a considerable delay in realizing this potential. This is possibly the result of a lack of interest by most academic research workers in industrial problems and of industry in fundamental solutions to problems that could be solved by other means, e.g., in this case titer improvement by mutation alone without using recombination. In the last decade, more interest has been shown by industry in new methods of penicillin titer improvement including recombination, possibly because of diminishing returns from other methods.

The genetic system of *A. nidulans* is in many ways ideal for a precise study of penicillin production from either a qualitative or a quantitative point of view (see Sect. B). With *P. chrysogenum*, this is not the case. The absence of a sexual cycle in this organism is a disadvantage but does not necessarily present major problems (see Table 1, part A). However, it can be seen from Table 1, part B, that highly mutated industrial strains, obligatory in commercially relevant work, restrict the literal extrapolation of work with *A. nidulans* to the commercial strains of *P. chrysogenum*. The development of the genetics of *P. chrysogenum* both from the fundamental point of view and for titer improvement falls readily into the historical eras mentioned in the introduction. Therefore, these studies will be discussed under I. Early Studies, and II. Later Studies.

I. Early Studies

The first attempts at a more detailed understanding of the parasexual cycle and genetic determination of penicillin production were made by Sermonti and co-workers (reviewed by SERMONTI 1959, 1961, 1969). Much of the work was empirically based as was the later work of Alikhanian and co-workers (ALIKHANIAN 1962; ALIKHANIAN and KAMENEVA 1961) and MACDONALD et al. (1963 a, b, c, 1964, 1965). This was emphasized in still later reviews by BALL (1973 b, 1978) and MACDONALD and HOLT (1976) and as a result, it was difficult to draw many definitive

Table 2. *p*-Fluorophenylalanine-induced haploid segregants from diploids od *P. chrysogenum* of general type Brw Nic × Whi Nic⁺ [a] showing parental genotype segregation in divergent strain crosses but not in sister strain crosses

Segregant class	Phenotype	Number of segregants	
		Sister strain cross[b]	Divergent strain cross[c]
Parental	Brw Nic	12	83
Parental	Whi Nic^+	48	128
Recombinant	Brw Nic^+	12	0
Recombinant	Whi Nic	51	0
Recombinant	Green spored	0	0

[a] Data presented by Morrison and Ball at the Second International Symposium on the Genetics of Industrial Microorganismem. Brw and Whi refer to brown and white spore color, respectively, the genes being located on chromosomes 1 and Nic refers to requirement for nicotinamide the gene being located on linkage group III (Ball 1971)

[b] Pooled data from five independently isolated diploids of the type described by Ball (1973a). One strain Brw Nic was common to all crosses

[c] Pooled data from eight independently isolated diploids between strain Brw Nic used in the crosses described in b. and a strain Whi Nic^+ independently derived from the Wisconsin series and supplied by Dr. K. D. MacDonald

conclusions. Later reviews have tended to reiterate many of the points made in the earlier ones.

Among the definitive conclusions drawn from this and other work were the facts that penicillin production was under nuclear control as judged by the heterokaryon test (MacDonald et al. 1963b) and that diploid synthesis rarely gave increases in penicillin titer. Unequivocal evidence as to whether segregants from diploids could give rise to penicillin titer improvement over both the immediate and prototrophic ancestors of a cross was not obtained. Also, it was not clear from most studies whether the recombinant phenotypes were haploid or diploid or whether any induced segregant was the product of intra-chromosomal (haploidization or nondisjunction) or interchromosomal recombination (mitotic crossing-over) (see Sect. A). In addition, the term "parental genome segregation" was introduced to explain the difficulty in obtaining recombinants; chromosome translocation was suggested as the reason (MacDonald 1968).

In the absence of reliable linkage data at the time, it seemed quite possible that orthodox linkage could explain many of these cases of parental genome segregation. However, later studies (Table 2) employing knowledge of the linkage map endorsed the principle of such parental genome segregation being due to causes other than linkage.

In the early work, a number of conclusions were drawn with regard to the dominance and recessivity of penicillin titer increasing mutations. Often an assumption was made that diploids with titers much lower than either parent indicated recessivity of all the titer-increasing genes in each parent. This could be an oversimplification since any interdependence of sequentially introduced titer-increasing genes would mean that only one of these, possibly the first one, would need to be recessive to prevent expression of the rest. Also, in later studies, the possibility that mitotic crossing-over or mutation could contribute to diploid titer variability was acknowledged in a study by MACDONALD (1964) of 68 diploids formed from the same parent strains which were themselves slightly divergent. In the same study diploids formed from virtually identical parent strains were found to exhibit considerable variability with the result that mutation as a cause of titer variability was favored. This idea was supported by the later studies of BALL (1973a) (see Sect. C.II), based on the analysis of segregants.

II. Later Studies

Many of the workers who contributed to the earlier studies with *P. chrysogenum* subsequently moved on to work with other organisms. However, various industrial workers were not allowed this privilege or even the advantage of working with wild-type *P. chrysogenum*. Instead, they attempted to capitalize on the early experiences and work with the reality of industrial strains in various ways. ELANDER (1967), ELANDER et al. (1973, 1976) and BALL (1971, 1973a, b), and BALL and AZEVEDO (1976) worked with sister strains, i.e., strains closely related in mutational lineage differing only in the qualitative markers for spore color and auxotrophy. BALL (1973a) constructed a genetic map and introduced single-step mutations for increases in penicillin titer so that crosses could be carried out without a high degree of parental divergence. The studies of CALAM et al. (1976) were more empirically based but several types of crosses were carried out together with the introduction of a selection line based on sequential mutation of a diploid.

In contrast with the earlier studies, these later studies were successful in producing recombinant strains with increased titers. ELANDER (1967) was able to show increases in titer through diploidization of sister strains. CALAM et al. (1976) produced increases in titer and sporulation by their sequential mutation of a diploid. BALL (1973a) increased the titer by recombination of single qualitative mutations for titer increase after creating and exploiting a genetic map. The approach adopted in this latter work using the genetic map was time consuming and is not necessarily the only way that industrial breeding should be carried out. However, it did illustrate a principle, namely that haploid recombinants with increased titer compared with the immediate and original parents could be produced. In this work, a number of problems outlined in Table 1 B were overcome. However, despite improving strain stability, segregants with a wide range of titers were produced, suggesting enhanced mutation via diploidization as discussed in Sect. C.I.

Certain workers with *A. nidulans* have suggested that the biometrical approach should be introduced with *P. chrysogenum* in studies of penicillin production. However, CATEN and JINKS (1976) point out that results from the parasexual cycle cannot always be compared with results from the sexual cycle even in *A. nidulans*, and there are no good examples in *A. nidulans* of exploitation of the parasexual cycle for biometrical studies. Their idea of chromosome substitution is very similar

Table 3. Some guidelines for using the parasexual cycle to increase penicillin yield. (Based on BALL 1973b)

1. Parent strains should be relatively stable for penicillin production
2. Parent strains should be divergent, i.e., products of independent mutation and selection lines that have been directed at increasing penicillin yield
3. Genetic markers should not modify penicillin yield either singly or when combined
4. Preferably all the genetic markers should be recovered from the parasexual cross
5. Methods for increasing the recombination frequency and improving detection of recombinants should be used, e.g. recombinogens to increase mitotic crossing-over and haploidization, and markers to screen and select the products of such events
6. Quantitative analyses of genetic variability affecting penicillin yield should be made on both parental and segregant population

to that employed by BALL (1973a) with *P. chrysogenum*. However, there are major problems that can be envisaged in attempting such chromosome substitution techniques in crosses between strains of *P. chrysogenum* that are highly divergent. These include parental genome segregation and reduced independent assortment of chromosomes possibly because of chromosome translocation (see Table 2). Nevertheless, recombination between strains of high divergence does occur to a limited extent particularly by mitotic crossing-over. The use of biometrical techniques to identify different titer distributions associated with different markers and genotypes could help in interpreting data and possibly in predicting future breeding strategies.

As a result of the accumulated experience with *P. chrysogenum*, it is possible to draw up a set of guidelines for breeding studies (Table 3).

A question that has been raised by CALAM et al. (1976) is the relevance of genetic mapping to industrial breeding. The foregoing discussion has hopefully answered this. In addition, the extensive indirect use of genetic mapping is worth emphasizing. For example, MORRISON and BALL (unpublished work) have used a genetic map (BALL 1971) to discover agents that induce different types of segregation which allowed them to obtain additional data on the order of markers on chromosome I. They exploited spore color markers as recessive screenable markers for detection of recombination events on chromosome I. The work is described below at length with data given in Table 4.

The materials and methods used were identical to those described by BALL (1971) unless otherwise stated. The recessive alleles for requirement of lysine, choline, and nicotinamide are indicated as *lys*-5, *cho*-1, and *nic*-1, respectively. Resistance to 8-aza adenine, a semidominant gene, is indicated as *aa*-1. The designations *y*-1 and *w*-2 indicate the mutant spore colors yellow and white, respectively, and *br*-1 and *br*-3 are independently isolated brown spore color mutants. Phenotypes are indicated by nonitalicized symbols with capital first letters, e.g., Br. Of the markers used in this work only *nic*-1 was not located on group I. Several diploids were synthesized. Diploid 1 was *br*-3 *lys*-5/*y*-1 *cho*-1 and was green spored. Diploid 2 was *br*-3 *lys*-5 *cho*-1/*w*-2 *aa*-1; *nic*-1 and was green spored. One of the parents of diploid 2, *br*-3 *lys*-5 *cho*-1 was a recombinant from diploid 1.

According to the method of BALL (1971) *p*-fluorophenylalanine (PFA) was used to induce haploidization of both diploids. In addition, gamma rays (γ) were used to induce recombination and segregation from diploid 1 by the following technique based on that of KÄFER (1963): Spore suspensions in water were irradiated with γ from a Co^{60} source (20,000 rad to give 1% survival). The surviving spores were plated onto complete medium to give 20

Table 4. Haploid and diploid segregants[a] from diploids 1 and 2

Diploid segregants		Haploid segregants	
Phenotypes		Genotypes	
Segregants from diploid 1			
Br Lys Cho^+	11	*br*-3 *lys*-5	68
Y Lys^+ Cho	4	*y*-1 *cho*-1	50
Br Lys Cho	0	*br*-3 *lys*-5 *cho*-1	3
Y Lys^+ Cho^+	21	*y*-1	14
Br Lys^+ Cho	1	*br*-3 *cho*-1	10
Y Lys Cho^+	3	*y*-1 *lys*-5	4
Br Lys^+ Cho^+	19	*br*-3	2
Y Lys Cho	0	*y*-1 *lys*-5 *cho*-1	0
	59		151
Segregants from diploid 2[b]			
Br Aa^+ Lys Cho	0	*br*-3 *lys*-5 *cho*-1	12
Br Aa^+ Lys Cho^+	6	*br*-3 *lys*-5	11
Br Aa^+ Lys^+ Cho^+	21	*br*-3	25
Br Aa Lys^+ Cho^+	4	*br*-3 *aa*-1	18
W Aa^+ Lys Cho	0	*w*-2 *lys*-5 *cho*-1	0
W Aa^+ Lys Cho^+	0	*w*-2 *lys*-5	0
W Aa^+ Lys^+ Cho^+	1	*w*-2	0
W Aa Lys^+ Cho^+	4	*w*-2 *aa*-1	95
	36		161

[a] Classified for group I markers for diploid 1 *br*-3 *lys*-5/*y*-1 *cho*-1 and diploid 2 *br*-3 *lys*-5 *cho*-1/*w*-2 *aa*-1; *nic*-1

[b] The low frequency of white spored recombinants from diploid 2 is unexplained, but might be due to growth disadvantage

colonies per plate, following incubation at 25 °C for 4 days. Sectors with mutant spore color were purified by spore platings and classified, only one sector per colony being tested. 5-Fluorouracil (FU) was used to treat diploid 2 by the following technique: FU at a final concentration of 3.9 μg/ml in complete medium agar was used. Spores were plated onto this medium such that 1% survived to give about five colonies per dish following incubation at 25 °C for 10 days. Sectors with mutant spore color were purified by spore platings and classified, only one sector per colony being tested. A third diploid, *br*-1 *cho*-1/*br*-3 *lys*-5 was synthesized. This was brown and sporogenous and, since no green diploids could be recovered from diploidization between *br*-1 *cho*-1 and *br*-3 *lys*-5, this result suggests that *br*-1 and *br*-3 are allelic. Previous work (Ball 1971) had indicated, following complementation and linkage studies, that *y*-1 and *br*-1 were closely linked. Therefore, it can be concluded that *y*-1 and *br*-3 are probably closely linked, a result of relevance to interpretation of segregation data from diploids 1 and 2 (see text and Table 4).

Following PFA treatment of diploid 1, all of the 17 segregants had parental genotypes (i.e., 7 *y*-1 *cho*-1 and 10 *br*-3 *lys*-5) as expected from a diploid carrying four group I markers. Similarly, following PFA treatment of diploid 2, 37 of the 39 haploid segregants had parental genotypes with respect to the group I markers (13 *br*-3 *lys*-5 *cho*-1, 24 *w*-2 *aa*-1, 1 *br*-3 *lys*-5, and 1 *w*-2 *aa*-1 *cho*-1).

Clearly from neither diploid 1 nor 2 could recombinants with respect to group I markers be readily induced with PFA. Therefore, diploids 1 and 2 were treated with γ and FU in or-

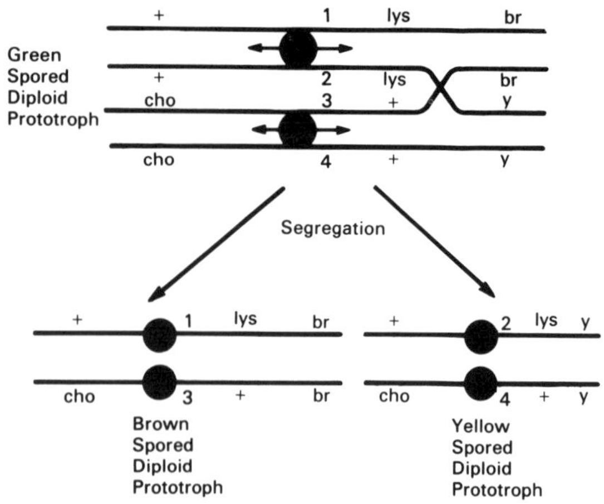

Fig. 2. Mitotic crossing-over in diploid *br*-3 *lys*-5/*y*-1 *cho*-1. Based on data in Table 4. The 4 chromatid stage of mitosis and mitotic crossing-over between *br*-3 and *lys*-5 is shown together with segregation of chromatids *1* with *3* and *2* with *4*. **Note:** All markers distal to the cross-over become homozygous and markers proximal to the cross-over remain heterozygous

der to increase the frequency of such recombinants and the results are shown in Table 1. Recombinant diploids and haploids were obtained.

The diploid segregant data from diploid 1 shown in Table 4 and Fig. 2 indicate that certain products of mitotic crossing-over namely yellow and brown prototrophs, occur at highest frequency. Clearly the auxotrophic markers *cho*-1 and *lys*-5 are not distal to the spore color markers. The other diploid recombinant classes from diploid 1 are the products of multiple events, e.g., mitotic crossing-over plus nondisjunction and, therefore, occur in low frequency. These diploid classes cannot be used to determine unambiguously marker order but the haploid segregant data help in such ordering. The haploid segregant data from diploid 1 are compatible with the gene order *br*-3/*y*-1 *lys*-5 *cho*-1. On the basis of this order, the *br*-3 and *y*-1 *lys*-5, *cho*-1 segregants would require at least two crossing-over events and would, therefore, occur in the lowest frequency, as shown in Table 1.

The data from diploid 2 are consistent with this gene order. None of the markers *aa*-1, *lys*-5 or *cho*-1 is distal to the segregating *br*-3 markers amongst the diploid segregants. Two main conclusions can be drawn from the diploid segregant data from diploid 2. First, Br Lys diploid segregants were readily isolated suggesting that the markers *br*-3 and *lys*-5 are on the same arm, the Br Lys recombinants being produced by recombination between *lys*-5 and the centromere. Secondly, the largest class, brown-spored diploid recombinant prototrophs, can be divided into those with the *aa*-1 marker and those without. This suggests that *aa*-1 is located between *lys*-5 and *br*-3. The haploid segregant data from diploid 2 support these conclusions. Thus, the gene order is probably *br*-3 *lys*-5 *cho*-1 because *br*-3, *cho*-1 segregants are absent, requiring a triple event for their occurrence. Similarly, *aa*-1 can be positioned between *br*-3 and *lys*-5 since no *br*-3 *lys*-5 *aa*-1 phenotypes were detected, requiring a triple event for their occurrence. Finally, *w*-2 is probably distal and not closely linked to *aa*-1 since a high frequency of brown spore colored resistant segregants were recovered, other work having shown that white spore color is epistatic to brown spore color. To sum up, this study together with previous published data, indicates that the gene order on linkage group I in *P. chrysogenum* is *br*-3/*y*-1, *w*-2, *aa*-1, *lys*-5, centromere, *cho*-1.

Recently NORMANSELL et al. (1979) have extended the earlier discussed studies on mutants impaired in penicillin biosynthesis in *A. nidulans* to a low-yielding strain of *P. chrysogenum*. They discovered five complementation groups (V, W, X,

Y, and Z) that were located on three chromosomes. Biochemical studies of intracellular peptides accumulated showed the absence of α-aminoadipoyl-cysteinyl-valine from mutants of group X, Y, and Z and interestingly the mutant from group X also lacked the ability to catalyze penicillin-acyl exchange. In addition, a mutant in group V lacked the latter activity but could form tripeptide. Mutants of group W possessed both properties and the suggestion was made that they could be blocked between tripeptide and isopenicillin N. Such studies exemplify the potential use of qualitative genetic analysis as discussed earlier. The realization of such potential in the improvement of high-yielding industrial strains is the next logical step.

D. Cephalosporium acremonium

Interest in *C. acremonium* and related fungi as β-lactam producers started with studies of penicillin N production in *Emericellopsis* species. Recombination studies were limited. One of few reports was that of FANTINI (1962) and FANTINI and OLIVE (1960) who were successful in demonstrating both the parasexual and sexual cycles in certain *Emericellopsis* species. Penicillin N production in sister strain sexual crosses was studied. Presumably there was little expectation of titer improvements arising from such a study but it did illustrate the profound effects of different types of markers on antibiotic production.

Following the isolation of cephalosporin C and its demonstration as an improvement over penicillin N for production of certain types of derived antibiotic, interest focused on its production by *C. acremonium*. Initial reports emphasized the difficulty in finding any type of recombination system in this organism. The first positive report was the claimed demonstration of the parasexual cycle by NÜESCH et al. (1973) but this report was not extensive. Subsequent comments by ELANDER et al. (1976) reemphasized the negative results and quoted others, e.g., MACDONALD (personal communication) as having similar negative results. The suggestion was made that diploids, if they occur in *C. acremonium*, might be unstable but further investigations of this possibility were not carried out.

The next key development in this field was the work of ANNÉ and PEBERDY (1976), who showed that protoplasts of *C. acremonium* could be prepared and fused with polyethylene glycol (PEG). Isolation of diploids and genetic analysis was not attempted. This was followed by HAMLYN and BALL (1979) who reported that protoplast fusion was a major advantage in genetic analysis in this organism compared with orthodox methods. Furthermore, they showed that following protoplast fusion nuclear fusion could be immediate and that segregants were readily obtained by rapid breakdown of this fusion product.

Total recombinant recovery could be achieved only by plating onto media which allowed direct selection of recombinants but not parental strains. Figure 3 summarizes the events that led up to this discovery. Initially, plating of the fused parents was onto MM and retesting was carried out on CM and MM at equivalent low-density plating. In this way, four different types of prototrophs were detected on the MM onto which the initial fusion mixture was plated. These were: (a) heterokaryons which on subsequent plating to CM and MM gave no growth on MM

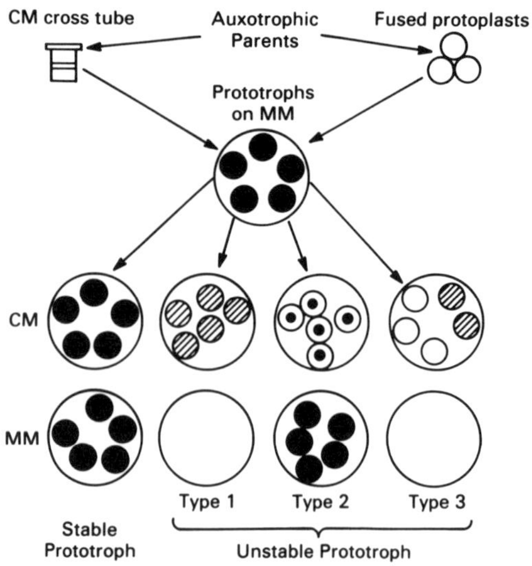

Fig. 3. Formation of different types of prototrophic strains following cell fusion in *C. acremonium*. *CM*, complete medium; *MM*, minimal medium. On plates: *solid black circles* indicate prototrophs; *hatched circles* indicate auxotrophs with parental requirements; *open circles* indicate recombinant auxotrophs. Note that *C. acremonium* does not have a readily detectable spore pigment and, therefore, spore color mutants are not available. Type 1 unstable prototrophs are putative heterokaryons and are obtained in most types of crosses, the exception being certain crosses between strains of highly divergent mutational origin. Type 2 unstable prototrophs were rarely obtained particularly as heterozygotes for more than one genetic marker, with the exception of crosses between strains of highly divergent mutational origin (see text). Type 3 unstable prototrophs and stable prototrophs were readily obtained in most crosses following protoplast fusion, but not by the conventional CM cross-tube method

and parental genotypes on CM; (b) stable prototrophs which gave the same number of colonies on MM as on CM; (c) unstable prototrophs which produced auxotrophic sectors on CM but gave prototrophic growth on MM; (d) mixed growth which on plating gave parental and recombinant types on CM and much less growth on MM. The latter category plus the fact that stable prototrophs could not be made to segregate and were cytologically like the parent strains supported the idea that the diploids in *C. acremonium* are unstable, the stable prototrophs being haploid recombinants.

Plating onto media selective for recombinants was carried out and the technical analogy with multiple factor crosses in streptomycetes was noted. This work was carried out with closely related derivatives of the low-yielding strain M8650. Additional studies with strains having a more divergent mutational ancestry gave heterozygotes at a higher frequency but these were very unstable. Figure 4 illustrates a possible explanation of such heterozygotes based on chromosome translocation which have a high probability of occurring in highly mutated divergent lines used as parents in crosses. A degree of stability is ensured by the balanced lethal condition in an analogous way to that suggested by MacDonald (1964) for *P. chrysogenum* diploid stabilization. Presumably it is still unstable due to escape from bal-

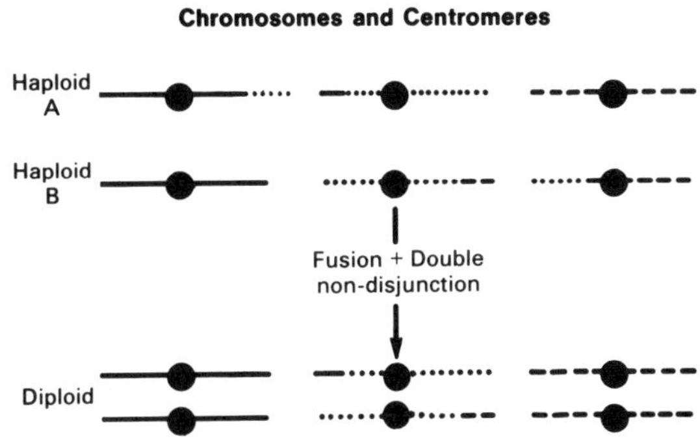

Fig. 4. Formation of a balanced lethal diploid due to chromosome translocation. Haploid A carries a reciprocal translocation between chromosomes I and II. Haploid B carries a reciprocal translocation between chromosomes II and III. Idea based on that previously suggested by BALL (1973 b)

anced lethality by crossing-over. From such a cross, it was possible to recombine the desirable properties of two strains namely growth rate and cephalorporin C synthesis from sulfate and in addition raise the cephalorporin C titer above that of either immediate or prototrophic parent.

E. Recombination Between Naturally Incompatible Fungi

The technique of protoplast fusion has opened up a large number of possibilities for overcoming natural barriers to genetic exchange [see 5th International Protoplast Symposium (1979), Szeged, Hungary; abstract book and full proceedings in press]. Protoplast fusion per se or protoplast fusion as a means to aid DNA uptake (transformation) has been used to cross such barriers. In studies relevant to β-lactam production by fungi several groups of workers have been active.

Where protoplast fusion per se is concerned the work of ANNÉ and PEBERDY (1976) in studying mainly intraspecies fusions provided very important background for the attempts at subsequent interspecies fusions. Following such fusions in a number of fungi including *P. chrysogenum* and *A. nidulans*, heterokaryons were formed following protoplast fusion and diploids arose as secondary sectors from such heterokaryons. DALES and CROFT (1977) were able to extend this earlier work with *A. nidulans* and were able to demonstrate heterokaryosis between pairs of previously incompatible strains. Also in later studies ANNÉ et al. (1976) showed recombination between different species, *Penicillium roquefortii* and *P. chrysogenum*. They showed recombination of the properties of penicillin production from *P. chrysogenum* and certain of the genes of *P. roquefortii*. KEVEI and PEBERDY (1977) obtained recombinants between *A. nidulans* and *Aspergillus rugulosus*.

The so-called hybrids generate strains that have genes from the two parent strains combined, i.e., recombinants. Furthermore, using master strains of *A. nidulans* marked on all eight chromosomes, KEVEI and PEBERDY (1979) were able to show independent chromosome segregation, suggesting considerable chromosome homology between *A. nidulans* and *A. rugulosus*. The latter two organisms are very closely related but such a relationship may not be required to cross wide taxonomic barriers in recombination experiments using protoplast fusion. The reader is referred to reviews by PEBERDY (1979, 1980) for discussion of related topics involving protoplasts. Recently, QUEENER and BALTZ (to be published) have debated the possible use of a hybrid between β-lactam producers *C. acremonium* and *P. chrysogenum*, should it be possible to obtain such a hybrid. They conclude on the basis of known biochemical specificities in these two organisms that it is unlikely that a cephalosporin molecule with an aromatic group at position 7 could result from such a hybrid. Other possibilities are also discussed including the manipulation of β-lactam fungi and actinomycetes. It is possible that to cross broad taxonomic barriers the technique of transformation is the most likely to succeed. The problem with filamentous fungi is to obtain a suitable vector that can be used to aid the introduction of foreign genes into these fungi. The recent demonstration of genetic transformation in yeast using a hybrid *Escherichia coli* yeast plasmid (BEGGS 1978; HINNEN et al. 1978; STRUHL et al. 1979) illustrates what might be achieved.

Acknowledgments. The author thanks the people cited in references for forwarding information on their work and Dr. J. MCCULLOUGH for his comments on the text.

References

Alikhanian SI (1962) Induced mutagenesis in the selection of microorganisms. Adv Appl Microbiol 4:1–48

Alikhanian SI, Kameneva SV (1961) Microbial genetics and its application to fermentation. Sci Rep Inst Super Sanita 1:454–463

Anné J, Peberdy JF (1976) Induced fusion of fungal protoplasts following treatment with polyethylene glycol. J Gen Microbiol 92:413–417

Anné J, Eyssen H, de Sommer P (1976) Somatic hybridization of *Penicillium roquefortii* with *Penicillium chrysogenum* after protoplast fusion. Nature 626:719–721

Ball C (1971) Haploidization analysis in *Penicillium chrysogenum*. J Gen Microbiol 66:63–69

Ball C (1973a) Improvement of penicillin productivity in *Penicillium chrysogenum* by recombination. In: Vaněk Hošťálek Z, Cudlín J (eds) Genetics of industrial microorganisms, vol 2, actinomycetes and fungi. Elsevier, Amsterdam New York London, p 227–237

Ball C (1973b) The genetics of *Penicillium chrysogenum*. Prog Ind Microbiol 12:47–72

Ball C (1978) Genetics in the development of the penicillin process. In: Hütter R, Leisinger T, Nüesch J, Wehrli W (eds) Antibiotics and other secondary metabolites, FEMS (Fed Eur Microbiol Soc) Symp, Academic Press, London, New York, San Francisco, pp 165–176

Ball C, Azevedo JL (1976) Genetic instability in parasexual fungi. In: MacDonald KD (ed) Second international symposium on the genetics of industrial microorganisms. Academic Press, London, New York, San Francisco, p 243

Beggs JD (1978) Transformation of yeasts by a replicating hybrid plasmid. Nature 275:104–109

Birkett JA, Roper JA (1977) Chromosome aberrations in *Aspergillus nidulans*. In: Smith JE, Pateman JA (eds) Genetics and physiology of aspergillus. Academic Press, London New York, p 293

Calam CT, Daglish LB, McCann EP (1976) Penicillin: Tactics in strain improvement. In: MacDonald KD (ed) Second international symposium on the genetics of industrial microorganisms. Academic Press, London New York, p 273

Caten CE, Jinks JL (1976) Quantitative genetics. In: MacDonald KD (ed) Second international symposium on the genetics of industrial microorganisms. Academic Press, London New York, p 93

Dales RBG, Croft JH (1977) Protoplast fusion and the isolation of heterokaryons and diploids from vegetatively incompatible strains of *Aspergillus nidulans*. FEMS Microbiol Lett 1:201–204

Ditchburn P, Holt G, MacDonald KD (1976) The genetic location of mutations increasing penicillin yield in *Aspergillus nidulans*. In: MacDonald KD (ed) Second international symposium on the genetics of industrial microorganisms. Academic Press, London New York, p 213

Edwards GFSTL, Holt G, MacDonald KD (1974) Mutants of *Aspergillus nidulans* impaired in penicillin biosynthesis. J Gen Microbiol 84:420–422

Elander RP (1967) Enhanced penicillin biosynthesis in mutant and recombinant strains of *Penicillium chrysogenum*. Abh Dtsch Akad Wiss (Berlin) 2:403–423

Elander RP, Espenshade MA, Pathak SG, Pan CH (1973) The use of parasexual genetics in an industrial strain improvement program with *Penicillium chrysogenum*. In: Vaněk Z, Hošťálek Z, Cudlín J (eds) Genetics of industrial microorganisms, vol 2, actinomycetes and fungi. Elsevier, Amsterdam New York London, p 239

Elander RP, Corum CJ, De Valeria H, Wilgus RM (1976) Ultraviolet mutagenesis and cephalosporin synthesis in strains of *Cephalosporium acremonium*. In: MacDonald KD (ed) Second international symposium on the genetics of industrial microorganisms. Academic Press, London New York, p 253

Fantini AA (1962) Genetics and antibiotic production of Emericellopsis species. Genetics 47:161–177

Fantini AA, Olive LS (1960) Sexual recombination in a homothallic antibiotic producing fungus. Science 132:1670

Hamlyn P, Ball C (1979) Recombination studies with *Cephalosporium acremonium*. In: Sebek OK, Laskin AI (eds) Genetics of industrial microorganisms. ASM Washington, p 185

Hinnen A, Hicks JB, Fink GR (1978) Transformation of yeast. Proc Natl Acad Sci USA 75:1929–1933

Holt G, MacDonald KD (1968a) Isolation of strains with increased penicillin yield after hybridization in *Aspergillus nidulans*. Nature 219:636–637

Holt G, MacDonald KD (1968b) Penicillin production and its mode of inheritance in *Aspergillus nidulans*. Antonie van Leeuwenhoek 34:409–416

Holt G, Edwards GFSTL, MacDonald KD (1976) The genetics of mutants impaired in the biosynthesis of penicillin. In: MacDonald KD (ed) Second international symposium on the genetics of industrial microorganisms. Academic Press, London New York, pp 199–211

Käfer E (1963) Radiation effects on mitotic recombination in diploids of *Aspergillus nidulans*. Genetics 48:27–45

Käfer E (1977) Meiotic and mitotic recombination in *Aspergillus* and its chromosomal aberrations. Adv Genet 19:33–124

Käfer E, Upshall A (1973) The pheontypes of the eight disomics and trisomics of *Aspergillus nidulans*. J Hered 64:35–38

Kevei F, Peberdy JF (1977) Interspecific hybridization between *Aspergillus nidulans* and *Aspergillus rugulosus* by fusion of somatic protoplasts. J Gen Microbiol 102:255–262

Kevei F, Peberdy JF (1979) Induced segregates in interspecifid hybrids of *Aspergillus nidulans* and *Aspergillus rugulosus* obtained by protoplast fusion. Mol Gen Genet 170:213–218

MacDonald KD (1964) Preservation of the heterozygous diploid condition in industrial microorganisms. Nature 204:404–405

MacDonald KD (1966) Differences in diploids synthesized between the same parental strains. Antonie von Leeuwenhoek 32:431–441

MacDonald KD (1968) The persistence of parental genome segregation in *Penicillium chrysogenum* after nitrogen mustard treatment. Mutat Res 5:302–305

MacDonald KD, Holt G (1976) Genetics of biosynthesis and overproduction of penicillin. Sci Prog 63:547–573

MacDonald KD, Hutchinson JM, Gillett WA (1963a) Isolation of auxotrophs of *Penicillium chrysogenum* and their penicillin yields. J Gen Microbiol 33:335–374

MacDonald KD, Hutchinson JM, Gillett WA (1963 b) Heterokaryon studies and the genetic control of penicillin and chrysogenum production in *Penicillium chrysogenum*. J Gen Microbiol 33:375–383
MacDonald KD, Hutchinson JM, Gillett WA (1963 a) Formation and segregation of heterozygous diploids between and wild-type strain and derivatives of high penicillin yield in *Penicillium chrysogenum*. J Gen Microbiol 33:335–394
MacDonald KD, Hutchinson JM, Gillett WA (1964) Properties of heterozygous diploids between strains of *Penicillium chrysogenum* selected for high penicillin yield. Antonie van Leeuwenhoek 33:209–224
MacDonald KD, Hutchinson JM, Gillett WA (1965) Heterozygous diploids of *Penicillium chrysogenum* and their segregation patterns. Genetics 36:378–397
Merrick MJ (1975 a) Hybridization and selection for increased penicillin titer in wild-type isolates of *Aspergillus nidulans*. J Gen Microbiol 91:278–286
Merrick MJ (1975 b) The inheritance of penicillin titer in crosses between lines of *Aspergillus nidulans* selected for increased productivity. J Gen Microbiol 91:287–294
Merrick MJ, Caten CE (1975) The inheritance of penicillin titer in wild-type isolates of *Aspergillus nidulans*. J Gen Microbiol 86:283–293
Normansell PJM, Normansell ID, Holt G (1979) Genetic and biochemical studies of mutants of *Penicillium chrysogenum* impaired in penicillin production. J Gen Microbiol 112:113–126
Nüesch J, Treichler HJ, Liersch M (1973) The biosynthesis of cephalosporin C. In: Vaněk Z, Hošťálek Z, Cudlín J (eds) Genetics of industrial microorganisms, vol 2, Actinomycetes and fungi. Elsevier, Amsterdam London New York, p 309
Peberdy JF (1979) Fungal protoplasts: Isolation, reversion and fusion. Ann Rev Microbiol 33:21–39
Peberdy JF (1980) Protoplast fusion in a tool for genetic manipulation and breeding in industrial microorganisms. Enzyme Microb Technol 2:23–29
Pontecorvo G, Sermonti G (1954) Parasexual recombination in *Penicillium chrysogenum*. J Gen Microbiol 11:94–104
Pontecorvo G, Roper JA, Hemmons LM, MacDonald KD, Butron AWJ (1953) The genetics of *Aspergillus nidulans*. Adv Genet 5:141–238
Queener SW, Baltz RH (to be published) Genetics of industrial microorganisms. Annu Rep Ferm Processes 3:5–45
Roper JA (1952) Production of heterozygous diploids in filamentous fungi. Experientia 8:14–15
Roper JA (1966) Mechanisms of inheritance: The parasexual cycle. In: Ainsworth GC, Sussman SS (eds) The fungi, vol 2. Academic Press, New York, p 589
Sermonti G (1959) Genetics of penicillin production. Ann NY Acad Sci 81:950–973
Sermonti G (1961) The parasexual cycle in *Penicillium chrysogenum* and its application to the production of penicillin. Sci Rep Inst Super Sanita 1:441–483
Sermonti G (1969) Genetics of antibiotic-producing microorganisms. Wiley, London New York
Simpson I, Caten CE (1977) Genetics of penicillin production in lines of *Aspergillus nidulans* selected through successive generations of mutagenic treatment. Microb Genet Bull 42:3–5
Simpson IN, Caten CE (1979 a) Induced quantitative variation for penicillin titer in clonal populations of *Aspergillus nidulans*. J Gen Microbiol 110:1–12
Simpson IN, Caten CE (1979 b) Recurrent mutation and selection for increased penicillin titer in *Aspergillus nidulans*. J Gen Microbiol 113:p209–217
Struhl K, Stinchcomb DT, Scherer S, Davis RW (1979) High frequency transformation of yeast: Autonomous replication of hybrid DNA molecules. Proc Natl Acad Sci USA 76:1035–1039
Upshall A, Käfer E (1974) Detection and identification of translocations by increased specific non-disjunction in *Aspergillus nidulans*. Genetics 76:19–31
Upshall A, Giddings B, Teow SC, Mortimore JD (1979) Novel methods of genetic analysis in fungi. In: Sebek OK, Laskin AI (eds) Genetics of industrial microorganisms. ASM, Washington, p 197

CHAPTER 5

Genetics of β-Lactam-Producing Actinomycetes

R. KIRBY

A. Introduction

The commercial usefulness of novel β-lactam antibiotics has turned the interests of the pharmaceutical industry towards the *Actinomycetales* as a possible source. This group of organisms has provided over the years a rich harvest of new antibiotics, but only recently has it been shown that they are able to produce β-lactam antibiotics (NAGARAJAN et al. 1971; NAGARAJAN 1972). This group of substances had been thought to be produced only by fungi up to that point.

The *Antinomycetales* are gram-positive filamentous bacteria which constitute a well-defined taxonomic group of organisms. In molecular and ultrastructural terms they are typical prokaryotes although their morphology belies this. During their life cycle they undergo a complex morphological differentiation (HOPWOOD 1967). When a spore germinates on solid medium, it produces one or two mycelial germ tubes which grow and divide to form a circular, loosely packed colony of much-branched septate mycelium. These mycelial cell units are multinucleate. As development progresses, white furry aerial mycelial branches are formed which grow vertically upwards from the colony. These then undergo a process of septation which ends with a rounding off process to give uninucleate (for the most part) spores (WILDERMUTH 1970; KALAKOUTSKI and AGRE 1976). This metamorphosis into spores is different from that of *Bacillus* as it does not seem to require any special conditions to trigger it and it occurs as a natural part of the life cycle. The spores of the *Actinomycetales* are not endospores. They are not highly resistant to environmental damage, but are merely slightly less vulnerable to such things as dessication compared to the cells of the vegetative mycelium (Fig. 1).

The *Actinomycetales* are ubiquitous in their distribution throughout the soil, although they do colonize other environments. For example, certain *Nocardia* are opportunist pathogens of man and there are examples of marine *Actinomycetales*. Approximately 85% of known antibiotics are produced by members of the *Actinomycetales;* the fungi which produce antibiotics are also soil organisms (HOPWOOD and MERRICK 1977; HOPWOOD 1978). Thus it is possible that soil provides an environment where antibiotic production is favored. Up to the present, except in a few specialized cases, it has proved difficult to show that antibiotics are produced in a natural environment. As a corollary, it has therefore proved equally difficult to show that antibiotic production has any selective advantage to the wild-type organism in its original ecosystem. The alternative hypothesis, that the production of antibiotics by these organisms through secondary metabolism is merely an example of the excretion of random waste products, is unlikely as it does not explain their preponderance and activity (HOPWOOD and MERRICK 1977).

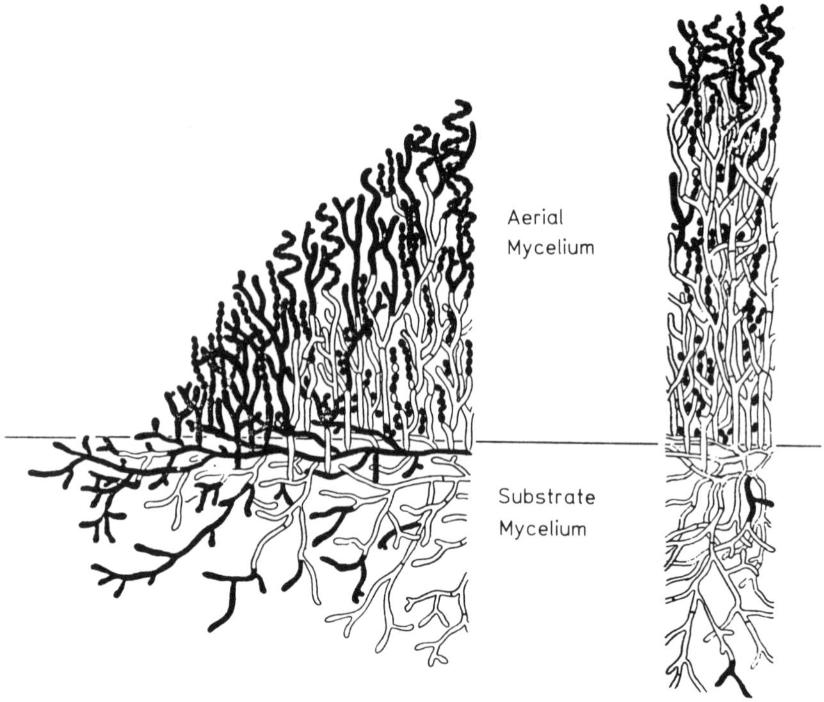

Fig. 1. Structure of a *Streptomyces* colony (HOPWOOD 1967)

It is against this background that we must consider the *Actinomycetales* which produce the β-lactam antibiotics and what their relationship is with each other and with the β-lactam-producing fungi. One may speculate that there may have been a single event or parallel evolution of similar pathways. It has been suggested that resistance plasmids found among the eubacteria originated from the *Actinomycetales* (FREEMAN et al. 1977). Since actinomycetes produce antibiotics, it is necessary that they have resistance mechanisms to cope with their own antibiotics (DEMAIN 1974). Our present knowledge is not enough to confirm or deny such an explanation by comparison of the mechanism, but the micro-environment of the soil may provide an ideal environment for such an exchange.

Despite their importance, the genetics of β-lactam antibiotic production in actinomycetes has remained a relatively backward area of study. This is in common with most other antibiotic-producing actinomycetes of commercial interest where genetic data are relatively scanty. There are two aspects to the genetics of antibiotic production: (1) the structural genes involved in the biosynthesis and (2) the control genes which are probably scattered about the various anabolic and catabolic pathways and regulate antibiotic production. The control genes are probably the major group which is affected in increasing titer in an organism while the structural genes obviously play a part in any attempt to modify the end product of the pathway (MERRICK 1975).

B. β-Lactam Antibiotics and the Actinomycetales

Until the late 1960 s, the β-lactam antibiotics were thought to be produced only by certain fungi. During the general search for novel antibiotics in the *Actinomycetales*, it became clear that this is not the case. Although not widely distributed like certain other antibiotics, β-lactam antibiotics are produced by a number of species (HIGGENS et al. 1974).

At this point, it is useful to consider the taxonomy of the actinomycetes. They form Part 17 of the prokaryotic bacteria as described in the Eighth Edition of Bergey's Manual of Determinative Bacteriology (PRIDHAM and TRESNER 1974). The two genera of interest to us are *Nocardia* and *Streptomyces;* it is these that produce the majority of antibiotics. The two genera are distinguished by cell wall composition; the *Streptomyces* genus is by far the larger of the two. As would be expected, the majority of species which produce β-lactam antibiotics are *Streptomyces* although one species of *Nocardia is known to do so* (NAGARAJAN 1972).

One problem is that the classification into subspecies and species, which is based on morphology and biochemical criteria, leaves something to be desired when considering whether one species is closely related to another. Even after using such a technique as phage typing, deciding where species start and end is difficult. The presence or absence of a restriction system can have a profound difference. Speciation refers in population genetics to the development of two distinct populations without genetic exchange between them. This is easy to define in the gross world of large plants and animals. In the soil, the microenvironment is such that

Table 1. Species of *Streptomyces* known to produce β-lactam antibiotics

Species of *Streptomyces*	Strain	β-Lactam antibiotics produced	References
S. griseus	NRRL 3851	Cephamycin	PARAG (1978)
S. cattleya	NRRL 8057	Thienamycin	
S. jumonjinensis	NRRL 5741	Penicillin N	KIRBY (unpublished results)
S. clavuligerus		Caphalosporin Clavulanic acid Penicillin N Cephamycin Olivanic acid	AHARONOWITZ and DEMAIN (1978) READING and COLE (1976) HIGGENS and KASTNER (1971)
S. lipmanii	NRRL 3584	Olivanic acid	GODFREY (1973)
S. olivaceus	ATCC 31126	Olivanic acid	BIX et al. (1979)
Nocardia uniformis var *tsuyamensis*	ATCC 21806	Penicillin N	NAGARAJAN (1972)
S. cremeus subsp. *auratilis*	ATCC 31358	PS-5	OKAMURA et al. (1978) OKAMURA et al. (1979)
S. fulvoviridis		Olivanic acid	OKAMURA et al. (1979)
S. lactamdurans		Cephamycins	STAPLEY et al. (1972)

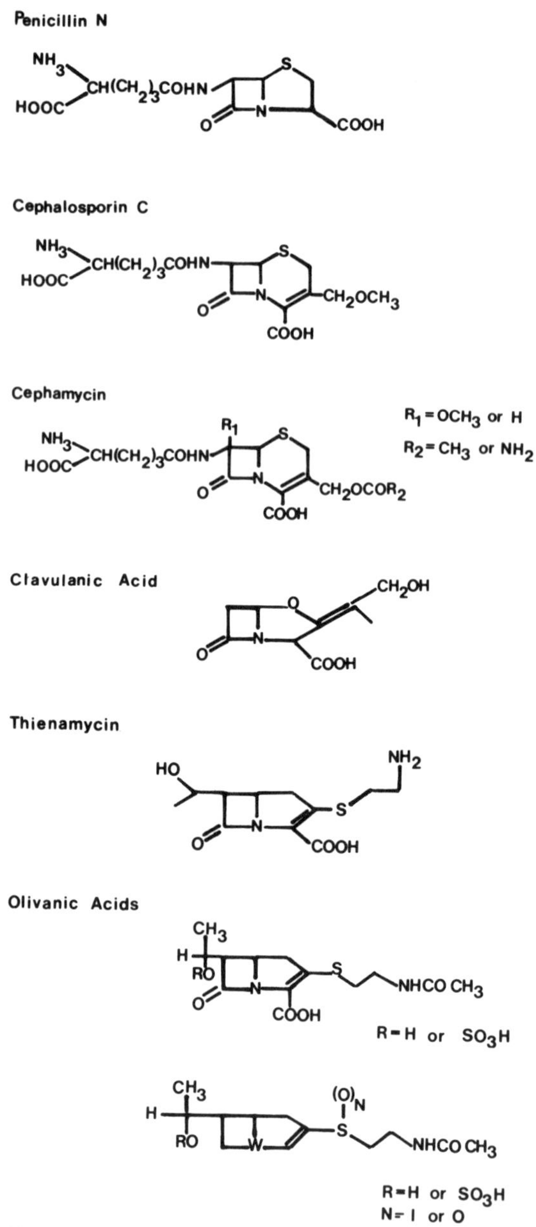

Fig. 2. β-Lactam antibiotic structures

widespread genetic exchange would seem unlikely and so this should increase the likelihood of speciation. The identification of closely similar species which can undergo genetic exchange supports diversification without necessarily the development of barriers to genetic exchange (HOPWOOD and WRIGHT 1973a, b; ALACEVIC 1963; LOMOVSKAYA et al. 1977; POLSINELLI and BERETTA 1966).

Even so, there is a widespread similarity of species throughout the world, although some species have only been isolated once. β-Lactam antibiotics are found in a diverse group of species. The actinomycetes which can produce β-lactam antibiotics as described in published research are shown in Table 1. Obviously this is by no means a complete list of known β-lactam producers. Industrial companies have probably isolated unpublished examples of other species. The list describes a large spectrum of actinomycete species and a broad spectrum of β-lactam antibiotics ranging from penicillin N to β-lactamase inhibitors and antibiotics, thienamycin, and clavulanic acid (Fig. 2).

An important aspect of antibiotic production in these species and a marked difference from the fungi is that in most cases the actinomycetes produce additional antibiotics completely different from β-lactams. For example, *Streptomyces clavuligerus* also produces tunicamycin and holomycin (KENIG and READING 1979). This is important when one begins the purification of the β-lactam antibiotics; it can also cause problems during the direct study of their production when using bioassays. In the latter case, changes in the production of one antibiotic could have an effect on other antibiotics, either masking or confusing the issue (KIRBY 1978 b).

C. Streptomyces Genetics

The genetics of *Streptomyces* has lagged somewhat behind the rapid advances in the genetics and molecular biology of eubacteria for a number of reasons. The first and foremost is that the direct transfer of techniques from eubacteria to actinomycetes has rarely been simple. This, combined with the relative manpower numbers in the two areas, makes progress slow although the prokaryotic nature of actinomycetes has been readily demonstrated (BRADLEY and LEDERBERG 1956; BRAENDLE and SZYBALSKI 1959). The pragmatic approach of most drug companies to yield improvement, involving the use of the well-tried but random approach of mutation and screening, has not helped to develop actinomycete genetics. This approach has produced little in the way of information on the secondary metabolic pathways of actinomycetes and fungi. It is now possible to look forward to the exploitation of the elegant techniques of molecular biology and genetic engineering based on recent work on the genetics of *Streptomyces*.

Most of the original work on the mechanisms of genetic modification and transfer in *Streptomyces* was and still is being carried out on *Streptomyces coelicolor* A3(2) by Hopwood and his colleagues. *S. coelicolor* A3(2) and its derivatives are probably more closely related to *Streptomyces violaceus-ruber* than to *S. coelicolor* (PRIDHAM and TRESNER 1974). However, in order to avoid causing confusion by changing from its commonly used name, and to continue the tradition established in the literature, I shall use this species name.

S. coelicolor A3(2) has a circular genetic map of over one hundred markers (HOPWOOD 1967). It is known to produce at least two distinct antibiotics, methylenomycin A and actinorhodin, neither of which is of commercial interest (RUDD and HOPWOOD 1979; KIRBY et al. 1975; KIRBY and HOPWOOD 1977; WRIGHT and HOPWOOD 1976a, b; RUDD and HOPWOOD 1978; HORNEMANN and HOPWOOD 1978). Using standard genetic methods involving the isolation of multiply marked strains and mutagenic treatments and crosses involving four or more genetic markers, it was possible to produce the circular gene genetic map (Fig. 3a). This had characteristically two large regions at 9 o'clock and 3 o'clock in which genetic markers were very sparse. This seems to be similar in other species. Either these regions are highly active during recombination, causing an elongation with respect to the remainder of the genetic map, or they are physically long but contain few markers (HOPWOOD 1967; HOPWOOD et al. 1973).

The level of genetic exchange in different crosses varied significantly. This led to the identification of a fertility system in this species. The fertility factor turned out to be a genetic element which was self-transmissible but unliked to the chromosomal markers of *S. coelicolor*, i.e., a plasmid. This was the first identification of a plasmid in *Streptomyces*. The plasmid was found to code for the production of and resistance to the antibiotic methylenomycin A. It was lost at an appreciable frequency and was transmitted to plasmid-less strains at high frequency. No linkage could be identified between the element and any chromosomal marker (VIVIAN 1971; HOPWOOD and WRIGHT 1973a, b; KIRBY et al. 1975; KIRBY and HOPWOOD 1977).

This so-called SCP1 plasmid was transmissible to other closely related species of *Streptomyces* and could be forced to integrate into the main chromosome to give a high frequency of chromosomal mobilization. It is with such an SCP1^{NF} strain that most of the chromosomal mapping of *S. coelicolor* was carried out. It was also possible to create modified SCP1 plasmids which carried pieces of the main chromosome including known chromosomal markers, i.e., plasmid-primes (HOPWOOD and WRIGHT 1976). The resemblance between the SCP1 plasmid of *S. coelicolor* and the well-studied plasmids of eubacteria is obvious.

The genetic mapping of *S. coelicolor* stimulated the production of maps of other species which were of much greater commercial interest than *S. coelicolor*. Figure 3b–d show examples of the maps produced. These are for *Streptomyces olivaceus*, which produces the β-lactam olivanic acid class, *S. clavuligerus*, a species which produces at least four different β-lactam antibiotics, and the NRRL8351 strain of *Streptomyces griseus* which a β-lactam antibiotic. How closely this latter strain is related to the streptomycin-producing *S. griseus* is not known but this illustrates the taxonomic problems that occur when strains identified as the same species produce totally different antibiotics. There is no information about the general applicability of the genetic map of a species to other isolates of that species which may vary significantly in the antibiotics that they produce. Attempts have been made to determine whether the general structure of all maps of *Streptomyces* is similar, but this has not been proved satisfactorily.

The identification of plasmid sex factors in *S. coelicolor* A3(2) may imply a similarity between these gram-positives and the gram-negative eubacteria. However, the widespread presence of heterokaryosis in *Streptomyces* (HOPWOOD et al. 1963; MATSELYUKH 1976; KIRBY 1978a), which may originate by a method not involving plasmid mobilization, would also suggest differences. In most cases of commercially important *Streptomyces*, once genetic exchange has been detected, little attempt has been made to study the mechanism in detail.

In the β-lactam producers, *S. clavuligerus*, *S. griseus*, and *S. olivaceus* are the only species for which genetic mape are available (KIRBY 1978a; PARAG 1978;

MALSELYUKH 1976). Heteroclones, partial diploids and heterokaryotes seem to be quite common in *Streptomyces*. Early work suggested that transduction occurs in *Streptomyces* (ALIKHANIAN et al. 1960). However, only recently has transduction of genes by bacteriophage been clearly demonstrated (STUTTARD 1979). This means that all three methods of transfer of genetic material between bacterial species have been demonstrated in *Streptomyces:* conjugation, transduction, and transformation. Transformation will be discussed later.

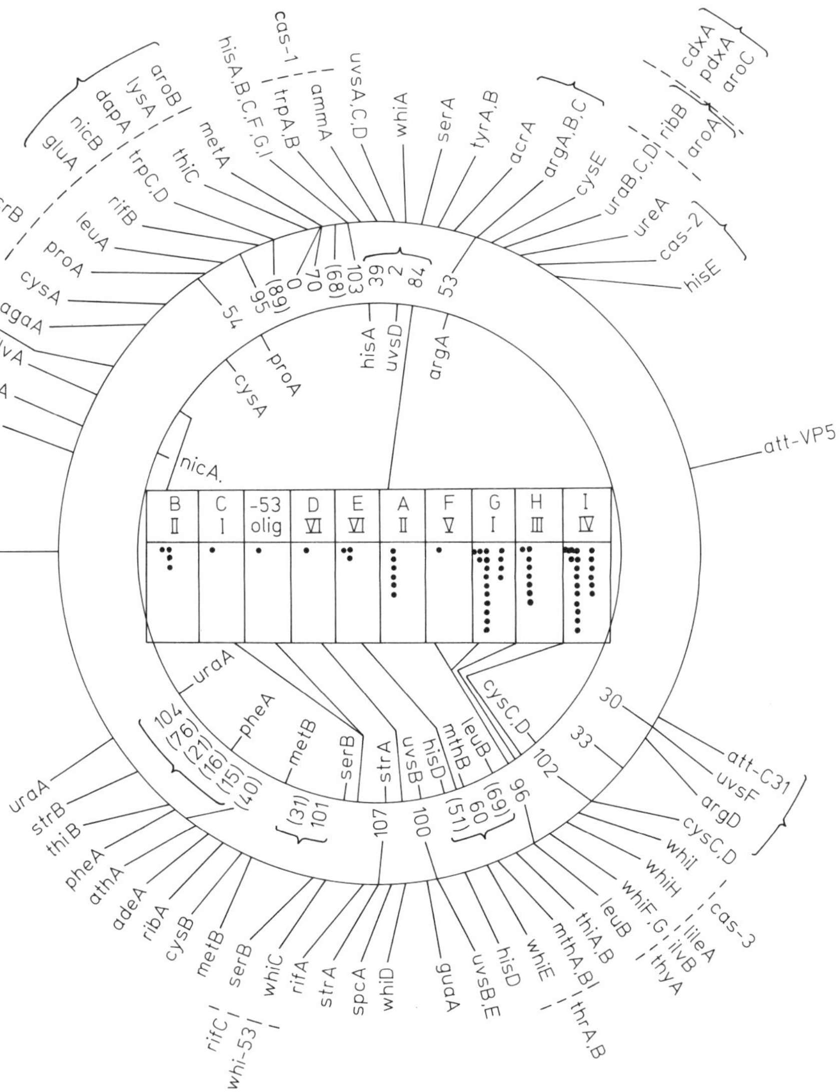

Fig. 3a

Fig. 3. a Genetic map of *Streptomyces coelicolor* A3(2) (HOPWOOD et al. 1973). **b** Genetc map of *Streptomyces olivaceus* (MALSELYUK 1976). **c** Genetic map of *Streptomyces clavuligerus* (KIRBY 1978a). **d** Genetic map of *Streptomyces griseus* (PARAG 1978)

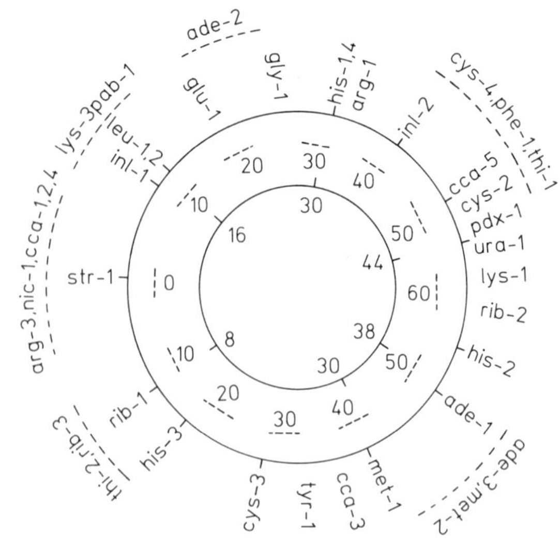

Fig. 3 b

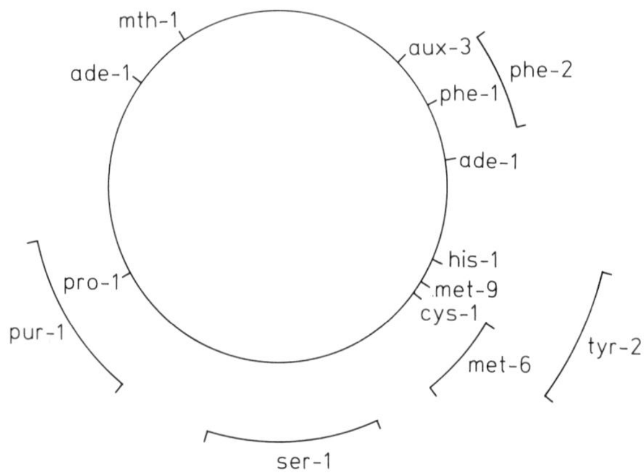

Fig. 3 c

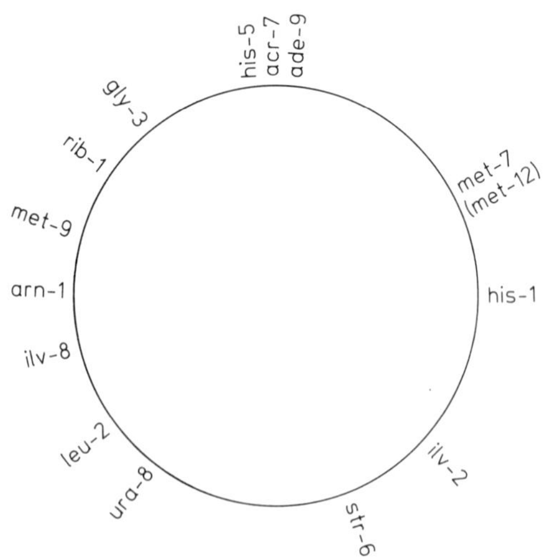

Fig. 3 d

I. Plasmids in Streptomyces

The genetic identification of an extrachromosomal element in *S. coelicolor* A3(2), which fitted the description of a bacterial plasmid, gave hope that the genetics and molecular biology of *Streptomyces* would resemble those of the better understood eubacteria (VIVIAN 1971). Since the concept of a plasmid is a purely genetic one, the initial failure to identify covalently closed circular DNA in *S. coelicolor* corresponding to SCP1 was not an obstacle to the development of plasmid studies in *Streptomyces* (SCHREMPF et al. 1975). Antibiotic production in *Streptomyces* is known in many cases to involve unstable systems and plasmide offer a possible explanation (AKAGAWA et al. 1975; BORONIN and SADOVNIKOVA 1972; CHANG et al. 1978; GREGORY and HUANG 1964b;KIRBY 1978b; OKANISHI et al. 1970; REDSHAW et al. 1979; SHAW and PIWOWARSKI 1977; YU-GU et al. 1978).

A brief description of the phenotype of the SCP1 plasmid is shown in Table 2. It proved impossible to isolate any mutants which directly affected methylenomycin A production and could be clearly shown to be chromosomal. A possible exception to this is the pleiotropic effect of certain "bald" (Bld^-) mutants on antibiotic production (MERRICK 1976). It was possible however to isolate mutants which failed to produce methylenomycin A which were plasmid linked. Cosynthesis between these mutants gave methylenomycin A, showing that a major part, if not all, of the genes coding for the pathway of synthesis of this antibiotic is carried of SCP1. These mutations also affected methylenomycin A resistance and plasmid transfer, showing that these too are plasmid-linked (KIRBY et al. 1975; WRIGHT and HOPWOOD 1976b; KIRBY and HOPWOOD 1977; HORNEMANN and HOPWOOD 1978).

The mycelial nature of *Streptomyces* makes the concept and analysis of such phenomena as entry exclusion and incompatibility in these species much more difficult than in eubacteria. The separation of surface phenomena from intracellular plasmid interaction is almost impossible as the transfer of plasmids takes place over days on solid agar compared to minutes in liquid culture with eubacteria. Using plasmid-primes carrying different chromosomal markers on the SCP1 plasmid, it was possible to show that the presence of one plasmid did inhibit the entry of a second. The plasmids used had the same origin and this would be expected from similar work in eubacteria (KIRBY 1976). However, as will be mentioned later, *S. coelicolor* contains a second plasmid which is compatable with SCP1 (BIBB et al. 1977).

Overall, there is a strong resemblance between SCP1 and many eubacterial plasmids involved in fertility and antibiotic resistance. Recent work has shown that SCP1 exists as physical cccDNA and is about 100 megadaltons (md) in size (West-

Table 2. The phenotype of the two plasmids of *Streptomyces coelicolor* A3(2)

Plasmid	Size (md)	Antibiotic production	Antibiotic resistance	Transfer	Lethal zygosis	Fertility factor	Plasmid primes	Episome
SCP1	100	Yes	Yes	Yes	Yes	Yes	Yes	Yes
SCP2	19.2	No	No	Yes	No	Poor	No	No
SCP2*	19.2	No	No	Yes	Yes	Yes	Yes	Probably

pheling, personal communication). If these plasmids are similar to the plasmids of *Pseudomonas aeruginosa* and *Agrobacterium tumefaciens*, which are also involved in complex processes, their size would be expected to be 100 md larger.

The first physical isolation of a plasmid from a *Streptomyces* species as cccDNA was accomplished by Schrempf et al. (1975) and this was a 19.2 md plasmid from *S. coelicolor* A3(2) (Kirby and Wotton 1979). This plasmid was present in all the strains of *S. coelicolor* A3(2) studied irrespective of the SCP1 plasmid status. No variation in size could be detected in SCP1$^+$, SCP1$^-$, SCP1^{NF}, and SCP1′ strains. In the case of the plasmid-primes, genetic evidence had shown that they carried quite large pieces of chromosomal DNA and thus should be easily detectable. Restriction enzyme analysis confirmed the absence of any relationship between the physical 19.2 md plasmid and SCP1 (Bibb et al. 1977).

The new plasmid, SCP2, was shown to be a fertility factor too, being responsible for the residual level of recombination found in SCP1$^-$ × SCP1$^-$ crosses. This was shown when a modified SCP2 was identified which gave an increased fertility and allowed the isolation of SCP2$^-$ strains. This modification was designated SCP2*. It would seem that this modification was not of the large-scale chromosomal insertion plasmid-prime type as no gross change in the restriction map has been noted. Nor was it due to plasmid integration, since the plasmid was still easily isolated as cccDNA and SCP2* was unlinked to chromosomal markers. One important factor in the distinction between SCP2 and SCP2* is that the transfer of SCP2* to an SCP2$^-$ strain produced a zone of "lethal zygosis" around the SCP2$^-$ colony. This lethal zygosis was also detected in the methylenomycin A zone produced by SCP1 strains. This "pock" formation provided an indirect selection for the SCP2* plasmid. It is possible that a mutational event could have resulted in the formation of SCP2* from SCP2 and this has caused derepression of transfer. Pock formation as an indirect selection allowed the development of the transformation technique in *Streptomyces*. The phenotype of SCP2 is described in relation to SCP1 in Table 2.

The physical isolation of the SCP2 plasmid and the development of transformation (see Sect. III) as a means of reintroducing DNA into the cell have led to the direct physical manipulation of *Streptomyces* genes using genetic engineering. It has not proved possible to induce SCP2 to replicate in *E. coli*. No direct selection for the SCP2 plasmid has yet come to hand and this is a necessary requirement for serious cloning of *Streptomyces* genes (see Sect. D. V). There is no certainty that SCP2* will express pock formation in other than species closely related to *S. coelicolor*. For that matter, there is no evidence to show that SCP2 will replicate in a wide range of *Streptomyces*. It is known to replicate only in *Streptomyces lividans*, *Streptomyces parvulus*, and *Streptomyces coelicolor*.

Plasmids have now been physically isolated in many species (Table 3). Table 3 also includes other examples which are specifically plasmid-like in their behavior but have not yet yielded to physical isolation. The latter can be quite difficult in eubacteria with plasmids larger than 100 md and the limit for *Streptomyces* using the Bibb et al. (1977) technique seems to be about 60 md. However an improved method by Westpheling (1980, personal communication) has allowed the identification of the SCP1 plasmid of *S. coelicolor* A3(2) as cccDNA of about 100 md. This method will hopefully allow the identification of the more difficult plasmids.

Table 3. Plasmids in *Streptomyces*

Microorganism	Physical plasmids	Functions	Genetic plasmids and their functions	References
S. ambofaciens	Yes	Spiramycin production and/or resistance	–	OMURA et al. (1979)
S. bikiniensis	–	–	Streptomycin production?	SHAW and PIWOWARSKI (1977)
S. clavuligerus	–	–	Control of holomycin production?	KIRBY (1978b)
S. coelicolor A3(2)	SCP1 100 md	Methylenomycin production	–	KIRBY and HOPWOOD (1977) WESTPHELING (1980, personal communication)
	SCP2 19.2 md	Fertility factor	–	SCHREMPF et al. (1975)
S. coelicolor	55 md	Unknown	–	SCHREMPF and GOEBEL (1978)
	8 md	Unknown	–	
S. fradiae	55 md	Unknown	Unstable neomycin resistance	
S. fradiae	22 md	Unknown	–	YAGASAWA et al. (1978)
	15 md	Unknown	–	
S. glaucescens	–	–	Melanin production	BAUMAN and KOCHER (1976)
S. griseus	–	–	Cephamycin production	PARAG (1979)
S. griseus	–	–	Streptomycin production	YU-GU et al. (1978)
S. hydroscopicus	–	–	Turimycin production	KAHLER and NOACK (1974)
S. jumoniensis	22 md	Tunicamycin	–	KIRBY et al. (1982)
	26 md	Resistance?	–	
S. kanamyceticus	Yes	Unknown	Kanamycin production	CHANG et al. (1978)
S. kasugaensis	6.7 md	Aureothricin production	–	
	30 md	Kasugamycin production	–	OKANISHI and UMEZAWA (1978)
	1.2 md	Unknown	–	TOYAMA et al. (1979)

Table 3 (continued)

Microorganism	Physical plasmids	Functions	Genetic plasmids and their functions	References
S. lipmanii	2 md	Unknown	–	Kirby et al. (1982)
S. lividans	SLP1 7.9 md	Lethal zygosis	–	Bibb et al. (1980)
S. olivaceus	3 md	Unknown	–	Kirby et al. (1982)
S. juniceus	17.3 md and 39.1 md	Viomycin production	–	Hayakawa et al. (1979)
S. reticuli	48 md	Leukomycin and melanin production	–	Schrempf and Goebel (1978)
S. rimosus	–	–	Oxytetracycline production (some genes)	Boronin and Mindlin (1971) Boronin and Sadovnikova (1972)
S. rimosus	–	–	Fertility factor	Friend et al. (1978)
S. rimosus	High G+C content	–	–	Kirby et al. (1982)
S. scabies	–	–	Tyrosinase production	Gregory and Huang (1964a, b)
S. venezuelae	18 md	–	Chloramphenicol production	Akagawa et al. (1975) Akagawa et al. (1979)
S. virginiae	Yes	Unknown	–	Canham et al. (1978)
Streptomyces sp. 2217-Gl	3.2 md 18.0 md	Unknown	–	Hayakawa et al. (1979a)
Streptomyces sp. 7068-CC	22.2 md 47.0 md	Unknown	–	Hayakawa et al. (1979a)
Streptomyces sp.	11.2 md (linear)	Unknown	–	Hayakawa et al. (1979b)

It must be borne in mind that there are even groups of plasmids in the eubacteria which have failed to yield physical evidence of their existence as cccDNA, e.g., RPI-I and the J group of plasmids.

Of specific interest among the plasmids that have been physically isolated so far are those from *Streptomyces fradiae*, one or more of which may code for neomycin resistance, and the plasmids from *Streptomyces jumonjinensis*, one of which may be involved in tunicamycin resistance. Both of these could lead to development of better cloning vehicles in *Streptomyces*. Other physical plasmids may be involved in antibiotic production but only in the case of methylenomycin A and SCP1 is this clearly known.

Recent work by BIBB et al. (1981) has demonstrated that cloning of genes related to antibiotic production in *Streptomyces* is possible. Essential to this was the identification of a means of transforming *Streptomyces* with cccDNA. Although *Thermoactinomyces vulgaris* was demonstrated to undergo transformation with crude DNA, it required a modification of the protoplast treatment with polyethylene glycol to obtain significant transformation. Up to 10% transformation was obtained with supercoiled DNA and success was also obtained with relaxed and linear DNA using SCP2* as the marker (BIBB et al. 1980). It has also proved possible to transfect using this method.

II. Plasmids in β-Lactam-Producing Streptomyces

Three of the *Streptomyces* known to produce β-lactam antibiotics have been shown to contain physical plasmids. These are *S. jumonjensis*, *Streptomyces lipmanii* and *S. olivaceus*. In the latter two cases, the plasmids are very small (2–3 md) and neither was initially found using cesium chloride ethidium bromide density gradients. They were detected on a number of occasions by using an electron microscope to examine grids made from the material taken from the gradient where the plasmid ought to have banded. No further studies have been carried and due to the problem of low copy number (KIRBY, unpublished results). In the case of *S. jumonjinensis*, a typical plasmid band was detected on a CsCl-EtBr gradient and was shown to contain two plasmids.

There is evidence for plasmids in two other β-lactam producing strains. In *S. griseus*, where a genetic map of the strain has been published, it has been suggested that cephamycin production is plasmid controlled or coded (PARAG 1978). In *S. clavuligerus*, no evidence for plasmid-encoded β-lactam is available; indeed there is evidence that one of the genes for clavulanic acid synthesis maps to the chromosome (R. KIRBY, unpublished results). Indirect evidence suggests that direct plasmid involvement is unlikely when compared to other *Streptomyces* since no instability of β-lactam production could be detected in *S. clavuligerus* for any of the various β-lactam antibiotics produced. There is however strong evidence in *S. clavuligerus* for a plasmid-like entity, which is involved in the production of a non-β-lactam antibiotic (KIRBY 1978b). Holomycin production is unstable in *S. clavuligerus* and the element which confers the ability to produce holomycin is self-transmissible and could be a sex factor. No reversion to holomycin production was or has been detected although no direct selection is available. However, the genes coding for holomycin synthesis are not carried on this element as it is possible to show that the plasmid-minus strains can still make holomycin in liquid culture. Thus the unstable plasmid-like entity which is self-transmissible and sex-factor-like is involved in the control of holomycin production. This seems to be quite complex; recent evidence seems to show that two other antibiotics are involved concomitantly with this element, i.e., tunicamycin and clavulanic acid (β-lactam); again, in a control function. Loss of the entity also seems to induce the same loss of ability to produce spores, but this is not clear cut. As no physical evidence is available to confirm the existence of this possible plasmid, it remains a possibility that it is not cccDNA but an unstable control element of the type which will be discussed later (S. Napier, personal communication).

D. Antibiotic Production in Actinomycetes

The actinomycetes in which the biochemistry and genetics of antibiotic production have been studied are those which produce industrially important antibiotics. Most of the commercial β-lactam antibiotics are produced by fungi and, although the search for novel β-lactam antibiotics is widespread in the actinomycetes, only little has been published on the biochemistry and genetics of β-lactam production in these species (BROWN et al. 1976; FAWCETT et al. 1976; HOLT et al. 1976; AHARHOWITZ and FRIEDRICH 1980). A study of the various genetic systems for antibiotic production should give some insight into the possibilities for β-lactam antibiotics.

The diversity of the β-lactam antibiotics produced by even a single actinomycete has led to a hypothesis as to the biochemical mechanism of antibiotic production. In the fungus *Cephalosporium acremonium*, the biochemical pathway has been suggested to run through a common ring closure enzyme and then through various enzymatic modification steps. Thus by starting with various different tripeptide substrates which can be acted on by the ring closure enzyme, and using the same postclosure modification enzyme, a variety of different β-lactam antibiotics could be produced. In the fungi, either the possible initial substrates are limited or the ring-closure enzymes are relatively specific. In the actinomycetes, this may not be the case and thus a wider variety of β-lactam antibiotics is found.

There are now specific examples of a number of different genetic systems for antibiotic production in *Streptomyces*. The simplest, an example of which is actinorhodin production by *S. coelicolor* A3(2), involves genes which are all chromosomal and closely linked in what could be an operon (RUDD and HOPWOOD 1979). This study was aided by the colored nature of actinorhodin, which simplified the isolation of actinorhodin-negative mutants (Act$^-$) and their mapping. No plasmid involvement has been detected.

Blocked mutants have been obtained which map in a gene cluster and form at least seven phenotypic classes on the basis of precursor/shunt pigments and cosynthesis. They all map between the two closely linked Cys D and gua A loci. Work has been carried on with an SCPI′ of this region to study complementation and dominance. The clustering may be a characteristic of bacterial antibiotic synthesis.

A second class is that in which all the genes involved in antibiotic synthesis are plasmid borne, as with methylenomycin A production by *S. coelicolor* A3(2) and

SCP1. Again this is quite simple and easy to study (KIRBY and HOPWOOD 1976). A third class involves a plasmid which seems to be involved in the control of antibiotic production but does not carry any genes directly involved in synthesis. Holomycin production by *S. clavuligerus* is an example of this; at least some of the synthesis genes seem to be chromosomal in this case (KIRBY 1978b). A fourth class is that in which part of the synthesis genes are chromosomal and part plasmid borne; oxytetracycline formation by *Streptomyces rimosus* is such a case. This is one of the more complicated systems studied (BORONIN and SADOVNIKOVA 1972). A final class, of which an example is yet to be clearly identified, is antibiotic production carried on or involving transposable genetic elements.

What little evidence there is suggests that β-lactam synthesis genes are chromosomal and control may be affected by either plasmids or transposable elements.

I. Unstable Genetic Systems in Streptomyces Which do not Involve Plasmids

Evidence is accumulating that in cases in *Streptomyces* where a phenotype can be shown to be unstable, plasmids are not involved. It is suggested that another type of unstable element is responsible. Most of the evidence has come from work on instability of antibiotic resistance but a relationship between this element and production is apparent too.

The evidence for this type of phenomenon was first detected in *S. coelicolor* A3(2). FREEMAN et al. (1977) showed that chloramphenicol (Cm) resistance in this species was unstable but, unlike plasmid-encoded resistance, the loss of resistance was reversible in a totally cyclic manner. Although the forward and reverse frequencies differed, no genetic information was lost. Equally important was a failure to show any linkage to chromosomal markers in *S. coelicolor* using conventional mapping techniques. This was puzzling and led to the question of the molecular explanation of this element in *S. coelicolor*.

No linkage could be detected with either of the two known plasmids of *S. coelicolor*, SCP1 and SCP2; nor could a physical change be detected in the case of the latter plasmid. Thus modification of these independent entities was eliminated. A completely satisfactory molecular model has not yet been put forward but a transposon type element would seem a likely possibility. Assuming the number of sites of insertion in the main chromosome are numerous enough (more than six scattered randomly around the chromosome) and the frequency of the event is great enough to ensure a random distribution of the insertions after the 10–20 days incubation needed to carry out the cross, no chromosomal linkage could be detected. By picking Cm^s clones immediately and carrying out the crosses, it was possible to show various chromosomal map locations for the resistance element. It is not clear whether these clonally studied events are due to random transposition or if they can cause insertional inactivation (SERMONTI et al. 1977, 1978, 1980). The work of FREEMAN et al. (1977) showed that insertional inactivation of chromosomal genes did not occur.

Two further examples have now been studied in detail. These are *S. griseus* and *S. bikiniensis* (KIRBY and LEWIS 1981). A number of other species are also candidates (FREEMAN and HOPWOOD 1978). In both species, streptomycin resistance is implicated.

The results with *S. bikiniensis* are more complex than with *S. coelicolor*. The instability was initially attributed to plasmid loss (SHAW and PIWOWARSKI 1977). However, further work has shown cyclic reversion and the induction of the Bld$^-$ (lack of aerial mycelium) phenotype. As auxotrophs are also induced at a frequency much higher than the mutation frequency, this supports an insertion hypothesis and the specificity would suggest either a specific location or a specific insertion (KIRBY and LEWIS 1981). This situation resembled the induction of Bld$^-$ Arg$^-$ clones in many *Streptomyces* species including β-lactam producers (MERRICK 1976; REDSHAW et al. 1979; KIRBY and O'REILLY 1979). Many of the putative plasmid negatives from *S. clavuligerus* lacked aerial mycelium and as reversion to antibiotic production could not be eliminated in this case, transposition could be involved. Thus, in general, the role of specific insertional events and transposons provides a useful model for *Streptomyces* instability and control which will be tested in the future (COHEN 1976; PTASHNE and COHEN 1974; FORD-DOOLITTLE and SAPIENZA 1980; FINCHAM and SASTRY 1974; ORGEL and Crick 1980).

The hypothesis concerning transposons in *Streptomyces* has been recently confirmed at the molecular level by the detection of a kanamycin resistance transposon and its cloning into *Escherichia coli* (DANILENKO et al. 1979).

II. Protoplast Fusion and Streptomyces

The development of protoplast formation and regeneration (OKANISHI et al. 1974) and protoplast fusion (HOPWOOD et al. 1977) has presented new possibilities for an approach to the classic genetic problems of industrial strains. Protoplast fusion was shown to occur between marked strains of *S. coelicolor* A3(2) in the presence of polyethylene glycol 1,000; dimethylsulphoxide can also be added as an aid to fusion. In the absence of the known sex factor of *S. coelicolor*, a recombination frequency of greater than 10% was detected regularly. Later work (HOPWOOD and WRIGHT 1978) showed that up to four strains could be fused at the same time and that multiple rounds of recombination occured. Exchange of genetic material also involved large pieces of chromosome and a higher level than normal of multiple cross-overs.

This development of genetic exchange within species at a level previously only obtainable in the presence of specific sex factors has led to its use to speed up the creation of new genetically marked strains. In order to do serious conventional mapping in a new species, triple auxotrophic strains must be obtained by repeated mutagenic treatment. This has two major disadvantages. First, it is slow, since indirect selection and testing on pools of supplements must accompany each mutagenesis. Second, if the species is a producer of a useful antibiotic, pleiotropic effects of any induced mutations and silent mutations can seriously affect antibiotic production, especially in strains developed for high-level production. This can now be overcome by using a one-step mutagenesis to collect a large pool of single auxotrophic mutations; this can be checked and any deleterous mutations eliminated from any manipulations. Pairs or even up to four different mutant strains can be crossed using protoplast fusion and multiple auxotrophs selected indirectly from the output of the cross. With a recombination frequency in the region of 10% and a high level of multiple cross-overs, only a few hundred clones need to be screened to find the required combination of auxotrophic mutations. As protoplast fusion does not break down normal genetic map relationships, such crosses can continue to be used to map any interesting genes.

This ability to introduce auxotrophs nonmutagenically into any strain means that high-yielding strains can now be crossed with genetically marked strains to introduce auxotrophic mutations. High-yielding strains can then be crossed, even in the absence of genetic markers, at a frequency high enough to ensure that recombinants can be detected after relatively few clones have been screened. Crosses without genetic markers may give very variable results especially after much mutagensis. This use of crosses between high-yielding strains will allow a wider genetic pool to be subjected to selection by conventional industrial techniques for an, as yet, new gene combination which gives yet higher yield. This method has been shown to be useful by the work of MERRICK (1975) on β-lactam production in the fungus *Aspergillus nidulans* using wild-type strains.

The second major possibility arising from protoplast fusion is derived from the ability of this method to overcome the normal limitation of interspecific mating. Thus there is no need for special mating mechanisms and direct contact between the genetic material of the two species is induced by protoplast fusion. Unfortunately, the results up to the moment have not been encouraging. Little genetic exchange seems to occur between species under the conditions of protoplast fusion. What does occur is limited to small areas of the chromosome (OCHI et al. 1979; HOPWOOD and WRIGHT 1979; R. KIRBY, unpublished results). Heterokaryons are very common and are very unstable, suggesting that homology between the chromosomes may be the problem. The use of UV irradiation to enhance recombination between DNA could be useful.

III. Transformation and Streptomyces

Although transformation was indentified as the method of genetic exchange for chromosomal genes in *T. vulgaris* at the beginning of the 1970s (HOPWOOD and WRIGHT 1972), only recently has a more general method of transforming DNA into *Streptomyces* been developed. This specifically involved plasmid DNA in the first case (BIBB et al. 1978). Using SCP2* and SLP1–SLP6 plasmid DNA, it has proved possible to obtain transformation frequencies of up to 10% or more using protoplasts and polyethylene glycol 1,000. Detection was achieved not by using a direct selection method but by using an indirect method to pick out the clones which gave zones of lethal zygosis which are induced by these plasmids. This method is a general one which will allow the transformation of plasmids both intraspecifically and interspecifically in *Streptomyces*. Since plasmids have been detected in β-lactam producing *Streptomyces* (see Table 3), this provides the means of manipulating the plasmids for a variety of purposes.

It has also proved to be possible to transfect *Streptomyces* protoplasts with bacteriophage DNA using this method (SUAREZ and CHATER 1980; KRUEGEL et al.

1980). This will now allow the development of a phage vector for in vitro genetic manipulation in a manner similar to which phage lambda has been used.

IV. Restriction and Modification Systems in Streptomyces

If one intends to transfer genetic material between strains or species of *Streptomyces*, it is essential to have some idea of the barriers due to restriction and modification systems acting on the DNA in these organisms. Chater and Wilde (1976) provided the first clear evidence for restriction and modification in *Streptomyces albus G* where a correlation between the restriction endonuclease enzyme Sal GI and restriction was shown. This is one of the few cases where a type II restriction enzyme has been shown to be responsible for a genetic restriction system. Further work has shown that the restriction mechanisms and their relationship with the bacteriophage are complex (Chater 1977; Chater and Carter 1978, 1979). It has proved possible to select mutants which fail to show restriction in *Streptomyces;* this hopefully will allow full genetic exchange to occur between these organisms (Chater and Wilde 1980).

Table 4. Restriction/modification of bacteriophage FF4 by *Streptomyces olivaceus* (OL328), *Streptomyces cattleya* (CA221) and *Streptomyces lipmanii* (LP326)

First host	Second host	Third host	Strain assayed against	Efficiency of plating relative to AL322
AL322	–	–	OL328	3.0×10^{-8}
AL322	OL328	–	OL328	7.1×10^{-2}
AL322	OL328	AL322	OL328	9.1×10^{-5}
AL322	–	–	CA221	1.8×10^{-7}
AL322	CA221	–	CA221	1.1×10^{-1}
AL322	CA221	AL322	CA221	5.9×10^{-7}
AL322	–	–	LP326	8.3×10^{-8}
AL322	LP326	–	LP326	5.5×10^{-5}
AL322	LP326	AL322	LP326	2.6×10^{-6}

Table 5. Similarilty of restriction/modification systems of bacteriophage FF4 in *Streptomyces olivaceus* (OL328), *Streptomyces cattleya* (CA221) and *Streptomyces lipmanii* (LP326)

First host	Second host	Strain assayed against	Efficiency of plating relative to AL322
AL322	OL328	OL328	2.4×10^{-1}
AL322	OL328	CA221	1.0×10^{-1}
AL322	OL328	LP326	4.1×10^{-3}
AL322	CA221	OL328	2.7×10^{-1}
AL322	CA221	CA221	3.5×10^{-2}
AL322	CA221	LP326	4.2×10^{-2}
AL322	LP326	OL328	2.2×10^{-1}
AL322	LP326	CA221	2.3×10^{-1}
AL322	LP326	LP326	2.8×10^{-2}

Restriction has been detected in three β-lactam-producing species of *Streptomyces* (FLETT et al. 1979). Of interest is that the restriction–modification systems of these species, *S. olivaceus*, *S. cattleya* and *S. lipmanii* have a similar specificity (Table 4 and 5). Although this does not eliminate the possibility of a hidden restriction system which does not affect phage FF4, it is hopeful that genetic exchange between these species may be relatively easy to obtain. It also raises the question of their taxonomic relatedness.

V. Genetic Engineering and Streptomyces

The identification of plasmids in *Streptomyces* as independently replicating extrachromosomal covalently closed circular DNA has opened up the possibility of their use for in vitro genetic manipulation. The plasmid DNA can be isolated in quite good yields and restricted using the available restriction endonucleases. SCP2 and SCP2* have been studied in the greatest detail and although the high G+C content of *Streptomyces* DNA affects the distribution of endonuclease sites on the DNA, useful sites have been found. For example, there are a large number of Sal I sites. Figure 4 shows the map of SCP2 and Table 6 gives the enzymes used, their recognition sites and the number of sites identified. The G+C ratio of the DNA based on the sample calculated from the recognition sites is approximately 70%, which agrees quite closely with the 73% estimated for *S. coelicolor* A3(2) (BENIGNI et al. 1975) using thermal denaturation. The sample is obviously biased. Other plasmids have been studied to a limited extent but are equally amenable to endonuclease digestion.

Transformation of the SCP2* DNA into *S. coelicolor* protoplasts, as described by BIBB et al. (1978), has allowed the reintroduction of such plamid DNA back into *Streptomyces* via protoplasts. The first example of in vitro genetic manipulation in

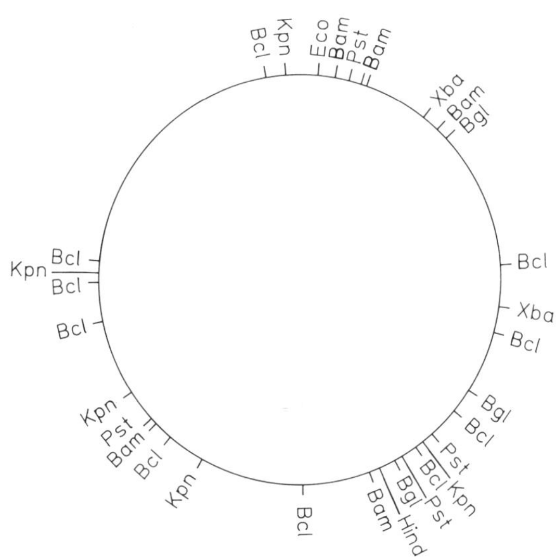

Fig. 4. Restriction enzyme map of the SCP2 plasmid (mol. wt = 19.2 md) of *Streptomyces coelicolor* A3(2) (KIRBY and WOTTON 1979)

Table 6. Restriction enzyme sites present in the SCP2 plasmid of *Streptomyces coelicolor* A3(2). (KIRBY and WOTTON 1979)

Restriction enzyme	Number of sites	Origin	Sequence recognized
Bam HI	4	*Bacillus amyloliquefaciens*	G/GATCC
Bcl I	10	*Bacillus caldolyticus*	T/GATCA
Bgl I	0	*Bacillus globigii*	CGG(N_4)/NGGC
Bgl II	3	*Bacillus globigii*	A/GATCT
Eco RI	1	*Escherichia coli* RYI3	G/AATTC
Eco RII	0	*Escherichia coli* R245	/CC$\frac{A}{T}$GG
Hind III	1	*Haemophilus influenzae*	A/AGCTT
Hpa I	1	*Haemophilus parainfluenzae*	GTT/AAC
Kpn I	5	*Klebsiella pneumoniae*	GGTAC/C
Pst I	4	*Providencia stuartii*	CTGCA/G
Rsp I	8	*Rhodopseudomonas sphaeroides*	CGATCG
Sma I	18	*Serratia marcescens*	CCC/GGG
Xba I	2	*Xanthomas badrii*	T/CTAGA

Streptomyces involved the cloning of the methylenomycin (Mm) A resistance gene from the SCP1 plasmid of *S. coelicolor* into SCP2* and SLP2. This was carried out by using a "shot-gun" technique to ligate total DNA from *S. coelicolor* SCP1* into these plasmids using the enzyme Pst I. The religated DNA was then transformed into the respective hosts, *S. coelicolor* and *S. lividans*. Selection for methylenomycin A resistance (Mm^r) was carried out using the antibiotic produced by *S. coelicolor* SCP1* on patch plates. A number of SCP2* Mm^r and SLP2 MM^r plasmids were obtained as well as cut-down plasmids which still showed lethal zygosis. The isolation of these plasmids provided one step towards developing a directly selectable *Streptomyces* cloning system.

The Mm^r plasmids have a number of disadvantages as a cloning vehicle. Firstly, methylenomycin A is not available in sufficient quantities to allow its use as an additive to selective plates and patches of SCP1* strains must be used to select Mm^r clones. Considering the diversity of antibiotics produced by the *Streptomyces* which are commercially available, it should be possible to clone such a resistance gene (see Sect. D). Secondly, the diversity of the strains in which either of the two Mm^r plasmids can replicate and express is not known except for a number of species closely related to *S. coelicolor*. Finally, the copy number of SCP2 is only one; SLP2 has a copy number of 4+ and may be more useful.

A possible alternative method of developing a cloning vehicle for *Streptomyces* would be based on using a modified phage: Essential to this is the identification and characterization of a temperate phage. For the purposes of industrial cloning as envisaged with the β-lactam producing *Streptomyces*, a temperate phage of wide host range is required. Such a phage is now being studied (CHATER and CARTER 1979). It is hoped that it will eventually be modified by restriction/ligation and mutation for use as a cloning vehicle (K. F. Chater, personal communication).

Another approach to the in vitro genetic manipulation of *Streptomyces* is to use the technology already available in the eubacteria. Two systems have been tried.

First, cloning vector plasmids from *E. coli* and *Bacillus subtilis* have been transformed into *Streptomyces* using the polyethylene glycol/protoplast method and selecting for the appropriate resistance markers. The most hopeful plasmids to use are those from gram-positives. pBR322 and pAyC184 do not transform into *S. cattleya*, *S. griseus*, or *S. albus* (R. Kirby, unpublished results). PK-545 and pUB110 do transform into *S. lactamdurans* (GRAY et al. 1980). pUB110 also transform into *S. cattleya* and *S. griseus* but are very unstable (R. Kirby, unpublished results).

Second, attempts have been made to clone *Streptomyces* DNA into *E. coli* using plasmid vectors and selecting for expression of the alien DNA in this environment. HORINOUCHI et al. (1980) failed to show any expression for various prototrophic markers from *S. fradiae*, *Streptomyces violaceoruber* and what is probably a *Streptomyces venezuelae* strain. They used a pBR322 vector in *E. coli* C600. This was a limited choice of genes and does not completely exclude interspecific expression with these species. However gram-positive to gram-negative expression seems to be poor in general. Another attempt by DANILENKO et al. (1979) to clone an antibiotic resistance marker from *Streptomyces kanamyceticus* in *E. coli* was successful. This marker proved to be highly unstable in the cloned form and relocated itself to the chromosome in a manner similar to a transposon. The molecular status of this unstable resistance element was shown to be similar to eubacterial transposons. If the unstable resistance marker can be handled, this can be a method of producing specific *Streptomyces* vectors. The most likely resistance genes to express in *E. coli* are those that are enzymatic rather than those that depend on membrane changes or structural changes. A failure to clone streptomycin resistance from *S. griseus* to *E. coli* by HORINOUCHI et al. (1980) is not explicable in this manners since resistance must be enzymatic (VALU and SZABO 1980).

E. The Genetics of β-Lactam Antibiotics and the Future

The problems of the antibiotic industry can be divided into three main areas: (1) increased yields of known useful antibiotics; (2) increased stability of the strains involved in antibiotic production; and (3) the identification and development of novel antibiotics. These problems are as important for β-lactam antibiotics as for any other group.

The major β-lactam antibiotics which are produced at the moment are still obtained from fungal fermentations. However new ones increasingly originate from *Streptomyces*, e.g., clavulanic acid and thienamycin. The opportunity to use classic genetics as well as protoplast fusion as part of a standard industrial mutation and selection program is intriguing How great will be the return from this innovation is not yet clear. With longer and longer times between discovery and marketing of novel antibiotics, the possibility is real.

The research on genetic instability in *Streptomyces* is now bearing fruit and transposon-like elements would seem to be a possible major factor. Plasmids probably still play a part but may be concerned with control and probably carry these elements too. How one could eliminate these unstable systems from *Streptomyces* is not clear. An understanding of their function will help and if they carry strong promotors and termination codons as in eubacteria, they will be useful for in vitro manipulation.

Many different species of *Streptomyces* produce similar antibiotics by what may be similar pathways. This is very true for the β-lactam antibiotics. Genetic manipulation using in vivo and in vitro techniques will allow the exchange of enzymes from one species to another. The exchange of precursor pathways with ring closure enzyme complexes of different specificities and the use of different modification enzymes for the terminal steps of the pathway could lead to novel antibiotics.

The genetics of the β-lactam producing *Streptomyces* may be on the brink of solving some of the problems facing the antibiotics industry. In the longer term, the cloning of the enzymes of the β-lactam pathway into an organism which can produce them in bulk could lead to their use on immobilized matrixes on a commercial level and eliminate batch culture fermentation altogether.

References

Aharonowitz Y, Demain AL (1978) Carbon catabolite regulation of cephalosporin production in *Streptomyces clavuligerus*. Antimicrob Agents Chemother 14:159–164

Aharonowitz Y, Friedrich CG (1980) Alanine dehydrogenase of the beta-lactam antibiotic producer *Streptomyces clavuligerus*. Arch Microbiol 125:137–142

Akagawa H, Okanishi M, Umezawa H (1975) A plasmid involved in chloramphenicol production in *Streptomyces venezuelae:* evidence from genetic mapping. J Gen Microbiol 90:336–346

Akagawa H, Okanishi M, Umezawa H (1979) Genetic and biochemical studies of chloramphenicol non-producing mutants of *Streptomyces venezuelae* carrying a plasmid. J Antibiot 32:610–620

Alacevic M (1963) Interspecific recombination in *Streptomyces*. Nature 197:1323

Alikhanian SI, Ilyina TS, Lomovskaya ND (1960) Transduction in *Actinomycetes*. Nature 188:245–246

Baumann R, Kocher HP (1976) Genetics of *Streptomyces glaucescens* and regulation of melanin production. In: MacDonald KD (ed) Second international symposium on the genetics of industrial microorganisms. Academic Press, London, pp 535–551

Benigni R, Petrov PA, Carere A (1975) Estimate of the genome size by renaturation studies in *Streptomyces*. Appl Microbiol 30:324–326

Bibb MJ, Freeman RF, Hopwood DA (1977) Physical and genetical characterisation of a second factor, SCP 2, for *Streptomyces coelicolor*. Mol Gen Genet 154:155–166

Bibb MJ, Ward JM, Hopwood DA (1978) Transformation of plasmid DNA into *Streptomyces* at high frequency. Nature 274:398–400

Bibb MJ, Schettel JL, Cohen SN (1980) A DNA cloning system for interspecific gene transfer in antibiotic producing *Streptomyces*. Nature 284:526–531

Box SJ, Hood JD, Spear SR (1979) Four further antibiotics related to olivanic acid produced by *Streptomyces olivaceus* – fermentation, isolation, characterisation, and biochemical studies. J Antibiot 32:1239–1247

Boronin AM, Mindlin SZ (1971) Genetic analysis of *Actinomyces rimosus* mutants with impaired synthesis of antibiotic (In Russian). Genetika 7:125–159

Boronin AM, Sadovnikova LG (1972) Elimination by acridine dyes of oxytetracyclin resistance in *Actinomyces rimosus* (In Russian). Genetika 8:174–176

Bradley SG, Lederberg J (1956) Heterokaryosis in *Streptomyces*. J Bacteriol 72:219–225

Braendle DH, Szybalski W (1959) Heterokaryotic compatability, metabolic cooperation and genetic exchange in *Streptomyces*. Ann NY Acad Sci 81:824–851

Brown AG, Butterworth D, Cole M, Hanscombe G, Hood JD, Reading C, Rolinson GN (1976) Naturally occuring beta-lactamase inhibitors with antimicrobial activity. J Antibiot 29:668–669

Canham PL, Michelson AM, Vining LC (1978) Plasmids and chloramphenicol production by Streptomyces species 3122a (Abstr). 3rd int symp genet ind micro-organisms, Madison, No 72, p 36

Chang LT, Behr DA, Elander PP (1978) Effects of plasmid-curing agents on the cultural characteristics and kanamycin formation in a production strain of *Streptomyces kanamyceticus* (Abstr). 3rd int symp genet ind micro-organisms, Madison, no 73, p 36

Chater KF (1977) A site-specific endodeoxyribonuclease from *Streptomyces albus* CMI 52766 sharing site specificity with *Providencia stuartii* endonuclease Pst I. Nucleic Acids Res 4:1989–1998

Chater KF, Carter AT (1978) Restriction of a bacteriophage in *Streptomyces albus* P (CMI 52766) by endonuclease Sal PI. J Gen Microbiol 109:181–185

Chater KF, Carter AT (1979) A new wide host-range temperate bacteriophage (R4) of *Streptomyces* and its interaction with some restriction-modification systems. J Gen Microbiol 115:431–442

Chater KF, Wilde LC (1976) Restriction of the bacteriophage of *Streptomyces albus* G involving endonuclease Sal I. J Bacteriol 128:644–650

Chater KF, Wilde LC (1980) *Streptomyces albus* G mutants defective in the Sal GI restriction-modification system. J Gen Microbiol 116:323–334

Cohen SN (1976) Transposable genetic elements and plasmid evolution. Nature 263:731–738

Danilenko VN, Yankovskii NK, Kalezhskii VE, Moshentseva VN, Sladkova IA, Kozlov YI, Fedorenko VA, Rebentish BA, Lomovskaya ND, Debabov VG (1979) Study of the structure and functioning of the kanamycin transposon of *Actinomycetes*, transferred in vitro to *E. coli* K12. Dokl Biol Sci 244:701–704

Demain AL (1974) How do antibiotic producing organisms avoid suicide? Ann NY Acad Sci 235:601–602

Fawcett PA, Usher JJ, Abraham EP (1976) Aspects of cephalosporin and penicillin biosynthesis. In: MacDonald KD (ed) 2nd International Symposium on the Genetics of Industrial Microorganisms. Academic Press, London New York San Francisco, pp 129–138

Fincham JRS, Sastry GRK (1974) Controlling elements in Maize. Ann Rev Genet 8:15–50

Flett F, Wotten SF, Kirby R (1979) A common host-specificity in the restriction and modification of a bacteriophage by three distinct *Streptomyces* species. J Gen Microbiol 110:465–467

Ford-Doolittle W, Sapienza C (1980) Selfish genes, the phenotype paradigm and genome evolution. Nature 284:601–603

Freeman RF, Hopwood DA (1978) Unstable naturally occuring resistance to antibiotics in *Streptomyces*. J Gen Microbiol 106:377–381

Freeman RF, Bibb MJ, Hopwood DA (1977) Chloramphenicol acetyltransferase-independent chloramphenicol resistance in *Streptomyces coelicolor* A3(2). J Gen Microbiol 98:453–465

Friend EJ, Warren JM, Hopwood DA (1978) Genetic evidence for a plasmid controlling fertility in an industrial strain of *Streptomyces rimosus*. J Gen Microbiol 106:201–206

Godfrey OW (1973) Isolation of regulatory mutants of the aspartic and pyruvic acid families and their effect on the antibiotic production in *Streptomyces lipmanii*. Antimicrob Agents Chemother 4:73–79

Gray O, Chang S, Wolf E (1980) The stable transfer and functional expression of *Staphylococcus aureus* neomycin resistance markers from pK-545 and pUB110 to *Streptomyces lactamdurans* by interspecific cell fusion and by transformation. Abstr 80th Annu Meeting Am Soc Microbiol, p 10

Gregory KE, Huang JCC (1964a) Tyrosinase inheritance in *Streptomyces scabies*. I Genetic recombination. J Bacteriol 87:1281–1286

Gregory KE, Huang JCC (1964b) Tyrosinase inheritance in *Streptomyces scabies*. II Induction of tyrosinase deficiency by acridine dyes. J Bacteriol 87:1287–1294

Hayakawa T, Otake N, Yonehara H, Tanaka T, Sakaguchi K (1979a) Isolation and characterisation of plasmids of *Streptomyces*. J Antibiot 32:1348–1350

Hayakawa T, Tanaka T, Sakaguchi K, Otake N, Yonehara H (1979b) A linear plasmid-like DNA in *Streptomyces* sp producing lankacidin group antibiotics. J Gen Appl Microbiol 25:255–260

Higgens CE, Kastner RE (1971) *Streptomyces clavuligerus sp. nov.*, a Beta-lactam antibiotic producer. Int J Syst Bacteriol 21:326–331

Higgens CE, Hamill RL, Sands TH, Hoehn MM, Davis NE, Nagarajan R, Boeck LD (1974) The occurence of deactoxycephalosporin C in fungi and streptomycetes. J Antibiot 27:298–300

Holt G, Edwards GFSTL, Macdonald KD (1976) The genetics of mutants impaired in the biosynthesis of penicillin. In: Macdonald KD (ed) Second international symposium on the genetics of industrial micro-organisms. Academic Press, London New York, pp 199–211

Hopwood DA (1967) Genetic analysis and genome structure in *Streptomyces coelicolor*. Bacteriol Rev 31:373–403

Hopwood DA (1978) Extrachromosomally determined antibiotic production. Annu Rev Microbiol 32:373–392

Hopwood DA, Merrick MJ (1977) Genetics of antibiotic production. Bacteriol Rev 41:595–635

Hopwood DA, Wright HM (1972) Transformation in *Thermoactinomyces vulgaris*. J Gen Microbiol 71:383–398

Hopwood DA, Wright HM (1973a) Transfer of a plasmid between *Streptomyces* species. J Gen Microbiol 77:187–195

Hopwood DA, Wright HM (1973b) A plasmid of *Streptomyces coelicolor* carrying a chromosomal locus and its interspecific transfer. J Gen Microbiol 79:331–342

Hopwood DA, Wright HM (1976) Genetic studies on SCP I-prime strains of *Streptomyces coelicolor* A3(2). J Gen Microbiol 95:107–120

Hopwood DA, Wright HM (1978) Bacterial protoplast fusion: recombination in fused protoplasts of *Streptomyces coelicolor*. Mol Gen Genet 162:307–317

Hopwood DA, Wright HM (1979) Factors affecting recombinant frequency in protoplast fusions of *Streptomyces coelicolor*. J Gen Microbiol III:137–143

Hopwood DA, Sermonti G, Spada-Sermonti I (1963) Heterozygote clones in *Streptomyces coelicolor*. J Gen Microbiol 30:249–260

Hopwood DA, Chater KF, Dowding DE, Vivian A (1973) Recent advances in *Streptomyces coelicolor* genetics. Bacteriol Rev 37:371–405

Hopwood DA, Wright HM, Bibb MJ, Cohen SN (1977) Genetic recombination though protoplast fusion in *Streptomyces*. Nature 268:171–174

Horinouchi S, Uozumi I, Beppu T (1980) Cloning of *Streptomyces* DNA into *E. coli*. Absence of heterospecific gene expression of *Streptomyces* genes in *E. coli*. Agric Biol Chem 44:367–382

Hornemann U, Hopwood DA (1978) Isolation and characterisation of desepoxy-4,5-didehydro-methylenomycin A. A precursor of the antibiotic methylenomycin A in SCP I$^+$ strains of *Streptomyces coelicolor* A3(2). Tetrahedron Lett 33:2977–2978

Kahan JS, Kahan FM, Goegelman R, Currie SA, Jackson M, Stapley O, Miller TW et al. (1979) Thienamycin, a new beta-lactam antibiotic. I Discovery, taxonomy, isolation, and physical properties. J Antibiot 32:1–12

Kalakoutskii LV, Agre NA (1976) Comparative aspects of development and differentiation in *Actinomycetes*. Bacteriol Rev 40:469–524

Kenig M, Reading C (1979) Holomycin and an antibiotic MM-19290 related to tunicamycin, metabolites of *Streptomyces clavuligerus*. J Antibiot 32:549–554

Kirby R (1976) Genetic studies on *Streptomyces coelicolor* plasmid one. PhD Thesis, University of East Anglia, Norwich, England

Kirby R (1978a) Genetic mapping of *Streptomyces clavuligerus*. FEMS Microbiol Lett 3:177–180

Kirby R (1978b) An unstable genetic element affecting the production of the antibiotic holomycin by *Streptomyces clavuligerus*. FEMS Microbiol Lett 3:283–286

Kirby R, Hopwood DA (1977) Genetic determination of methylenomycin synthesis by the SCP I plasmid of *Streptomyces coelicolor* A3(2). J Gen Microbiol 98:239–252

Kirby R, Lewis E (1981) Unstable genetic elements affecting streptomycin resistance in the streptomycin producing organisms *Streptomyces griseus* NCIB8506 and *Streptomyces bikiniensis* ISP5235. J Gen Microbiol 122:351–355

Kirby R, O'Reilly C (1979) Genetic instability in *Streptomyces cattleya*. Proceedings of the Society for General Microbiology 6:172

Kirby R, Wotton S (1979) Restriction studies on the SCP 2 plasmid of *Streptomyces coelicolor* A3(2). J Gen Microbiol 6:321–324

Kirby R, Wright LF, Hopwood DA (1975) Plasmid-determined antibiotic synthesis and resistance in *Streptomyces coelicolor*. Nature 254:265–267

Kirby R, Lewis E, Botha C (1982) A survey of *Streptomyces* species for covalently closed circular (ccc) DNA using a variety of methods. FEMS Microbiol Lett 13:79–82

Kruegel H, Fiedler G, Noack D (1980) Transfection of protoplasts of *Streptomyces lividans* 66 with actinophage SH-10 DNA. Mol Gen Genet 117:297–300

Lomovskaya ND, Voeykoya TA, Mkrtumian NM (1977) Construction and properties of hybrids obtained in interspecific crosses between *Streptomyces coelicolor* A3(2) and *Streptomyces griseus* Kr15. J Gen Microbiol 98:187–198

Matselyukh BP (1976) Structure and function of the *Actinomyces olivaceus* genome. In: Macdonald KD (ed) Second international symposium on the genetics of industrial micro-organisms. Academic Press, London New York, pp 553–563

Merrick MJ (1975) Hybridisation and selection for increased penicillin titre in wild-type isolates of *Aspergillus nidulans*. J Gen Microbiol 91:278–286

Merrick MJ (1976) A morphological and genetic mapping study of bald colony mutants of *Streptomyces coelicolor*. J Gen Microbiol 96:299–315

Nagarajan R (1972) Beta-lactam antibiotics from *Streptomyces*. In: Flynn EH (ed) Cephalopsporins and penicillins; chemistry and biology. Academic Press, New York, pp 636–661

Nagarajan R, Boeck LD, Gorman M, Hamill RC, Higgins CE, Hoehn MM, Stark WM, Whitney JG (1971) Beta-lactam antibiotics from *Streptomyces*. J Am Chem Soc 93:2308–2310

Ochi K, Hitchcock JM, Katz E (1979) High-frequency fusion of *Streptomyces parvulus* or *Streptomyces antibioticus* protoplasts induced by polyethylene glycol. J Bacteriol 139:984–992

Okamura K, Hirata S, Koki K, Hori K, Skibamoto N, Okamura Y, Okabe R et al. (1979) PS-5, a new beta-lactam antibiotic. I Taxonomy of the producing organism, isolation, and physio-chemical properties. J Antibiot 32:262–271

Okamura K, Hirata S, Okamura Y, Fukagawa Y, Shimauchi Y, Ishikura T, Lein J (1978) PS-5, a new beta-lactam antibiotic from *Streptomyces*. J Antibiot 31:480–482

Okamura K, Sakamoto M, Fukagawa Y, Ishikura T (1979) PS-5, a new beta-lactam antibiotic. III Synergistic effects and inhibitory activity against a beta-lactamase. J Antibiot 32:280–304

Okanishi M, Ohta T, Umezawa H (1970) Possible control of formation of aerial mycelium and antibiotic production in *Streptomyces* by episomic factors. J Antibiot 23:45–47

Okanishi M, Suzuki K, Umezawa H (1974) Formation and reversion of *Streptomyces* protoplasts: cultural conditions and morphological study. J Gen Microbiol 80:389–400

Okanishi M, Umezawa H (1978) Plasmids involved in antibiotic production in *Streptomycetes*. Genetics of the *Actinomycetales*. Proceedings of the international colloquium at the Forschungsinstitut Borstel. Ed: Freerksen E, Tárnok I, Thumin JH. Fischer, Stuttgart, pp 19–36

Omura S, Ikeda H, Kita C (1979) The detection of a plasmid in *Streptomyces ambofaciens* KA-1028 and its possible involvement in spiramycin production. J Antibiot 32:1058–1060

Orgel LE, Crick FHC (1980) Selfish DNA: the ultimate parasite. Nature 284:604–607

Parag Y (1978) Genetic recombination in *Streptomyces griseus*. J Bacteriol 183:1027–1031

Polsinelli M, Beretta M (1966) Genetic recombination in crosses between *Streptomyces aureofaciens* and *Streptomyces rimosus*. J Bacteriol 91:63–68

Pridham TG, Tresner HG (1974) The Streptomycetes. Bergey's manual of determinative bacteriology 8th edition. Williams and Wilkins, Baltimore

Ptashne M, Cohen SN (1974) Occurence of insertion sequences (IS) regions on the plasmid deoxyribonucleic acid as direct and inverted nucleotide sequence duplications. J Bacteriol 122:776–781

Reading C, Cole M (1976) Clavulanic acid, a beta-lactamase inhibiting beta-lactam from *Streptomyces clavuligerus*. J Chem Soc Commun 19:266–267

Redshaw PA, McCann PA, Pentella MA, Pogell BM (1979) Simultaneous loss of multiple differentiated functions in aerial mycelium negative isolates of *Streptomyces*. J Bacteriol 137:891–899

Rudd BAM, Hopwood DA (1978) Genetics of actinorhodin biosynthesis in *Streptomyces coelicolor* A3(2). Abstr 3rd int symp genet ind micro-organisms, Madison, no 19, p 10

Rudd BAM, Hopwood DA (1979) Genetics of actinorhodin biosynthesis by *Streptomyces coelicolor* A3(2). J Gen Microbiol 114:35–43

Schrempf H, Goebel W (1978) Plasmids in *Streptomyces*. Abst int symp genet ind micro-organisms, Madison, no 80, p 40

Schrempf H, Bujard H, Hopwood DA, Goebel W (1975) Isolation of covalently closed circular deoxyribonucleic acid from *Streptomyces coelicolor* A3(2). J Bacteriol 121:416–421

Sermonti G, Petris A, Micheli M, Lanfaloni L (1977) A factor involved in chloramphenicol resistance in *Streptomyces coelicolor* A3(2): its transfer in the absence of the fertility factor. J Gen Microbiol 100:347–353

Sermonti G, Petris A, Micheli M, Lanfaloni L (1978) Chloramphenicol resistance in *Streptomyces coelicolor* A3(2) – possible involvement of a transposable element. Mol Gen Genet 164:99–103

Sermonti G, Lanfaloni L, Micheli MR (1980) A jumping gene in *Streptomyces coelicolor* A3(2). Mol Gen Genet 177:453–458

Shaw PD, Piwowarski J (1977) Effect of ethidium bromide and acriflavine on streptomycin production by *Streptomyces bikiniensis*. J Antibiot 30:404–408

Stapley EO, Jackson M, Hernandez S, Zimmerman SB, Currie SA, Mochales S, Mata JM, Woodruff HB, Hendlin D (1972) Cephamycins, a new family of beta-lactam antibiotics. I. Production by *actinomycetes* including *Streptomyces lactamdurans* sp. Antimicrob Agents Chemother 2:122–131

Stuttard C (1979) Transduction of auxotrophic matkers in a chloramphenicol producing strain of *Streptomyces*. J Gen Microbiol 110:479–482

Suarez JE, Chater FF (1980) Polyethylene glycol-assisted transfection of *Streptomyces* protoplasts. J Bacteriol 142:8–14

Toyama H, Okanishi M, Umezawa H (1979) Cleavage maps of the plasmids in *Streptomyces kasugaensis*. Jpn J Genet 54:471

Valu G, Szabo G (1980) Streptomycin sensitivity of ribosomes isolated from a streptomycin producing *Streptomyces griseus*. Acta Microbiol Acad Sci Hung 26:207–212

Vivian A (1971) Genetic control of fertility in *Streptomyces coelicolor* A3(2): plasmid involvement in the interconversion of UF and IF strains. J Gen Microbiol 69:353–364

Wildermuth JG (1970) Development and organisation of the aerial mycelium in *Streptomyces coelicolor*. J Gen Microbiol 60:43–50

Wright LF, Hopwood DA (1976a) Identification of the antibiotic determined by the SCP I plasmid of *Streptomyces coelicolor* A3(2). J Gen Microbiol 95:96–106

Wright LF, Hopwood DA (1976b) Actinorhodin is a chromosomally determined antibiotic in *Streptomyces coelicolor* A3(2). J Gen Microbiol 96:289–297

Yu-gu S, Ke-suing D, Min L, Ying-fang Z, Nai-quam Y (1978) Genetic evidence of the presence of plasmid in *Streptomyces griseus* and its relationship with the biosynthesis of streptomycin. Acta Microbiol Sin 18:195–201

Yagisawa M, Huang TSR, Davies J (1978) The possible role of plasmids in neomycin biosynthesis and modification. Abstr int symp genet ind microorganisms, Madison, no 73, p 37

CHAPTER 6

Biosynthesis of β-Lactam Antibiotics

A. L. DEMAIN

A. Introduction

The discovery of penicillin by FLEMING (1929) and its development by the Oxford group (FLOREY et al. 1949) began the antibiotic era. The success of this β-lactam antibiotic led the way for the development of all other antibiotics. As will be described later in this chapter, new and more effective β-lactam antibiotics are being discovered now, over 50 years after Fleming's initial discovery.

A number of natural hydrophobic penicillins are formed by *Penicillium chrysogenum*, depending on the acids (R-CO) present in the medium or made by the cells:

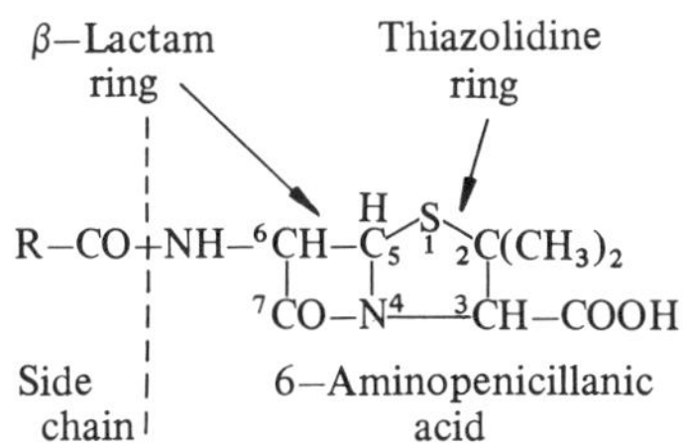

Addition of side-chain precursors is standard procedure today in order to increase the total production of penicillins and to direct the fermentation toward a single penicillin such as benzylpenicillin (penicillin G) or the acid-stable phenoxymethylpenicillin (penicillin V).

Although hydrophobic penicillins are made by many species of fungi, *P. chrysogenum* remains the choice for industrial production. No hydrophobic penicillin is made by prokaryotic microorganisms. All natural and biosynthetic hydrophobic penicillins made by fungi are susceptible to the action of penicillin β-lactamase which catalyzes the opening of the β-lactam ring, thereby destroying all biological activity.

The hydrophobic penicillins exhibit a high degree of activity against gram-positive organisms but are much less active against gram-negative organisms. A completely different type – a hydrophilic penicillin showing equivalent activity against both classes of microorganisms – is penicillin N, a penicillin possessing a D-α-aminoadipyl side chain, i.e., (D-4-amino-4-carboxy-*n*-butyl)-penicillin:

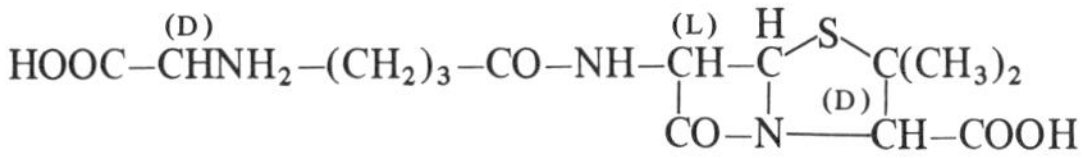

The fungus best known for production of penicillin N is *Cephalosporium acremonium;* it is also known in the literature as *Cephalosporium* sp, *Acremonium chryso-*

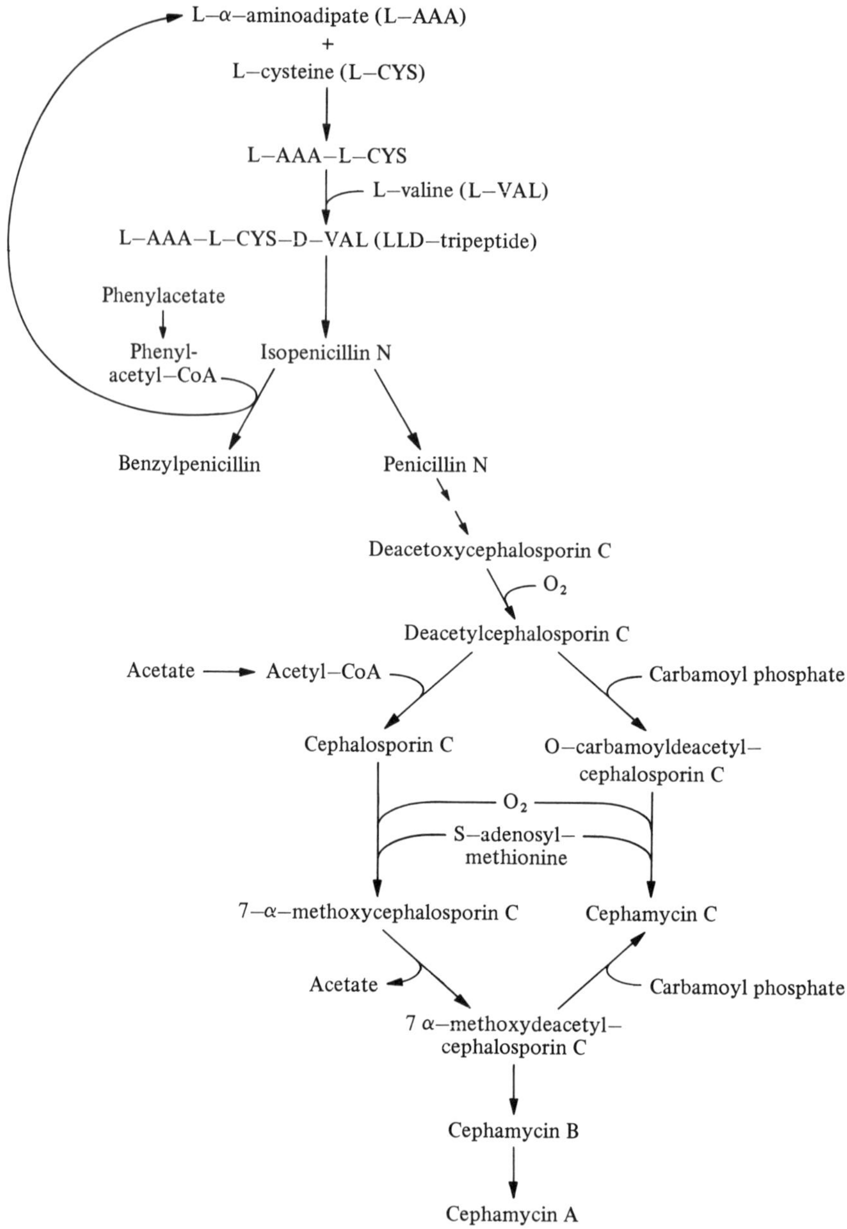

Fig. 1. Composite pathway of penicillin and cephalosporin biosynthesis in molds and actinomycetes. The left branch at isopenicillin N is the hydrophobic branch; the right branch is the hydrophilic branch. The existence of the monocyclic β-lactam has not yet been confirmed and thus is enclosed in brackets. (Modified from DEMAIN 1981)

genum, and *Acremonium strictum*. In addition to fungi, streptomycetes also produce this hydrophilic penicillin.

During their studies on the purification of penicillin N from broths of *C. acremonium*, NEWTON and ABRAHAM (1955) noted the presence of another antibiotic in their crude preparations. It was named cephalosporin C, the structure of which is as follows (ABRAHAM and NEWTON 1961):

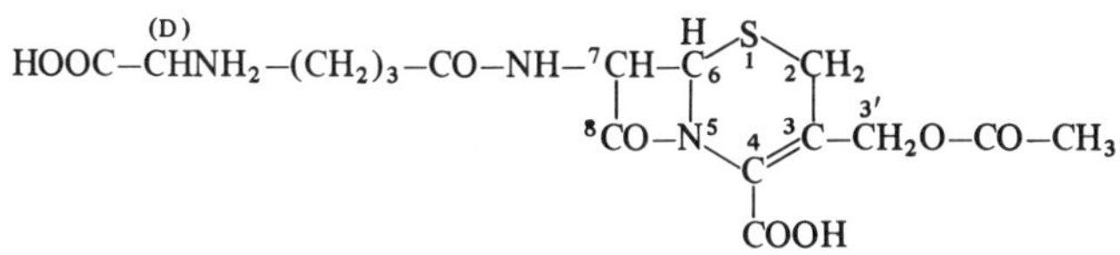

Cephalosporin C resembles the penicillins in having an acyl side-chain attached to an amino group of a double-ring nucleus. The side chain is identical to that of penicillin N, i.e. D-α-aminoadipic acid. Although both penicillins and cephalosporins have the four-membered β-lactam moiety, cephalosporin C possesses a six-membered dihydrothiazine ring instead of the five-membered thiazolidine ring characteristic of the penicillins. The nucleus of cephalosporin C is called 7-aminocephalosporanic acid (7-ACA).

Although cephalosporin C contains the β-lactam ring, which is the site of staphylococcal penicillin β-lactamase action, it is a poor substrate for the enzyme. This stability is a function of the dihydrothiazine ring. Cephalosporin C, although resistant to penicillin β-lactamase, is hydrolyzed by cephalosporin β-lactamase. The terms penicillin β-lactamase and cephalosporin β-lactamase are used only for convenience. In reality, the β-lactamases constitute a family of enzymes with a wide spectrum of activities on penicillins and cephalosporins.

An overall picture of penicillin and cephalosporin biosynthesis is shown in Fig. 1. This is a composite picture constructed from data obtained from many microorganisms and will be discussed later in this chapter. No single microorganism can carry out the entire series of reactions. However, all can carry out the initial series of steps to isopenicillin N. The pathway then branches. The short branch to the left is that carried out by *Penicillium* and other fungi which produce extracellular hydrophobic β-lactams. The right hand branch is found in producers of hydrophilic β-lactam antibiotics; these are fungi such as *Cephalosporium* and the actinomycetes. The fungi proceed only to cephalosporin C whereas the actinomycetes can go much further in their production of cephalosporins including the 7-methoxy forms known as cephamycins.

B. Hydrophobic β-Lactam Antibiotics

I. Biosynthetic Precursors

The early fermentation media for production of hydrophobic penicillins by *P. chrysogenum* contained corn steep liquor, lactose, side-chain precursor, surface-active agent, and mineral salts. In later years, the lactose was replaced by slow feeding of glucose. The submerged fermentation displays a growth phase followed by a stage of product formation. The hydrophobic antibiotic is excreted as it is formed and very little can be found inside mycelia.

When it was found that phenylacetate could stimulate both the formation of total penicillins and the formation of benzylpenicillin at the expense of other penicillins, it became obvious that the limiting factor in biosynthesis was the synthesis of the side-chain precursor. The most efficiently used precursor is phenylacetic acid or one of its derivatives. Direct proof of the incorporation of phenylacetate into penicillin was obtained with various labeled phenylacetate molecules (BEHRENS et al. 1948; CRAIG et al. 1951; GORDON et al. 1953; SEBEK 1953; HALLIDAY and ARNSTEIN 1956).

After the discovery that penicillin N was formed by *C. acremonium*, many workers tried to force *P. chrysogenum* to produce this hydrophilic antibiotic by supplementation of the medium with α-aminoadipic acid, but all attempts failed. Similarly, feeding of phenylacetic acid to cultures of *C. acremonium* did not yield benzylpenicillin. Although this was a puzzle for many years, we can now understand these observations (see C.III).

The β-lactam-thiazolidine ring nucleus common to all penicillins can be conceived as a condensation product of L-cysteine and D-valine. Indeed, cysteine and valine are the precursors of the nucleus although valine enters the biosynthetic path as the L form. Condensation of these two moieties however requires the participation of another amino acid, L-α-aminoadipic acid.

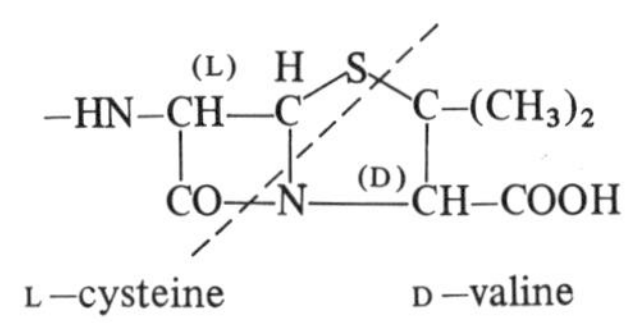

The addition of cysteine to fermentations containing inorganic sulfate did not increase penicillin production since the endogenous production of cysteine was not limiting. However, with starved mycelial suspensions, a stimulation of penicillin biosynthesis by cysteine occurred in the presence of lactose, phenylacetate, buffer and mineral salts (DEMAIN 1956). In such a system, *S*-ethyl-DL-cysteine inhibited antibiotic synthesis; this effect was reversed by L-cystine. Synthesis was also inhibited by α-methyl-DL-cystine (ARNSTEIN and MARGREITER 1958).

Direct evidence for the incorporation of cysteine was obtained by isotopic studies. It was demonstrated (STEVENS et al. 1953) that L-cysteine, but not D-cysteine, is utilized in preference to inorganic sulfate as a surce of sulfur for the penicillin molecule. Work by Arnstein's group (ARNSTEIN and GRANT 1954a, b; ARNSTEIN and CRAWHALL 1957) proved conclusively that the intact cyst(e)ine molecule is incorporated into penicillin. Upon addition of cystine to a penicillin fermentation in idiophase, the amino acid was immediately incorporated into penicillin at a linear rate (STEVENS et al. 1956).

Recent studies with various types of labelled cyst(e)ine have shown that the C-3 of L-cysteine is incorporated into C-5 of penicillin with overall retention of stereochemistry (MORECOMBE and YOUNG 1975; YOUNG et al. 1977; HUDDLESTON et al. 1978) and that α,β-dehydrocysteine-containing compounds are not intermediates (BYCROFT et al. 1975).

As in the case of cysteine, valine addition failed to stimulate penicillin synthesis. Even with starved mycelia, valine did not stimulate the rate of penicillin formation in the presence of lactose and phenylacetate. However, in a system composed of L-cystine, phenylacetate, and salts, the addition of L-valine stimulated the rate of antibiotic production by starved resting cells (DEMAIN 1956). D-valine, on the other hand, inhibited penicillin synthesis. The addition of α-methyl-DL-valine was inhibitory to penicillin formation, and its action was reversed by L-valine. Another inhibitor of antibiotic synthesis is DL-isoleucine, which may be considered a structural analogue of valine (ARNSTEIN and MARGREITER 1958).

The use of ^{14}C-labeled valine provided direct evidence for the incorporation of the valine carbon skeleton into penicillin. DL-valine-γ,γ-^{14}C enters the valine moiety of the antibiotic (ARNSTEIN and GRANT 1954a) and the addition of carboxyl-labeled DL-valine resulted in the production of penicillin labeled in its carboxyl group (STEVENS et al. 1954). The intact carbon chain of valine is used for penicillin biosynthesis (ARNSTEIN and CLUBB 1957). Various forms of chirally labelled valine have been incorporated into penicillin (NEUSS et al. 1973; ABERHART and LIN 1974). Overall retention of configuration at the β-carbon of L-valine was observed during formation of the ring system. Incorporation of valine deuterated in the methyl carbons (ABERHART et al. 1974) revealed that the methyl groups are not modified, thus eliminating a β,γ-unsaturated valinyl peptide as a possible intermediate.

Although the valine moiety of penicillin is of the D-configuration, the stimulation of synthesis by the L-form and the inhibitory effect of D-valine indicated L-valine to be the actural precursor. Comparative studies on the incorporation of labeled L- and D-valine have further proven the role of L-valine in penicillin biosynthesis (ARNSTEIN and MARGREITER 1958; STEVENS et al. 1956; ARNSTEIN and CLUBB 1957). Although there is an inversion from L-valine to D-valine during biosynthesis, the amino group is retained (STEVENS and DELONG 1958; BOOTH et al. 1976; ABERHART et al. 1974).

DEMAIN (1957) found that lysine is a potent inhibitor of penicillin synthesis by *P. chrysogenum*. Since the fungal biosynthetic pathway to lysine involves α-aminoadipic acid as an intermediate, attempts were made to reverse lysine inhibition with the latter. α-Aminoadipic acid not only reversed the inhibitory effect of lysine, but also stimulated penicillin synthesis in the absence of added lysine (SOMERSON et al. 1961). About the same time, Arnstein and coworkers (ARNSTEIN et al. 1960; ARNSTEIN and MORRIS 1960) observed the formation of an intracellular labeled tripeptide, δ-(α-aminoadipyl)-cysteinyl-valine (ACV) uppon addition of L-valine-^{14}C to *P. chrysogenum* and BAUER (1970) reported the production of ACV by cell-free extracts. The structure of the tripeptide in *P. chrysogenum* is δ-(L-α-aminoadipyl)-L-cysteinyl-D-valine(LLD-ACV) (ADRIAENS et al. 1975; CHAN et al. 1976). Additional peptides detected in broths of *P. chrysogenum* but whose biosynthetic significance is doubtful include α-aminoadipyl-alanyl-valine, α-aminoadipyl-serinylvaline, α-aminoadipyl-serinyl-isodehydrovaline (NEUSS et al. 1980) and peptides containing α-aminoadipic acid and valine (AVANZINI and VALENTI 1980).

The above facts indicated that L-α-aminoadipic acid is involved in the initial peptide-forming steps. That it remains attached throughout the entire process by which the nucleus is formed was strongly suggested by the discovery (HALE et al.

1953; Flynn et al. 1962; Cole and Batchelor 1963) that in media devoid of precursors, *P. chrysogenum* produces the hydrophilic penicillin, isopenicillin N, which contains L-α-aminoadipic acid as its side-chain. Although isopenicillin N was found in both mycelia and broth filtrates in precursor-free fermentations, its usual location is intracellular, where it predominates over hydrophobic penicillins. As it did with the hydrophobic penicillins, lysine inhibited production of isopenicillin N and α-aminoadipic acid supplementation stimulated its production (Goulden and Chattaway 1968). The major compound which accumulated in precursor-free fermentation broths was the penicillin nucleus, 6-aminopenicillanic acid (6-APA). The close structural relationship between ACV, isopenicillin N and benzylpenicillin strongly suggested that the first two are intermediates in the biosynthesis of benzylpenicillin and other hydrophobic penicillins. The initial reaction of penicillin biosynthesis appears to be the condensation of L-cysteine and L-α-aminoadipic acid to form L-α-aminoadipyl-L-cysteine (Arnstein and Morris 1960). L-valine is presumably converted to the D-form during activation and is then added to form LLD-ACV.

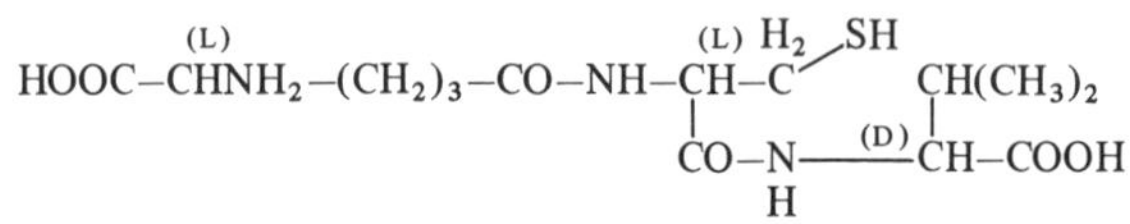

δ–(α–aminoadipyl) cysteinylvaline

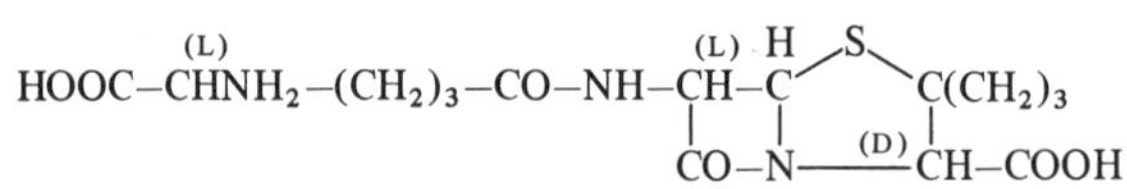

Isopenicillin N

Cyclization of LLD-ACV to isopenicillin N has been observed with cell-free extracts of *P. chrysogenum* (Meesschaert et al. 1980). In this study, the investigators noted the presence of a presumed intermediate which they believe to be a β-lactam-containing monocyclic intermediate 1-(1-D-carboxy-2-methylpropyl)-3-L-(5-L-aminoadipamide)-4-L- mercapto-azetidin-2-one.

The pathway of lysine biosynthesis in fungi is shown in Fig. 2. The pathway in *P. chrysogenum* has not yet been studied in detail, but it is known that early-blocked lysine auxotrophs can use α-aminoadipate for growth. Goulden and Chattaway (1968) found that a lysine auxotroph blocked before α-aminoadipate cannot make penicillin in the presence of lysine unless α-aminoadipate is also added. Conversely, a mutant blocked after aminoadipate made penicillin when lysine alone was added. Nash et al. (1974) found that such a late blocked mutant incorporates ^{14}C-α-aminoadipic acid into isopenicillin N, LLD-ACV and other unidentified peptides. These data established a role for α-aminoadipate in benzylpenicillin biosynthesis.

The picture that emerges from many studies on lysine inhibition and repression of penicillin biosynthesis (see Chap. 7) is that lysine and penicillin are products of a branched biosynthetic pathway, the branch occurring at α-aminoadipate or its adenylate. The expected decrease in L-α-aminoadipate in the amino acid pool upon lysine addition results in the depression of penicillin biosynthesis. High lysine con-

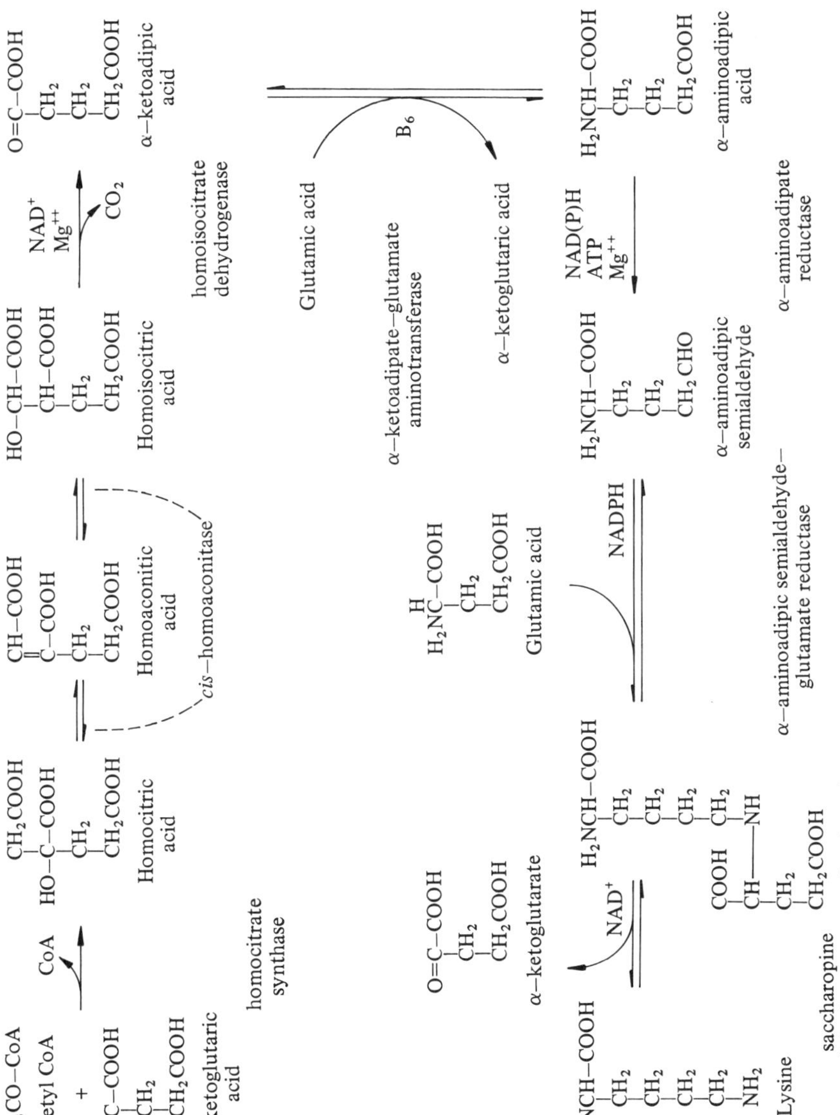

Fig. 2. Pathway of lysine biosynthesis in fungi. (DEMAIN 1974)

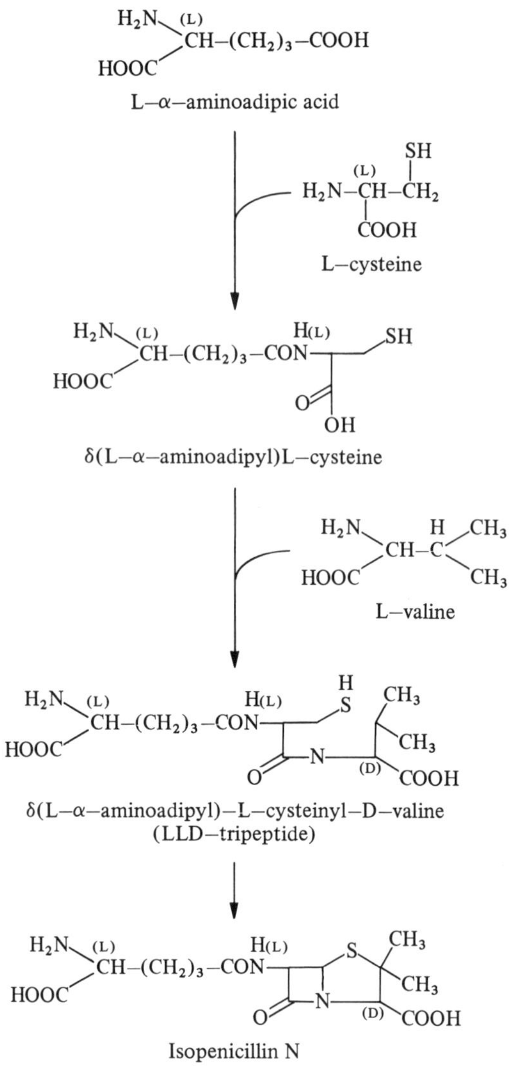

Fig. 3. The early common steps of penicillin and cephalosporin biosynthesis in molds and actinomycetes. (Modified from Demain 1981)

centrations also interfere with cephalosporin production in *Paecilomyces persicinus* (D'AMATO and PISANO 1976) and *C. acremonium* (MEHTA et al. 1979).

The above data indicate that penicillin biosynthesis up to the stage of intracellular isopenicillin N can be represented as shown in Fig. 3. The final step shown in Fig. 4 is described in the next section.

II. Terminal Biosynthetic Reaction

The discovery of the accumulation of the penicillin nucleus in fermentation broths without added side-chain precursor was made by KATO (1953) and confirmed by DEMAIN (1959). BATCHELOR et al. (1959) later isolated the compound and found it to be 6-APA.

6-APA is the major penicillin derivative accumulating in precursor-free fermentations of penicillin-producing fungi (KITANO et al. 1975a); it has not been found in broths of fungi which do not produce penicillins (COLE 1966). Despite these facts, I doubt that 6-APA has a direct role in the do novo biosynthesis of benzylpenicillin. For example, WOLFF and ARNSTEIN (1960) failed to observe a clear precursor–product relationship between 6-APA and benzylpenicillin. 6-APA is probably a shunt metabolite derived by deacylation (MURAO 1955; ERICKSON and BENNETT 1965) of isopenicillin N in the absence of side-chain precursor. Thus the terminal reaction of benzylpenicillin synthesis is most likely an exchange of the L-aminoadipic acid side-chain of isopenicillin N for phenylacetic acid from phenylacetyl-coenzyme A (CoA) (Fig. 4). Such acyltransferase activity was reported by LODER (1972) in crude extracts of *P. chrysogenum*, i.e. she found labeled benzylpenicillin to be produced from ^{14}C-phenylacetate, CoA and isopenicillin N; phenylacetyl-CoA is presumably the true acyl donor. Penicillin acyltransferase is intracellular and present in all penicillin-producing fungi. Phenylacetyl-CoA arises from phenylacetate and coenzyme A by the action of a side-chain-activating enzyme; the appearance of this enzyme precedes rapid penicillin formation and declines at the same time as does the penicillin production rate in fermentations (BRUNNER et al. 1968). In the absence of phenylacetyl-CoA, isopenicillin N is pre-

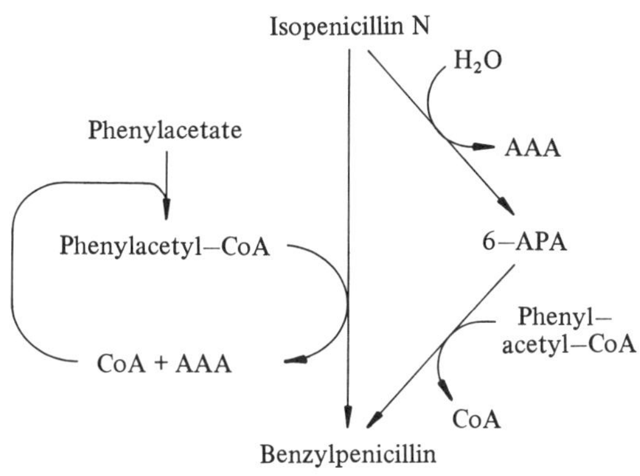

Fig. 4. The hydrophobic branch from isopenicillin N to benzylpenicillin in *Penicillium* and some other fungi. This branch does not occur in cephalosporin-producing fungi such as *Cephalosporium*, *Paecilomyces*, and *Emericellopsis* or in the actinomycetes. (DEMAIN 1981)

sumably hydrolyzed to 6-APA by penicillin acyltransferase. Although VANDERHAEGHE et al. (1968) failed to observe hydrolysis of isopenicillin N to 6-APA by extracts of *P. chrysogenum*, this result was not considered to be conclusive (DEMAIN 1974) and indeed the reaction was later demonstrated by ABRAHAM (1977). 6-APA may be converted to benzylpenicillin if phenylacetyl-CoA becomes available. This proposal implicates isopenicillin N as the true immediate precursor of the hydrophobic penicillins and 6-APA acylation as a salvage pathway. The finding of LODER (1972) and FAWCETT et al. (1975) that extracts can convert isopenicillin N (but not penicillin N) to benzylpenicillin is consistent with the above proposal but it still must be established whether the conversion is direct or involves a prior hydrolysis of isopenicillin N to 6-APA, especially since the extracts used were also capable of phenylacetylating free 6-APA.

Since L-α-aminoadipate is obligatory for penicillin synthesis but is eliminated in the acyltransferase reaction, it should be required only in very low amounts. FRIEDRICH and DEMAIN (1978) indeed found that only low concentrations of α-aminoadipate are required for penicillin biosynthesis. Thus α-aminoadipate is apparently recycled during penicillin biosynthesis and at least ten molecules of penicillin can be formed per molecule of α-aminoadipate supplied. However some of the released α-aminoadipate is lost to the medium as shown by the isolation of high concentrations of extracellular 6-oxo-piperidine-2-carboxylic acid, the lactam of cyclized α-aminoadipate (BRUNDIDGE et al. 1980).

The importance of penicillin acyltransferase for penicillin biosynthesis is indicated by the observation that only those acyl groups present as side-chains in natural penicillins can function as acyl donors irrespective of whether the acyl donor is a penicillin or a CoA ester (SPENCER 1968; GATENBACK and BRUNSBERG 1968; SPENCER and MAUNG 1970). Furthermore, the dynamics of enzyme formation correlate with those of penicillin formation (PRUESS and JOHNSON 1967). Specific activity of the enzyme is greater in media supporting high penicillin production. Acyltransferase is absent from fungi which do not produce penicillin and is present at higher levels in superior penicillin-producing mutants than in their predecessors.

C. Hydrophilic β-Lactam Antibiotics

Although the hydrophilic penicillin N never became an antibiotic of commercial importance, its biosynthesis is of interest since penicillin N is related to both the hydrophobic penicillins and the cephalosporins, i.e. it possesses the 6-APA nucleus of the hydrophobic penicillins and the side chain of all natural cephalosporins, D-α-aminoadipic acid. Penicillin N and cephalosporins are produced by species of the fungi *Scopulariopsis*, *Diheterospora*, *Arachnomyces*, *Anixiopsis*, *Spiroidinium*, *Emericellopsis*, *Paecilomyces*, and *Cephalosporium* (KITANO et al. 1974; HIGGENS et al. 1974; PISANO and VELOZZI 1974). They are also formed by many species of actinomycetes (NAGARAJAN et al. 1971; STAPLEY et al. 1972; KITANO 1977). Microorganisms capable of producing hydrophobic penicillins such as benzylpenicillin cannot produce cephalosporin C or penicillin N. A major difference between the organisms which produce hydrophobic penicillins (e.g., *Penicillium*) and those that produce hydrophilic β-lactams (e.g., *Cephalosporium*) is that the latter group fails to respond to the addition of side-chain precursors.

Table 1. Natural cephamycins made by actinomycetes. (Modified from CASSIDY 1981)

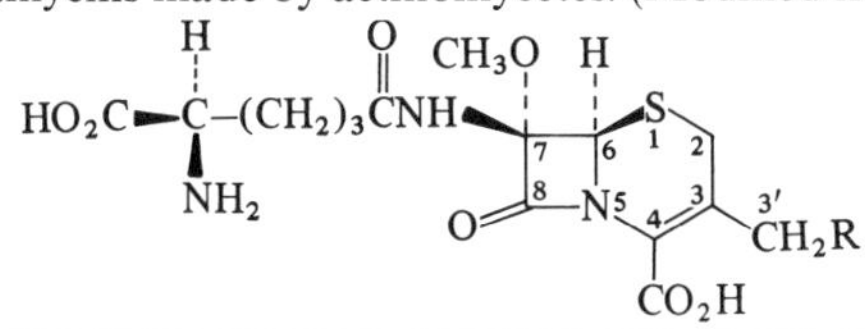

Name	R	Producing organisms
Cephamycin C (A-16886 B)	$—OCONH_2$	*S. albogriseolus, S. clavuligerus, S. filipensis, S. inositovorus, S. jumonjinensis, N. lactamdurans, S. todorominensis, S. wadayamensis*
A-16884 A	$—OCOCH_3$	*S. lipmanii*
Cephamycin A	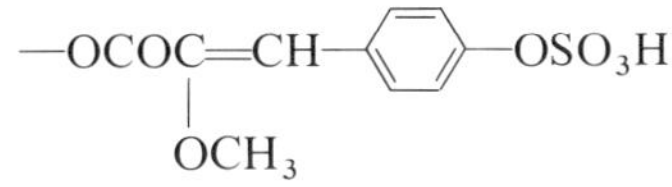	*Streptomyces chartreusis, S. cinnamonensis, S. fimbriatus, S. griseus, S. halstedii, S. heteromorphus, S. panayensis, S. rochei, S. viridochromogenes*
Cephamycin B	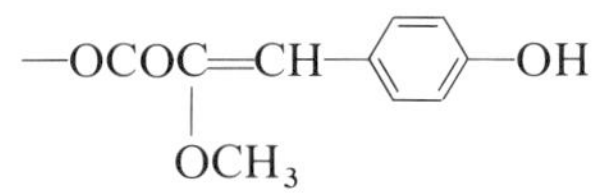	
C-2801 X	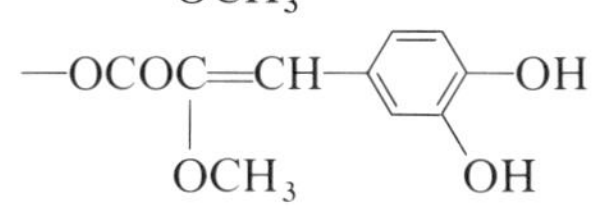	*S. heteromorphus, S. panayensis*
7-Methoxy-deacetyl-cephalosporin C	—OH	*S. chartreusis*
WS-3442 D	—H	*S. wadayamensis*

The fungal cephalosporins include cephalosporin C, deacetoxycephalosporin C and deacetylcephalosporin C. The streptomycete cephalosporins additionally include cephalosporins modified with a methoxy group at C-7 (cephamycins) (Table 1) and/or an acetoxy, carbamoyl or substituted cinnamoyl group attached to carbon 3′. The presence of the methoxy group at C-7 confers high resistance to β-lactamases and increases activity against gram-negative and anaerobic pathogens (STAPLEY et al. 1979).

Deacetylcephalosporin C is usually found in broths of fungi and streptomycetes which produce cephalosporin C (KITANO et al. 1976a; KANZAKI and FUJISAWA 1976). Although deacetylcephalosporin C is an intermediate (see below), studies on the kinetics of labeling show that most of it is formed by hydrolysis of cephalosporin C (ABRAHAM et al. 1965). It had been postulated that the hydrolysis may be a nonenzymatic reaction (HUBER et al. 1968); however, nonenzymatic deacylation cannot account for the large amount of deacetylcephalosporin C produced (KOCECNY et al. 1973). More likely, deacetylation is carried out by the cephalosporin C acetylhydrolase found in *C. acremonium* (FUJISAWA et al. 1973; HINNEN and NÜESCH 1976). The fungus also is thought to contain a β-lactamase ("arylamidase") which degrades cephalosporins but not penicillins (DENNEN et al. 1971).

The overall biosynthetic path to hydrophilic β-lactams can be seen in Figs. 1, 3, 5, and 6. Evidence supporting this scheme is described below.

I. Early Biosynthetic Steps

Cephalosporin C is a derivative of α-aminoadipic acid, cysteine, valine, and acetate. Although addition of α-aminoadipic acid to *C. acremonium* failed to stimulate cephalosporin C formation, added DL-α-aminoadipic acid-2-^{14}C labeled the antibiotic almost exclusively in the side chain (TROWN et al. 1963a). As expected, mycelial lysine was also labeled. Exogenous α-aminoadipic acid was only poorly taken up, however.

The endogenous formation of α-aminoadipic acid in fungi occurs by the lysine biosynthetic pathway previously discussed (Fig. 2). This pathway and the operation of the tricarboxylic acid cycle account for the labeled carbon atoms of the antibiotic when the fungus was fed acetate labeled in C-1 or C-2 or α-ketoglutarate labeled in C-5 with ^{14}C or ^{13}C (TROWN et al. 1962, 1963b; NEUSS et al. 1971). The 7-ACA moiety of cephalosporin C is formed from L-cysteine, L-valine, and acetate as indicated by labeling experiments (TROWN et al. 1962, 1963a; DEMAIN 1963; NEUSS et al. 1971). Valines with chiral ^{13}C labels were specifically incorporated into cephalosporin C; (2 RS, 3R) [4-^{13}-C] valine labeled C-2 of the dihydrothiazine ring wheres (2S, 3S) [4-^{13}C] valine labeled the exocyclic methylene carbon attached to C-3 of this ring in cephalosporin C and the α-methyl carbon of penicillin N (NEUSS et al. 1973; KLUENDER et al. 1973). There was net inversion at position 2 and net retention at position 3 of L-valine as it was incorporated into penicillin N and cephalosporin C (NEUSS et al. 1973; KLUENDER et al. 1973; BALDWIN et al. 1973). Exogenous D-valine failed to dilute out the radioactivity incorporated from L-valine-1-^{14}C (WARREN et al. 1967).

Studies on the streptomycete cephalosporins (INAMINE and BIRNBAUM 1972; WHITNEY et al. 1972) indicated that the biosynthetic precursors are similar to those involved in the fungal formation of cephalosporin C, i.e. cysteine, valine and α-aminoadipic acid. Since α-aminoadipic acid is not an intermediate of lysine biosynthesis in procaryotes, it must be derived by lysine degradation (KERN et al. 1980). The pathway involves epsilon deamination to L-1-piperideine-6-carboxylate by L-lysine ε aminotransferase, presumably followed by an NAD-linked enzymatic oxidation to L-α-aminoadipate. Thus label from radioactive lysine was incorporated into streptomycete cephalosporins but not into fungal cephalosporin C. As one would expect, a streptomycete mutant deficient in lysine breakdown did not produce cephalosporins (CARVER and GODFREY 1974). In contrast to the situation in fungal synthesis of cephalosporins, α-aminoadipate formation is rate-limiting in the biosynthesis of cephamycin C and thus addition of α-aminoadipic acid stimulates production of cephamycin C by *Nocardia* (previously *Streptomyces*) *lactamdurans*.

C. acremonium and *P. persicinus* produce the intermediate of penicillin biosynthesis, LLD-ACV (LODER and ABRAHAM 1971a, b; FAWCETT et al. 1976a, b; ENRIQUEZ and PISANO 1977). Neither LLD-ACV nor penicillin is taken up by *Cephalosporium* mycelia when added to suspensions. ^{14}C-labeled L-cysteine, L-valine, and L-α-aminoadipate were incorporated into the tripeptide and into the β-lactam antibiotics although they failed to increase the rate of antibiotic formation. The L-form of α-aminoadipate is a precursor of LLD-ACV, penicillin N and cephalosporin C, but the D-form is not (WARREN et al. 1967a; LODER and ABRAHAM 1971a). The precursor of the D-valine moiety of the tripeptide and penicillin N is L-valine, not the D-form; D-valine, in fact, inhibits penicillin N production. The most likely possibility for inversion of L-valine to the D form is that it occurs during valine activation prior to incorporation into LLD-ACV, in the same way that L-phenylalanine is converted by *Bacillus brevis* to the D-phenylalanine moiety of gramicidin S. Studies employing a mutant of *C. acremonium* blocked at the LLD-ACV stage and DL- and L-[1-^{14}C-3-^{3}H] valines showed that the configuration of C-3 of valine is retained during biosynthesis of the tripeptide (BALDWIN and WAN 1981).

For many years, the steps of penicillin N and cephalosporin C biosynthesis were very difficult to elucidate due to the lack of a cell-free system. In early attempts to develop such a system, a particulate fraction from cells broken by ultrasonic treatment or by grinding with sand or alumina failed to synthesize detectable antibiotic (ABRAHAM 1974; FAWCETT et al. 1976a, b) but was able to incorporate ^{14}C-DL-valine into LLD-ACV when incubated with δ-(L-α-aminoadipyl)-L-cysteine (LODER and ABRAHAM 1971b). This dipeptide was detected in actinomycetes which produce β-lactams (ABRAHAM 1977). No labeling took place if δ-(D-α-aminoadipyl)-L-cysteine or free D-α-aminoadipate plus L-cysteine were added to the disrupted cells in place of the above dipeptide. No incorporation of ^{14}C-DL-α-aminoadipate into tripeptide occurred in the presence of L-cys-D-val, L-cys-L-val or L-cysteine plus L-valine. When labelled L-valine was converted into LLD-ACV, only the α-proton was lost, eliminating the possibility of dehydrovaline as an intermediate (HUANG et al. 1975).

Antibiotic-negative mutants of *C. acremonium* accumulate five kinds of peptides, all of which are disulfides (KANZAKI and FUJISAWA 1976; SHIRAFUJI et al. 1979). They are (a) LLD-ACV dimer, (b) the disulfide of LLD-ACV and methanethiol, (c) the disulfide of LLD-ACV and *N*-acetyl-LLD-ACV, (d) the dimer of *N*-acetyl-LLD-ACV, and (e) the disulfide of *N*-acetyl-LLD-ACV and methanethiol. The significance of these compounds in antibiotic biosynthesis is unknown; they could merely be shunt metabolites of LLD-ACV or the disulfides might play a role in ring formation (BALDWIN and WAN 1979).

II. Formation of the Bicyclic Ring Structure

The inability of the above disrupted cell preparation (LODER and ABRAHAM 1971b) to synthesize antibiotic suggested that one (or more) of the enzymes responsible for biosynthesis of β-lactam antibiotics is part of an unstable complex which is destroyed by drastic treatment. ABRAHAM et al. (1965) reasoned that the conversion of cells into protoplasts followed by gentle lysis might preserve the integrity of the enzymes. DUNCAN and NEWTON (1970) observed incorporation of DL-valine-1-^{14}C into a compound with the properties of penicillin N or isopenicillin N by protoplasts of *C. acremonium*. They also described incorporation into this "antibiotic" and into a crude peptide complex (thought to contain peptides involved in antibiotic synthesis) by sonicated protoplasts. Conversion of L-[^{14}C]-valine to the "antibiotic" by a cell-free lyzed protoplast preparation was observed by BOST and DEMAIN (1977); no incorporation into cephalosporins was observed.

ABRAHAM (1977) reported that incubation of lyzed protoplasts with DL-[^{14}C]-valine, δ-(L-α-aminoadipyl)-L-cysteine, ATP and an energy-generating system yielded the above "antibiotic." The same lyzed protoplast system weakly incorporated LLD-ACV (but not the LLL- or DLD-tripeptides) into the "antibiotic" (FAWCETT et al. 1976 a, b). If LLD-ACV was used in the tritiated form, its α-valinyl proton was retained during ring formation; this again showed that formation of the C-S bond does not involve an α,β-dehydrovaline intermediate. Conversion of LLD-ACV to "antibiotic" was also demonstrated with extracts of *S. clavuligerus* (ABRAHAM 1977).

Along with LLD-ACV, LODER and ABRAHAM (1971 a, b) detected in *C. acremonium* the formation of tetrapeptides which appeared to be δ-(α-aminoadipyl)-cysteinylvalyl-glycine and the corresponding β-hydroxyvaline tetrapeptide. Tetrapeptides were also found in *P. persicinus* although the glycine was thought to be N terminal, rather than C terminal (ENRIQUEZ and PISANO 1979). The significance of the glycine residue is not known at this point.

Neither 7-ACA nor 6-APA appears to be involved in the biosynthesis of cephalosporin C or penicillin N. In an experiment in which L-valine was converted by *C. acremonium* mycelia to intracellular LLD-ACV, penicillin N, cephalosporin C, and deacetylcepahosporin C, no 7-ACA or 6-APA was formed (WARREN et al. 1967 b). Direct experiments on the effect of exogenous 7-ACA have not been successful since it does not penetrate the mycelium (ABRAHAM et al. 1965); free 7-ACA has never been detected in a microbial broth. The origin of the trace concentrations of 6-APA sometimes found in *C. acremonium* broths (COLE and ROLINSON 1961; LEMKE and NASH 1972) is probably not penicillin N since the penicillin acylase of this organism cannot hydrolyze penicillin N (COLE and ROLINSON 1961; CLARIDGE et al. 1963). This suggested the possibility that isopenicillin N was the source of 6-APA. Although isopenicillin N had never been reported in broths or mycelia of *C. acremonium*, it would have been difficult to differentiate it from penicillin N which it resembles chemically and physically. Indeed it is now known (KONOMI et al. 1979) that the "antibiotic" produced by the above cell-free systems from valine or LLD-ACV (DUNCAN and NEWTON 1970; FAWCETT 1976 a, b; BOST and DEMAIN 1977) is predominantly isopenicillin N.

Cell-free extracts prepared from *C. acremonium* protoplast lysates and subsequently frozen and thawed were found to convert LLD-ACV (but not LLL-ACV) to a penicillinase-labile antibiotic. The latter was detected by its activity against a β-lactam supersensitive bacterium; none of the cephalosporins was produced (KONOMI et al. 1979). Since the same extracts could convert penicillin N to deacetoxycephalosporin C (see below), it was obvious that the penicillinase-labile antibiotic produced was not penicillin N. As indicated by its antibacterial activity against four bacteria, the antibiotic was found to be isopenicillin N. Independent evidence supporting this conclusion was obtained using various labelled LLD-ACV molecules (O'SILLIVAN et al. 1979 a; BALDWIN et al. 1980 b; BEHADUR et al. 1981). No free intermediate [such as the monocyclic intermediate claimed to occur in *P. chrysogenum* (MEESSCHAERT et al. 1980)] was detected during the course of this conversion. The cyclization reaction as catalyzed by crude extracts was stimulated by Fe^{2+} but not by ATP or α-ketoglutarate (SAWADA et al. 1980 a); reducing agents such as ascorbate and dithiothreitol also were stimulatory (ABRAHAM et al. 1980).

The enzyme carrying out the reaction initially appeared to be membrane-bound, i.e. activity was stimulated by sonication or the surfactant, Triton X-100

(Sawada et al. 1980a). However, more recent studies using preparations prepared by grinding with glass beads (Abraham et al. 1980) or by sonication (Kupka et al. 1983b) indicate the activity to be soluble. It is probable that the earlier preparations (Sawada et al. 1980a) contained unlyzed protoplasts which were subsequently broken upon sonication or exposure to the surfactant. In an antibiotic-non-producing mutant, the enzyme reached its peak specific activity after growth ceased and then rapidly disappeared. However, in two antibiotic-producing strains, cyclization activity appeared during growth (Abraham et al. 1980; Shen, Kupka and Demain, unpublished work). The biosynthetic pathway up to the isopenicillin N stage is described in Fig. 3.

The cyclase enzyme (isopenicillin N synthetase) has been partially purified and shown to react not only with the LLD-tripeptide but also with an analogue tripeptide in which D-valine has been replaced by D-isoleucine; the product is antibiotically active (Abraham et al. 1980; Bahadur et al. 1981). However, tripeptides in which the aminoadipate moiety was replaced by glutamate or the cysteine replaced by aminobutyrate, serine or alanine were not converted to active products.

III. Epimerization of Isopenicillin N to Penicillin N

Conversion of isopenicillin N to penicillin N (Fig. 5) is catalyzed by an epimerase which isomerizes the L-aminoadipic acid side chain to the D-configuration. This activity was discovered in fresh cell-free extracts of *C. acremonium* by Konomi et al. (1979). It was noted that such freshly prepared extracts could convert LLD-tripeptide to a cephalosporin but with frozen–thawed extracts, the sequence stopped at isopenicillin N. Thus, this activity is very labile in cell-free extracts. Isopenicillin N was also converted to the cephalosporin by fresh, but not by frozen–thawed, extracts (Konomi and Demain, unpublished). The existence of the epimerase and its extreme lability have been confirmed (Baldwin et al. 1981b; Jayatilake et al. 1981). It is probable that microorganisms like *Penicillium*, which produce hydrophobic penicillins, lack this epimerase and instead, transacylate the isopenicillin N to hydrophobic penicillins. On the other hand, organisms like *Cephalosporium*, which produce only hydrophilic β-lactams, would lack acyltransferase activity. This indeed was demonstrated years ago in *Emericellopsis glabra* (Pruess and Johnson 1967).

IV. Conversion of Penicillin N to Cephalosporin C

Production of both penicillin N and cephalosporin C by a single microorganism is an interesting phenomenon. Both antibiotics contain the D-α-aminoadipic acid side chain and production of both is stimulated by methionine (see Chap. 7). From time to time, investigators have wondered whether penicillin N is a precursor of cephalosporin C but until recently no evidence had been found to support such a possibility. Instead, the view was often expressed (e.g., Demain 1974) that penicillin N and cephalosporin C are products of a branched biosynthetic pathway.

Despite the above viewpoint, two facts caused some concern about the branched pathway hypothesis. First, the chemical transformation of a penicillin into a cephalosporin had been accomplished in the early 1960s (Morin et al. 1963).

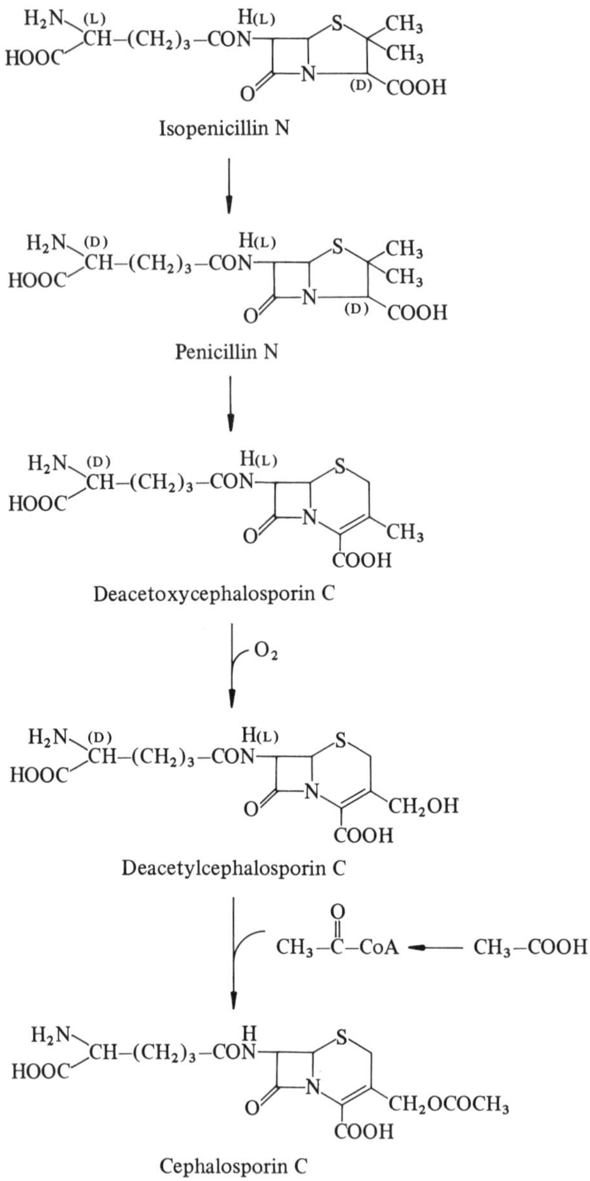

Fig. 5. The hydrophilic branch from isopenicillin N as far as cephalosporin C in *Cephalosporium* and actinomycetes. This is as far as *Cephalosporium* can proceed in the branch whereas the actinomycetes proceed further. The branch does not occur in *Penicillium* and other fungi which produce hydrophobic penicillins. (DEMAIN 1981)

Second was the isolation of penicillin N–positive, cephalosporin C–negative mutants as well as mutants which could produce neither antibiotic; however no penicillin N-negative, cephalosporin C-positive mutant was ever found (STAUFFER et al. 1966; LEMKE and NASH 1972). Finally it was discovered by KOHSAKA and DEMAIN (1976) that protoplast lysates of *C. acremonium* could convert penicillin N (but not penicillin G or 6-APA) to an antibiotic which was resistant to penicillinase. The reaction was stimulated by an energy-generating system and intensive aeration and inhibited by cyanide. Extracts of mutants blocked in the formation of penicillin N and cephalosporins were able to carry out this conversion but mutants which produced only penicillin N in fermentations yielded inactive extracts (YOSHIDA et al. 1978). The product of the conversion was found to be deacetoxycephalosporin C (YOSHIDA et al. 1978; BALDWIN et al. 1980a, c; MILLER et al. 1981) which had earlier been observed in broths of many β-lactam producing fungi and streptomycetes (KITANO et al. 1974, 1975b, 1976a; HIGGENS et al. 1974). Although *C. acremonium* normally produces only low concentrations (0.1 g/liter) of deacetoxycephalosporin C, a cephalosporin C nonproducing mutant accumulated increased levels (1.5 g/liter) of this intermediate (QUEENER et al. 1974).

An important breakthrough was that of HOOK et al. (1979) showing that the ring-expansion enzyme (deacetoxycephalosporin C synthetase) was markedly stimulated by Fe^{2+} and ascorbic acid, known stimulators of dioxygenases. BALDWIN et al. (1980c) demonstrated the incorporation of ^{3}H and ^{14}C from singly and doubly labelled penicillin N molecules into deacetoxycephalosporin C. The optimum concentrations of Fe^{2+} and ascorbate were found to be 0.04 m*M* and 0.67 m*M* respectively (SAWADA et al. 1979). In the presence of these cofactors, it was found that an ATP regeneration system was unnecessary, the concentration of ATP could be markedly reduced, and the activity of the cell-free system was 60–70-fold improved in rate over an earlier (YOSHIDA et al. 1978) system. Like the isopenicillin N synthetase, the ring-expansion activity in a nonproducing mutant reached its peak specific activity after growth ceased and then rapidly disappeared. Although α-ketoglutarate showed no stimulation of activity in crude extracts of an antibiotic-negative mutant of *C. acremonium* (HOOK et al. 1979; SAWADA et al. 1979), recent studies by FELIX et al. (1981) using ether-permeabilized cells of another *C. acremonium* mutant have revealed α-ketoglutarate stimulation. The α-ketoglutarate effect has been confirmed (KUPKA et al. 1983a) using purified enzyme from an antibiotic-positive strain.

The mutant used by FELIX et al. (1981) is peculiar. It was isolated as a cephalosporin C-negative mutant overproducing penicillin N. By present concepts, it should not possess ring-expansion activity but indeed it does. Of further curiosity is the finding reported in the same paper that ring-expansion activity could not be found in the cephalosporin C-producing parent or in a tripeptide-accumulating mutant. These puzzling findings await clarification.

In the first studies on ring-expansion (KOHSAKA and DEMAIN 1976), the activity appeared to be soluble, but later work (SAWADA et al. 1980b) suggested that it was membrane-bound, i.e., the activity in protoplast lysates of a nonproducing mutant was removed by Millipore filters and was increased by sonication or by Triton X-100 addition. Recent studies using sonic extracts prepared from the antibiotic-producing parent again indicate the activity to be soluble (KUPKA et al. 1983a). It is now felt that incomplete lysis of protoplasts or poor protoplast formation had led to the results suggesting a membrane location.

The mechanism involved in the ring-expansion reaction is still unknown. Apparently the intermediate formation of β-sulfoxides or β-acetoxymethyl-penicillin N does not occur (BALDWIN et al. 1980a). Also 7-β(5D-aminoadipo)-3β-hydroxy-3α-methyl-cepham-4-carboxylic acid, which has been isolated from broths of *C. acremonium*, is not an intermediate. Likewise, 7β-(5D-aminoadipamido)-3-exomethylene cepham-4α-carboxylic acid is not involved in the conversion (MILLER et al. 1981; BALDWIN et al. 1981a) although it does inhibit the reaction.

Deacetoxycephalosporin C is hydroxylated to deacetylcephalosporin C by an α-ketoglutarate-linked dioxygenase (LIERSCH et al. 1976; FUJISAWA et al. 1977; BREWER et al. 1977b). Mutants have been isolated from a deacetylcephalosporin C producer which produce only deacetoxycephalosporin C (FUJISAWA et al. 1975a). Such mutants lack the dioxygenase activity (LIERSCH et al. 1976). The enzymatic conversion, catalyzed by cell-free extracts from *C. acremonium* and *S. clavuligerus* (TURNER et al. 1978), is optimal near pH 7.0; α-ketoglutarate, ascorbate, dithiothreitol and Fe^{2+} stimulate the reaction. The enzyme catalyzes incorporation of oxygen from molecular oxygen into deacetylcephalosporin C (TURNER et al. 1978; STEVENS et al. 1975). The in vitro lability of the dioxygenase is presumably the reason that the cell-free conversion of penicillin N stops at the deacetoxycephalosporin C stage.

The role of deacetylcephalosporin C as a precursor of cephalosporin C was further supported by the isolation of cephalosporin C nonproducing mutants which form deacetylcephalosporin C as their sole extracellular antibiotic (FUJISAWA et al. 1973, 1975b). These mutants lack acetyl CoA; deacetylcephalosporin C acetyltransferase (FUJISAWA et al. 1973; FUJISAWA and KANZAKI 1975; LIERSCH et al. 1976). This enzymatic conversion of deacetylcephalosporin C to cephalosporin C is the terminal reaction in cephalosporin-producing fungi.

V. Formation of Additional Cephalosporins by Actinomycetes

Although the fungi stop at cephalosporin C, the actinomycetes can convert both cephalosporin C and deacetylcephalosporin to additional cephalosporins including cephamycins (i.e., 7-methoxy cephalosporins) as shown in Fig. 6.

In the actinomycete cephalosporins, the side chain attached to the C-3′ methyl is acetoxy, carbamoyl or some other group. In *S. clavuligerus*, O-carbamoyl transferase is responsible for catalyzing transfer of a carbamyol group from carbamoyl phosphate to deacetyl-7-α-methoxycephalosporin C forming cephamycin C (BREWER et al. 1977a, 1980).

Fig. 6. The latter part of the hydrophilic branch in actinomycetes. This is a composite scheme in which parts are present in the different strains. *Solid arrows* indicate that the reaction has been observed in cell-free extracts. *Dashed lines* are hypothetical. All the compounds shown have been detected in one actinomycete or another. *SAM*, *S*-adenosylemethionine. (Modified from DEMAIN 1981)

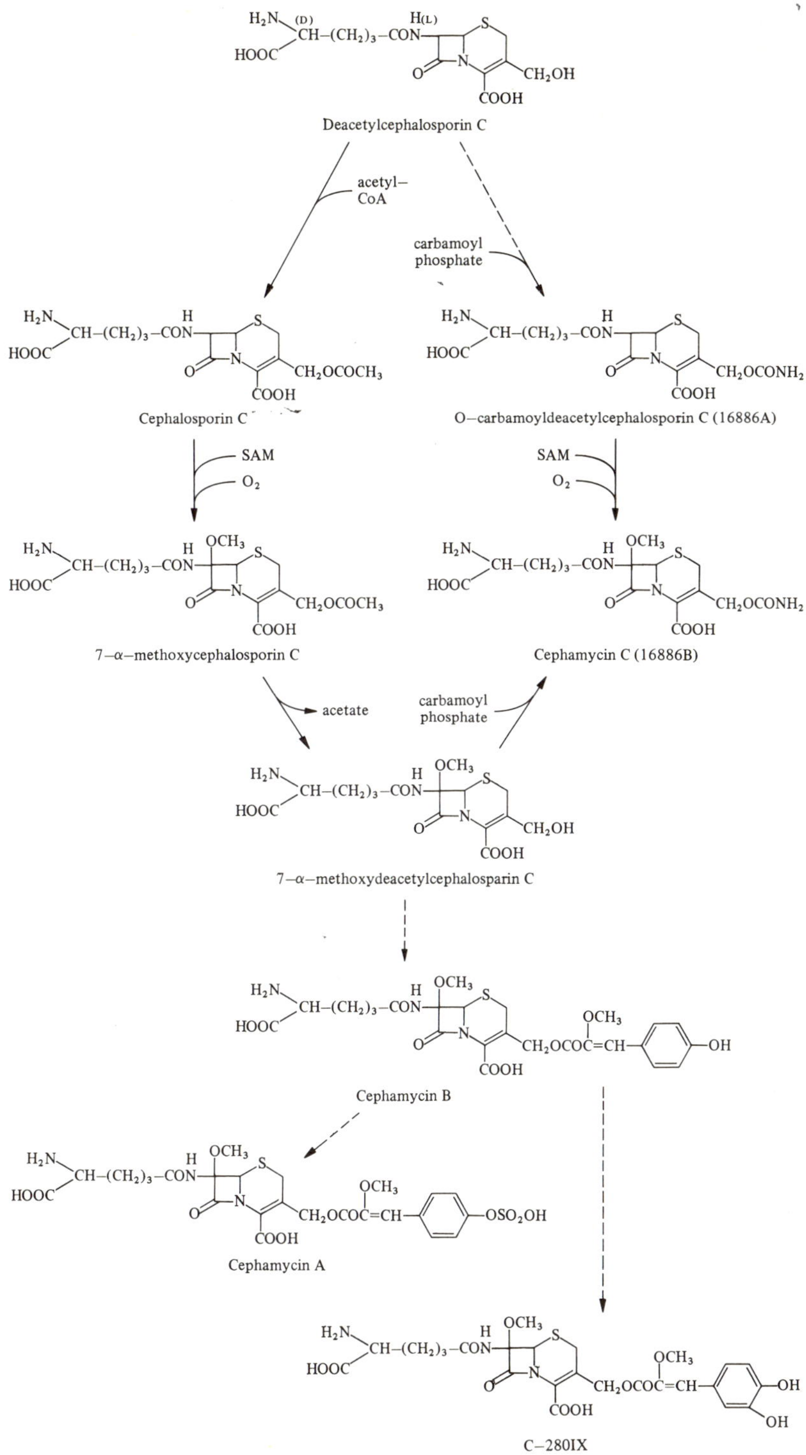
Deacetylcephalosporin C
acetyl–CoA
carbamoyl phosphate
Cephalosporin C
O–carbamoyldeacetylcephalosporin C (16886A)
SAM
O2
7–α–methoxycephalosporin C
Cephamycin C (16886B)
acetate
7–α–methoxydeacetylcephalosparin C
Cephamycin B
Cephamycin A
C–2801X

The 7-methoxy group of the cephamycins comes from methionine (WHITNEY et al. 1972) and molecular oxygen (O'SULLIVAN et al. 1979 b). Cell-free extracts of *S. clavuligerus* convert cephalosporin C and O-carbamoyldeacetylcephalosporin C into-α-methoxy derivatives in the presence of *S*-adenosylmethionine, α-ketoglutarate, Fe^{2+} and a reducing agent such as ascorbate (O'SULLIVAN and ABRAHAM 1980). The system, which apparently contains a dioxygenase and a methyltransferase, failed to methoxylate deacetylcephalosporin C and acted only slightly on deacetoxycephalosporin C. This indicates that the 7-α-methoxy group is introduced only after the complete cephalosporin molecule, including the side chain linked to C-3, is formed.

D. Antibiotic Production by Pairs of Blocked Mutants

A major problem in studying β-lactam biosynthesis has been the inability to obtain antibiotic production by mixed cultures of blocked mutants. For example, LEMKE and NASH (1972) obtained four *C. acremonium* mutants blocked at the tripeptide stage and two mutants blocked in tripeptide formation but when pairs were grown together, no antibiotics were produced. Only when a heterokaryon was prepared between the two classes of mutants was penicillin N produced (NASH et al. 1974). A breakthrough was recently accomplished by MAKINS et al. 1980). Whereas mixed intact mycelia of different blocked mutant classes of *Aspergillus nidulans* failed to make penicillin, pairs of osmotically fragile mycelia did achieve complementation. The treated mycelia were prepared with lytic enzymes and the production buffer contained polyoxin and 2-deoxyglucose to prevent cell-wall regeneration.

E. Novel β-Lactam Antibiotics

A number of novel antibiotics have been discovered with mutants of the organisms described above or with related strains. In addition, completely unrelated microbes have been shown to produce monocyclic β-lactams. These novel antibiotics are described below.

I. Fungal Products

Paecilomyces carneus was found to produce 6-(5-hydroxy-*n*-valeramido)-penicillanic acid (KITANO et al. 1976c) along with penicillin N, deacetoxycephalosporin C, deacetylcephalosporin C, and cephalosporin C. The new compound is evidently produced from penicillin N by an enzyme system liberating CO_2 and NH_3:

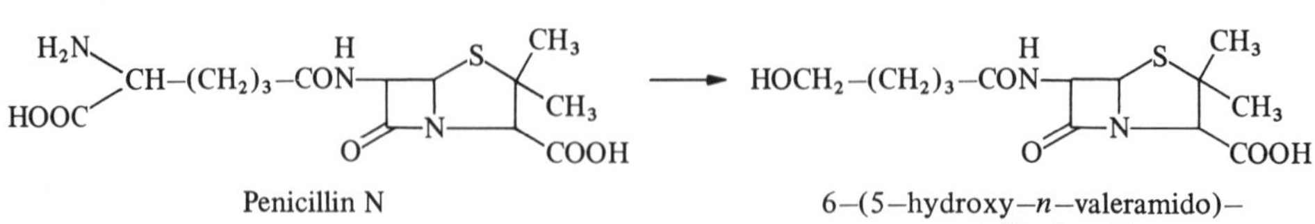

Penicillin N

6-(5-hydroxy-*n*-valeramido)-penicillanic acid

A lysine auxotroph of *C. acremonium*, which cannot form α-aminoadipic acid because of the early block in the lysine biosynthetic pathway, produces 6-(D)-{[(2-amino-2-carboxyl)-ethylthio]-acetamido}-penicillanic acid upon supplementation with the aminoadipic acid analogue, L-*S*-carboxymethylcysteine (TROONEN et al. 1976). This is the only known "biosynthetic" penicillin produced by *Cephalosporium*. Presumably a modified tripeptide is formed which can be converted to an analogue of penicillin N but, because of the specificity of the ring expansion enzyme, cannot be converted to a cephalosporin. The new antibiotic has a sulfur atom replacing CH_2 in penicillin N.

(see formula 1, p. 210)

A mutant of *C. acremonium*, which produces penicillin N and deacetoxycephalosporin C but only a trace of cephalosporin C, was found to accumulate *N*-acetyldeacetoxycephalosporin C (TRAXLER et al. 1975). This compound presumably arises as a shunt metabolite by acetylation of deacetoxycephalosporin C when the normal hydroxylation to deacetylcephalosporin C is blocked:

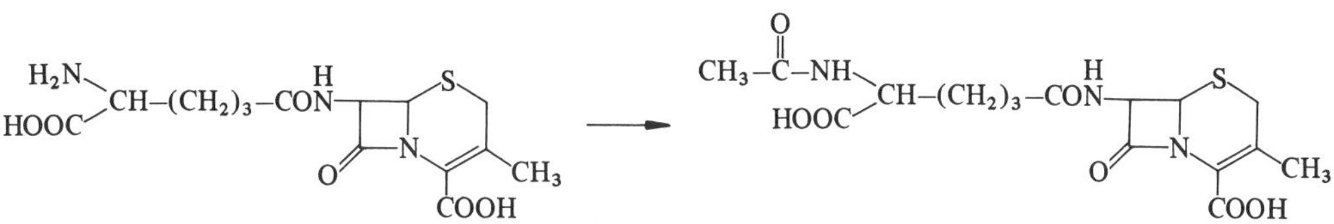

Deacetoxycephalosporin C — *N*-acetyldeacetoxycephalosporin C

Cephalosporium chrysogenum and mutant strains of *Cephalosporium polyaleurum* and *C. acremonium* produce (in addition to cephalosporin C, deacetylcephalosporin C, and deacetoxycephalosporin C) compounds with glutaric acid replacing D-α-aminoadipic acid (KITANO et al. 1976b). These very weak derivatives are probably produced by oxidative deamination (or transamination), followed by decarboxylation, of cephalosporin C and its two preceding biosynthetic intermediates.

(see formula 2, p. 211)

A mutant strain of *C. acremonium* produces the following weakly active modified cephalosporin, which is probably the result of a reaction between deacetylcephalosporin C (or cephalosporin C) and penicillamine (KANSAKI et al. 1976):

(see formula 3, p. 212)

D-Penicillamine is a breakdown product of penicillin N and could accumulate in *Cephalosporium* broths. A related derivative, the 3-methyl-thiomethyl-cephem compound, is produced by another *C. acremonium* mutant (KANZAKI et al. 1974):

(see formula 4, p. 212)

This could arise from deacetylcephalosporin C reacting with methanethiol (methyl mercaptan), a product from methionine produced by the enzyme, methionase (KANZAKI and FUJISAWA 1976).

A mutant blocked in the conversion of deacetylcephalosporin C to cephalosporin C produced a new compound in addition to deacetylcephalosporin C (FU-

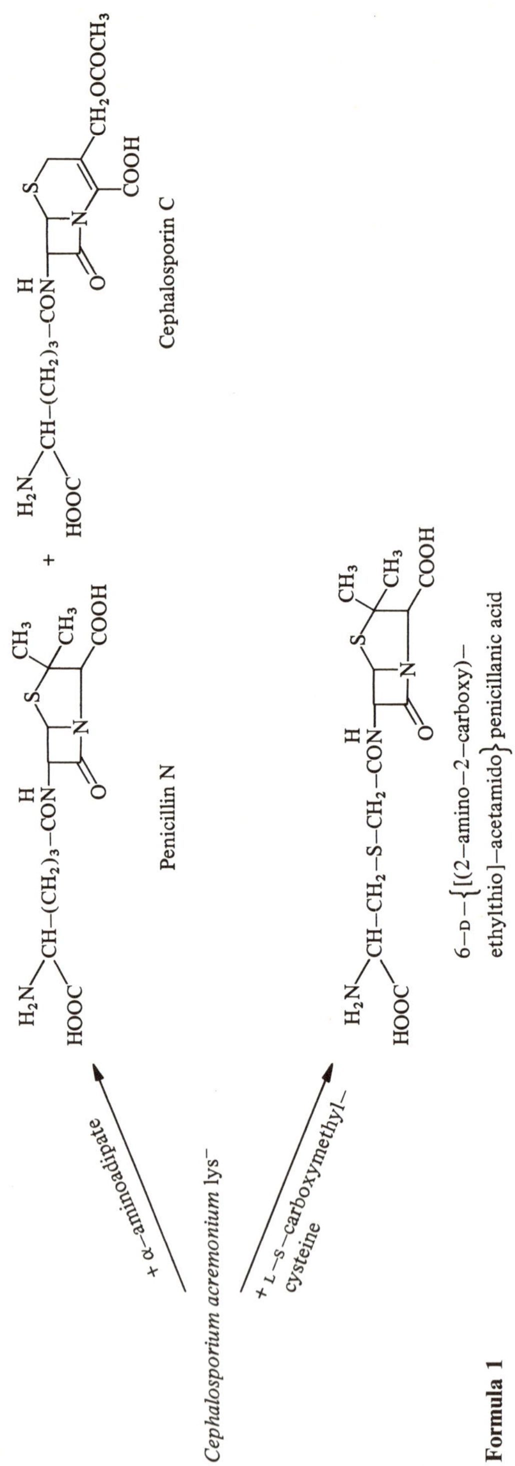
Penicillin N
Cephalosporin C
6–D–{[(2–amino–2–carboxy)–
ethylthio]–acetamido} penicillanic acid
Cephalosporium acremonium lys⁻
+ α–aminoadipate
+ L–S–carboxymethyl–
cysteine

Formula 1

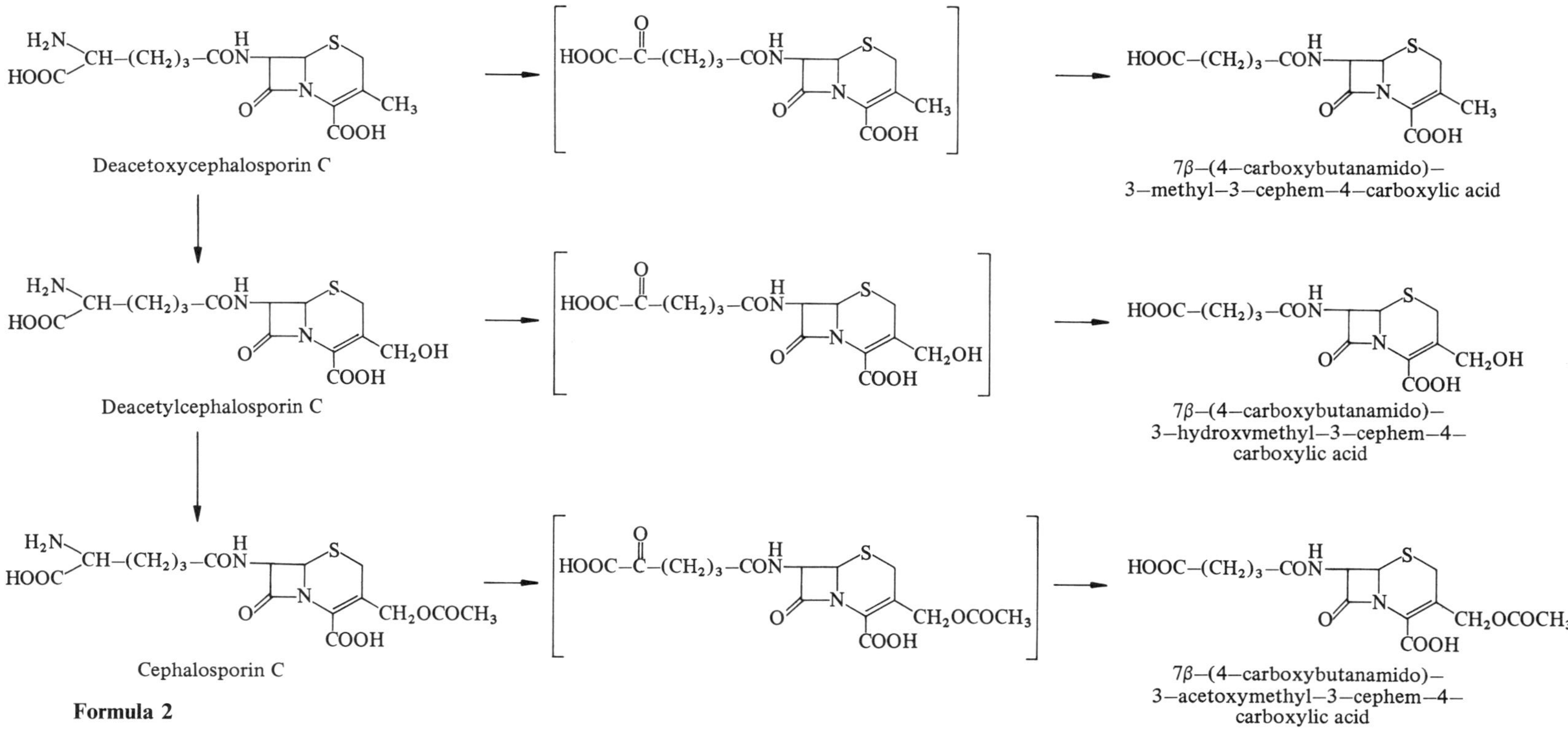
Deacetoxycephalosporin C
Deacetylcephalosporin C
Cephalosporin C
7β–(4–carboxybutanamido)–
3–methyl–3–cephem–4–carboxylic acid
7β–(4–carboxybutanamido)–
3–hydroxvmethyl–3–cephem–4–
carboxylic acid
7β–(4–carboxybutanamido)–
3–acetoxymethyl–3–cephem–4–
carboxylic acid

Formula 2

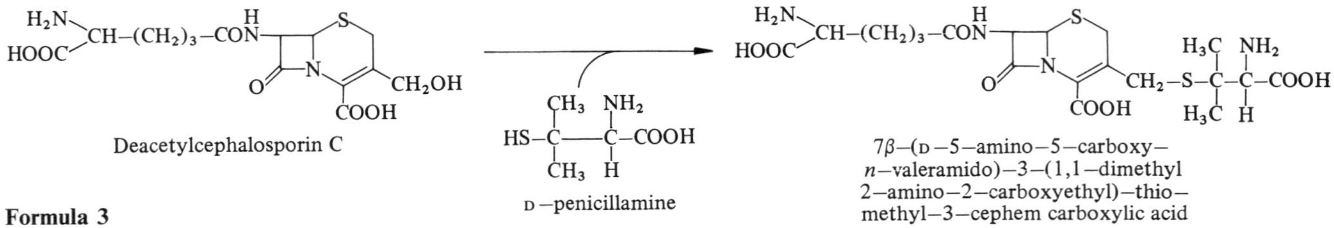

Formula 3

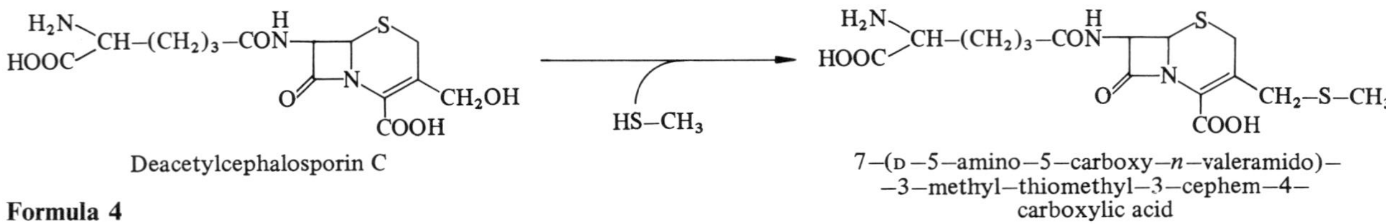

Formula 4

JISAWA and KANZAKI 1975). It is probably formed by an oxidation of the CH_2OH group of the dihydrothiazine ring to the aldehyde followed by opening of the β-lactam ring by a chemical reaction:

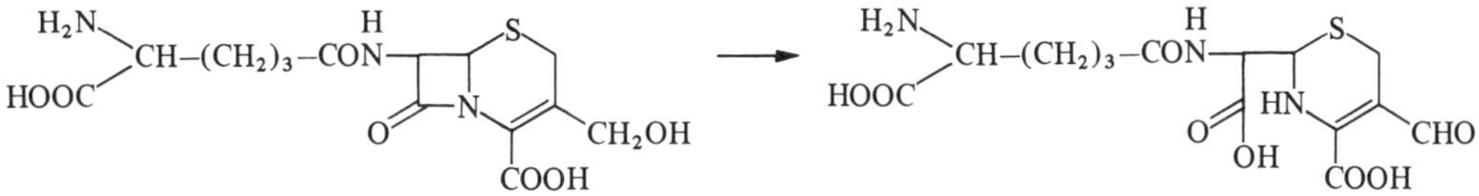

Deacetylcephalosporin C

D-5-amino-5-carboxyvaleramido-(5-formyl-4-carboxy-2H, 3H, 6H-tetrahydro-1, 3-thiazinyl) glycine

II. Actinomycete Products

Cephamycin production by *Streptomyces oganonensis* is susceptible to modification of the side-chain attached to the C-3′ methyl group by directed biosynthesis (OSONO et al. 1980).

In addition to its production of penicillin N and cephalosporins, *S. clavuligerus* produces a weak antibiotic, clavulanic acid, which however is an extremely potent irreversible inhibitor of a broad-spectrum of β-lactamases (HOWARTH et al. 1976; BROWN et al. 1976; READING and COLE 1977):

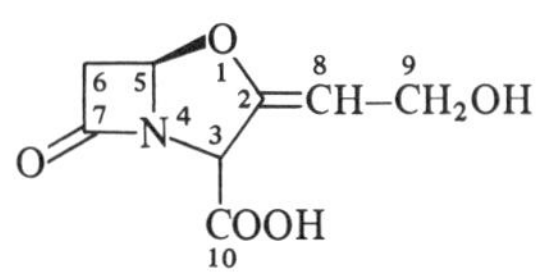

Clavulanic acid

Obvious in this penicillin-like structure is the lack of any side chain at C-6, and oxygen substituting for sulfur in the five-membered ring.

Biosynthetic studies (ELSON and OLIVER 1978; STIRLING and ELSON 1979) using ^{14}C and ^{13}C-labeled precursors indicate that carbons 5, 6, and 7 of the β-lactam ring can come from glycerol or a late intermediate of the TCA cycle, and probably is close to phosphoenolpyruvate. Carbons 9, 8, 2, 3, and 10 of the oxazolidine ring appear to be derived from glutamate:

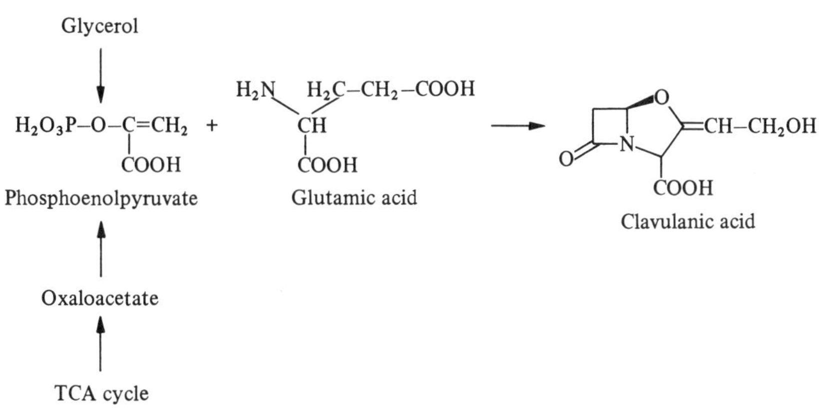

In addition to clavulanic acid, three related structures have been obtained from *S. clavuligerus* (BROWN et al. 1979):

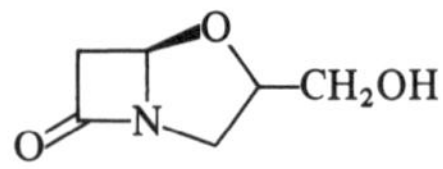

2–hydroxymethylclavan

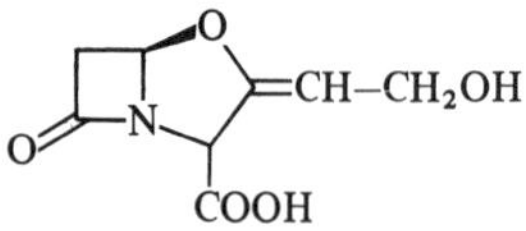

Clavulanic acid

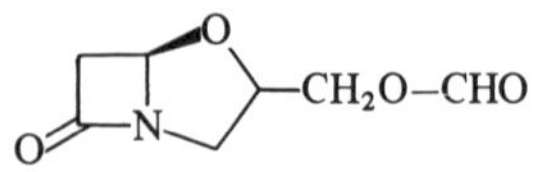

2–formyloxymethylclavan

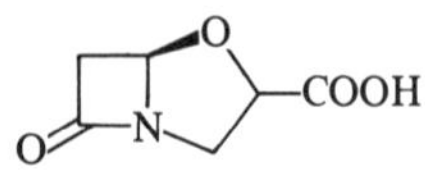

methylclavan –2–carboxylate

Surprisingly these three compounds lack β-lactamase inhibitory activity and antibacterial action but have activity versus fungi, particularly fungal plant pathogens.

Streptomyces cattleya produces a novel β-lactam antibiotic, thienamycin, which contains carbon instead of sulfur in the five-membered ring (KAHAN et al. 1979):

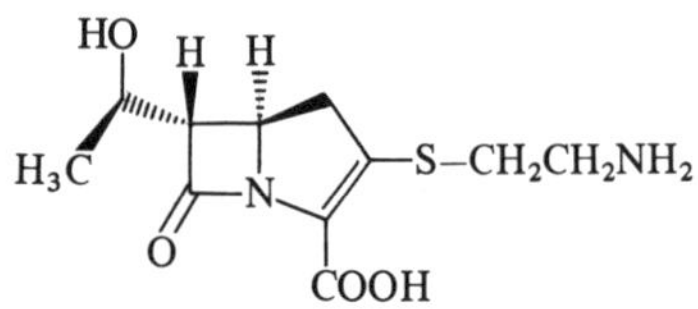

This broad spectrum antibiotic is probably the most potent, nontoxic, natural agent ever discovered. Although it is extremely unstable, more stable derivatives have been produced by semisynthesis. It inhibits cell-wall biosynthesis as do the penicillins and cephalosporins and is relatively resistant to β-lactamase. ALBERS-SCHÖNBERG et al. (1976) reported that the ring system is derived from acetate and glutamate. Glutamate apparently is the precursor of the five-carbon ring while acetate supplies C6-7.

The discovery of thienamycin led the way to an "explosion" of new antibiotic discoveries. These compounds are grouped under the name of carbapenems and have various degrees of activity as broad-spectrum antibiotics and β-lactamase inhibitors.

Included in this group are six epithienamycins produced by *Streptomyces flavogriseus* (STAPLEY et al. 1981; CASSIDY et al. 1981). These are epimeric to thienamycin at at least one of the asymmetric centers and contain other structural modifications.

Closely related to thienamycin is the antibiotic PS-5 produced by *Streptomyces cremeus* subsp. *auratilis* (OKAMURA et al. 1978):

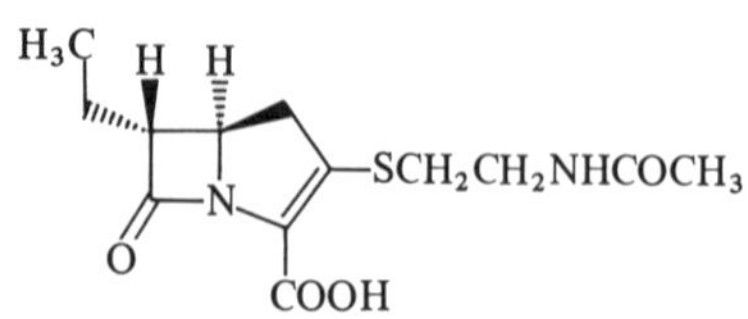

Two mutants of *S. cattleya* produce *N*-acetylthienamycin and dehydroxythienamycin respectively instead of thienamycin (ROSI et al. 1981). This suggests that the terminal reactions in the thienamycin pathway are as follows:

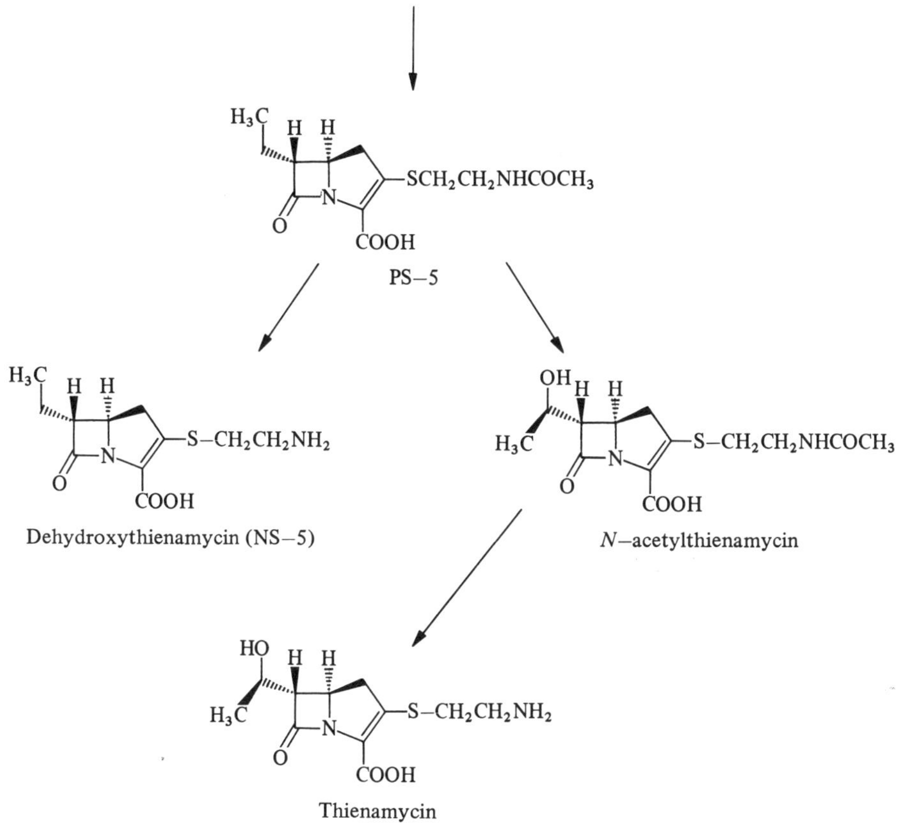

PS-5, as mentioned above, is a product of *S. cremeus* but might be a thienamycin precursor in *S. cattleya*. Dehydroxythienamycin (called NS-5) can also be produced by treating PS-5 with L-aminoacylase from porcine kidney, D-amino acid acylase from *Streptomyces olivaceus*, or cells of *Pseudomonas* sp strain 1158 (FUKAGAWA et al. 1980).

Other related compounds known as olivanic acids are produced by *S. olivaceus* and *Streptomyces fulvoviridis* (BROWN et al. 1977; CORBETT et al. 1977; MAEDA et al. 1977; BOX et al. 1979). Some are identical to epithienamycins (CASSIDY et al. 1981):

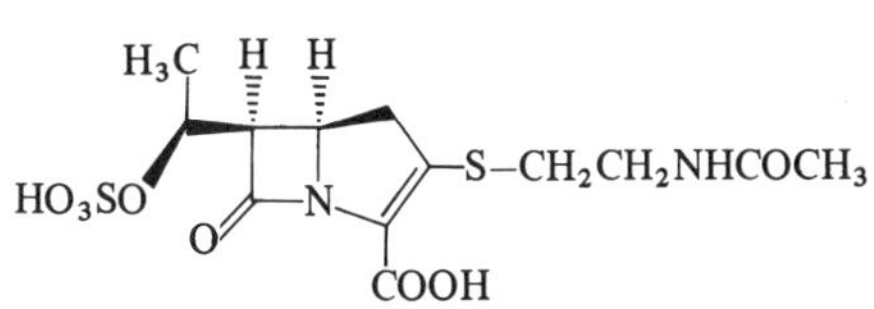

MM17880; epithienamycin F

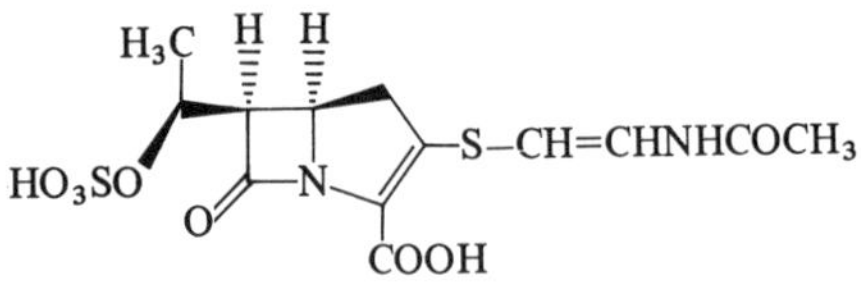

MM13902; epithienamycin E

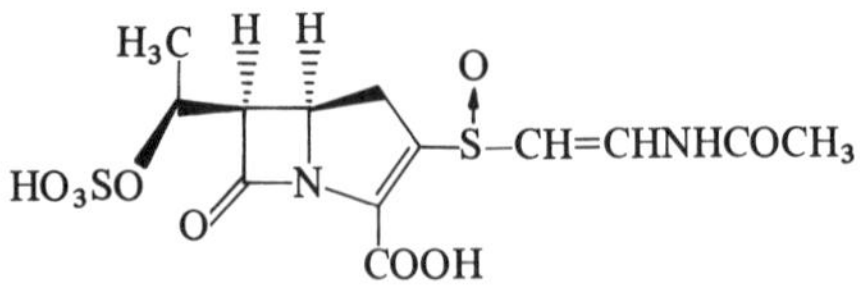

MM4550

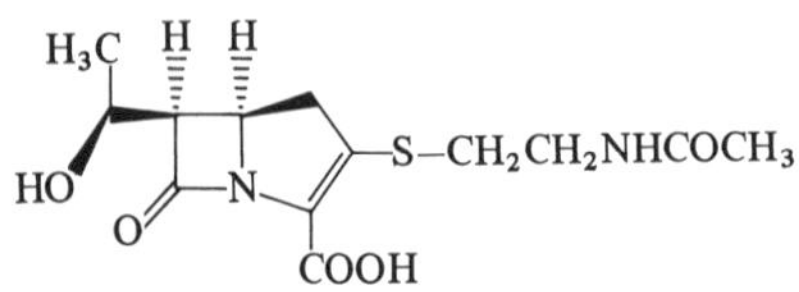

MM22380; epithienamycin A

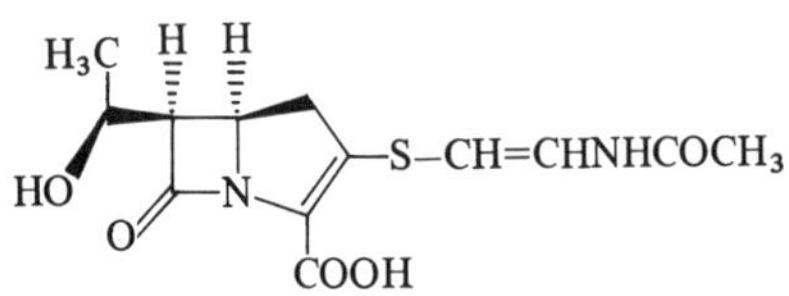

MM22382; epithienamycin B

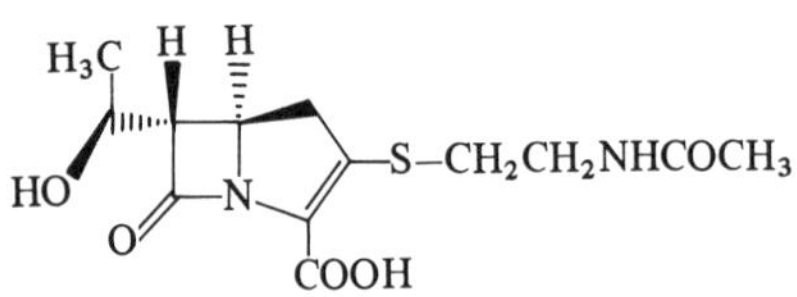

MM22381; epithienamycin C

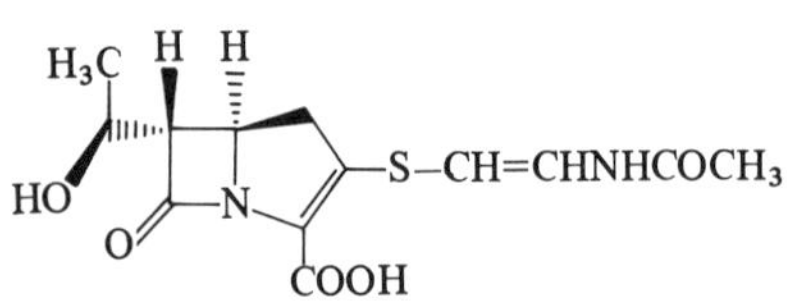

MM22383; epithienamycin D

Dimethyl carbapenems are produced by *Streptomyces griseus* subsp. *cryophilus* (IMADA et al. 1980); they are called C-19393 S_2 and H_2 and are identical to the carpetimycins (NAKAYAMA et al. 1981).

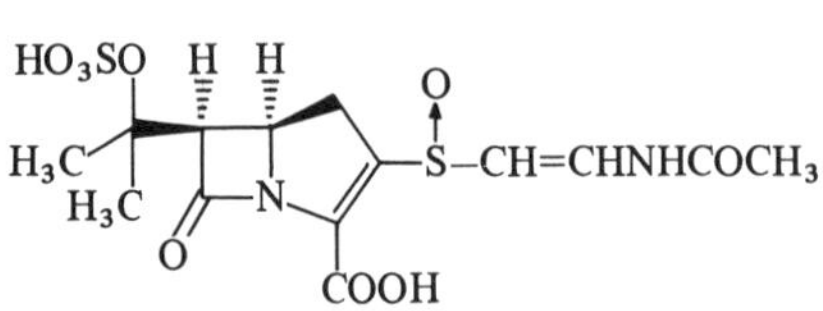

C–19393 S_2; carpetimycin B

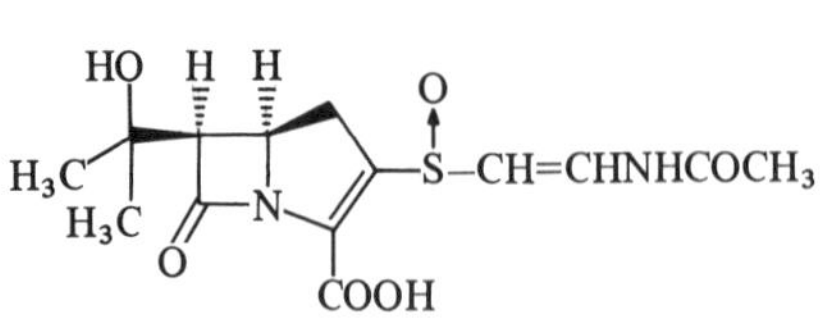

C–19393 H_2; carpetimycin A

Studies using a blocked mutant of *S. olivaceus* (Box et al. 1979) showed that the addition of MM22382 led to the production of MM13902 and MM4550, the addition of MM22380 yielded MM17880, MM13902, and MM4550, and the addition of MM13902 or MM17880 led to no detectable product. As a result the authors postulated the following biosynthetic sequence:

(see formula 5, p. 218)

A series of very different β-lactam antibiotics, called nocardicins, are produced by *Nocardia uniformis* subsp. *tsuyamanensis* (Aoki et al. 1976; Hashimoto et al. 1976; Hosada et al. 1977a). Nocardicin A is a unique β-lactam compound because of its monocyclic structure, good activity against gram-negative bacteria and poor gram-positive activity, much better in vivo than in vitro activity, and its stability to acid, base and β-lactamase. As expected from β-lactam antibiotics, nocardicin A inhibits cell-wall formation and is relatively nontoxic.

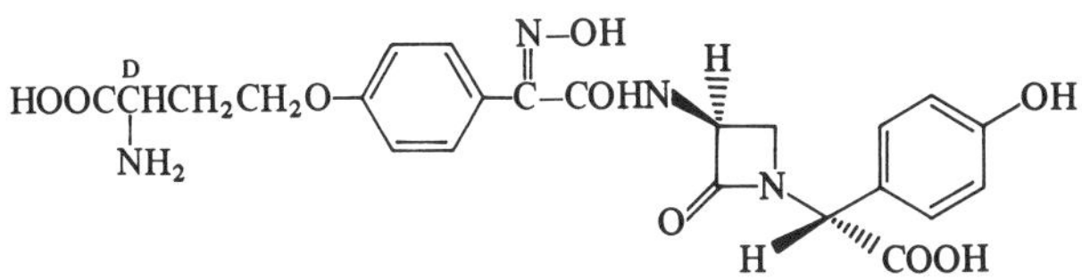

At present, seven natural nocardicins are known (A through G) but only A has a high degree of antibacterial activity. Biosynthetic studies using ^{14}C-amino acids revealed the incorporation of radioactivity from uniformly labeled L-tyrosine, L-serine, glycine, and L-homoserine (Hosada et al. 1977b). In addition, L-tyrosine, *p*-hydroxyphenylpyruvic acid, DL-*p*-hydroxymandelic acid and L-*p*-hydroxyphenylglycine stimulated antibiotic production. From these observations, Hosada et al. (1977b) have proposed the following biosynthetic pathway:

(see formula 6, p. 219)

III. Products of Unicellular Bacteria

Recently two new species of *Pseudomonas (acidophila* and *mesoacidophila)* were found to produce different novel monocyclic β-lactam antibiotics (Imada et al. 1981). These are sulfazecin and isosulfazecin. The structure of sulfazecin contains D-glutamate in unit A and D-alanine in unit B. In

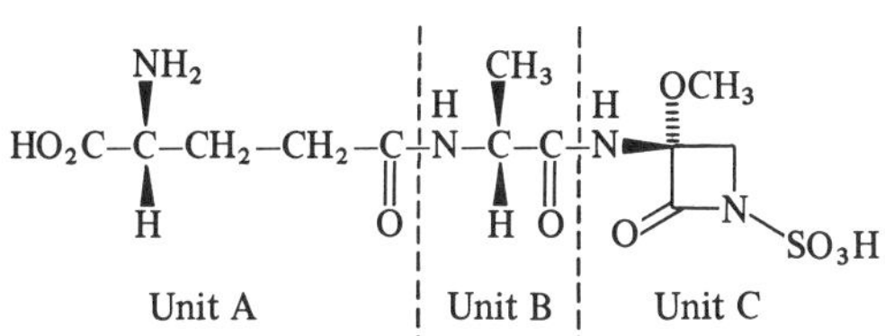

isosulfazecin, L-alanine replaces D-alanine. The antibiotics were detected using β-lactam-supersensitive mutants of *P. aeruginosa* and *E. coli*. Independently, another group (Sykes et al. 1981) isolated seven similar compounds from strains of *Aceto-*

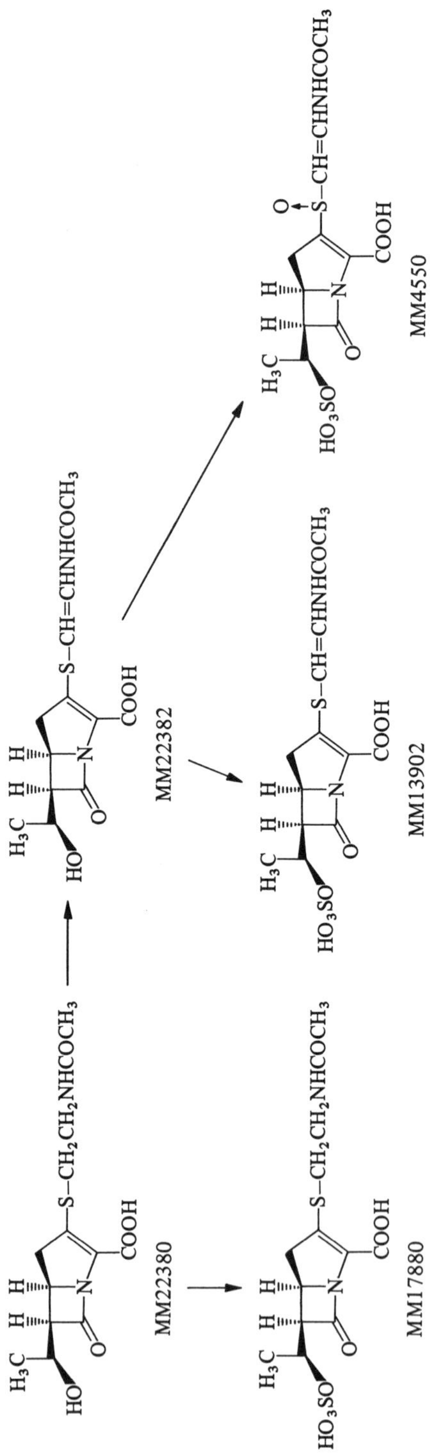
MM22380
MM17880
MM22382
MM13902
MM4550
S–CH2CH2NHCOCH3
S–CH=CHNHCOCH3
COOH
HO3SO
H3C

Formula 5

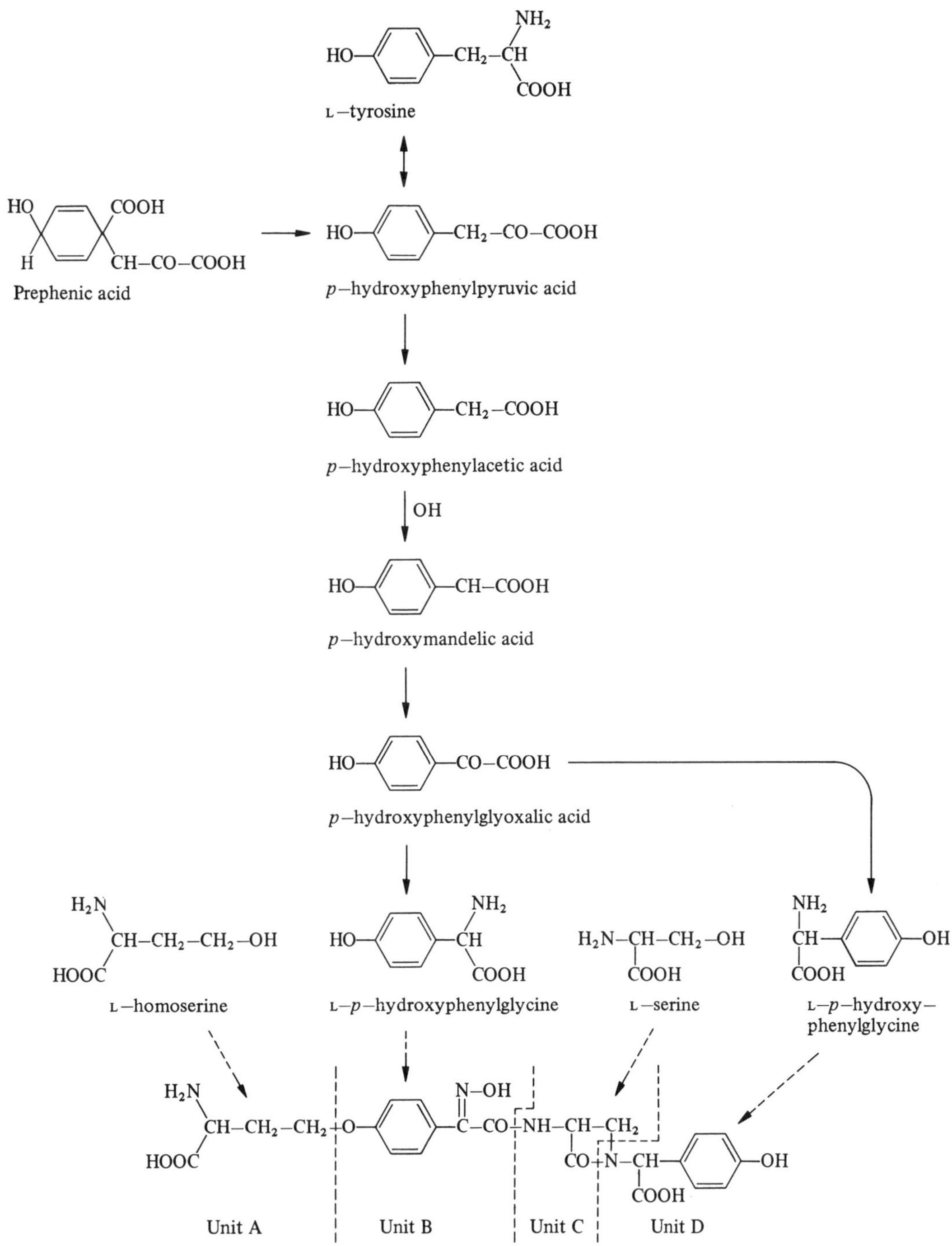

Formula 6 Nocardicin A

bacter sp, *Chromobacterium violaceum* and *Agrobacterium radiobacter*. In addition to sulfazecin produced by *Acetobacter* sp., the following were isolated:

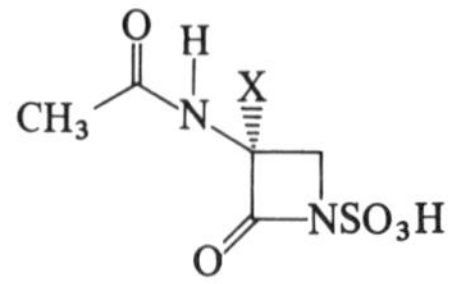

(from *C. violaceum*)

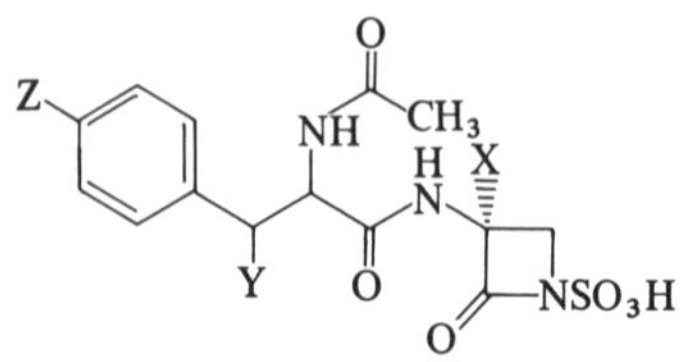

(from *A. radiobacter*)

where X is H or OCH_3, Y is H, OH or OSO_3, and Z is H, OH or OSO_3H.

The entire group has been named monobactams.

Production of monobactams appears to involve serine as the source of the carbon atoms of the β-lactam ring and methionine as the source of the methoxy group (Imada, personal communication, O'SULLIVAN et al. 1982).

Acknowledgments. This work was supported by NIH grant A1-16640 and by NSF grant DAR 79-19493.

References

Aberhart DJ, Chu JY-R, Neuss N, Nash CH, Occolowitz J, Huckstep LL, De La Higuera N (1974) Retention of valine methyl hydrogens in penicillin biosynthesis. J Chem Soc Chem Commun:564–565

Aberhart DJ, Lin LJ (1974) Studies on the biosynthesis of β-lactam antibiotics. 1. Stereospecific synthesis of *(2RS,3S)*-[4,4,4-$^2H_3$]-, *(2RS,3S)*-[4-^{3}H]-, *(2RS,3R)*-[4-^{3}H]-, and *(2RS,3S)*-[4-^{13}C]-valine. Incorporation of *(2RS,3S)*-[4-^{13}C]-valine into penicillin V. J Chem Soc Perkin Trans 1:2320–2326

Abraham EP (1974) Biosynthesis and enzymic hydrolysis of penicillins and cephalosporins. University of Tokyo Press, Tokyo

Abraham EP (1977) β-Lactam antibiotics and related substances. Jpn J Antibiot 30:S1-S25

Abraham EP, Huddleston JA, Jayatilake GS, O'Sullivan J, White RL (1980) Conversion of δ-(L-α-aminoadipyl(-L-cysteinyl-D-valine to isopenicillin N in cell-free extracts of *Cephalosporium acremonium*. In: Gregory GI (ed) Recent advances in the chemistry of β-lactam antibiotics. Royal Society of Chemistry, London, pp 125–134

Abraham EP, Newton GGF (1961) The structure of cephalosporin C. Biochem J 79:377–393

Abraham EP, Newton GGF, Warren SC (1965) Problems relating to the biosynthesis of peptide antibiotics. In: Vanek Z, Hostalek Z (eds) Biogenesis of antibiotic substances. Czech Acad Science, Prague, pp 169–194

Adriaens P, Meesschaert B, Wuyts W, Vanderhaeghe H, Eyssen H (1975) Presence of δ-(L-α-aminoadipyl)-L-cysteinyl-D-valine in fermentations of *Penicillium chrysogenum*. Antimicrob Agents Chemother 8:638–642

Albers-Schönberg G, Arison BH, Kaczka E, Kahan FM, Kahan JS, Lago B, Maise WM, Rhodes RE, Smith JL (1976) Thienamycin. A new β-lactam antibiotic. 3. Structure determination and biosynthetic data. Abstract 229, 16th Intersci Conf Antimicrob Ag Chemother, Chicago

Aoki H, Sakai H-I, Kohsaka M, Konomi T, Hosoda J, Kubochi Y, Iguchi E, Imanaka H (1976) Nocardicin A, a new monocyclic β-lactam antibiotic. 1. Discovery, isolation and characterization. J Antibiot (Tokyo) 29:492–500

Arnstein HRV, Clubb ME (1957) The biosynthesis of penicillin. Comparison of valine and hydroxyvaline as penicillin precursors. Biochem J 65:618–627

Arnstein HRV, Crawhall JC (1957) The biosynthesis of penicillin. 6. A study of the mechanism of the formation of the thiazolidine-β-lactam rings, using tritium-labelled cystine. Biochem J 67:180–187

Arnstein HRV, Grant PT (1954a) The biosynthesis of penicillin. The incorporation of cystine into penicillin. Biochem J 57:360–368

Arnstein HRV, Grant PT (1954b) The biosynthesis of penicillin. The incorporation of some amino acids into penicillin. Biochem J 57:353–359

Arnstein HRV, Margreiter H (1958) The biosynthesis of penicillin. 7. Further experiments on the utilization of L- and D-valine and the effect of cysteine and valine analogues on penicillin biosynthesis. Biochem J 68:339–348

Arnstein HRV, Morris D (1960) The structure of a peptide, containing α-aminoadipic acid, cysteine, and valine, present in the mycelium of *Penicillium chrysogenum*. Biochem J 76:357–361

Arnstein HRV, Artman N, Morris D, Toms EJ (1960) Sulfur-containing amino acids and peptides in the mycelium of *Penicillium* chrysogenum. Biochem J 76:353–357

Avanzini F, Valenti P (1980) Peptide presence constituted by α-aminoadipic acid (α-AAA) and valine in *P. chrysogenum* fermentation broth. Abstracts 6th international ferm symp, London, Ontario, 20–25 July 1980, p 18

Bahadur G, Baldwin JE, Field LD, Lehtonen EMM, Usher JJ, Vallijo CA, Abraham EP, White RL (1981) Direct ^{1}H N.M.R. observation of the cell-free conversion of δ-(L-α-aminoadipyl)-L-cysteinyl-D-valine and δ-(L-α-aminoadipyl)-L-cysteinyl-D-(−)-isoleucine into penicillins. J Chem Soc Chem Commun 917–919

Baldwin JE, Wan TS (1979) Penicillin biosynthesis: a model for carbon and sulphur bond formation. J Chem Soc Chem Commun 249–250

Baldwin JE, Wan TS (1981) Penicillin biosynthesis. Retention of configuration at C-3 of valine during its incorporation into the Arnstein tripeptide. Tetrahedron 37:1589–1595

Baldwin JE, Lolliger J, Rastetter W, Neuss N, Huckstep LC, De La Higuera N (1973) Use of chiral isopropyl groups in biosynthesis. Synthesis of *(2RS,3R)*)-[4-^{13}C] valine. J Am Chem Soc 95:3796–3797

Baldwin JE, Jung M, Singh P, Wan T, Haber S, Herchen S, Kitchin J, Demain AL, Hunt NA, Kohsaka M, Konomi T, Yoshida M (1980a) Recent biosynthetic studies on β-lactam antibiotics. Philos Trans R Soc Lond B Biol Sci 298:169–172

Baldwin JE, Johnson BL, Usher JJ, Abraham EP, Huddleston JA, White RL (1980b) Direct N.M.R. observation of cell-free conversion of (L-α-amino-δ-adipyl)-L-cysteinyl-D-valine into isopenicillin N. J Chem Soc Chem Commun 1271–1273

Baldwin JE, Chakravarti B, Jung M, Patel NJ, Singh PD, Usher JJ, Vallejo C (1981a) On the possible role of the 3-methylene isomer of deacetoxycephalosporin C in the biosynthesis of cephalosporin. J Chem Soc Chem Commun 934–936

Baldwin JE, Keeping JW, Singh PD, Vallejo CA (1981b) Cell-free conversion of isopenicillin N into deacetoxycephalosporin C by *Cephalosporium acremonium* mutant M-0198. Biochem J 194:649–651

Baldwin JE, Singh PD, Yoshida M, Sawada, Demain AL (1980c) Incorporation of ^{3}H and ^{14}C from [6α-^{3}H] penicillin N into deacetoxycephalosporin C. Biochem J 186:889–895

Batchelor FR, Doyle FP, Nayler JHC, Rolinson GN (1959) Synthesis of penicillin: 6-aminopenicillanic acid in penicillin fermentations. Nature 183:257–258

Bauer K (1970) Zur Biosynthese der Penicilline: Bildung von 5-(2-Aminoadipyl)-cysteinyl-valin in Extrakten von *Penicillium chrysogenum*. Z Naturforsch [B] 25:1125–1129

Behrens OK, Corse J, Jones RG, Kleinderer EC, Soper QF, Van Abelle FR, Larson LM, Sylvester JC, Haines WJ, Carter HE (1948) Biosynthesis of penicillins. 2. Utilization of deuterophenylacetyl-N^{15}-DL-valine in penicillin biosynthesis. J Biol Chem 175:756–769

Booth H, Bycroft BW, Wels CM, Corbett K, Maloney AP (1976) Application of ^{15}N pulsed Fourier transformation nuclear magnetic resonance spectroscopy to biosynthetic studies; incorporation of L-[^{15}N]-valine into penicillin G. J Chem Soc Chem Commun 110–111

Bost PE, Demain AL (1977) Studies on the cell-free biosynthesis of β-lactam antibiotics. Biochem J 162:681–687

Box SJ, Hood JD, Spear SR (1979) Four further antibiotics related to olivanic acid produced by *Streptomyces olivaceus:* fermentation, isolation, characterization, and biosynthetic studies. J Antibiot (Tokyo) 32:1239–1247

Brewer SJ, Boyle TT, Turner MK (1977a) The carbamoylation of the 3-hydroxymethyl group of 1α-methoxy-7β-(5-δ-aminoadipamido)-3-hydroxymethylceph-3-em-4- carboxylic acid (desacetyl-7-methoxycephalosporin C) by homogenates of *Streptomyces clavuligerus.* Biochem Soc Trans. 5:1026–1029

Brewer SJ, Farthing JE, Turner MK (1977b) The oxygenation of the 3-methyl group of 7-β(5-D-aminoadipamido)-3-methylceph-3-em-4-carboxylic acid (desacetoxycephalosporin C) by extracts of *Acremonium chrysogenum.* Biochem Soc Trans 5:1024–1025

Brewer SJ, Taylor PM, Turner MK (1980) An adenosine triphosphate-dependent carbamoyl-phosphate-3-hydroxymethylcephem *O*-carbamoyl-transferase from *Streptomyces clavuligerus.* Biochem J 185:555–564

Brown AG, Butterworth D, Cole M, Hanscomb G, Hood JD, Reading C, Rolinson GN (1976) Naturally occurring β-lactamase inhibitors with antibacterial activity. J Antibiot (Tokyo) 29:668–669

Brown AG, Corbett DF, Eglington AJ, Howarth TT (1977) Structures of olivanic acid derivatives MM4450 and MM1392; two new, fused β-lactams isolated from *Streptomyces olivaceus.* J Chem Soc Chem Commun 523–525

Brown D, Evans JR, Fletton RA (1979) Structures of three novel β-lactams isolated from *Streptomyces clavuligerus.* J Chem Soc Chem Commun 282–283

Brundidge SP, Gaeta FCA, Hook DJ, Sapino C Jr, Elander RP, Morin RB (1980) Association of 6-oxo-piperidine-2-carboxylic acid with penicillin V production in *Penicillium chrysogenum* fermentations. J Antibiot (Tokyo) 33:1348–1351

Brunner R, Roehr M, Zinner M (1968) Zur Biosynthese des Penicillins. Hoppe-Seyler's Z Physiol Chem 349:95–103

Bycroft BS, Wels CM, Corbett K, Lowe DA (1975) Incorporation of [α-^{2}H] and [α-^{3}H]-L-cystine into penicillin G and the location of the label using isotope exchange and ^{3}H nuclear magnetic resonance. J Chem Soc Chem Commun 123

Carver D, Godfrey OW (1974) Isolation of a mutant blocked in lysine catabolism and its effect on antibiotic synthesis in *Streptomyces lipmanii.* Annual meeting of the american society of microbiology [Abstr], 12–17 May 1974, Chicago, p 19

Cassidy PJ (1981) Novel naturally occurring β-lactam antibiotics – a review. Dev Ind Microbiol 22:181–209

Cassidy PG, Albers-Schonberg G, Goegelman RT, Miller T, Arison B, Stapley EO, Bernbaum J (1981) Epithienamycins. 2. Isolation and structure assignment. J Antibiot (Tokyo) 34:637–648

Chan JA, Huang F-C, Sih CJ (1976) The absolute configuration of the amino acids in δ-(α-aminoadipyl)-cysteinylvaline from *Penicillium chrysogenum.* Biochemistry 15:177–180

Claridge CA, Luttinger RJ, Lein J (1963) Specificity of penicillin amidases. Proc Soc Exp Biol Med 113:1008–1012

Cole M (1966) Formation of 6-aminopenicillanic acid, penicillins, and penicillin acylase by various fungi. Appl Microbiol 14:98–104

Cole M, Batchelor FR (1963) Aminoadipylpenicillin in penicillin fermentations. Nature 198:383–384

Cole M, Rolinson GN (1961) 6-Aminopenicillanic acid. 2. Formation of 6-aminopenicillanic acid by *Emericellopsis minima* (Stolk) and related fungi. Proc R Soc Lond B Biol Sci 154:490–497

Corbett DF, Eglington AJ, Howarth TT (1977) Structure elucidation of MM17880, a new fused β-lactam antibiotic isolated from *Streptomyces olivaceus;* a mild β-lactam degradation reaction. J Chem Soc Chem Commun 953–954
Craig JT, Tindall JB, Senkus M (1951) Determination of penicillin by using C^{13} isotope as a tracer. Anal Chem 23:332–333
D'Amato RF, Pisano MA (1976) A chemically defined medium for cephalosporin C production by *Paecilomyces persicinus.* Antonie Van Leeunwenhoek J Microbiol Serol 42:299–308
Demain AL (1956) Inhibition of penicillin formation by amino acid analogs. Arch Biochem Biophys 64:74–79
Demain AL (1957) Inhibition of penicillin formation by lysine. Arch Biochem Biophys 67:244–246
Demain AL (1959) The mechanism of penicillin biosynthesis. Adv Appl Microbiol 1:23–47
Demain AL (1963) L-Valine: a precursor of cephalosporin C. Biochem Biophys Res Commun 10:45–48
Demain AL (1974) Biochemistry of penicillin and cephalosporin fermentations. Lloydia 37:147–167
Demain AL (1981) Biosynthetic manipulations in the development of β-lactam antibiotics. In: Salton MRJ, Shockman GD (eds) β-lactam antibiotics: mode of action, new developments and future prospects. Academic Press, New York, pp 567–583
Dennen DW, Allen CC, Carver DD (1971) Arylamidase of *Cephalosporium acremonium* and its specificity for cephalosporin C. Appl Microbiol 21:907–915
Duncan M, Newton GGF (1970) Preparation and some properties of protoplasts from *Cephalosporium* sp. Acta Fac Med Univ Brun 37:129–136
Elson SW, Oliver RS (1978) Studies on the biosynthesis of clavulanic acid. Incorporation of ^{13}C-labelled precursors. J Antibiot (Tokyo) 31:586–592
Erickson RC, Bennet RE (1965) Penicillin acylase activity of *Penicillium chrysogenum.* Appl Microbiol 13:738–742
Enriquez LA, Pisano MA (1979) Isolation and nature of intracellular alpha-aminoadipic acid-containing peptides from *Paecilomyces persicinus* P-10. Antimicrob Agents Chemother 16:392–397
Fawcett PA, Usher JJ, Abraham EP (1975) Behavior of tritium-labelled isopenicillin N and 6-aminopenicillanic acid as potential penicillin precursors in an extract of *Penicillium chrysogenum.* Biochem J 151:741–746
Fawcett PA, Usher JJ, Abraham EP (1976a) Aspects of cephalosporin and penicillin biosynthesis. In: Macdonald KD (ed) Second international symposium on the genetics of industrial microorganisms. Academic Press, New York, pp 129–138
Fawcett PA, Usher JJ, Huddleston JA, Bleaney RC, Nisbet JJ, Abraham EP (1976b) Synthesis of δ-(α-aminoadipyl)cysteinylvaline and its role in penicillin biosynthesis. Biochem J 157:651–660
Felix HR, Peter HH, Treichler HJ (1981) Microbiological ring expansion of penicillin N. J Antibiot (Tokyo) 34:567–575
Fleming A (1929) On the antibacterial action of a *Penicillium,* with special reference to their use in the isolation of *B. influenzae.* Br J Exp Pathol 10:226–236
Florey HW, Chain EB, Heatley NG, Jennings MA, Sanders AG, Abraham EP, Florey ME (1949) Antibiotics, vol 2. Oxford University Press, London
Flynn EH, McCormick MH, Stamper MC, DeValeria H, Godzeski CW (1962) A new natural penicillin from *Penicillium chrysogenum.* J Am Chem Soc 84:4594–4595
Friedrich CG, Demain AL (1978) Uptake and metabolism of α-aminoadipic acid by *Penicillium chrysogenum.* Wis 54-1255. Arch Microbiol 119:43–47
Fujisawa Y, Kanzaki T (1975a) Occurrence of a new cephalosporin in a culture broth of a *Cephalosporium acremonium* mutant. J Antibiot (Tokyo) 28:372–378
Fujisawa Y, Kanzaki T (1975b) Role of acetyl CoA: deacetylcephalosporin C acetyltransferase in cephalosporin C biosynthesis by *Cephalosporin acremonium.* Agric Biol Chem 39:2043–2048
Fujisawa Y, Shirafuji H, Kida M, Nara K, Yoneda M, Kanzaki T (1973) New findings on cephalosporin C biosynthesis. Nature New Biol 246:154–155

Fujisawa Y, Kitano T, Kanyaki T (1975 a) Accumulation of deacetoxycephalosporin C by a deacetylcephalosporin C negative mutant of *Cephalosporium acremonium*. Agric Biol Chem 39:2049–2055

Fujisawa Y, Shirafuji H, Kida M, Nara K, Yoneda M, Kanzaki T (1975 b) Accumulation of deacetylcephalosporin C by cephalosporin C negative mutants of *Cephalosporium acremonium*. Agric Biol Chem 39:1295–1301

Fujisawa Y, Kikuchi M, Kanzaki T (1977) Deacetylcephalosporin C synthesis by cell-free extracts of *Cephalosporium acremonium*. J Antibiot (Tokyo) 30:775–777

Fukagawa Y, Kubo K, Ishikura T, Kuono K (1980) Deacetylation of PS-5, a new β-lactam compound. 1. Microbial deacetylation of PS-5. J Antibiot (Tokyo) 33:543–549

Gatenback S, Brunsberg U (1968) Biosynthesis of penicillin. 1. Isolation of 6-aminopenicillanic acid acyltransferase from *Penicillium chrysogenum*. Acta Chem Scand 22:1059–1061

Gordon M, Pan SC, Virgona A, Numerof P (1953) Biosynthesis of penicillin. I. Role of phenylacetic acid. Science 118:43

Goulden SA, Chattaway FW (1968) Lysine control of α-aminoadipate and penicillin synthesis in *Penicillium chrysogenum*. Biochem J 110:55–56

Hale CW, Miller GA, Kelly BK (1953) Hydrophilic penicillins produced by *Penicillium chrysogenum*. Nature 172:545–546

Halliday WJ, Arnstein HRV (1956) The biosynthesis of penicillin. 4. The synthesis of benzylpenicillin by washed mycelium of *Penicillium chrysogenum*. Biochem J 64:380–384

Hashimoto M, Konomi T, Kamiya T (1976) Nocardicin A, a new monocyclic β-lactam antibiotic. 2. Structure determination of nocardicins A and B. J Antibiot (Tokyo) 29:890–901

Higgens CE, Hamil RL, Sands TH, Hoehn MM, Davis NE, Nagarajan R, Boeck LD (1974) The occurrence of deacetoxycephalosporin C in fungi and streptomycetes. J Antibiot (Tokyo) 27:298–300

Hinnen A, Nuesch J (1976) Enzymatic hydrolysis of cephalosporin C by an extracellular acetylhydrolase of *Cephalosporium acremonium*. Antimicrob Agents Chemother 9:824–830

Hook DJ, Chang LT, Elander RP, Morin RB (1979) Stimulation of the conversion of penicillin N to cephalosporin by ascorbic acid, α-ketoglutarate, and ferrous ions in cell-free extracts of strains of *Cephalosporium acremonium*. Biochem Biophys Res Commun 87:258–265

Hosada J, Konomi T, Tani N, Aoki H, Imanaka H (1977 a) Isolation of new nocardicins from *Nocardia uniformis* subsp. *tsuyamanensis*. Agric Biol Chem 41:2013–2020

Hosada J, Tani N, Konomi T, Ohsawa S, Aoki H, Imanaka H (1977 b) Incorporation of ^{14}C-amino acids into nocardicin A by growing cells. Agric Biol Chem 41:2007–2012

Howarth TT, Brown AG, King TJ (1976) Clavulanic acid, a novel β-lactam isolated from *Streptomyces clavuligerus;* X-ray crystal structure analysis. J Chem Soc Chem Commun:266–267

Huang F-C, Chan JA, Sih CJ, Fawcett P, Abraham EP (1975) The nonparticipation of α,β-dehydrovalinyl intermediates in the formation of δ-(L-α-aminoadipyl)-L-cysteinyl-D-valine. J Am Chem Soc 97:3858–3859

Huber FM, Baltz RH, Caltrider PG (1968) Formation of desacetylcephalosporin C in cephalosporin C fermentation. Appl Microbiol 16:1011–1014

Huddleston JA, Abraham EP, Young DW, Morecombe DJ, Sen PK (1978) The stereochemistry of β-lactam formation in cephalosporin biosynthesis. Biochem J 169:705–707

Imada A, Nozaki Y, Kintaka K, Okonogi K, Kitano K, Harada S (1980) C-19393 and H_2, new carbapenem antibiotics. 1. Taxonomy of the producing strain, fermentation, and antibacterial properties. J Antibiot (Tokyo) 33:1417–1424

Imada A, Kitano K, Kintaka K, Muroi A, Asai M (1981) Sulfazecin and isosulfazecin, novel β-lactam antibiotics of bacterial origin. Nature 289:590–591

Inamine E, Birnbaum J (1972) Cephamycin C biosynthesis: isotope incorporation studies. Abstr Annual meeting of the american society of microbiology, 23–28 April 1972, Philadelphia, p 12

Jayatilake S, Huddleston JA, Abraham EP (1981) Conversion of isopenicillin N into penicillin N in cell-free extracts of *Cephalosporium acremonium*. Biochem J 194:645–647

Kahan JS, Kahan FM, Goegelman R, Currie SA, Jackson M, Stapley EO, Miller TW, Miller AK, Hendlin D, Mochales S, Hernandez S, Woodruff HB, Birnbaum J (1979) Thienamycin. A new β-lactam antibiotic. 1. Discovery, taxonomy, isolation, and physical properties. J Antibiot (Tokyo) 32:1–12

Kanzaki T, Fujisawa Y (1976) Biosynthesis of cephalosporin. Adv Appl Microbiol 20:159–201

Kanzaki T, Fukita T, Shirafuji H, Fujisawa Y, Kitano K (1974) Occurrence of a 3-methylthiomethylcephem derivative in a culture broth of *Cephalosporium* mutant. J Antibiot (Tokyo) 27:361–362

Kanzaki T, Fukita T, Kitano K, Katamoto K, Nara K, Nakao Y (1976) Occurrence of a novel cephalosporin compound in the culture broth of a *Cephalosporium acremonium* mutant. J Ferment Technol 54:720–725

Kato K (1953) Occurrence of penicillin-nucleus in culture broths. J Antibiot Ser (Tokyo) 6:130–136

Kern BA, Hendlin D, Inamine E (1980) L-lysine ε-aminotransferase involved in cephamycin C synthesis in *Streptomyces lactamdurans*. Antimicrob Agents Chemother 17:679–685

Kitano K (1977) Studies on the production of β-lactam antibiotics. Ph. D. thesis, Osaka University, Osaka, Japan

Kitano K, Kintaka K, Suzuki S, Katamoto K, Nara K, Nakao Y (1974) Production of cephalosporin antibiotics by strains belonging to the genera *Arachnomyces*, *Anixiopis*, and *Spiroidium*. Agric Biol Chem 38:1761–1762

Kitano K, Kintaka K, Katamoto K, Nara K, Nakao Y (1975a) Occurrence of 6-aminopenicillanic acid in culture broths of strains belonging to the genera *Thermoascus*, *Gymnoscus*, *Polypaecilum*, and *Malbranchea*. J Ferment Technol 53:339–346

Kitano K, Kintaka K, Suzuki S, Katamoto K, Nara K, Nakao Y (1975b) Screening of microorganisms capable of producing β-lactam antibiotics. J Ferment Technol 53:327–338

Kitano K, Kintaka K, Suzuki S, Katamoto K, Nara K, Nakao Y (1976a) Screening of microorganisms capable of producing β-lactam antibiotics from *n*-paraffins. J Ferment Technol 54:683–695

Kitano K, Fujisawa Y, Katamoto K, Nara K, Nakao Y (1976b) Occurrence of 7β-(4-carboxybutanamido)-cephalosporin compounds in the culture broth of some strains of the genus *Cephalosporium*. J Ferment Technol 54:712–719

Kitano K, Kintaka K, Suzuki S, Katamoto K, Nara K, Nakao Y (1976c) A novel penicillin produced by strains of the genus *Paecilomyces*. J Ferment Technol 54:705–711

Kluender H, Bradley CH, Sih CJ, Fawcett P, Abraham EP (1973) Synthesis and incorporation of (2S,3S) [4-^{13}C]-valine into β-lactam antibiotics. J Am Chem Soc 95:6149–6150

Kocecny J, Felber E, Gruner J (1973) Kinetics of the hydrolysis of cephalosporin C. J Antibiot (Tokyo) 26:135–141

Kohsaka M, Demain AL (1976) Conversion of penicillin N to cephalosporin(s) by cell-free extracts of *Cephalosporium acremonium*. Biochem Biophys Res Commun 70:465–473

Konomi T, Herchen S, Baldwin JE, Yoshida M, Hunt NA, Demain AL (1979) Cell-free conversion of δ-(L-α-aminoadipyl)-L-cysteinyl-D-valine to an antibiotic with the properties of isopenicillin N in *Cephalosporium acremonium*. Biochem J 184:427–430

Kupka J, Shen Y-Q, Wolfe S, Demain AL (1983a) Partial purification and properties of the α-ketoglutarate-linked ring-expansion enzyme of β-lactam biosynthesis in *Cephalosporium acremonium*. FEMS Microbiol Lett (in press)

Kupka J, Shen Y-Q, Wolfe S, Demain AL (1983b) Studies on the ring-cyclization and ring-expansion enzymes of β-lactam biosynthesis in *Cephalosporium acremonium*. Can J Microbiol (in press)

Lemke PA, Nash CH (1972) Mutations that affect antibiotic synthesis by *Cephalosporium acremonium*. Can J Microbiol 18:255–259

Liersch M, Nuesch J, Treichler HJ (1976) Final steps in the biosynthesis of cephalosporin C. In: Macdonald KD (ed) Second international symposium on the genetics of industrial microorganisms. Academic Press, New York, pp 179–195

Loder PB (1972) Postepy Hig Med Dosw 26:493–500

Loder PB, Abraham EP (1971 a) Isolation and nature of intracellular peptides from a cephalosporin C-producing *Cephalosporium* sp. Biochem J 123:471–476

Loder PB, Abrahm AP (1971 b) Biosynthesis of peptides containing α-aminoadipic acid and cysteine in extracts of a *Cephalosporium* sp. Biochem J 123:477–482

Maeda K, Takahashi S, Sezaki M, Iinuma K, Naganawa H, Kondo S, Ohno M, Umezawa H (1977) Isolation and structure of a β-lactamase inhibitor from *Streptomyces.* J Antibiot (Tokyo) 30:770–772

Makins JF, Holt G, Macdonald KD (1980) Co-synthesis of penicillin following treatment of mutants of *Aspergillus nidulans* impaired in antibiotic production with lytic enzymes. J Gen Microbiol 119:397

Mehta RJ, Speth JL, Nash CH (1979) Lysine stimulation of cephalosporin C synthesis in *Cephalosporium acremonium.* Eur J Appl Microbiol Biotechnol 8:177–182

Meesschaert B, Adriaens P, Eyssen H (1980) Studies on the biosynthesis of isopenicillin N with a cell-free preparation of *Penicillium chrysogenum.* J Antibiot (Tokyo) 33:722–730

Miller RD, Huckstep LL, McDermott JP, Queener SW, Kukolja S, Spry DO, Elzey TK, Lawrence SM, Neuss N (1981) High performance liquid chromatography (HPLC) of natural products. 4. Isolation of a new cepham derivative from the broth of *Cephalosporium acremonium* and its role in the biosynthesis of cephalosporin C in the cell-free system. J Antibiot (Tokyo) 34:984–993

Morecombe DJ, Young DW (1975) Synthesis of chirally labeled cysteines and the steric origin of C(5) in penicillin biosynthesis. J Chem Soc Chem Commun:198–199

Morin RB, Jackson BG, Mueller RA, Lavagnino ER, Scanlon WB, Andrews SL (1963) Chemistry of cephalosporin antibiotics. 3. Chemical correlation of penicillin and cephalosporin antibiotics. J Am Chem Soc 85:1896–1897

Murao S (1955) Studies on penicillin-amidase. 2. Research on conditions of producing penicillin amidase. J Agric Chem Soc Jpn 29:400–403

Nagarajan R, Boeck LD, Gorman M, Hamill RL, Higgens CH, Hoehn MM, Stark WM, Whitney JG (1971) β-Lactam antibiotics from *Streptomyces.* J Am Chem Soc 93:2308–2310

Nakayama M, Kimura S, Tanabe S, Mizoguchi T, Watanabe I, Mori T, Miyahara K, Kawasaki T (1981) Structures and absolute configuration of carpetimycins A and B. J Antibiot (Tokyo) 34:818–823

Nash CH, De La Higuera N, Neuss N, Lemke PA (1974) Application of biochemical genetics to the biosynthesis of β-lactam antibiotics. Dev Ind Microbiol 15:114–123

Neuss N, Nash CH, Baldwin JE, Lemke PA, Grutzner JB (1973) Incorporation of (2RS,3R) [4-^{13}C] valine into cephalosporin C. J Am Chem Soc 95:3797

Neuss N, Miller RD, Affolder CA, Nakatsukosa W, Mabe J, Huckstepp LL, De la Higuera N, Hunt AH, Occolowitz J, Gilham JH (1980) High performance liquid chromatography (HPLC) of natural products. 3. Isolation of new tripeptides from the fermentation broth of *P. chrysogenum.* Helv Chim Acta 63:1119–1129

Neuss N, Nash CH, Lemke PA, Grutzner JB (1971) The use of ^{13}C nmr. (CMR) spectroscopy in biosynthetic studies of β-lactam antibiotics. 1. The incorporation of [1-^{13}C]- and [2-^{13}C]-sodium acetate and DL-[1-^{13}C]- and DL-[2-^{13}]-valine into cephalosporin C. Proc R Soc S Lond B Biol Sci 179:2337–2339

Newton GGF, Abraham EP (1955) Cephalosporin C, a new antibiotic containing sulfur and D-α-aminoadipic acid. Nature 175:548

Okamura K, Hirata S, Okumura Y, Fukagawa Y, Shimanchi Y, Kouno K, Ishikura T, Lein J (1978) PS-5, a new β-lactam antibiotic from *Streptomyces.* J Antibiot (Tokyo) 31:480–482

Osono T, Watanabe S, Saito T, Gushima H, Murakami K, Tokohashi I, Yamaguchi H, Sasaki T, Susaki K, Tokamera S, Miyoshi T, Oka Y (1980) Oganomycins, new 7-methoxycephalosporins produced by precursor fermentation with heterocyclic thiols. J Antibiot (Tokyo) 33:1074–1078

O'Sullivan J, Abraham EP (1980) The conversion of cephalosporins to 7 α-methoxycephalosporins by cell-free extracts of *Streptomyces clavuligerus.* Biochem J 186:613–616

O'Sullivan J, Bleaney RC, Huddleston JA, Abraham EP (1979 a) Incorporation of ^{3}H from δ-(L-α-amino-[4,5-^{3}H]adipyl)-L-cysteinyl-D-[4,4-^{3}H] valine into isopenicillin N. Biochem J 184:421–426

O'Sullivan J, Aplin RT, Stevens CM, Abraham EP (1979 b) Biosynthesis of 7-α-methoxycephalosporin. Incorporation of molecular oxygen. Biochem J 179:47–52
O'Sullivan J, Gillum AM, Aklonis CA, Souser ML, Sykes RB (1982) Biosynthesis of monobactam compounds; origin of the carbon atoms in the β-lactam ring. Antimicrob. Agents Chemother 21:558–564
Pisano MA, Velozzi EM (1974) Production of cephalosporin C by *Paecilomyces persicinus* P-10. Antimicrob Agents Chemother 6:447–451
Pruess DL, Johnson MJ (1967) Penicillin acyltransferase in *Penicillium chrosygenum*. J Bacteriol 94:1502–1508
Queener SW, Capone JJ, Radue AB, Nagarajan R (1974) Synthesis of deacetoxycephalosporin C by a mutant of *Cephalsporium acremonium*. Antimicrob Agents Chemother 6:334–337
Reading C, Cole M (1977) Clavulanic acid: a beta-lactamase-inhibiting beta-lactam from *Streptomyces clavuligerus*. Antimicrob Agents Chemother 11:852–857
Rosi D, Droze ML, Kuhrt MF, Terminello L, Came PE, Daum SJ (1981) Mutants of *Streptomyces cattleya* producing *N*-acetyl and dehydro carbopenems related to thienamycin. J Antibiot (Tokyo) 34:341–343
Sawada Y, Hunt NA, Demain AL (1979) Further studies on microbiological ring expansion of penicillin N. J Antibiot (Tokyo) 32:1303–1310
Sawada Y, Baldwin JE, Singh PD, Solomon NA, Demain AL (1980 a) Cell-free cyclization of δ-(L-α-aminoadipyl)-L-cysteinyl-D-valine to isopenicillin N. Antimicrob Agents Chemother 18:465–470
Sawada Y, Solomon NA, Demain AL (1980 b) Stimulation of the cell-free β-lactam ring expansion reaction by sonication and Triton X-100. Biotechnol Lett 2:43–48
Sebek OK (1953) Biosynthesis of C^{14}-labelled benzylpenicillin. Proc Soc Exp Biol Med 84:170–172
Shirafuji H, Fujisawa Y, Kida M, Kanzaki T, Yoneda M (1979) Accumulation of tripeptide derivatives by mutants of *Cephalosporium acremonium*. Agric Biol Chem 43:155–160
Somerson NL, Demain AL, Nunheimer TD (1961) Reversal of lysine inhibition of penicillin production by α-aminoadipic acid. Arch Biochem Biophys 93:238–241
Spencer B (1968) The biosynthesis of penicillins: acylation of 6-amino-penicillanic acid. Biochem Biophys Res Commun 31:170–175
Spencer B, Maung C (1970) Multiple activities of penicillin acyltransferase of *Penicillium chrysogenum*. Biochem J 118:29–30
Stapley EO, Jackson M, Hernandez S, Zimmerman SB, Currie SA, Mochalis S, Mahta JM, Woodruff HB, Hendlin D (1972) Cephamycins, a new family of β-lactam antibiotics. 1. Production by actinomycetes, including *Streptomyces lactamdurans* sp. n. Antimicrob Agents Chemother 2:122–131
Stapley EO, Birnbaum J, Miller AK, Wallick H, Hendlin D, Woodruff HB (1979) Cefoxitin and cephamycins: microbiological studies. Rev Inf Dis 1:73–87
Stapley EO, Cassidy P, Tunac J, Monaghan RL, Jackson M, Hernandez S, Zimmerman SB, Mahta JM, Currie SA, Dovryt D, Hendlin D (1981) Epithienamycins – novel β-lactams related to thienamycin. I. Production and antibacterial activity. J Antibiot (Tokyo) 34:628–636
Stauffer JF, Schwartz LJ, Brady CW (1966) Problems and progress in a strain selection program with cephalosporin-producing fungi. Dev Ind Microbiol 7:104–113
Stevens CM, Vohra P, Inamine E, Roholt OA Jr (1953) Utilization of sulfur compounds for the biosynthesis of penicillins. J Biol Chem 205:1001–1006
Stevens CM, Vohra P, Delong CW (1954) Utilization of valine in the biosynthesis of penicillins. J Biol Chem 211:297–300
Stevens CM, Inamine E, Delong CW (1956) The rates or incorporation of L-cysteine and D- and L-valine in penicillin biosynthesis. J Biol Chem 219:405–409
Stevens CM, Delong CW (1958) Valine metabolism and penicillin biosynthesis. J Biol Chem 230:991–999
Stevens CM, Abraham EP, Huang F-C, Sih CJ (1975) Incorporation of molecular oxygen at C-17 of cephalosporin C during its biosynthesis. Fed Proc 34:625

Stirling I, Elson SW (1979) Studies on the biosynthesis of clavulanic acid. 2. Chemical degradations of ^{14}C-labelled clavulinic acid. J Antibiot (Tokyo) 32:1125–1129

Sykes RB, Cimarusti CM, Bonner DP, Bush K, Floyd DM, Georgopapadakou NH, Koster WH, Liu WC, Parker WL, Principe PA, Rathnum ML, Slusarchyk WA, Trejo WH, Wells JS (1981) Monocyclic β-lactam antibiotics produced by bacteria. Nature 291:489–491

Turner MK, Farthing JE, Brewer SJ (1978) The oxygenation of [3-methyl-^3H] desacetoxycephalosporin C [7β-(5-D-aminoadipamido)-3-methylceph-3-em-4-carboxylic acid] to [3-*hydroxymethyl*-^3H] desacetylcephalosporin C by 2-oxoglutarate-linked dioxygenases from *Acremonium chrysogenum* and *Streptomyces clavuligerus*. Biochem J 173:839–850

Traxler P, Treichler HJ, Nuesch J (1975) Synthesis of *N*-acetyldeacetoxycephalosporin C by a mutant of *Cephalosporium acremonium*. J Antibiot (Tokyo) 28:605–606

Troonen H, Roelants P, Boon B (1976) RIT 2214, a new biosynthetic penicillin produced by a mutant of *Cephalosporium acremonium*. J Antibiot (Tokyo) 29:1258–1267

Trown PW, Abraham EP, Newton GGF, Hale CW, Miller GA (1962) Incorporation of acetate into cephalosporin C. Biochem J 84:157–166

Trown PW, Smith B, Abraham EP (1963 a) Biosynthesis of cephalosporin C from amino acids. Biochem J 86:284–291

Trown PW, Sharp M, Abraham EP (1963 b) α-Oxoglutarate as a precursor of the D-α-aminoadipic residue in cephalosporin C. Biochem J 86:280–284

Vanderhaeghe H, Claesen M, Vlietinck A, Parmentier G (1968) Specificity of penicillin acylase of *Fusarium* and of *Penicillium chrysogenum*. Appl Microbiol 16:1557–1563

Warren SC, Newton GGF, Abraham EP (1967 a) Use of α-aminoadipic acid for the biosynthesis of penicillin N and cephalosporin C by a *Cephalosporium* sp. Biochem J 103:891–901

Warren SC, Newton GGF, Abraham EP (1967 b) The role of valine in the biosynthesis of penicillin N and cephalosporin C by a *Cephalosporium* sp. Biochem J 103:902–912

Whitney JD, Brannon DR, Mabe JA, Wicker KJ (1972) Incorporation of labeled precursors into A16886B, a novel β-lactam antibiotic produced by *Streptomyces clavuligerus*. Antimicrob Agents Chemother 1:247–251

Wolff EC, Arnstein HRV (1960) The metabolism of 6-aminopenicillanic acid and related compounds by *Penicillium chrysogenum* and its possible significance for penicillin biosynthesis. Biochem J 76:375–381

Yoshida M, Konomi T, Kohsaka M, Baldwin JE, Herchen S, Singh P, Hunt NA, Demain AL (1978) Cell-free ring expansion of penicillin N to deacetoxycephalosporin C by *Cephalosporium acremonium* CW-19 and its mutants. Proc Natl Acid Sci USA 75:6253–6257

Young DW, Morecombe DJ, Sen PK (1977) The stereochemistry of β-lactam formation in penicillin biosynthesis. Eur J Biochem 75:133–147

CHAPTER 7

Regulation of Biosynthesis of β-Lactam Antibiotics

J. F. MARTIN and Y. AHARONOWITZ

A. Introduction

The biosynthetic pathways of β-lactam antibiotics are known to a certain extent, although only a few of the enzymes involved have even been partially studied. Likewise, little is known of the regulatory mechanisms that control gene expression in relation to β-lactam biosynthesis. However from the point of view of increasing antibiotic yields, knowledge of these regulatory mechanisms will be extremely helpful for the selective removal of bottlenecks in the biosynthetic pathways by genetic manipulation.

B. Carbon Catabolite Regulation

Glucose is the best carbon and energy source for growth of many chemoheterotrophic microorganisms. Glucose promotes growth of antibiotic-producing microorganisms but decreases the biosynthesis of many different antibiotics (MARTIN and DEMAIN 1980) and many other secondary metabolites (DEMAIN et al. 1979; HOSTALEK 1980). This phenomenon, which was initially named the "glucose effect," is now understood in terms of carbon catabolite regulation (MAGASANIK 1961; REVILLA et al. 1980). There is evidence supporting a broad mechanism of catabolite regulation probably related to the specific growth rate of the culture. Nutritional conditions that support a high specific growth rate result in a decrease of antibiotic biosynthesis. Carbon catabolite regulation of antibiotic biosynthesis may offer a survival advantage to the cells. Since antibiotics are potent inhibitors, their production is delayed until most of the carbon source has been utilized and therefore growth has already occurred.

In a medium containing glucose plus a second carbon source, glucose is generally used first, thereby suppressing antibiotic biosynthesis. When glucose is depleted, the second carbon source is used and antibiotic formation occurs. However, in certain cases the regulatory effect may be exerted by carbon sources which are preferred for growth over glucose (KOMINEK 1972). Carbon catabolite regulation of antibiotic biosynthesis is a general mechanism controlling the biosynthesis of antibiotics belonging to widely different biosynthetic groups (MARTIN and DEMAIN 1980).

I. Regulation of the Biosynthesis of Fungal β-Lactams by Glucose

Early studies on media development for penicillin production indicated that di-, oligo-, or polysaccharides were better carbon sources than glucose for penicillin production (SOLTERO and JOHNSON 1953). Apparently, by limiting the availability of glucose, the growth rate was reduced. The same phenomenon occurs in the case of cephalosporin C (MATSUMURA et al. 1978).

The diphasic utilization of glucose and sucrose was initially reported in *Cephalosporium acremonium* (DEMAIN 1963; MATSUMURA et al. 1978). We have found similar results in penicillin fermentations (REVILLA, LOPEZ-NIETO and MARTIN, to be published).

The precise molecular mechanism of carbon catabolite regulation of penicillin biosynthesis is unknown, although there appears to be a close relationship to the energetic metabolism of the cell. Recent studies on glucose regulation of penicillin biosynthesis in *Penicillium chrysogenum* indicate that in the presence of 2.5% (140 m*M*) glucose, no significant levels of penicillin are produced during the first 72 h of fermentation. After the glucose is exhausted penicillin biosynthesis resumes, although at a lower specific rate. When increasing levels of glucose are used, the onset of antibiotic biosynthesis occurs in each case after glucose has been depleted (ANTEQUERA and MARTIN, unpublished work). It is interesting to note that glucose regulation of penicillin (ANTEQUERA and MARTIN, unpublished work) and cephalosporin production (KUENZI 1980; ZANCA and MARTIN, unpublished work) is strongly enhanced by phosphate. Inorganic phosphate itself has little or no effect on β-lactam biosynthesis at concentrations up to 100 m*M*.

Glucose represses but does not inhibit incorporation of (^{14}C)valine into penicillin (REVILLA et al. 1981). The overall activity of the enzymes involved in β-lactam biosynthesis is repressed by glucose. Derepression occurs after glucose is exhausted. Maximum activity occurs during the initial phase of antibiotic biosynthesis and decreases thereafter (REVILLA, ANTEQUERA, and MARTIN, unpublished work). No inhibition of enzyme activity was observed in *P. chrysogenum*. All decreases in penicillin biosynthesis were due to repression. However in *C. acremonium*, there seems to be both repression and inhibition of β-lactam synthesizing enzymes (ZANCA and MARTIN, unpublished work).

Other carbon sources exert different effects on the incorporation of (^{14}C)valine into penicillin. Biosynthesis of penicillin as measured by the incorporation of valine into penicillin was optimal in lactose as the carbon source. Sucrose, fructose, or galactose exert a repression effect similar to that of glucose, suggesting that *P. chrysogenum* has an active invertase. Polymeric carbon sources such as dextrins or starch exert a smaller repression effect. Nonmetabolizable structural analogs of glucose such as 3-*O*-methylglucoside and β-*O*-methylglucoside do not exert repression of penicillin biosynthesis. These results suggest that the repression effect is exerted not by glucose itself, but by a product of glucose catabolism (Fig. 1). However, repression of penicillin biosynthesis is exerted by 2-deoxyglucose, an analogue of glucose which is taken up into the cell and phosphorylated but not metabolized further (REVILLA, LOPEZ-NIETO, and MARTIN, to be published). This suggests that a phosphorylated intermediate of sugar metabolism may be the intracellular effector mediating glucose control of penicillin biosynthesis.

The mechanism of carbon catabolite regulation of inducible catabolic enzymes (e.g., β-galactosidase) is well known in enteric bacteria. It involves cyclic adenosine 3′-5′-monophosphate (c-AMP) as a positive effector (PASTAN and PERLMAN 1970). c-AMP and a c-AMP receptor protein (CRP) form a complex which binds to the

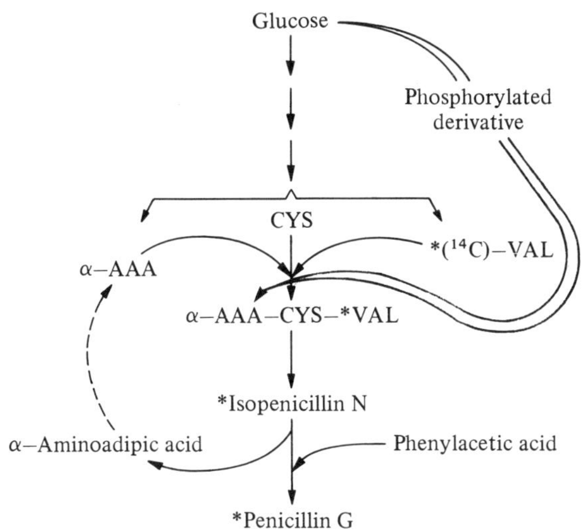

Fig. 1. Enzyme level at which carbon catabolite regulation is exerted. The amino acids α-aminoadipic acid, cysteine, and valine are formed from glucose (or from other carbon sources). A phosphorylated glucose derivative appears to be the intracellular effector. The effector seems to act by blocking the formation of the tripeptide (see text)

promotor site of the operon; binding of the complex to the DNA stimulates the initiation of the transcription by RNA polymerase. Glucose inhibits the formation of c-AMP from ATP by the enzyme, adenylate cyclase, thereby resulting in decreased transcription of carbon catabolite-sensitive operons (see reviews by PAIGEN and WILLIAMS 1970; PASTAN and ADHYA 1976). c-AMP does not appear to be involved in carbon catabolite regulation of penicillin biosynthesis. Addition of exogenous c-AMP or dibutyryl c-AMP does not reverse glucose repression of penicillin biosynthesis (REVILLA et al. 1980). However further evidence of c-AMP uptake is needed before any firm conclusion can be drawn.

It seems likely that carbon catabolite regulation affects the central enzymes of penicillin biosynthesis involved in the formation of the β-lactam nucleus. Very recent results suggest that glucose represses the formation of the α-aminoadipylcysteinylvaline tripeptide (ACV) in *P. chrysogenum* (REVILLA, LOPEZ-NIETO, and MARTIN, to be published). Glucose repression is not reversed in vivo by the component amino acids. It is also known that the degradative conversion of cephalosporin to deacetylcephalosporin C, a reaction which is normally carried out by the producer *C. acremonium*, is repressed by glucose, maltose or sucrose but not by succinate or glycerol (HINNEN and NUESCH 1976).

II. Carbon Catabolite Regulation of the Biosynthesis of β-Lactams by Actinomycetes

Actinomycetes produce large number of antibiotics having the β-lactam nucleus. Most of them are believed to be synthesized by pathways similar to those of penicillin and cephalosporin C (MARTIN 1981). Control of cephalosporin biosynthesis by the carbon source has been studied by AHARONOWITZ and DEMAIN (1978) in *Streptomyces clavuligerus*. This strain produces the cephalosporin 7-(5-amino-5-carboxyvaleramido)-3-carbamoyloxmethyl-3-cephem-4-carboxylic acid together with cephamycin C, clavulanic acid and penicillin N.

S. clavuligerus was found capable of utilizing starch, maltose or glycerol as sole carbon source for growth but incapable of using glucose. In addition, it grew on succinate, α-ketoglutarate or fumarate. The growth on carbohydrates and glycerol was much more extensive than growth on the organic acids. When *S. clavuligerus* cell were grown on glycerol or maltose, the specific production of cephalosporins decreased as concentration of the carbon source was increased above the growth-limiting concentration. Even though specific production of the antibiotics decreased upon increasing glycerol or maltose concentrations, a critical level of biomass was needed for high volumetric production of cephalosporins. The amount of maltose and glycerol to which cells were exposed affected the relationship between growth and production phases. At low concentrations, production appeared to be associated with growth. However, at non-growth-limiting concentrations, a distinct separation between growth and production phases could be observed. When organic acids such as succinate and α-ketoglutarate were used as single carbon sources, specific production was high and associated with growth. It seems therefore that the organic acids utilized as carbon sources for growth were relatively poorer carbon sources than maltose or glycerol, thus, providing growth-limiting conditions. These results suggest that some type of carbon catabolite control exists over antibiotic production in *S. clavuligerus*. The specific regulatory mechanisms operating at the molecular level on cephalosporins production by the carbon source in *S. clavuligerus* are yet to be elucidated.

C. Nitrogen Metabolite Regulation

The capacity of a given culture to synthesize β-lactam antibiotics has been generally considered genetically independent from its physiological state in respect to nitrogen metabolism. However, several reports indicate that β-lactam antibiotic biosynthesis, both in fungi and actinomycetes, is subject to nitrogen metabolite regulation (AHARONOWITZ 1980).

S. clavuligerus is capable of utilizing nitrogen for growth from a wide spectrum of compounds including ammonium salts, amino acid, and urea. However, its capacity to produce cephalosporins is strongly suppressed by the presence of excess ammonia. The negative effect of excess ammonia was observed when ammonia served as the sole nitrogen source or when added to an amino acid (AHARONOWITZ and DEMAIN 1979). Similarly, nitrogen source control operates on the production of cephamycin C by *Streptomyces cattleya* (LILLEY et al. 1981). In this culture, high titers were achieved in nitrogen-limited environments but repression of production occurred in nitrogen-sufficient cultures. Furthermore, in an ammonium-limited chemostat culture of *S. cattleya*, maximum cephamycin C synthesis occured at the low specific growth rates at which ammonium utilization rates were much reduced. The ammonia effect in *S. clavuligerus* expressed itself early during the growth phase and could not be attributed to a specific inhibition of activity of antibiotic-forming enzymes (AHARONOWITZ and DEMAIN 1979). Whether it operates at the level of specific antibiotic biosynthetic gene expression or at the level of primary metabolism is not yet established. In this regard, it has been suggested that control mechanisms operating at the level of primary nitrogen metabolism may also determine the efficiency of the antibiotic biosynthetic machinery mainly by affecting the availability of the amino acid precursors required for the biosynthesis of β-lactam antibiotics. The possible involvement of glutamine synthetase (GS), a key enzyme in general nitrogen metabolism, and other regulatory gene products operating in procaryotes (TYLER 1978) have attracted the attention of several groups. Thus, the correlation between GS activity and production of β-lactam antibiotics has been investigated in different producing cultures. AHARONOWITZ (1979) has shown that the highest specific cephalosporin production was obtained under those growth conditions that led to high GS activity.

When cells were grown on media containing ammonium in excess, both GS activity and specific antibiotic production decreased. When the kinetics of GS synthesis during the growth cycle of *S. clavuligerus* was studied, the GS activity reached a peak during the late stages of growth, always when ammonia was depleted from the medium. In the case of *S. cattleya*, WAX and SNYDER (1980) observed similar kinetics for GS and thienamycin production; there was a dramatic peak of GS activity at about the time that antibiotic synthesis commenced. This peak activity lasted for a short period and a sharp drop-off was observed. Whether modification of GS is taking place in streptomycetes, like that found in enteric bacteria, is not yet conclusively established. SHUSTER and AHARONOWITZ (unpublished works) could not detect adenylylated forms of GS in *S. clavuligerus* extracts, neither by treatment with snake venom phosphodiesterase nor by the assay of enzyme activity in cells grown under different physiological conditions. However, STREICHER and TYLER (1981) observed an adenylylated GS form in *S. cattleya*. The existence of a GS modification mechanism in *S. cattleya*, yet of unknown nature, was suggested by WAX and SNYDER (1980), as indicated by the loss of GS activity after "ammonium shock." This latter observation was confirmed in *S. clavuligerus* (SHUSTER and AHARONOWITZ, unpublished work).

Very recently SANCHEZ et al. (1980) have reported inhibition of penicillin biosynthesis in *P. chrysogenum* by high levels of NH_4. The ammonium effect was correlated with low levels of glutamine synthetase. Cells grown in low NH_4 concentration accumulated higher concentrations of glutamine in the free pool of amino acids and lower concentrations of glutamate. In contrast, increasing the concentration of NH_4 led to a decreased glutamine pool, increased glutamate concentration and poor antibiotic production. The important role of glutamine in the synthesis of penicillin could be further seen by using a cycloheximide-containing resting cell system of *P. chrysogenum* (SANCHEZ et al. 1980). Feeding the resting-cells with a limiting concentration of glutamine resulted in higher penicillin synthesis than in glutamate- or ammonium-supplemented systems.

In this regard, the results obtained in *Neurospora crassa* (ESPIN et al. 1979) are of special interest. A mechanism for the degradation of exogenous glutamine to glutamate and the resynthesis of internal glutamine and other amino acids has been proposed. This cycle might serve for the utilization of carbon and nitrogen for the

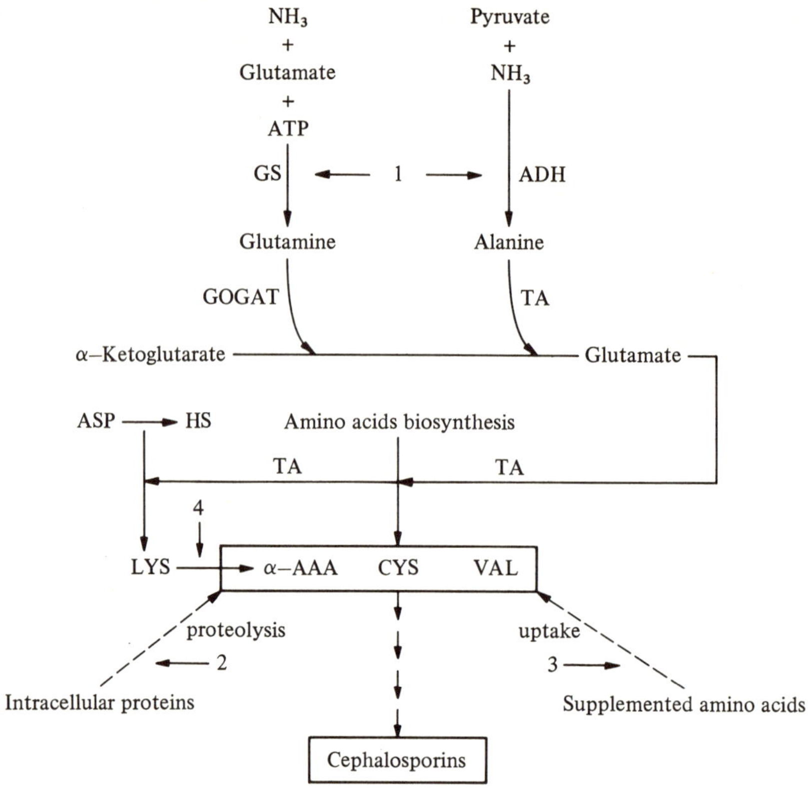

Fig. 2. Possible sites of interaction between primary nitrogen metabolism and cephalosporin biosynthesis (*numbered arrows*). *GS*, glutamine synthetase; *ADH*, alanine dehydrogenase; *GOGAT*, glutamate synthase; *TA*, transamination; *ASP*, aspartate; *HS*, homoserine; *LYS*, lysine; α-*AAA*, α-aminoadipate; *CYS*, cysteine; *VAL*, valine. (Aharonowitz 1979)

synthesis of amino acids in general and, in the case of *P. chrysogenum*, might affect the availability of the specific precursors required for penicillin biosynthesis.

Extracellular proteolytic activity in *S. clavuligerus* was also shown to be regulated by nitrogen (Aharonowitz 1979). When grown on asparagine as the sole nitrogen source, antibiotic production followed an increase in the total extracellular proteolytic activity; ammonium in excess drastically repressed both cephalosporin and extracellular protease formation. The same relationship was reported for serine proteases and cephamycin C production in *Streptomyces lactamdurans* (Ginther 1979). It was found that antibiotic production and serine protease formation were coordinately regulated.

From the experiments described above, it appears that signals from nitrogen metabolism elicit effects on β-lactam antibiotic production. The exact level at which these signals operate and their nature are not yet determined. The use of mutants, impaired in the different steps of nitrogen metabolism, for studies on antibiotic synthesis might contribute to the elucidation of this interesting phenomenon.

The study of nitrogen metabolite regulation in β-lactam antibiotic synthesis may be approached from any of the aspects mentioned previously (AHARONOWITZ 1980): nitrogen control at the level of the catabolism of nitrogen-containing compounds; regulation at the biosynthetic level by controlling the intracellular levels of glutamine and glutamate, the major source of amino groups in the cell; transport of nitrogen metabolites; modulation of intracellular concentration of free metabolites; protein turnover and degradation; and the regulation of antibiotic "synthetases" (Fig. 2).

D. Regulation at the Level of Sulfur Metabolism

The sulfur atom possessed by penicillins and cephalosporins is derived from cysteine. Radioactively labeled cysteine molecules have been shown to be incorporated into penicillin (ARNSTEIN and GRANT 1954), cephalosporin C (TROWN et al. 1963) and cephamycins produced by *Streptomyces* (WHITNEY et al. 1972). Attempts have been made to find any regulatory effect of the pathways leading to cysteine or pathways involved in sulfur metabolism in general on the synthesis of penicillin and cephalosporin. In order to better understand the results obtained, let us briefly summarize different alternatives for cysteine biosynthesis as have been proposed for fungal systems (UMBARGER 1978; TREICHLER et al. 1979) (Fig. 3). Cysteine may be derived from the reaction between sulfide and *O*-acetylserine catalyzed by *O*-acetylserine sulfhydrylase (cysteine synthase), step 7. In a different path, cysteine can be derived via the "reverse" transsulfuration pathway in which the sulfur of methionine is transferred to cysteine via a sequence of reactions, steps 13–17, including *S*-adenosylmethionine, *S*-adenosylhomocysteine, homocysteine and cystathionine as intermediates. In analogy to the first alternative, the incorporation of sulfide via homocysteine synthase (step 9) could be shown. In this latter reaction, *O*-acetyl-L-homoserine is the substrate and L-homocysteine is the product. As a result, this pathway provides a mechanism for incorporating sulfur into methionine (and hence cysteine) when cysteine sulfhydrylase (step 7) is missing. The efficiency with which any of these alternatives operates, in different organisms, is genetically determined, and coordinate control mechanisms regulating sulfur metabolism will determine the preferred substrate and pathway. Thus, the role of each sulfur compound in regulation of β-lactam antibiotic formation might differ for different producing strains. For example, sulfur for penicillin production in *P. chrysogenum* is obtained mainly from sulfate reduction (SEGAL and JOHNSON 1963). In this organism, the transsulfuration pathway has been considered to have a minor role only. This conclusion stems from a study on penicillin production by industrial *Penicillium* strains (SEGAL and JOHNSON 1961). In contrast, the sulfur atom for the β-lactam antibiotics formed by *C. acremonium* is considered to derive preferentially from methionine via the reverse transsulfuration pathway (CALTRIDER and NISS 1966; NUESCH et al. 1973). Furthermore, methionine has been found to stimulate the production of both penicillin N and cephalosporin C by *C. acremonium.*

Such observations raised the questions of whether methionine is obligatory for the conversion of sulfate to cephalosporin C in the *C. acremonium* system, and whether the role of methionine is regulatory or as a precursor. In order to answer

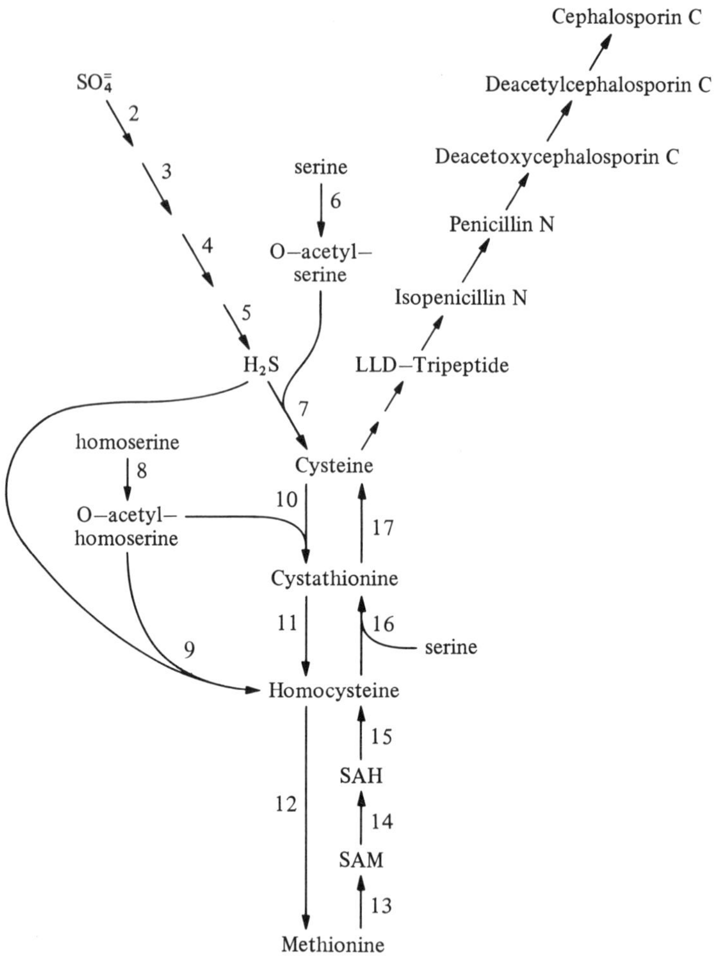

Fig. 3. The methionine-cysteine biosynthetic pathway and its involvement in β-lactam biosynthesis. (MARTIN and DEMAIN 1980)

this question *C. acremonium* strains carrying mutations in the sulfur metabolic pathways have been obtained and the effect of these mutations on antibiotic production has been studied.

One line of mutants was selected in which the pathway between sulfate and cysteine (steps 1–7) was blocked. By such an interference, a competitve effect of inorganic sulfate in cysteine production could be eliminated. The significance of these mutations has been interpreted by using data accumulated both in antibiotic producers and other fungal systems. In *Neurospora* and yeast, the uptake of sulfate and its conversion to sulfide was shown to be under the control of methionine rather than cysteine (UMBARGER 1978). In yeast, these enzymes of sulfate assimilation were strongly derepressed when methionine was limiting and repressed when methionine was in excess (UMBARGER 1978). Thus, in mutants blocked between sulfate and cysteine, such a possible interference could be eliminated. Several mutational studies in β-lactam-producing organisms have exploited this approach. DREW and DEMAIN (1975a) isolated a mutant of *C. acremonium*, 274-1, which could not grow on sulfate but did respond to cysteine, cysthathionine, homocysteine, and methionine. Cephalosporin C production by strain 274-1 was fully stimulated by methionine. However, intermediates between methionine and cephalosporin C were unable to fully replace methionine for stimulation of antibiotic biosynthesis. The fact that the stimulatory activity of the sulfur amino acids decreased as they became metabolically more distant from methionine and closer to cephalosporin C indicated the relative unimportance of sulfur donation to the phenomenon of methionine stimulation of cephalosporin C formation.

The function of cysteine synthase(*O*-acetyl-L-serine sulfhydrylase; step 7) in the biosynthesis of cephalosporin C was studied using a *C. acremonium* strain with a 75% reduced cysteine synthase activity (LIERSCH et al. 1980). Some antibiotic production was achieved in the mutant and the parental strains when SO_4^{2-} was used as the sulfur source; methionine stimulated antibiotic synthesis about 5-fold in both strains. When cysteine synthase activity was impared, methionine could still be formed from sulfate due to the diversion of sulfur to methionine via *O*-acetylhomoserine sulfhydrylase (step 9) yielding homocysteine. This latter enzyme was repressed by high concentrations of exogenous methionine but was stimulated by an excess of sulfate (TREICHLER et al. 1979). This observation would explain why mutants in which the alternative route is operating (steps 8 and 9) have an increasing cephalosporin C productivity from sulfate and a rather restricted tolerance to methionine. Support for this explanation comes from the study of a *C. acremonium* mutant (KOMATSU et al. 1975) which displayed potency levels more than twofold that of the parent in the presence of sulfate, but its productivity was severely inhibited by the addition of more than 0.5% methionine to the medium, a concentration that gave high cephalosporin C production with the parent. Support for the obligatory involvement of methionine in cephalosporin C biosynthesis comes from a study done with a mutant blocked in the transsulfuration pathway from cysteine to methionine when the pathway from sulfate to cysteine to cephalosporin C remains open (DREW and DEMAIN 1975b). When grown at a level of methionine just able to support optimum growth, cephalosporin C formation could not be detected; the culture should have been fully capable of converting sulfate to cysteine and then to cephalosporin C. Only when methionine was supplied in excess, was the synthesis of the antibiotic allowed. This observation suggests that cysteine must be first converted into methionine by transsulfuration, before it can stimulate antibiotic formation. This point was further examined by DREW and DEMAIN (1975a) by using a double mutant (Strain 11-8), blocked not only in the pathway from cysteine to methionine but also in the pathway from sulfate to cysteine. This mutant did not produce cephalosporin when grown in excess cysteine and enough methionine to support growth. However, addition of methionine in excess stimulated antibiotic production. Furthermore, the use of excess norleucine (a non-sulfur structural analog of methionine) could replace excess methionine in stimulation of cephalosporin C production in this mutant. These results provide strong evidence that methionine plays a regulatory role in cephalosporin C production rather than merely serving as a source of sulfur. Two mutants isolated by TREICHLER et al.

(1979), defective in steps 8 and 9, provide further evidence compatible with the results of Drew and Demain. The mutant blocked in step 8 grew on methionine, homocysteine, and cystathionine but not on cysteine or inorganic sulfur sources; the mutant was not stimulated by excess cysteine or sulfate in a medium containing a low but growth-sufficient concentration of methionine. The second mutant deficient in step 9 was depressed in cephalosporin synthesis from sulfate but not from methionine.

TREICHLER et al. (1979) have expanded the study of the influence of the different biosynthetic routes to cysteine on cephalosporin C and penicillin production in *C. acremonium* and *P. chrysogenum* respectively. Their main hypothesis is that cystathionine-γ-lyase activity (step 17) is crucial for the effect of the sulfur source on antibiotic biosynthesis. A mutant of *C. acremonium* blocked in step 17 was isolated which could not grow on methionine, homocysteine, and cystathionine but grew on cysteine and on inorganic sulfur source. The loss of the cystathionine-γ-lyase activity had a drastic influence on antibiotic formation; cephalosporin C production was not stimulated by methionine and was poorer even when compared to the wild strain in the absence of exogenous methionine. The expression of cystathionine-γ-lyase was further investigated in both *C. acremonium* and *P. chrysogeneum* with respect to the sulfur source (GYGAX et al. 1980). When grown for 72 h with inorganic sulfur compounds, the enzyme activity was quite similar in both strains. However, when grown on methionine, the level of the *C. acremonium* enzyme increased twofold whereas that of *P. chrysogenum* still remained at the same level. In the *C. acremonium* system the cystathionine-γ-lyase activity was proportional to cephalosporin C formation. These correlations of the enzyme activity with cephalosporin C production and differential expression of the enzyme activity in both strains were in good agreement with the difference in cysteine biosynthetic pathways of these two organisms (GYGAX et al. 1980). A somewhat different hypothesis was favored by DREW and DEMAIN (1977); they felt that methionine acts as an inducer of one or more of the specific β-lactam synthetases. A mutant strain (H) of *C. acremonium* was isolated (DREW and DEMAIN 1975c) blocked between step 2 and 8 and also in step 17. Since such a mutant should not be able to convert cystathionine to cysteine (it grows on cysteine), its antibiotic production should not be stimulated by methionine unless the methionine effect is expressed on the cephalosporin-forming enzymes. Indeed a methionine dipeptide (used instead of methionine to overcome the permeation problem) stimulated cephalosporin production. Thus, a controversy still exists and further studies are necessary to settle it. A better understanding of the specific sequence of enzyme activities leading to the β-lactam antibiotics is required. In this regard the increase in both tripeptide cyclase and ring-expansion activities in *C. acremonium* grown with methionine or norleucine (SAWADA et al. 1980c) strongly supports a regulatory role for methionine.

Stimulation of cystathionine-γ-lyase in methionine-induced cultures of *C. acremonium* has been also proven by Zanca and Martin (unpublished work). The methionine effect is broader than previously thought, affecting also enzymes involved in the biosynthesis of valine, another component amino acid of penicillin and cephalosporin. It seems that methionine induces a whole set of enzymes involved in cephalosporin biosynthesis (Zanca and Martín, unpublished work).

Sulfur metabolism in the β-lactam antibiotic-producing actinomycetes and its regulatory consequences on production of the antibiotics are now being studied (ROMERO, LIRAS and MARTIN, unpublished work).

E. Lysine Metabolism and Antibiotic Biosynthesis

The interest in the effect of lysine metabolism on β-lactam antibiotic biosynthesis started with the observation made by BONNER (1947) that 25% of the lysine-requiring mutants of *Penicillium notatum* failed to produce penicillin. DEMAIN (1957) found 10 years later that lysine was a potent inhibitor of penicillin synthesis in *P. chrysogenum*. In attempts to reverse the lysine inhibitory effect, it was found that α-aminoadipic acid (α-AAA) could reverse the inhibitory effect of lysine and furthermore, stimulated penicillin synthesis in the absence of added lysine (SOMERSON et al. 1961). Additional evidence of the role of α-AAA in β-lactam antibiotic synthesis was provided by ARNSTEIN et al. (1960) who detected the formation of a tripeptide (α-aminoadipyl)-cysteinyl-valine in the mycelium of *P. chrysogenum*. Later, LODER and ABRAHAM (1971) isolated the same tripeptide from the mycelium of *C. acremonium*, studied its structure and found it to have the LLD configuration. The same peptide was found to be present in *S. clavuligerus* [together with the dipeptide, (α-aminoadipyl)-cysteine (ABRAHAM 1978)], *Streptomyces griseus*, and *S. lactamdurans* (LIRAS and MARTIN, unpublished work). In parallel to these findings, a β-lactam antibiotic was found to contain L-α-AAA as its side chain. This hydrophilic penicillin, named isopenicillin N, was isolated from *P. chrysogenum* (FLYNN et al. 1962). Labeled α-AAA was shown to be the precursor for cephalosporin C (WARREN et al. 1967). The involvement of α-AAA in penicillin and cephalosporin formation was finally demonstrated directly by using the tripeptide as a precursor for antibiotic synthesis in cell-free systems both from fungi and streptomycetes (ABRAHAM 1978).

I. Control by Lysine of the Biosynthesis of Fungal β-Lactams

According to the information listed above, it could be expected that regulation of the pathway leading to α-AAA would influence directly the synthesis of β-lactam antibiotics. The metabolic relationship between lysine and α-AAA in fungi and streptomycetes differs significantly. The lysine pathway in fungi starts from α-ketoglutarate. Homocitrate is formed by condensation of the α-ketoglutarate with acetyl-CoA by the action of homocitrate synthase (EC 4.1.3.21). Homocitrate is converted into α-ketoadipate by a series of reactions (Fig. 4). α-Ketoadipate is converted to α-AAA in a transamination reaction. During the conversion of α-AAA to lysine, it is first activated, reduced to a semialdehyde which then accepts an amino group from glutamate in a covalently linked transfer involving saccharopine as an intermediate. The oxidative cleavage of saccharopine yields lysine (UMBARGER 1978). Thus, in fungi, α-AAA is an intermediate in the lysine biosynthetic pathway.

Since α-AAA, or its activated form, appeared to be a branch point between the lysine and the penicillin biosynthetic pathways (PIRT 1969), it was proposed that

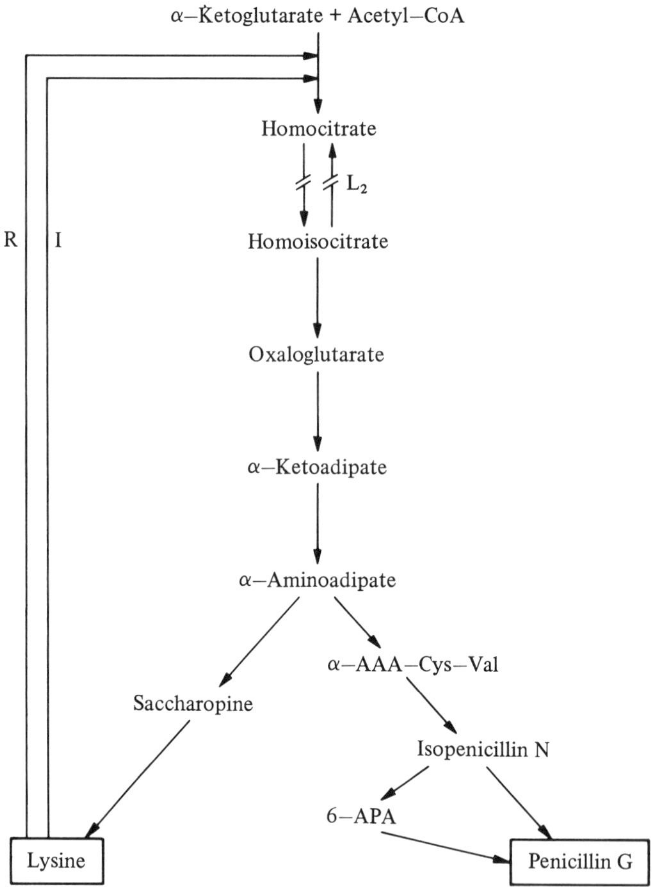

Fig. 4. Regulation by lysine of the biosynthesis of penicillin at the homocitrate synthase level in *P. chrysogenum*. *R*, repression; *I*, inhibition; L_2 is a mutant block. (LUENGO et al. 1980)

lysine inhibition of penicillin synthesis is due to feedback effects on its own biosynthesis, i.e. inhibition of an early step in the common part of the pathway. Such an inhibition would be expected to result in a deficiency of α-AAA needed for penicillin formation (DEMAIN 1974). Lysine decreases both the incorporation of (^{14}C)valine into penicillin and the excretion of homocitrate by a lysine auxotroph blocked in the lysine pathway after homocitrate (MASUREKAR and DEMAIN 1972; LUENGO et al. 1980).

The use of lysine auxotrophs of *P. chrysogenum* enabled DEMAIN and MASUREKAR (1974) to show an in vivo feedback inhibition of homocitrate synthase by lysine both in the growth and the production phase of the fungus. FRIEDRICH and DEMAIN (1977) supported these findings by showing that the addition of homocitrate in resting cultures could reverse the lysine inhibition of penicillin biosynthesis.

In fungi, like *Neurospora crassa* and yeasts, the control of carbon flow over the lysine biosynthetic pathway occurs in part via an inhibition and/or repression of the condensing enzyme, homocitrate synthase (MARAGOUDAKIS et al. 1967; HOGG and BROQUIST 1968; TUCCI 1969; TUCCI and CECI 1972; GAILLARDIN et al. 1976). However early attempts to show the in vitro inhibition of homocitrate synthase by 20 mM lysine in crude extracts of the penicillin producer *P. chrysogenum* were unsuccessful (MASUREKAR and DEMAIN 1974a). Recently we have shown that lysine both feedback inhibits homocitrate synthase activity and represses its synthesis in *P. chrysogenum* (LUENGO et al. 1980). Neither penicillin nor 6-aminopenicillanic acid exerted any effect at the homocitrate synthase level. Maximum homocitrate synthase activity in cultures of *P. chrysogenum* AS-P-78 was found at 48 h, coinciding with the phase of high rate of penicillin biosynthesis (LUENGO et al. 1980).

The possibility of inhibiting penicillin production by genetically increasing the intracellular lysine concentration was investigated in lysine analog-resistant strains (MASUREKAR and DEMAIN 1974b). Among these mutants, lysine regulatory mutants of *P. chrysogenum* which excreted lysine were found to be deficient in production of penicillin; a revertant to analog sensitivity recovered the ability to produce penicillin. LUENGO et al. (1979) were interested in the relevance of these findings to industrial strains and investigated the possibility that industrial mutant strains of *P. chrysogenum* have lost sensitivity to lysine inhibition of penicillin synthesis during the strain-improvement process. The inhibitory effect was compared in a low-penicillin-producing (Wis 54-1255) and a high-producing (AS-P-78) strain. Lysine inhibited total penicillin synthesis to a similar extent in both strains. However, in the high-producing strain, the onset of penicillin synthesis occurred even at a high lysine concentration, whereas in the low-producing strain lysine had to be depleted before penicillin production commenced. The homocitrate synthase activity was assayed in cell-free extracts of *P. chrysogenum* Wis 54-1255, the lys$^-$ auxotroph L_2 and the high penicillin producer AS-P-78 (MARTIN et al. 1979a; LUENGO et al. 1979). When Wis 54-1255 was grown in complex medium with daily 50 mM lysine additions, the enzyme activity was 52% less than the activity of control cultures. In a defined medium, the inhibition was complete and no antibiotic could be detected. Similar results were obtained with the auxotrophic mutant. The sensitivity of homocitrate synthesis to lysine inhibition as measured in cell-free extracts of the high-penicillin-producing strain AS-P-78 was identical.

The need for α-AAA to form the tripeptide precursor for penicillin biosynthesis and the regulatory effects imposed by lysine on its formation raised the question as to what extent α-AAA is required in penicillin biosynthesis. The currently accepted mechanism of penicillin biosynthesis postulates the release of α-AAA in the final step in the formation of the hydrophobic penicillins (DEMAIN 1979) (Fig. 1). If this is true, then α-aminoadipate should be required only in very low amounts, as long as transport into mycelium is effective and degradation is not extensive. However very high concentrations of exogenous α-AAA had been used to demonstrate its effect in penicillin formation with resting and growing cells of *P. chrysogenum* (SOMERSON et al. 1961; FRIEDRICH and DEMAIN 1977). More recently, however, FRIEDRICH and DEMAIN (1978) have shown that a relatively low concentration of added α-AAA is required for optimum penicillin biosynthesis. An external DL-α-AAA concentration of 0.01 mM was enough to yield about 50% of the maximum penicillins synthesis rate. Raising the exogenous concentration 10 times resulted in a maximum rate of penicillin formation. The low amount of α-AAA required for optimun antibiotic formation was presumably due to its relatively slow degradation and to its reuse after being released from penicillin N in the final steps of benzylpenicillin synthesis. It was concluded that about ten molecules of penicillin were produced per molecule of intracellular α-AAA (FRIEDRICH and DEMAIN 1978). This is in agreement with the finding by GOULDEN (1969) that the molar amount of intra-plus-extracellular α-AAA in a high-producing mutant of *P. chrysogenum* was considerably lower than the molar amount of penicillin produced.

REVILLA and MARTIN (unpublished work) have found recently that α-AAA stimulates the incorporation of (^{14}C)valine into penicillin by resting cells of *P. chrysogenum*. This effect is specific for α-AAA and is not produced by the other constituent amino acids valine and cysteine, suggesting that penicillin biosynthesis is sometimes limited by α-AAA.

The effect of lysine on accumulation of cephalosporin C by *C. acremonium* was investigated by MEHTA et al. (1979). Lysine added to a defined medium at a concentration of 1 mg/ml enhanced the production of cephalosporin C. The lysine effect was accompanied by a delayed differentiation to arthrospores followed by more extensive mycelial fragmentation. However, high lysine concentrations reduced the synthesis of cephalosporin C. In a resting cell system, the lysine inhibition was relieved by supplementation of the medium with 1–2 mg/ml of α-AAA. Again this reversal supports the hypothesis that lysine restricts the availability of α-AAA required for β-lactam biosynthesis. The stimulatory effect of low lysine concentrations on cephalosporin biosynthesis by *C. acremonium* could be related to sparing of endogenous pools of α-AAA for lysine biosynthesis (MEHTA et al. 1979). Caution should be taken, however, in interpreting results obtained with high-producing strains of *Penicillium* or *Cephalosporium* since most of these strains have been drastically altered by mutation treatments.

II. Lysine Effect in Actinomycetes

In contrast to the fungal biosynthetic pathway, lysine in bacteria is derived from 2,6-diaminopimelic acid (DAP) and serves as a precursor for α-AAA. Whole cell hydrolysates of the β-lactam antibiotic producer *S. clavuligerus* have been shown to contain L-DAP (HIGGENS and KASTNER 1971) and purified cell wall preparations to include the L,L-DAP isomer (KIRNBERG and AHARONOWITZ, unpublished work).

These findings have suggested that the DAP pathway for lysine biosynthesis is operative in streptomycetes and is the origin of the α-AAA side chain of the β-lactam antibiotics produced by them. In order to examine the involvement of lysine in the synthesis of the α-AAA side chain, labeled lysine and α-AAA were added to fermentations of *S. clavuligerus* (WHITNEY et al. 1972). The incorporation of labeled DL-lysine into cephamycin C and its recovery as the α-AAA side chain indicated that the origin of the α-AAA is different from that in *C. acremonium*. KIRKPATRICK et al. (1973a) investigated this problem in detail. They isolated a lysine-requiring mutant, LA-423 of *Streptomyces lipmanii*, which was defective in DAP decarboxylase. The mutant accumulated large quantities of DAP in its free amino acid pools when starved of lysine, suggesting some control of lysine over an earlier step(s) in the path. The wild type and the mutant strain could accumulate α-AAA

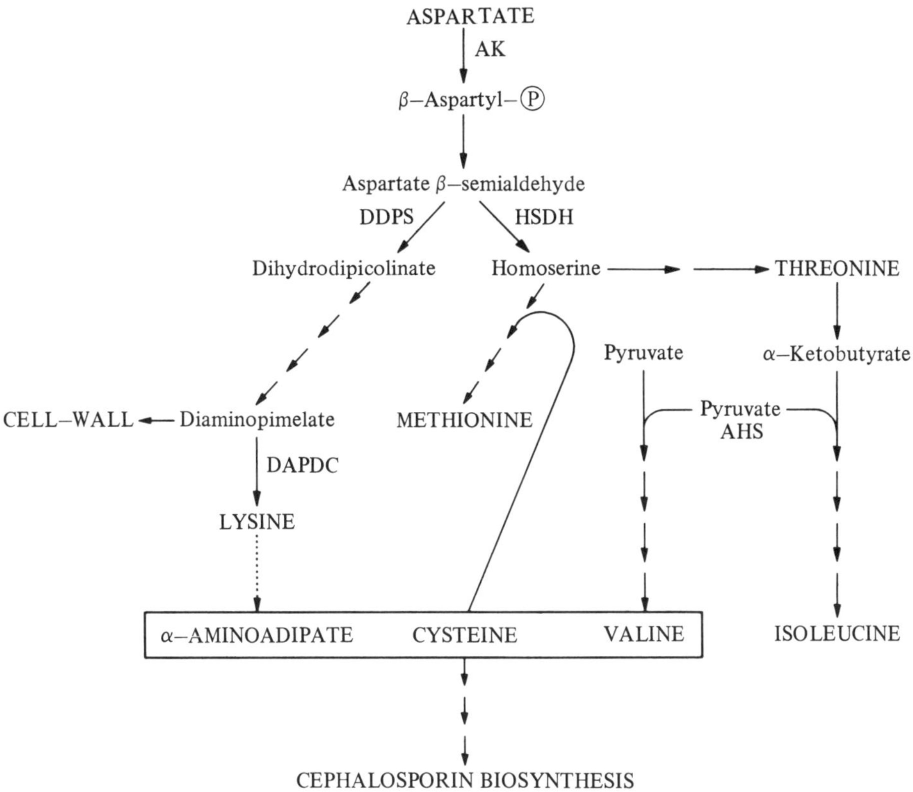

Fig. 5. Interrelationships between the aspartic acid family of amino acids and β-lactam antibiotic biosynthesis by *Streptomyces*. Conversion of lysine into α-aminoadipate (*dotted arrow*) is carried out by lysine ε-aminotransferase

in the intracellular pool when 1 mg lysine per milliliter growth medium was supplied. Antibiotic was produced by either strain, but only when it was supplied with high levels of lysine. Furthermore, incorporation of label from L-lysine could be detected in antibiotic products. The DAP decarboxylase activity of *S. lipmanii* was inhibited by lysine but repression could not be observed. Finally, the incorporation of (^{14}C)aspartic acid into DAP concluded the evidence for the operation of the DAP pathway for lysine biosynthesis in *S. lipmanii*. These observations together with the observation made by WHITNEY et al. (1972) have supported the hypothesis that α-AAA, in the prokaryotic β-lactam antibiotic producers, is a catabolic product of lysine. Preliminary evidence that an aminotransferase is involved in the conversion of L-lysine to α-AAA for the synthesis of β-lactam antibiotics by *S. lipmanii* was presented by KIRKPATRICK et al. (1973b). Quite recently KERN et al. (1980) and LIRAS et al. (1982) conclusively demonstrated an L-lysine/α-ketoglutarate ε-aminotransferase in *S. lactamdurans* (Fig. 5), a commercially important producer of cephamycin C. This enzyme was shown to catalyze the first reaction in the conversion of L-lysine to L-α-AAA. The product of the reaction was found to be L-1-piperideine-6-carboxylate. When the aminotransferase activity was followed during a fermentation, peak activity occurred very early in the fermentation at a time when cell growth was exponential and no cephamycin C synthesis was detected. Later in the fermentation, the enzyme disappeared rapidly as cephamycin C synthesis began. This latter fact suggests that a pool of α-AAA may be formed early in the fermentation and later drawn upon for antibiotic synthesis. Such an observation has not yet been reported. However, INAMINE et al. (1980) determined the intracellular pools of α-AAA in cultures of differing productivity; they found the productive capacity of the organisms to increase coordinately with the α-aminotransferase activity, and the intracellular pool of α-AAA to increase in the same way. Studies on the aminotransferase in *S. lactamdurans* have shown that the enzyme is subject to feedback inhibition by α-AAA but its synthesis is not affected; however the presence of α-AAA in the culture medium led to a more rapid decay of the enzyme (INAMINE et al. 1980). The investigations of the pathway leading to lysine and α-AAA in streptomycetes, discussed above, suggest at least two targets for regulation of the flow of carbon to α-AAA; DAP decarboxylase (KIRKPATRICK et al. 1973a) and L-lysine ε-aminotransferase (KERN et al. 1980). Interference in both their activities or their biosyntheses should lead to interference in antibiotic formation. As the metabolic interrelationship between lysine and α-AAA differ between fungi and actinomycetes, it is of great interest to study whether regulatory effects exerted at the early stages of lysine biosynthesis would affect antibiotic synthesis by the actinomycetes and in which direction.

MENDELOVITZ and AHARONOWITZ (1980) have approached this question in the β-lactam antibiotic producer, *S. clavuligerus*. When lysine, AAA and DAP were added to chemically defined medium at 10 m*M* concentration, the production of antibiotic was increased about twofold. This fact suggested that upon bypassing feedback effects on enzymes involved in lysine biosynthesis, lysine metabolic intermediates and catabolic products might increase in the intracellular free pool, concomitantly producing an increase in antibiotic synthesis. The pathway of lysine biosynthesis and its regulation in *S. clavuligerus* was investigated. It was found that the first enzyme in the path, aspartokinase (AK) is subject to concerted feedback inhibition by lysine and threonine. Dihydrodipicolinate (DDP) synthetase, the first specific enzyme of lysine biosynthesis, was not inhibited by lysine and was partially inhibited by high concentrations of AAA and DL-DAP. The biosynthesis of DDP synthetase was slightly decreased upon addition of 10 m*M* DAP; no other amino acids had any effect. These results suggested that an important control over the carbon flow to lysine is exerted through AK activity. Mutants resistant to the lysine-analog S-(2-aminoethyl)cysteine (AEC) were isolated. In about 75% of these mutants, the AK activity was deregulated, as assayed in vitro, and could not be inhibited by the concerted effect of lysine and threonine. Among these mutants, a large number produced significantly higher amount of antibiotic, ranging from 1.5 to 8 times more than that found in wild-type fermentations. The composition of intracellular free amino acid pools of the wild type and two mutant strains was examined. The main difference between the mutants and the parent strain was a dramatic elevation in the concentration of DAP in extracts of the mutants (MENDELOVITZ and AHARONOWITZ, to be published).

The reason why DAP accumulated instead of lysine or α-AAA was probably due to the inhibition of the DAP-decarboxylase by lysine, as has already been proposed by KIRKPATRICK et al. (1973a). Such a regulation over DAP decarboxylase is important for the cell in order to enable cell wall formation. This suggests that DAP-decarboxylase activity might be rate-limiting step in the formation of the cephamycins. This work examplifies the possible use of simple genetic and biochemical methods in strain-development programs. The isolation of lysine analog-resistant mutants in the fungal and actinomycete systems had two different rationales and led to opposite results. *P. chrysogenum* mutants, resistant to lysine antimetabolite, overproduced lysine and were underproducers of penicillin (MASUREKAR and DEMAIN 1974b). On the other hand, lysine analog–resistant mutants of *S. clavuligerus* were found to accumulate DAP and to overproduce cephamycin (MENDELOVITZ and AHARONOWITZ 1980).

F. Control of β-Lactam Specific Enzymes at the Level of Secondary Metabolism

Very little is known about the enzymes of the specific pathways for biosynthesis of penicillin, cephalosporin or cephamycins leading from the constituent amino acids α-AAA, cysteine and valine to the final β-lactam molecules (see Chap. 5). It is not surprising, therefore, that little, if any, experimental work has been done on regulatory mechanisms controlling these enzymes. In vitro studies are required to characterize the effectors controlling specific enzymes involved in β-lactam biosynthesis.

Genetic evidence first reported by LEMKE and NASH (1972) suggested that mutants unable to produce penicillin fell into two classes: those that were able to synthesize the tripeptide and those that were not (NASH et al. 1974). Genetic investigations on penicillin biosynthesis have been carried out in *P. chrysogenum* and *Aspergillus nidulans* (NORMANSELL et al. 1979; MAKINS et al. 1980). The latter microorganism elaborates much less penicillin than the former, but the formal genetics of *A. nidulans* is much better understood.

Twelve nonproducing or very low-producing mutants of *P. chrysogenum* have been classified in at least five complementation groups with respect to penicillin production (groups V, W, X, Y, and Z). Most mutants belonged to group Y. Mutants belonging to groups X, Y, and Z appeared to be unable to form the tripeptide ACV, so they appeared to be early blocked mutants. Mutants of groups V and W, which appeared to be able to produce ACV but not penicillin, could be blocked either at some stage in the cyclization of the tripeptide to form the nucleus or in the acyltransferase terminal reaction. Extracts of mutants of groups W, Y, and Z were able to catalyze a penicillin–acyl exchange reaction; a mutant of group V showed only a trace of activity and a mutant from group X completely lacked this ability.

It seems therefore that at least three enzymes (and probably four or more) are involved in the conversion of the constituent amino acids into penicillin. These include the tripeptide synthetase that forms the ACV tripeptide, tripeptide cyclase that forms the isopenicillin N nucleus possibly in two steps, an acyltransferase reaction that exchanges the phenylacetyl residue for the α-AAA side chain existing in isopenicillin N. A "racemase" that converts isopenicillin N into penicillin has been found in *C. acremonium* (KONOMI et al. 1979). Some of these enzymes have been partially characterized in vitro (DEMAIN 1981).

I. Possible Control Mechanisms at the Tripeptide Synthetase Level

A cell-free system of *C. acremonium* has been described which is capable of carrying out the biosynthesis of the ACV tripeptide (LODER and ABRAHAM 1971a, b; FAWCETT et al. 1976a, 1976b). ACV was first observed in *P. chrysogenum*, but it has also been found in *C. acremonium* (LODER and ABRAHAM 1971a, b; FAWCETT et al. 1976a) as well as in *S. clavuligerus*, *S. lipmanii* (ABRAHAM 1977; O'SULLIVAN and ABRAHAM 1981), *S. griseus*, and *S. lactamdurans* (LIRAS and MARTIN, unpublished work).

Little is known about the regulation at the tripeptide synthetase level. A particulate fraction of sonicated cells incorporated DL-(^{14}C)valine into ACV when incubated with the dipeptide (L-α-aminoadipyl)-L-cysteine (LODER and ABRAHAM 1971a, b), but no incorporation took place if free L-α-AAA plus cysteine were added to the cell extract. No incorporation of (^{14}C)valine occurred when (D-α-aminoadipyl)-L-cysteine was used. Moreover DL-(^{14}C)-α-AAA was not incorporated into ACV in the presence of L-cys-D-val, L-cys-L-val or L-cysteine plus L-valine. All these results point to a specific sequence of attachment of amino acids to form the tripeptide. It therefore seems likely that specific effectors may alter the ability of tripeptide synthetase to form the tripeptide. Recent results indicate that the formation of tripeptide is reduced by leucine and isoleucine. Furthermore, the tripeptide-forming activity is greatly stimulated in vivo by cycloheximide, indicating that blocking protein synthesis saves amino acids for tripeptide formation (LOPEZ-NIETO, REVILLA and MARTIN, unpublished work).

An interesting result is the observation that carbon catabolite regulation by glucose blocks tripeptide formation in *P. chrysogenum* (REVILLA, LOPEZ-NIETO and MARTIN, to be published).

Little is known about the regulation of the enzymes involved in the conversion of ACV to cephalosporin C except the observation that growth in methionine or isoleucine appears to induce the tripeptide cyclase (SAWADA et al. 1980b; KONOMI et al. 1979) and the ring-expansion enzyme (BALDWIN et al. 1980; HOOK et al. 1979; KOHSAKA and DEMAIN 1976; SAWADA et al. 1979, 1980a; YOSHIDA et al. 1978) (see below).

1. Control of the Cyclization of the Tripeptide

Enzyme extracts prepared by gentle lysis of protoplasts of *Cephalosporium acremonium* showed a weak activity which was able to convert the ACV tripeptide with the LLD configuration into a penicillin (FAWCETT et al. 1976b). The reaction proceeded without hydrolysis of the tripeptide (O'SULLIVAN et al. 1979b). A direct conversion of the ACV tripeptide into penicillin N was suggested initially. However, recent evidence showed that in *Cephalosporium acremonium* the product of the cyclization step is isopenicillin N which is later converted into penicillin N (KONOMI et al. 1979; O'SULLIVAN et al. 1979b). The "racemase" system of *Cephalosporium acremonium* which isomerizes the L-α-aminoadipate side chain of isopenicillin N to the D configuration of penicillin N seems to be extremely labile, and therefore nothing is known about its substrate specificity and regulation (KONOMI et al. 1979; DEMAIN 1981). The nature of the intermediates between the ACV tripeptide and isopenicillin N remained obscure for many years. Recently, MESSCHAERT et al. (1980) obtained preliminary evidence suggesting that the ACV tripeptide is first converted into a monocyclic β-lactam without a dehydrovalinyl intermediate. This proposed monocyclic β-lactam has the chemical structure of 1-(1-D-carboxyl-2-methylpropyl)-3-L-(S-L-aminoadipamide)-4-L-mercaptoazetidin-2-one.

Preliminary evidence indicates that cyclase activity also exists in *P. chrysogenum* (MESSCHAERT et al. 1980) and *Streptomyces clavuligerus* (O'SULLIVAN and ABRAHAM 1980).

The specificity of the cyclase system seems to be quite high since labeled α-aminoadipyl-cysteinyl-valine having the configuration LLL and DLD were not converted into isopenicillin (FAWCETT et al. 1976b).

Little is known about the regulation of the activity of the tripeptide cyclase. The activity of the *C. acremonium* enzyme was stimulated by ferrous ion, suggesting that it is an oxidative system. Optimal activity was obtained at 80 μM ferrous sulfate. In fermentations of an antibiotic negative mutant, the peak of activity was obtained after growth ceased and as occurs with many other enzyme activities it leveled off an decreased sharply thereafter (SAWADA et al. 1980b).

2. Control of the Ring-Expansion System

It is now well established that the five-membered ring of penicillin N is expanded by cell-free extracts of *Cephalosporium* to form deacetoxycephalosporin C (KOSHAKA and DEMAIN 1976). Mutants blocked in the ring-expansion system which accumulate penicillin N and are unable to produce cephalosporin C have been isolated (YOSHIDA et al. 1978; SHIRAFUJI et al. 1979). The product of the ring-expansion system has been definitively identified as deacetoxycephalosporin C (YOSHIDA et al. 1978; BALDWIN et al. 1980).

Regarding its regulation, the ring-expansion system is strongly stimulated by Fe^{2+} and ascorbate (HOOK et al. 1979; SAWADA et al. 1979). These are well-known cofactors of dioxygenases which suggested that the ring-expansion system, as the cyclase activity, is an oxidative system. Since the enzyme is stimulated by 2-oxoglutarate and manganese the system behaves as a 2-oxoglutarate-dependent dioxygenase (FELIX et al. 1981). The formation and disappearance of the ring-expansion system follows the same time course as the cyclase system (SAWADA et al. 1980).

The specificity of the ring expansion enzyme is high since penicillin N but not penicillin G or 6-APA could be recognized by the enzyme.

II. Control of Penicillin Acyltransferase

The last step of penicillin biosynthesis involves the exchange of the α-AAA side chain of isopenicillin N for a phenylacetyl residue, probably activated in the form of phenylacetyl-CoA. The enzyme appears to be able to deacetylate isopenicillin N into 6-APA and to convert 6-APA into penicillin G by acetylation with phenylacetyl-CoA.

The presence of acylase and acyltransferase activity in *P. chrysogenum* and other producers of β-lactam antibiotics has been extensively reviewed by VANDAMME

(1977). There is no doubt of the involvement of acyltransferase in the conversion of isopenicillin N into penicillin G. Isopenicillin N, but not penicillin N, is a substrate for *Penicillium* acyltransferase. Enzyme extracts of *P. chrysogenum* also convert 6-APA into penicillin G. 6-APA appears however to be a shunt metabolite of the penicillin biosynthetic pathway and its role in penicillin biosynthesis is by no means clear.

The possible regulatory mechanisms controlling penicillin acyltransferase have not been studied in detail. It has been reported that the synthetic capability of penicillin acylase was enhanced by using energy-rich side-chain precursors such as phenylacetylglycine and analogs, but this has not been confirmed by further studies. It is well established that addition of phenylacetic or phenoxyacetic acid directs the penicillin fermentation toward the formation of penicillin G or penicillin V and in addition greatly stimulates penicillin formation with respect to unsupplemented fermentations. Although this has been taken as an example of induction of penicillin-synthesizing enzymes, it is not clear whether this stimulation is simply due to a precursor effect.

III. Regulation of Late Enzymes in Cephalosporin and Cephamycin Biosynthesis

Deacetoxycephalosporin C, the product of the ring expansion reaction, is converted by hydroxylation into deacetylcephalosporin C by an α-ketoglutarate linked dioxygenase both in *Cephalosporium acremonium* (FUJISAWA et al. 1977) and *Streptomyces clavuligerus* (TURNER et al. 1978). The enzyme incorporates oxygen from molecular oxygen into deacetylcephalosporin C at an optimal pH of 7.0. It is activated by 2-oxoglutarate, ascorbate, dithiothreitol, and ferrous ions and appears to be quite unstable (LIERSCH et al. 1976).

It is very interesting to note that similar oxidative enzymes are involved in the cyclization reaction of the tripeptide to isopenicillin N, the ring expansion of penicillin N to deacetoxycephalosporin C and the hydroxylation of deacetoxycephalosporin C to deacetylcephalosporin C. All these enzymes may form an enzyme complex with similar regulatory properties thus facilatating the internal diffusion of intermediates.

The hydroxylation reaction depends very strongly on NADH and to a lesser extent on NADPH as cofactors. The enzyme shows a high specificity since neither cephalosporin C nor deacetylcephalosporin C could be used as substrates instead of deacetoxycephalosporin C, while 7-aminodeacetoxycephalosporanic acid could be recognized with about 50% of the hydroxylating activity.

The last intermediate in cephalosporin C biosynthesis, deacetylcephalosporin C, is acetylated using acetyl-CoA as acyl donor. The enzyme acetyl-CoA: deacetylcephalosporin C *O*-acetyltransferase has been characterized in extracts of *C. acremonium* (LIERSCH et al. 1976; FELIX et al. 1980). The enzyme is not very specific with respect to the substituents in the 7-amino group, since it is able to acetylate 7-aminodeacetylcephalosporanic acid (7-ADCA) and other derivatives.

The activity of the transacetylase is subject to feedback regulation. It is 100% inhibited by the final product of the reaction, cephalosporin C and by other semisynthetic cephalosporins and to a lesser extent by deacetoxycephalosporin C and penicillin N (LIERSCH et al. 1976).

Several other late reactions are known to occur during cephamycin biosynthesis in *Streptomyces*. Cephamycin C can be further transformed by enzymes which introduce either an acetoxy, carbamoyl, or some other moiety at the C-3 methyl group (BREWER et al. 1980) or a methoxy group at the C-7 position of the cephem nucleus (WHITNEY et al. 1972; O'SULLIVAN et al. 1979a).

Cell-free extracts of *Streptomyces* have been prepared which can carry out the transfer of the carbamoyl group from carbamoyl phosphate (BREWER et al. 1980). Introduction of the methoxy group requires the presence of S-adenosylmethionine, 2-oxoglutarate, Fe^{2+}, and a reducing agent such as ascorbate, suggesting that the system contains a methyltransferase and a dioxygenase (O'SULLIVAN and ABRAHAM 1980).

Nothing is known about the regulation of the α-ketoglutarate-linked dioxygenase converting deacetoxycephalosporin C to deacetylcephalosporin C or of the late reactions yielding cephamycins in actinomycetes (BREWER et al. 1980; O'SULLIVAN et al. 1979a, b; O'SULLIVAN and ABRAHAM 1980).

G. End-Product Regulation

Feedback control of biosynthetic reactions is an important mechanism of control of cell economy. However, for some time it was doubtful whether feedback control of antibiotic biosynthesis was of any significance in the degree of antibiotic production, due to the lack of knowledge of the enzymes involved. Recently, however, it has become evident that several antibiotics inhibit their own biosynthesis. Examples of feedback regulation of antibiotic biosynthesis include chloramphenicol, aurodox, cycloheximide, staphylomycin, ristomycin, puromycin, fungicidin, candihexin, and mycophenolic acid (see reviews by MARTIN 1978; MARTIN and DEMAIN 1980).

GORDEE and DAY (1972) claimed that penicillin inhibits its own biosynthesis. Although the significance of the data has been challenged (NESTAAS and DEMAIN 1981), recent use of a resting cell system that measures the incorporation of (^{14}C)valine into penicillin showed that high levels of exogenous penicillin fully inhibit de novo penicillin synthesis (REVILLA et al. 1978; MARTIN et al. 1979b). The concentration of exogenous penicillin required for complete inhibition depended upon the antibiotic level usually attained by each producer strain. Exogenous concentrations of 600 μg penicillin per milliliter fully inhibited penicillin synthesis by the low-producing strain Wis 54-1255, which normally produces 600 μg penicillin per milliliter. A high-producing strain, AS-P-78, which produces more than 5,000 μg penicillin per milliliter, required about 10,000 μg exogenous penicillin per milliliter to get complete inhibition of penicillin synthesis.

It has been observed that exogenous penicillin decreases the incorporation of (^{14}C)valine into penicillin when added at the time of inoculation, but has less or no effect when added later (REVILLA et al. 1978; MARTIN et al. 1979b). This appears to be due to a decreased uptake of exogenous penicillin as the fermentation proceeds. Exogenous penicillin may act by inhibiting the excretion of endogenously formed penicillin as the fermentation proceeds since it does not inhibit either homocitrate synthase, the first enzyme of the lysine biosynthetic pathway or tripeptide synthetase (REVILLA, LOPEZ-NIETO, and MARTIN, unpublished work).

Recently it has been suggested that the degradation of exogenous penicillin during the fermentation may account for the reduction in penicillin titers after addition of exogenous penicillin (NESTAAS and DEMAIN 1981). This is not the case in the work of MARTIN et al. (1979b) since the effect of de novo penicillin biosynthesis was measured by the incorporation of (^{14}C)valine into penicillin. Moreover, labeled penicillin added to the fermentation was degraded to the extent of only 15%–20% during a 96-h fermentation, which cannot explain the feedback effect which under some conditions amounts to a 100% reduction of penicillin biosynthesis.

End-product regulation by cephalosporin of the transacetylase activity of *C. acremonium* converting deacetylcephalosporin C into cephalosporin C has been described above.

H. Summary and Future Outlook

In the last few years, experiments with broken cell systems, especially with lysates of protoplasts of *C. acremonium* and *S. clavuligerus* have provided some insight of the biosynthesis of β-lactam antibiotics. Further studies in vitro are required for establishing unequivocally the regulatory mechanisms that control the biosynthesis of β-lactam antibiotics, and the effectors involved.

References

Abraham EP (1977) β-Lactam antibiotics and related substances. Jpn J Antibiot [Suppl] 30:S1–S26

Abraham EP (1978) Developments in the chemistry and biochemistry of β-lactam antibiotics. In: Hütter R, Leisinger T, Nuesch J, Wehrli W (eds) Antibiotics and other secondary metabolites. Academic Press, London, p 141

Aharonowitz Y (1979) Regulatory interrelationships of nitrogen metabolism and cephalosporin biosynthesis. In: Sebek OK, Laskin AI (ed) Genetics of industrial microorganisms. American Society of Microbiology, Washington DC, p 210

Aharonowitz Y (1980) Nitrogen metabolite regulation of antibiotic biosynthesis. Annu Rev Microbiol 34:209–233

Aharonowitz Y, Demain AL (1978) Carbon catabolite regulation of cephalosporin production in *Streptomyces clavuligerus*. Antimicrob Agents Chemother 14:159–164

Aharonowitz Y, Demain AL (1979) Nitrogen nutrition and regulation of cephalosporin production in *Streptomyces clavuligerus*. Can J Microbiol 25:61–67

Arnstein HRV, Grant PT (1954) The biosynthesis of penicillin. The incorporation of some amino acids into penicillin. Biochem J 57:353–359

Arnstein HRV, Artman M, Morris D, Toms EJ (1960) Sulfur-containing amino acids and peptides in the mycelium of *Penicillium chrysogenum*. Biochem J 76:353–357

Baldwin JE, Singh PD, Yoshida M, Sawada Y, Demain AL (1980) Incorporation of ^{3}H and ^{14}C from (6α-^{3}H)penicillin N and (10-^{14}C, 6α-^{3}H)penicillin N into deacetoxycephalosporin C. Biochem J 186:889–895

Bonner D (1947) Studies on the biosynthesis of penicillin. Arch Biochem 13:1–9

Brewer SJ, Taylor PM, Turner MK (1980) An adenosine triphosphate dependent carbamoyl-3-hydroxymethylcephem O-carbamoyltransferase from *Streptomyces clavuligerus*. Biochem J 185:555–564

Caltrider PG, Niss HF (1966) Role of methionine in cephalosporin synthesis. Appl Microbiol 14:746–753

Demain AL (1957) Inhibition of penicillin formation by lysine. Arch Biochem Biophys 67:244–245

Demain AL (1963) Synthesis of cephalosporin C by resting cells of *Cephalosporium sp.* Clin Med 70:2045–2051

Demain AL (1974) Biochemistry of penicillin and cephalosporin fermentations. Lloydia 37:147–167

Demain AL (1981) Biosynthetic manipulations in the development of β-lactam antibiotics. In: Salton MRJ, Shockman GD (eds) β-Lactams, mode of action, new developments and future perspectives. Academic Press, New York, p 567

Demain AL, Masurekar PS (1974) Lysine inhibition of *in vivo* homocitrate synthesis in *Pencillium chrysogenum.* J Gen Microbiol 82:143–151

Demain AL, Kennel YM, Aharonowitz Y (1979) Carbon catabolite regulation of secondary metabolism. In: Bull AT, Ellwood DC, Ratledge C (eds) Microbial technology: current state, future prospects, vol 29. Cambridge University Press, Cambridge, p 163

Drew SW, Demain AL (1975a) Production of cephalosporin C by single and double sulfur auxotrophic mutants of *Cephalosporium acremonium.* Antimicrob Agents Chemother 8:5–10

Drew SW, Damain AL (1975b) The obligatory role of methionine in the conversion of sulfate to cephalosporin C. Eur J Appl Microbiol 2:121–128

Drew SW, Demain AL (1975c) Stimulation of cephalosporin production by methionine peptides in a mutant blocked in reverse transulfuration. J Antibiot 28:889–895

Drew SW, Demain AL (1977) Effect of primary metabolites on secondary metabolism. Annu Rev Microbiol 31:343–356

Espin G, Palacios R, Mora J (1979) Glutamine metabolism in nitrogen-starved conidia of *Neurospora crassa.* J Gen Microbiol 115:59–68

Fawcett PA, Usher JJ, Abraham EP (1976a) Aspects of cephalosporin and penicillin biosynthesis. In: Macdonald KD (ed) Second international symposium on the genetics of industrial microorganisms. Academic Press, New York, p 129

Fawcett PA, Usher JJ, Hudleston RC, Bleany RC, Nisbet JJ, Abraham EP (1976b) Synthesis of δ(α-aminoadipyl)-cysteinylvaline and its role in penicillin biosynthesis. Biochem J 157:651–660

Felix HR, Nuesch J, Wehrli W (1980) Investigation of the two final steps on the biosynthesis of cephalosporin C using permeabilized cells of *Cephalosporium acremonium.* FEMS Microbiol Lett 8:55–58

Flynn EH, McCormick MH, Stamper MC, De Valeria H, Godzeski DW (1962) A new natural penicillin from *Penicillium chrysogenum.* J Chem Soc 84:4594

Friedrich CG, Demain AL (1977) Homocitrate synthase as the crucial site of the lysine effect on penicillin biosynthesis. J Antibiot 30:760–761

Friedrich CG, Demain AL (1978) Uptake and metabolism of α-aminoadipic acid by *Penicillium chrysogenum* Wis 54-1255. Arch Microbiol 119:43–47

Fujisawa Y, Kikuchi M, Kanzaki T (1977) Deacetylcephalosporin C synthesis by cell-free extracts of *Cephalosporium acremonium.* J Antibiot 30:775–777

Gaillardin CM, Poirier L, Heslot H (1976) A kinetic study of homocitrate synthase activity in the yeast *Saccharomycopsis lipolytica.* Biochim Biophys Acta 432:390–406

Ginther L (1979) Sporulation and the production of serine protease and cephamycin C by *Streptomyces lactamdurans.* Antimicrob Agents Chemother 150:522–526

Gordee EZ, Day LE (1972) Effect of exogenous penicillin on penicillin biosynthesis. Antimicrob Agents Chemother 1:315–322

Goulden SA (1969) Some aspects of metabolic control in *Penicillium chrysogenum.* Ph. D. thesis, University of Leeds

Gygax D, Dobeli N, Nuesch J (1980) Correlation between β-lactam antibiotics production and γ-cystathionase activity. Experientia 36:487

Higgens CE, Kastner RE (1971) *Streptomyces clavuligerus* sp. nov., a β-lactam antibiotic producer. Int J Syst Bacteriol 21:326–331

Hinnen A, Nuesch J (1976) Enzymatic hydrolysis of cephalosporin C by an extracellular acetylhydrolase of *Cephalosporium acremonium.* Antimicrob Agents Chemother 9:824–830

Hogg RW, Broquist HP (1968) Homocitrate formation in *Neurospora crassa* in relation to lysine biosynthesis. J Biol Chem 243:1839–1845

Hook DJ, Chang LT, Elander RP, Morin RB (1979) Stimulation of the conversion of penicillin N to cephalosporin by ascorbic acid, α-ketoglutarate, and ferrous ions in cell-free extracts of *Cephalosporium acremonium*. Biochem Biophys Res Commun 87:258–265

Hostalek Z (1980) Catabolite regulation of antibiotic biosynthesis. Folia Microbiol (Praha) 25:445–450

Inamine E, Kern BA, Hendlin D (1980) Paper presented at Ann. Mtg. Am. Soc. Microbiol., Miami. 11–16 May 1980

Kern BA, Hendlin D, Inamine E (1980) L-Lysine ε-aminotransferase involved in cephamycin C synthesis in *Streptomyces lactamdurans*. Antimicrob Agents Chemother 17:679–685

Kirpatrick JR, Doolin JL, Godfrey OW (1973a) Lysine biosynthesis in *Stretomyces lipmanii*. Implication in antibiotic biosynthesis. Antimicrob Agents Chemother 4:542–550

Kirpatrick JR, Godfrey OW, Doolin LE (1973b) The role of lysine in antibiotic biosynthesis in *Streptomyces lipmanii*. Abstr Annu Meet Am Soc Microbiol E74:13

Kohsaka M, Demain AL (1976) Conversion of penicillin N to cephalosporins by cell-free extracts of *Cephalosporium acremonium*. Biochem Biophys Res Commun 70:465–473

Komatsu KI, Mizuno M, Kodira R (1975) Effect of methionine on cephalosporin C and penicillin N production by a mutant of *Cephalosporium acremonium*. J Antibiot (Tokyo) 28:881–888

Kominek LA (1972) Biosynthesis of novobiocin by *Streptomyces niveus*. Antimicrob Agents Chemother 1:123–134

Konomi T, Herchen S, Baldwin JE, Yoshida M, Hunt NA, Demain AL (1979) Cell-free conversion of δ-(L-α-aminoadipyl)-L-cysteinyl-D-valine into an antibiotic with the properties of isopenicillin N in *Cephalosporium acremonium*. Biochem J 184:427–430

Kuenzi MT (1980) Regulation of cephalosporin synthesis in *Cephalosporium acremonium* by phosphate and glucose. Arch Microbiol 128:78–81

Lemke P, Nash C (1972) Mutations that affect antibiotic synthesis by *Cephalosporium acremonium*. Can J Microbiol 18:255–259

Liersch M, Nuesch J, Treichler HJ (1976) Final steps in the biosynthesis of cephalosporin C. In: MacDonald KD (ed) Second international symposium on the genetics of industrial microorganisms. Academic Press, New York, p 179

Liersch M, Treichler HJ, Nuesch J (1980) Correlation between cysteine synthase activity and cephalosporin C production in *Cephalosporium acremonium*. Experientia 36:487

Lilley G, Clark AE, Lawrence GC (1981) Control of the production of cephamycin C and thienamycin by *Streptomyces cattleya* NRRL 8057. J Chem Tech Biotechnol 31:127–134

Liras P, Castro JM, Martin JF (1982) Production of cephamycin by *S. lactamdurans* NRRL 3802 and Amy$^-$ variants. Abstracts IVth international symposium on genetics of industrial microorganisms. Kyoto, p 112

Loder PB, Abraham EP (1971a) Isolation and nature of intracellular peptides from a cephalosporin C-producing *Cephalosporium* sp. Biochem J 123:471–476

Loder PB, Abraham EP (1971b) Biosynthesis of peptides containing α-aminoadipic acid and cysteine in extracts of *Cephalosporium* sp. Biochem J 123:477–482

Luengo JM, Revilla G, Villanueva JR, Martin JF (1979) Lysine regulation of penicillin biosynthesis in low-producing and industrial strains of *Penicillium chrysogenum*. J Gen Microbiol 115:207–211

Luengo JM, Revilla G, Lopez-Nieto MJ, Villanueva JR, Martin JF (1980) Inhibition and repression of homocitrate synthetase by lysine in *Penicillium chrysogenum*. J Bacteriol 144:869–876

Magasanik B (1961) Catabolite repression. Cold Spring Harbor Symp. Quant. Biol. 26:249–250

Makins JF, Holt G, MacDonald KD (1980) Cosynthesis of penicillin following treatment of mutants of *Aspergillus nidulans* impaired in antibiotic production with lytic enzymes. J Gen Microbiol 119:397–404

Maragoudakis ME, Holmes H, Strassman M (1967) Control of lysine biosynthesis in yeast by a feedback mechanism. J Bacteriol 93:1667–1680

Martin JF (1978) Manipulation of gene expression in the development of antibiotic production. In: Leisinger T, Hutter R, Nuesch J, Wehrli W (eds) Antibiotics and other secondary metabolites: biosynthesis and production. Academic Press, London, p 19
Martin JF (1981) Biosynthesis of metabolic products with antimicrobial activities: β-lactam antibiotics. In: Schaal KP, Pulverer G (eds) Actinomycetes. Fischer, Stuttgart, p 417
Martin JF, Demain AL (1980) Control of antibiotic biosynthesis. Microbiol Rev 44:230–251
Martin JF, Luengo JM, Revilla G, Villanueva JR (1979) Biochemical genetics of the β-lactam antibiotic biosynthesis. In: Sebek OK, Laskin AI (eds) Genetics of industrial microorganisms. American Society for Microbiology, Washington D.C., p 83
Masurekar PS, Demain AL (1972) Lysine control of penicillin biosynthesis. Can J Microbiol 18:1045–1048
Masurekar PS, Demain AL (1974a) Insensitivity of homocitrate synthase in extracts of *Penicillium chrysogenum* to feedback inhibition by lysine. Appl Microbiol 28:265–270
Masurekar PS, Demain AL (1974b) Impaired penicillin production in lysine regulatory mutants of *Penicillium chrysogenum*. Antimicrob Agents Chemother 6:366–368
Matsumura M, Imanaka T, Yoshida T, Taguchi H (1978) Effect of glucose and methionine compsumption rates on cephalosporin C production by *Cephalosporium acremonium*. J Ferment Technol 56:345–353
Mendelovitz S, Aharonowitz Y (1980) Cephalosporin production by *Streptomyces clavuligerus* mutant possessing a deregulated aspartokinase activity. Abstr sixth int ferment symp, 20–25 July 1980, London, Canada. National Research Council Publications
Meesschaert B, Adriaens P, Eyssen H (1980) Studies on the biosynthesis of isopenicillin N with a cell-free preparation of *Penicillium chrysogenum*. J Antibiot 33:722–730
Mehta RJ, Speth JL, Nash CH (1979) Lysine stimulation of cephalosporin C synthesis in *Cephalosporium acremonium*. Eur J Appl Microbiol Biotechnol 8:177–182
Nash C, De La Higuera N, Neuss N, Lemke PA (1974) Application of biochemical genetics to the biosynthesis of β-lactam antibiotics. Dev Ind Microbiol 15:114–123
Nestaas E, Demain AL (1981) Influence of penicillin instability on interpretation of feedback regulation experiments. Eur J Appl Microbiol Biotechnol 12:170–172
Normansell PJ, Normansell ID, Holt H (1979) Genetic and biochemical studies of mutants of *Penicillium chrysogenum* impaired in penicillin production. J Gen Microbiol 112:113–126
Nuesch J, Treichler HJ, Liersch M (1973) The biosynthesis of cephalosporin C. In: Vanek Z, Hostalek Z, Cudlin J (eds) Genetics of industrial microorganisms, vol 2. Academia, Prague, p 309
O'Sullivan J, Abraham EP (1980) The conversion of cephalosporins to 7-α-methoxycephalosporins by cell-free extracts of *Streptomyces clavuligerus*. Biochem J 186:613–616
O'Sullivan J, Abraham EP (1981) Biosynthesis of β-lactam antibiotics. In: Corcoran JW (ed) Antibiotics IV. Biosynthesis. Springer, Berlin Heidelberg New York, p 101
O'Sullivan J, Aplin RT, Stevens CM, Abraham EP (1979a) Biosynthesis of 7-α-methoxycephalosporin. Incorporation of molecular oxygen. Biochem J 179:47–52
O'Sullivan J, Bleany RC, Huddleston JA, Abraham EP (1979b) Incorporation of ^{3}H from δ[L-α-amino(4,5-^{3}H)adipyl]-L-cysteinyl-D-(4,4-^{3}H) valine into isopenicillin N. Biochem J 184:421–426
Paigen K, Williams B (1970) Catabolite repression and other control mechanisms in carbohydrate utilization. Adv Microb Physiol 4:251–324
Pastan I, Adhya S (1976) Cyclic adenosine 5′-monophosphate in *Escherichia coli*. Bacteriol Rev 40:527–551
Pastan I, Perlman R (1970) Cyclic adenosine monophosphate in bacteria. Science 169:339–344
Pirt SJ (1969) Microbial growth and product formation. Symp Soc Gen Microbiol 19:199–221
Pogell BM, Sankaran L, Redshaw PA, McCann PA (1976) Regulation of antibiotic biosynthesis and differentiation in *Streptomyces*. In: Schlessinger D (ed) Microbiology 1976. American Society for Microbiology, Washington DC, p 543
Revilla G, Luengo JM, Martin JF (1978) End-product regulation of penicillin biosynthesis. Abstr first Eur congr biotechnol, Interlaken, p 3/51–3/52

Revilla G, Luengo JM, Villanueva JR, Martin JF (1981) Carbon catabolite repression of penicillin biosynthesis. In: Vezina C, Singh K (eds) Advances in biotechnology, vol III. Pergamon Press, Toronto, p 155

Sanchez S, Paniagua L, Mateos RC, Lara F, Mora J (1980) Nitrogen regulation of penicillin biosynthesis in *Penicillium chrysogenum*. In: Vezina C, Singh K (eds) Advances in biotechnology, vol III. Pergamon Press, Toronto, p 147

Sawada Y, Hunt NA, Demain AL (1979) Further studies on microbiological ring expansion of penicillin N. J Antibiot 32:1303–1310

Sawada Y, Solomon NA, Demain AL (1980a) Stimulation of the cell-free ring expansion of penicillin N by sonication and triton X-100. Biotechnol Lett 2:43–48

Sawada Y, Baldwin JE, Singh PD, Solomon NA, Demain AL (1980b) Cell-free cyclization of δ-(L-α-aminoadipyl)-L-cysteinyl-D-valine to isopenicillin N. Antimicrob Agents Chemother 18:465–470

Sawada Y, Konomi T, Solomon NA, Demain AL (1980c) Increase in activity of β-lactam synthetases after growth of *Cephalosporium acremonium* with methionine or norleucine. FEMS Microbiol Lett 9:281–284

Segal IH, Johnson MJ (1961) Accumulation of intracellular inorganic sulfate by *Penicillium chrysogenum*. J Bacteriol 81:91–98

Segal IH, Johnson JM (1963) Intermediates in inorganic sulphate utilization by *Penicillium chrysogenum*. Arch Biochem Biophys 103:216–226

Soltero FV, Johnson MJ (1953) Effect of the carbohydrate nutrition on penicillin production by *P. chrysogenum* Q-176. Appl Microbiol 1:52–57

Somerson NL, Demain AL, Nunheimer TD (1961) Reversal of lysine inhibition of penicillin production by α-aminoadipic acid. Arch Biochem Biophys 93:238–241

Streicher SL, Tyler B (1981) Regulation of glutamine synthetase by adenylylation in the gram-positive bacterium *Streptomyces cattleya*. Proc Natl Acad Sci USA 78:229–233

Treichler HJ, Liersch M, Nuesch J, Dobeli H (1979) Role of sulfur metabolism in cephalosporin C and penicillin biosynthesis. In: Sebek OK, Laskin AI (eds) Genetics of industrial microorganisms. American Society for Microbiology, Washington DC, p 97

Trown PW, Smith B, Abraham EP (1963) Biosynthesis of cephalosporin C from amino acids. Biochem J 86:284–291

Tucci AF (1969) Feedback inhibition of lysine biosynthesis in yeasts. J Bacteriol 99:624–625

Tucci AF, Ceci LN (1972) Control of lysine biosynthesis in yeasts. Arch Biochem Biophys 153:751–754

Turner MK, Farthing JE, Brewer SJ (1978) The oxygenation of (3-methyl-^{3}H)deacetoxycephalosporin C to (3-hydroxymethyl-^{3}H)deacetyl cephalosporin C by 2-oxoglutarate linked dioxygenases from *Acremonium chrysogenum* and *Streptomyces clavuligerus*. Biochem J 173:839–850

Tyler B (1978) Regulation of the assimilation of nitrogen compounds. Annu Rev Biochem 47:1127–1162

Umbarger HE (1978) Amino acid biosynthesis and its regulation. Annu Rev Biochem 47:533–606

Vandamme ET (1977) Enzymes involved in β-lactam antibiotic biosynthesis. Adv Appl Microbiol 21:89–123

Warren SC, Newton GGF, Abraham EP (1967) Use of α-aminoadipic acid for the biosynthesis of penicillin N and cephalosporin C by a *Cephalosporium* sp. Biochem J 103:891–901

Wax R, Snyder L (1980) Glutamine synthetase of *Streptomyces cattleya*. Annu meet Am soc microbiol [Abstr] American Society for Microbiology Publications. Washington DC, p 107

Whitney JG, Brannon DR, Mabe JA, Wicker KJ (1972) Incorporation of labelled precursors into A16886B, a novel β-lactam antibiotic produced by *Streptomyces clavuligerus*. Antimicrob Agents Chemother 1:247–251

Yoshida M, Konomi T, Kohsaka M et al. (1978) Cell-free ring expansion of penicillin N to deacetoxycephalosporin C by *Cephalosporium acremonium* CW-19 and its mutants. Proc Natl Acid Sci USA 75:6253–6257

CHAPTER 8

Biochemical Engineering and β-Lactam Antibiotic Production

D.-G. Mou

A. Introduction

Technologically, biochemical engineering is an essential discipline concerned with fermentation production of antibiotics. It is by its exercise that the principles outlined under biochemistry, microbiology, and chemical engineering are put into commercial practice. In theory, all antibiotics can be produced by three different fermentation systems: batch, fed-batch, and continuous. The development of a batch process demands little engineering design and much empirical and experimental work. Many of the low-volume and high-cost antibiotics are believed to be produced by this type of process, in which the entire nutrient supply is present initially. Additions during the run may include acid and/or base for pH control, antifoam agents, biosynthetic precursors, and water. For some high-volume and low-cost products, the concern over manufacturing productivity and cost control frequently presses for the better engineered fed-batch process originally designed for penicillin production. In this case, the sugar concentration is kept low by controlled addition of the supply according to a programmed schedule. This enables external manipulation of some of the key biological events while tighter control is exerted on raw material usage. Frequently, a feedback mechanism is employed by operating from a measurement of a certain biochemical parameter such as dissolved oxygen concentration, pH, or carbon dioxide concentration. Fed-batch systems approach the biochemical conditions obtained in steady-state processes, except that cellular activities are more uniform (narrower "age" distribution) and the cell and product concentrations increase continously in the former.

A continuous process operates under steady-state conditions. That is, the concentration of all nutrients, cell density, excretion products, and microbiological parameters such as cell growth rate, morphology, and macromolecular composition remain constant. A selected balance is obtained between input and outflow of all the contributing components in the production vessel. For the steady-state conditions to be maintained, such systems have to be controlled by relatively complex equipment, and in-depth understanding of the fermentation kinetics is often necessary. If specific conditions are required during certain periods of the growth cycle to maximize the efficiency of cellular synthesis, multiple-vessel systems become necessary. The cells then pass from vessel to vessel, the conditions being different in each. In a simple two-stage system, the first vessel normally cultivates the cellular mass and biosynthetic "capacity" of the individual cell, and the second optimizes the productivity and substrate-conversion efficiency. This has the disadvantage of subjecting cells to some shock as nutrient and product concentrations, pH, temperature, and other conditions may change suddenly at the moment of transfer. Other factors that bar most of the continuous processes from industrial practice include contamination hazard, strain degeneration, unacceptable trade-off of substrate-conversion efficiency, and costly recovery of the low-potency broth.

Antibiotic production processes share certain basic features of all fermentation processes. The essential ones are raw-material storage/batching, sterilization, reaction-vessel construction, culture maintenance, seed-culture production, monitoring of feeds, temperature, pH, and foam control, cell separation, and gaseous/solid/liquid effluent disposal. Special features of antibiotic fermentation include the use of complex slow-releasing particulate nutrients for carbon and nitrogen, kinetics of product accumulation, filamentous type of cell growth at the fermentation stage, and costly product extraction and purification at the recovery stage.

Because of the relatively easier success with strain improvement, much effort is usually devoted to fermentation process development and little is directed to study of product recovery. After all, the maximum possible recovery efficiency can go no higher than 100%, whereas the fermentation yield improvements of tens or hundreds of that are not unusual. Aside from what is contributed by better genetic makeup, this success depends on theoretical understanding of the biosynthetic pathway(s) and fermentation kinetics. Owing to the differences in medium complexity, broth rheology, and geometric scale, the engineering practice of this understanding is frequently difficult. Although laboratory investigation under relatively defined conditions may aid the situation, a pilot plant capable of simulating as many features as possible of the production-scale equipment is necessary for most purposes. It is here that the confidence in scaling up new strains and processes can be properly established.

Because of these peculiar complications, process development work often emphasizes an individual's specific experience and results in laborious trial-and-error experimental routines. From shake-flask discovery to production-scale materialization, the compounded efforts of many individuals in different scientific disciplines are involved. However successful in improving the fermentation productivity and/or economy, these efforts often stop at superficial understanding of the final experimental results, and must be repeated time and again whenever a key process variable such as the producing strain or the complex nutrient source is varied. With subjective personal observations short-circuiting communication and an indirect dependent variable such as broth titer being the absolute scale for strain/process evaluation, this development exercise can become extremely time-consuming. On the other hand, the frequently refined production protocol is often so specific and strict that it usually discriminates against new production strains or process conditions. To improve communication and to start some kind of reciprocal approach between the development laboratory and the manufacturing plant, one needs to demonstrate a generalized methodology that would allow quantitative interpretation in the laboratory and thus aid the production scale-up by providing scientific rationale and justified expectation.

Hence, for the simple reason of practicality, the present chapter will not review each individual fermentation process used for production of β-lactam antibiotics. Instead, it will formulate a generalized methodology for process development, with the fed-batch penicillin fermentation as an example. The relatively comprehensive understanding of this fermentation allows a critical and accurate analysis of our findings. Furthermore, the experimental data obtained from Panlabs' high-yielding *Pencillium chrysogenum* strain P-2 also provide a realistic insight into the engineering of a modern production strain. For an up-to-date review of fermentations of β-lactam antibiotics, see the paper by ELANDER and AOKI (to be published). SWARTZ's (1979) paper is highly recommended for techniques useful for analyzing the economics of a fermentation process. Also, the review article by QUEENER and SWARTZ (1979) on penicillin manufacturing makes an exhaustive review unnecessary here.

To fulfill the stated objective of this chapter, answers to the following questions will be explored:

1. What are the key process parameters that can be readily addressed by existing technology?
2. Can a complex medium be simplified to enable realistic process interpretation?
3. What motivates the use of computer-coupled fermentors for antibiotic fermentation process development?
4. What is involved in generating a successful computer-based methodology for on-line growth control?
5. How are improvements of tank productivity and overall substrate-conversion efficiency linked to on-line growth control by computer?
6. Can corn-steep liquor in production media be replaced by glucose?

B. Penicillin Fermentation – Current Status

Fleming's original strain of *Penicillium notatum* produced only a few milligrams of penicillin per liter, but today's production strains approach broth potencies of penicillin G close to 30 g/liter, i.e., 50,000 Oxford units/ml (SWARTZ 1979). This improvement, according to DEMAIN (1973), was initially due to advances in the art of submerged fermentation (1941–1946) and later due to successful mutagenesis carried out by the testing of random survivors, as well as morphological and color mutants (1946–1969). Panlabs' 1973 P-2 strain produced 8.3 g/liter, and its most recent P-15 produces 29.4 g/liter of penicillin G (as the potassium salt) (SWARTZ 1979). Note, however, that high-producing strains, although superior to their parent in penicillin production under one particular condition (such as a batch fermentation in shake flasks), are not necessarily superior under a different condition (such as a glucose fed-batch fermentation in a mechanically agitated deep tank) and vice versa. Alteration of the genotypic makeup of the new isolate may call for different environmental conditions to allow the expression of improved cellular productivity. Hence, without extensive "screening" for the matching process condition for a particular mutant, one may find that often it is not the laboratory scientist but rather the established fermentation conditions that screen for the superior culture. This is why process scale-down is just as important as scale-up (AIBA et al. 1973).

To establish priorities for fermentation process development, Swartz at the Eli Lilly Company has presented an updated economic analysis of the penicillin G fermentation (SWARTZ 1979). Parts of his results are summarized in Table 1, which shows that penicillin production cost is associated mostly with the fermentation step. For a fully depreciated plant, sugar and precursor consumptions account for

Table 1. Analysis of penicillin manufacturing cost. (Swartz 1979)

	(% of total)
Fermentation cost	
Raw materials	
Glucose	12
Precursor	11
Others	5
Utility	12
Labor/supervision	3
Maintenance/laboratory	9
Fixed charges	21
Plant overhead	6
Purification cost	
Direct production cost	13
Fixed charge/plant overhead	8
	100

more than a third of the total fermentation cost. Their efficient conversion into penicillin is therefore an important process objective to consider.

To follow glucose consumption in penicillin fermentation, Cooney (1979) has presented a simple mechanistic model. His calculation indicates that during a 126-h fermentation of Panlabs' strain P-2, 70%, 26%, and 4% of total glucose consumed is directed to growth, maintenance, and penicillin synthesis, respectively. Had this been Panlabs' modern strain P-15 and had the growth curve and fermentation cycle time remained the same, the results would have been a glucose distribution of 52%, 38%, and 10% toward growth, maintenance, and penicillin synthesis, respectively. This calculation is based on the reported P-15 overall conversion yield ($\bar{Y}_{P/S}$) of 0.12 g penicillin G per gram glucose consumed (Swartz 1979). On the other hand, if the (average) maintenance demand (g glucose/g cells per hour) and the fermentation growth/production curves are known for a particular culture, the economic coefficient in converting glucose to penicillin ($\bar{Y}_{P/S}$) can also be estimated. A sample calculation based on a simplified growth curve is illustrated in Table 2. Here we borrow the maintenance glucose demand (m) figure of 0.022 g/g per hour of *P. chrysogenum* Wis. 54-1255 published by Righelato et al. (1968). The resulting overall conversion yield of 0.17 g penicillin/g glucose is higher than the 0.12 g/g claimed for strain P-15. However, this could be due to the relatively short cycling time used in the calculation. If the production phase is extended for 60 h more, the maintenance demand would increase to 103 g glucose/liter and the overall conversion yield would drop to 0.138 g/g glucose.

Penicillin fermentation objectives can be better described by the following two equations of total antibiotic accumulation and total substrate consumption:

$$\int dP = \int X \cdot q_{\text{pen}} \cdot dt\,, \tag{1}$$

$$\int dS = \int X \cdot \left(\frac{\mu}{Y_{X/S}} + m + \frac{q_{\text{pen}}}{Y_{P/S}} \right) \cdot dt\,, \tag{2}$$

Table 2. Estimation of "maximum" overall conversion yield of glucose to penicillin

1. Growth demand – cells grow in the fast-growth phase to *20 g/liter* at *30 h* and then grow linearly to double their concentration at *126 h*.
   Observed maximum growth yield ($Y_{X/S}$) = 0.48 g/g
   glucose consumed for growth (S_X) = 40/0.48
   = 83.3 g/liter

2. Production demand – final penicillin concentration is that of Panlabs' P-15 strain, *30 g/liter*.
   Theoretical conversion yield of glucose to penicillin ($Y_{P/S}$) = 1.2 g/g (COONEY and ACEVEDO 1977)
   Glucose consumed for penicillin synthesis (S_P) = 30/1.2 = 25 g/liter

3. Maintenance demand – the average maintenance demand is assumed to be negligible during the fast-growth phase and *0.022 g/g cells per hour* during the production phase.
   $$\text{Glucose consumed for cell maintenance } (S_m) = m \int_{30}^{126} X\,dt = (0.022)\left[\frac{(20+40)(126-30)}{2}\right] = 63.4 \text{ g/liter}$$

4. Total demand for glucose = $S_X + S_P + S_m$
   = 83.3 + 25 + 63.4
   = 171.7 g/liter

5. "Maximum" overall conversion
   Yield of glucose to penicillin = 30/171.7
   = 0.17 g penicillin g glucose

(All concentration figures are based on final harvest volume)

where $Y_{X/S}$ is the observed maximum growth yield and $Y_{P/S}$ is the theoretical conversion yield of glucose to penicillin (COONEY and ACEVEDO 1977). Improvement of q_{pen} obviously would bring proportionally higher broth titer and volumetric productivity. For a specific production demand, this also means reduction of cell concentration X, which in turn could be translated by Eq. (2) into reduced sugar demand for cell growth and maintenance and thus improved overall conversion yield of glucose to penicillin ($\bar{Y}_{P/S} = \int dP / \int dS$). Reduced cell concentration also implies lowered broth viscosity and enhanced bulk mixing and mass transfer and nullifies demands for extra agitator power and cooling capacity. Table 3 clearly illustrates the net accomplishment of strain improvement in achieving higher tank productivity and efficient substrate conversion.

It now becomes clear that improvement of the economics of penicillin production has to rely on (a) the increase of broth potency and (b) the decrease of cell growth and/or maintenance demand for glucose relative to the amount of penicillin produced. Although the industrial mutation/screening program has scored well for the former in the past, an objective selection for the latter is particularly beneficial today, considering the keen competition and rising cost of raw material.

To maximize the growth yield, $Y_{X/S}$ (g cells/g glucose), one considers the effects of strain, carbohydrate source, precursor toxicity, inoculum, broth sugar concen-

Table 3. Improvement of penicillin fermentation during 1950–1978

P. chrysogenum strain	Medium	Total utilization of (g/liter)		Volume (liter)	Control method[a]	t[b]	X[b]	P[b]	$\bar{Y}_{P/S}$[b]	G[b]	Reference
		Sugars	N source								
Wis. Q-176	Complex	Lactose, 30 glucose, 10	CSL solids, 40	15	*a*+*b*	105	19[c]	1,820	0.010	17	Brown and Peterson (1950)
Wis. 49-133	Complex	Lactose, 40	CSL solids, 30	15	*b*	120	26[c]	1,850	0.011	15	Anderson et al. (1953)
Wis. Q-176	Defined	Glucose, 34	Ammonia N, 2.4	15	*a*+*d*	114	23[c]	1,774	0.021	16	Hosler and Johnson (1953)
Wis. 49-133	Complex	Lactose, 30 glucose, 5	CSL solids, 30	15	*c*	90	–	1,610	0.011	18	Davey and Johnson (1953)
Wis. 49-133	Complex	Glucose, 40	CSL solids, 30	15	*c*	83	–	1,520	0.009	18	Davey and Johnson (1953)
P 5005 (Squibb)	Complex(?)	Reducing sugar, 65	(?)	25(?)	?	120	32	5,300	–	44	Donovick (1960)
HA-6 (Hindustan)	Complex	Lactose, 40	Peanut meal, 30 CSL, 5	1,200	*b*	112	–	3,440	0.020	31	Chaturbhuk et al. (1961)

HA-6 (Hindustan)	Complex	Sucrose, 66	Peanut meal, 30 CSL, 5	1,200	*d*	158	–	4,500	0.019	29	CHATURBHUK et al. (1961)
ICI strain A	Defined	Glucose, 84	Ammonia, ?	7	*a*+*d*	120	30	7,500	0.036	63	WRIGHT and CALAM (1968)
ICI strain B (?)	Complex	Lactose+ glucose+ oil, 42	CSL, ?	20	*b*+*e*	147	40	11,200	–	76	CALAM and RUSSELL (1973)
Panlab's 1973 strain P-2	Complex	Sugars+ vegetable oil, ?	?	Production scale	*b*+*e*(?)	158	–	13,800	0.034	87	SWARTZ (1979)
Panlabs' 1974 strain P-7	Complex	Sugars+ vegetable oil, ?	?	Production scale	*b*+*e*(?)	185	–	26,800	0.061	145	SWARTZ (1979)
Panlabs' 1978 strain P-15	Complex	Sugars+ vegetable oil, ?	?	Pilot scale	*b*+*e*(?)	183	–	49,000	0.081	268	SWARTZ (1979)

[a] *a*, pH control; *b*, intermittent feeding of phenylacetic acid (PAA); *c*, continuous feeding of PAA; *d*, continuous feeding of sugar and PAA; *e*, continuous feeding of sugar

[b] *t*, fermentation period (h); *X*, final cell concentration (g/liter); *P*, final penicillin G titer (u/ml); $\bar{Y}_{P/S}$, overall conversion efficiency of carbon substrates [g 6-APA carbon produced/g substrate carbon consumed (assuming CSL solids and peanut meal contain 35% carbon)]; *G*, volumetric productivity (u/ml per hour)

[c] Back-calculated from mycelial nitrogen concentration by assuming a cellular nitrogen content of 6.5%

tration, specific growth rate, and environmental conditions such as dissolved oxygen, temperature, and pH. Sugar polymers such as starch may decrease the biomass and antibiotic yields by limiting the growth. Excess glucose in the broth can result in transient concentration buildup of organic acid(s) (Pirt and Callow 1960; Wright and Calam 1968), such as gluconic acid, which may interrupt the metabolic events crucial to antibiotic production. An exponentially growing mycelial culture has higher and more uniform growth activity and hence a better growth yield than a slow-growing pelleting culture. Tests done by Calam (1976) showed that in fermentations initiated with poor inocula and followed by slow growth, sugar was used less efficiently, resulting in more CO_2 and less cell mass production per unit amount of sugar consumed. The importance of this early growth was well stated by Hockenhull (1963). "Unless the early mycelial growth is optimal, it is extremely unlikely that the best yield will be attained and far more likely that the rate of product formation will remain well below its potential in spite of all efforts to alter it." The fulfillment of this criterion of optimal early growth is the major reason why corn-steep liquor and other complex nutrients are used at high concentrations in antibiotic fermentation media (Pirt and Righelato 1967).

To sustain the specific penicillin production rate q_{pen} and thus reach for higher broth titer, various approaches have been proposed. When oxygen becomes limiting during the production phase, a repeated "draw-off" of the fermentation followed by replacement with fresh nutrient solution can prolong penicillin production (Ryu and Humphrey 1972). Pan et al. (1972) found that pH-mediated sugar feed can maintain the fast production rate longer. Squires (1972) proposed a similar procedure by using dissolved oxygen level (DO) as the primary process variable to control sugar feed. Since pH and DO increases are results of growth deterioration, these empirical methods do not control the growth but merely respond to it. An approach to quantitative control of cell growth is therefore more desirable. To maintain a quasi-steady-state penicillin production (i.e., constant q_{pen}), Ryu and Humphrey (1972, 1973) suggested the need to meet the critical specific oxygen demand of the culture, while others proposed to control the specific growth rate at or above a critical level μ_c (Pirt and Righelato 1967; Righelato et al. 1968; Young and Koplove 1972). Note, however, that these experimental observations are derived mainly from continuous-culture studies. There are basic differences between the batch (or fed-batch) and continuous fermentation kinetics. One crucial fact is that the maximum q_{pen} in batch or fed-batch culture is usually higher than that observed in a chemostat (Pirt and Righelato 1967; Wright and Calam 1968), and this holds true in both defined and complex media. Also, the μ_{max} experienced in batch experiments is significantly higher than the range of dilution rates normally covered by continuous-culture experiments.

In summary, growth rate is believed to determine the rate and amount of antibiotic production, as well as a major portion of the culture demand for carbon and energy. Process productivity and conversion efficiency are therefore directly associated with effective cell growth monitoring and control. The missing link now is a quantitative methodology to manipulate growth so that a desired growth curve for antibiotic production and substrate conservation can be derived and subsequently confirmed in a production vessel.

C. Growth Monitoring and Control – Method of Approach

I. Formulation of a Realistic Medium

For external control of cell density and growth rate, it is desirable to have a starting fermentation medium which contains as little carbon-energy supply as possible. Thus, most published production media containing high concentrations of corn-steep liquor (CSL) and/or lactose are not suitable here. Although no defined medium is available to provide satisfactory growth and production, a less than 1% supplementation of CSL in an otherwise defined medium (see Table 4) does produce realistic results when used for the cultivation of Panlabs' strain P-2 (Mou and Cooney 1983a). With external glucose addition, this medium can support more than 400 g (dry basis) of cell growth. The amounts of CSL carbon and nitrogen used contribute less than 1% and 2% respectively of the total carbon and nitrogen consumed in the fermentation. Continuous feed of precursor phenylacetic acid supports penicillin G synthesis in this medium.

For an analysis of the cell growth data, three approaches can be applied in the present system: the use of (1) empirical correlations, (2) physiological models, and (3) carbon-balancing equation. Successful analyses made in each of the three categories are summarized in the following section.

Table 4. A semidefined penicillin production medium used for glucose fed-batch fermentation in a 15-liter fermentor[a]

	(g/Tank)
Cerelose	Continuous addition
Phenylacetic acid	Continuous addition
Corn-steep liquor	42.5
$(NH_4)_2SO_4$	42.5
$MgSO_4$	8.6
$CaSO_4 \cdot 2H_2O$	3.8
KH_2PO_4	34.0
K_2HPO_4	30.0
NaCl	4.3
$FeSO_4 \cdot 7H_2O$	3.4
$MnSO_4 \cdot H_2O$	0.34
$ZnSO_4 \cdot 7H_2O$	0.26
$CuSO_4 \cdot 5H_2O$	0.07
Dow chemical P-2000 antifoam	5.00

(pH adjusted to 6.5 with NaOH after sterilization)

[a] Seed medium contained corn-steep liquor, 32 g/liter; cerelose, 21 g/liter; $MgSO_4$, 2.4 g/liter; Na_2SO_4, 3 g/liter; and P-2000, 0.5 g/liter; presterilization pH was adjusted to 6.0 with NaOH. Tank liquid after inoculation was $\sim$7.5 liters

II. Growth Monitoring

1. Empirical Correlations

a) Carbon Dioxide Growth Yield – Y_{CO_2}

The experimental correlation between total cell mass and total CO_2 production in the semidefined medium is shown in Fig. 1. A CO_2 yield coefficient of 35.8 g cells per mol CO_2 produced is observed when specific growth rate is near μ_{max}. Based on the results of five glucose fed-batch experiments, it has a standard deviation of ± 1.1 g/mol CO_2. This yield coefficient remained relatively constant when substantial amount of gluconic acid accumulated under the condition of high residual glucose concentration. The CO_2 yield was also not sensitive to a high CSL concentration when glucose was fed to meet the growth demand (Mou and Cooney 1983a). Nevertheless, excess phenylacetic acid addition can sharply reduce the CO_2 growth yield (Mou 1979).

b) Ammonia Nitrogen Growth Yield – Y_{NH_3}

The experimental correlation between total cell growth and total NH_3 added to maintain constant pH during the logarithmic growth in the semidefined medium is shown in Fig. 2. It shows a constant NH_3 nitrogen growth yield of 11.3 g cells per g NH_3 nitrogen added. This figure agrees well with the measured cellular nitrogen content of $\sim 9\%$ (see Fig. 4). Because NH_3 nitrogen addition is a more direct measurement of cell mass synthesis in the present medium, conditions affecting $Y_{X/S}$ and Y_{CO_2}, such as changes of pH or temperature or growth rate and the onset of endogenous metabolism, may be less damaging to the correlation between NH_3 and growth. The observation of no obvious effect of phenylacetic acid addition on the value of Y_{NH_3} supports the above statement. Y_{NH_3} is, however, susceptible to the accumulation of acidic metabolite in the broth. Because of inherent limitations in pH sensing and control, Y_{NH_3} is also less desirable than CO_2 growth correlation for calculating the instantaneous cell growth rate.

2. Physiological Model – Respiratory Quotient

Consistent correlations between respiratory quotient (RQ) and the cell growth activity were also observed in the fed-batch experiments (Mou and Cooney unpublished work). When glucose was the growth-limiting substrate, fast-growth-phase cultures ($\mu \geqq 0.04$ h^{-1}) had an RQ of 1.06–1.07. The production-phase RQ varied as functions of the specific growth rate as well as the concentration of the complex nitrogen-containing nutrient in the media. A specific growth rate of 0.014 h^{-1} could keep the RQ constant at 1.06, and a zero growth rate resulted in a steady decrease of RQ to as low as 0.89.

Since the energy metabolism of fat and protein normally result in an RQ of 0.8 or below (1.0 for glucose), the drop in fermentation RQ can sometimes be looked upon as an indicator of shift in carbon-energy supply (Giese 1973). The endogenous metabolic activities responsible for biomass turnover (mostly cell protein) (Trinci and Righelato 1970) are believed to have contributed to the above pro-

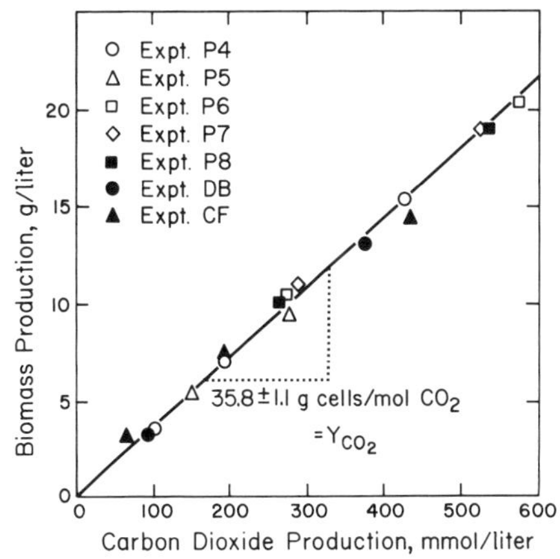

Fig. 1. Experimental correlation between biomass production and carbon dioxide production of *Penicillium chrysogenum* strain P-2 in the logarithmic-growth phase. Experiments P4–P8 were fed-batch experiments with the semidefined medium. Experiment DB was a batch fermentation charged with 40 g/liter glucose at the start. Experiment CF was a fed-batch fermentation with 60 g/liter corn-steep liquor in the starting medium. (MOU and COONEY 1983a)

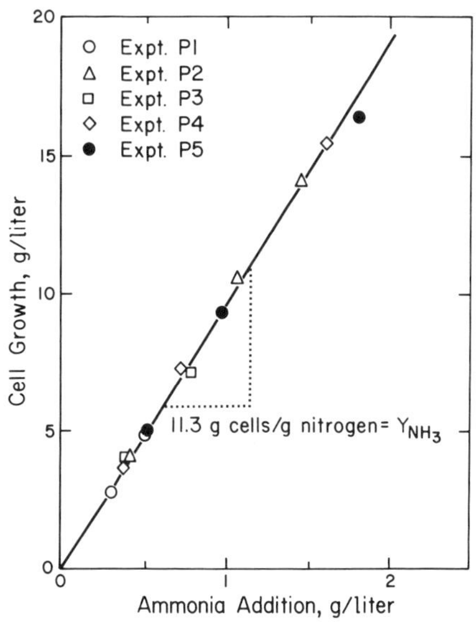

Fig. 2. Experimental correlation between biomass production and NH_3 addition (for pH control) in the fast-growth phase of fed-batch fermentations with the semidefined medium and *Penicillium chrysogenum* strain P-2. (MOU and COONEY 1983a)

duction phase observations. Since exogenous substrate limitation would step up endogenous biomass turnover, the reduction of RQ in the production phase could reflect the magnitude of cell growth rate shift-down in the transition phase. In a fermentation utilizing mixed carbon-energy sources, it also signals the onset of protein and/or lipid metabolism.

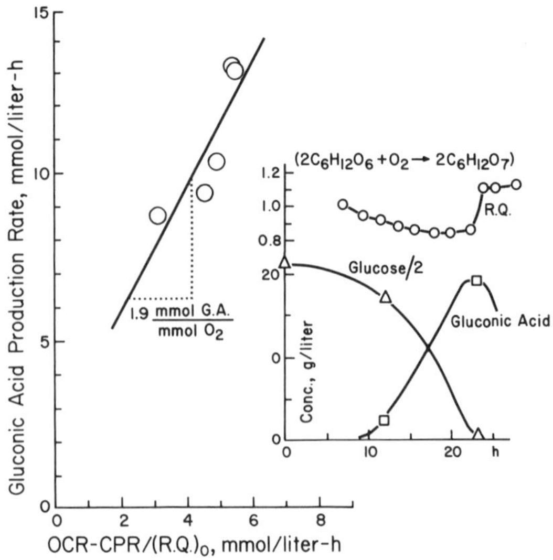

Fig. 3. Experimental correlation between the gluconic acid production rate and the respiratory state of *Penicillium chrysogenum* strain P-2. *Insert* shows the changes of respiratory quotient, glucose, and gluconic acid concentrations during the fermentation. *OCR*, oxygen consumption rate; *CPR*, CO_2 production rate; $(RQ)_0$, cellular respiratory quotient when acid production is near zero. (Mou and Cooney unpublished work)

Furthermore, fermentation RQ is useful in predicting cell metabolite accumulation when the reaction stoichiometry involves either CO_2 production (Wang et al. 1977) or oxygen consumption. It is therefore not surprising that gluconic acid production by *P. chrysogenum* (Mason and Righelato 1976), a one-step reaction involving glucose and oxygen, can be quantitatively followed by the RQ data. The experimental results from a batch fermentation started with 40 g/liter glucose in the semidefined medium give a yield constant of 1.9 mmol gluconic acid produced per millimole O_2 consumed (Fig. 3). This is close to the theoretical value of 2. As a result, the following equation can be used as a physiological model for on-line calculation of gluconic acid production:

$$\text{Gluconic acid production rate, mmol/h}$$
$$= \{O_2 \text{ consumption rate, mmol/h}\}\left[1 - \frac{RQ}{[RQ]_0}\right]\cdot 2, \tag{3}$$

where $[RQ]_0$ is the RQ of cell growth without coproduction of gluconic acid. In the glucose fed-batch penicillin fermentation, the reduction of RQ in the fast-growth phase could also indicate the overfeeding of glucose – a necessary condition for gluconic acid accumulation.

3. Carbon-Balancing Equation

The elemental-balancing technique is probably the only option that is convenient to use, and it is least susceptible to process variations, such as changes in produc-

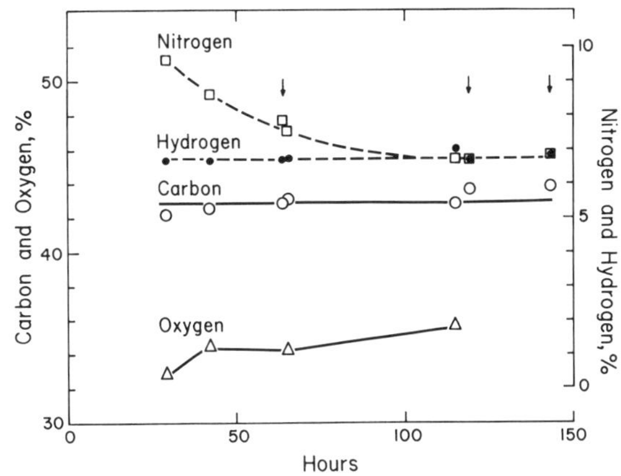

Fig. 4. Variation of cell elemental composition (expressed as wt% of dry weight) of *Penicillium chrysogenum* strain P-2 in fed-batch penicillin fermentation using the semidefined medium. Samples were taken from two separate fermentations; *arrows* indicate samples taken from one fermentation. Both experiments had μ_{gr} of 0.09 h^{-1} in the first 30 h. Afterward, μ_{pr} was kept at $\sim 0.005\ h^{-1}$ in one experiment and $\sim 0.008\ h^{-1}$ in the other. (MOU and COONEY 1983a)

tion strain, fermentation pH, temperature, or substrate. Hence, unlike the empirical approaches, it does not rely upon repetitious experiments to precede the investigation of each specific fermentation condition. Details of this approach have been discussed by COONEY et al. (1977).

The elemental composition of C, H, O, and N of Panlabs' strain P-2 is shown in Fig. 4. Since carbon is the major element in cell mass and the cellular carbon content remains relatively constant throughout the fermentation, it is possible to calculate the cell growth by carbon balance (MOU and COONEY 1983a). Table 5 summarizes the carbon balancing results of seven glucose fed-batch experiments – the first four used the semidefined medium and the other three a more complex medium containing ten times more CSL. The near 100% recovery of the total substrate carbon provides the foundation for a growth calculation using the carbon-balancing equation:

$$X_t = \frac{C_S + C_{PAA} + C_I - C_{CO_2} - C_{pen} - C_p - C_x}{x_c}, \tag{4}$$

where

C_S = carbon in substrates consumed ($= C_{glu} + C_{CSL}$)
C_{PAA} = carbon in penicillin G precursor fed
C_I = carbon in inoculum
C_p = carbon in side-products such as gluconic acid
C_x = carbon in unidentified soluble products
x_c = cellular carbon content (%/100)

Side-products accumulation (C_p) can be assumed to be negligible under glucose-limited growth conditions, and C_x can be measured by total organic carbon assay of the broth supernatant. C_{CO_2} can be measured continuously by a gas analyzer or

Table 5. Examination of total carbon recovery in computer-aided fed-batch penicillin fermentations

Expt. No.[a]	t (h)	C_{glu} (g)	C_{CSL} (g)	C_{PAA} (g)	C_{IN}[b] (g)	C_{cells}[c] (g)	C_{CO_2} (g)	C_{pen} (g)	C_x (g)	C_{OUT} (g)	Recovery (%)
1	137	571	6	41	630	151	408	30	58	647	102.7
4	96	600	6	26	644	207	366	32	59	664	103.1
5	126	596	6	42	656	202	378	39	42	661	100.8
6	137	600	6	42	660	202	357	41	47	647	98.0
	(Total				2,590)	(Total				2,619)	
7	117	472	57	37	578	180	345	38	48	611	105.7
8	137	516	57	43	628	176	332	40	51	599	95.4
9	187	400	57	53	522	136	328	42	43	549	105.2
	(Total				1,728)	(Total				1,759)	(101.6 ± 3.8)

[a] Expts. 2 and 3 are left out here because their broth samples were not assayed for C_x

[b] C_{IN} includes seed-medium carbon of 12 g

[c] Weights of freeze-dried cells are used here (2% lower than weights of hot-air-dried cells)

a mass spectrometer. C_S and C_{PAA} can be monitored by weighing the feed vessels with load cells or electronic scales and maintaining their residual concentration in the broth near zero. Penicillin production can be continuously assessed by using either an autoanalyzing device or an empirical simulation equation (MOU and COONEY 1983a). The application of this carbon-balancing method in the penicillin fermentation is also supported by the experimental data of MCCANN and CALAM (1972) and those of MASON and RIGHELATO (1976). Since CO_2 carbon is the major product of fermentation, particular attention should be given to air flow rate and off-gas CO_2 concentration measurements in order to reduce calculation error. The widespread use of complex nutrients in the production media presents a major obstacle to the application of the carbon-balancing equation for real-time growth calculation under industrial fermentation conditions. This is particularly true during the fast-growth and early production phases when complex organic nutrients are the primary carbon source for growth.

III. Growth Control in Fed-Batch Fermentation

Although some of the growth correlations discussed above have been common knowledge for years, their application for on-line monitoring and control of growth has rarely been demonstrated. Frequently, the studies have ended at the curve-fitting stage. The use of complex fermentation media containing nonbiomass solids at high concentration is one obvious reason for not bothering with growth measurement and control. To do this, starting media are charged with enough readily utilizable nutrient to carry the growth at a high rate into the production phase. Once the production phase is underway, empirical indicators such as the time trends of broth pH and dissolved oxygen (DO) are used to control the sugar feed (PAN et al. 1972; SQUIRES 1972). The rate of sugar addition, when governed by pH and/or DO changes, is thought to meet the culture demand necessary for optimal penicillin production. However, because of the time lag between the onset of glucose starvation and the detection of consequent pH and DO increases, the objective of supplying glucose to meet metabolic needs is not totally fulfilled. A successful fermentation should therefore be aimed at quantitative control of growth and consequently minimizing these undesirable pH and/or DO fluctuations to the infinitesimal. This approach requires knowledge of the instantaneous biomass concentration and a predetermined growth curve for maximized product accumulation. In the present model system, glucose is fed in the fast-growth phase primarily to support the growth demand and in the transition and production phases to satisfy first the maintenance demand and second the needs for growth and product synthesis.

1. Control Strategy

The instantaneous specific growth rate μ_t in the fast-growth phase can be calculated as frequently as every 15 min by using the CO_2 production rate data. When Y_{CO_2} is known, cell concentration X_t can be calculated from the total CO_2 production at time t. It can otherwise be calculated from overall carbon balancing if residual glucose concentration is kept low by independent means. In the transition (every 15 min) and production phases (every 30 min), because of the onset of en-

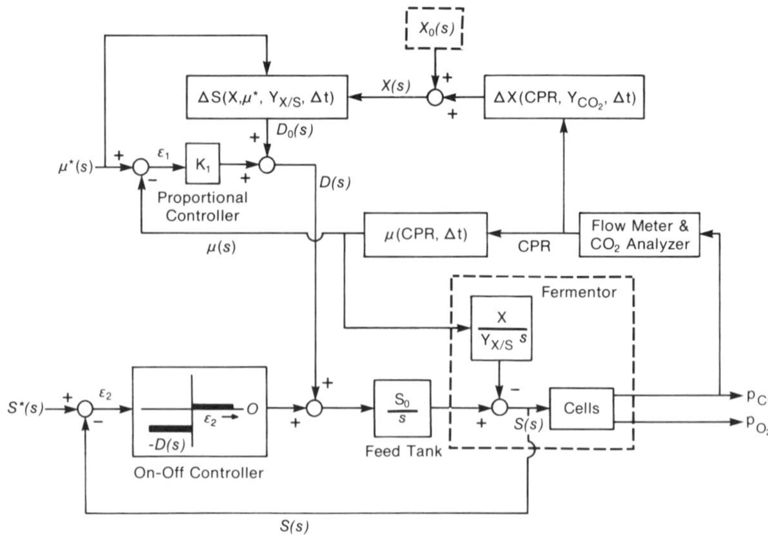

Fig. 5. Block diagram of a feed-forward modification of feedback control of glucose feed for constant cell growth rate during the fast-growth phase of fed-batch penicillin fermentation. X_o, cell concentration; D, additional glucose demand for the next time increment; S_o, glucose concentration in feed solution; S, residual glucose concentration. p_{CO_2}, partial pressure of CO_2 in spent air; p_{O_2}, partial pressure of O_2 in spent air. (Mou and Cooney 1983a)

dogenous metabolism, overall carbon balancing should be the sole choice for X_t and μ_t calculations.

To define the cell growth curve, the following control set points need to be specified at the beginning of each experiment: the fast-growth-phase growth rate $\mu^{\star}_{gr}$; cell concentration at the end of the fast-growth phase $X^{\star}_{tr}$; and the production-phase growth rate $\mu^{\star}_{pr}$. During the fermentation, real-time cell concentration and growth rate can be continually assessed and compared with the set points by an on-line computer. The glucose feed rate is then adjusted to narrow the discrepancy in growth rate or to switch growth to production. An example block diagram of maximizing the growth rate in the fast-growth phase is shown in Fig. 5. Details of the on-line calculation and control and the related experimental results are published elsewhere (Mou and Cooney 1983a). Some of the key experiments are summarized in the following section.

2. Manipulation of Cell Growth Curve by On-Line Controlled Glucose Feed

a) Variation of Production-Phase Growth Rate (μ_{pr})

In four experiments with $\mu^{\star}_{gr}$ set at μ_{max}, $X^{\star}_{tr}$ set at 20 g/liter, and $\mu^{\star}_{pr}$ set at 0, 0.006, 0.010, and 0.015 h^{-1}, we obtained the computer-controlled cell growth curves shown in Fig. 6. The actual production-phase growth rates obtained are 0, 0.006, 0.009, and 0.014 h^{-1}, respectively. Logarithmic cell growth at a high rate to ~ 20 g/liter was accurately reproduced in each experiment. The high growth rate compares well with the μ_{max} of 0.12 h^{-1} observed in batch fermentation ex-

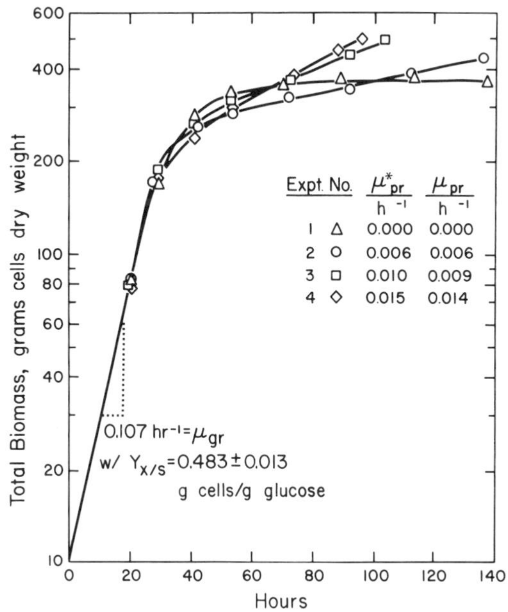

Fig. 6. Computer-controlled *Penicillium chrysogenum* P-2 growth curves in fed-batch fermentations using the semidefined medium. Growth curves were drawn by connecting the experimentally measured total dry cell weights in the fermentor indicated by the open symbols. $\mu^{\star}_{pr}$, set point of specific growth rate in production phase, μ_{pr}, actual specific growth rate in production phase; μ_{gr}, actual specific growth rate in fast-growth phase. (Mou and Cooney 1983a)

periments. Nonetheless, the residual glucose concentration was kept below 1 g/liter under all conditions. The efficient use of glucose is reflected by the high and consistent growth yield observed, 0.48 ± 0.01 g/g glucose. Furthermore, constant production-phase growth rates were maintained near the set points by the computer.

b) Variation of Cell Concentration (X_t)

Ability to control the production-phase cell density would help the study of the effects of mass transfer and/or nutrient limitation on antibiotic production. This can be achieved simply by changing the set point of $X^{\star}_{tr}$ within the capacity of the fermentor to supply oxygen. One such example (Expt. 5) with $X^{\star}_{tr}$ set at 10 g/liter is shown in Fig. 7. The computer-coupled fermentor accurately reproduced the cell growth rates in Expt. 4, but with the production-phase cell density reduced by half, as predicted.

c) Variation of Growth Rate of Fast-Growth Phase (μ_{gr})

To examine the effect of μ_{gr} on q_{pen}, a cell growth curve with low growth rate in the fast-growth phase needs to be produced. Hence, Expt. 6 was run with $\mu^{\star}_{gr}$ set at 0.05 h^{-1}. To compare the production results with Expt. 4 and 5, $\mu^{\star}_{pr}$ is again set at 0.015 h^{-1} and $X^{\star}_{tr}$ is set at 20 g/liter to obtain comparable cell density in the transition and production phases. The resulting cell growth curve obtained by computer control is compared with that of Expt. 4 in Fig. 8. The observed growth rates

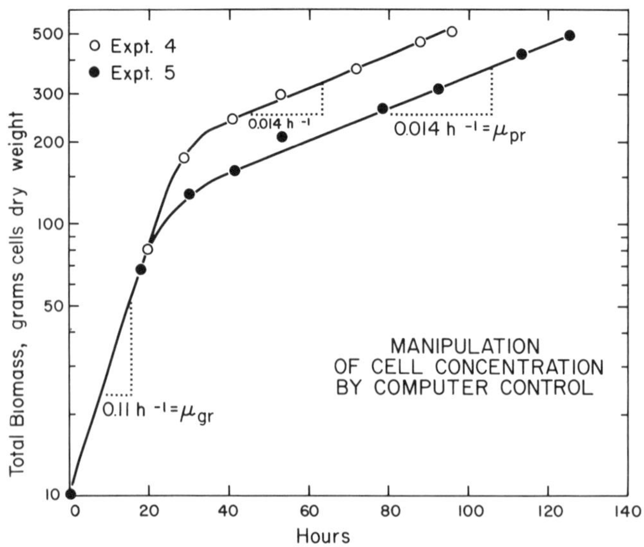

Fig. 7. Fed-batch growth kinetics of *Penicillium chrysogenum* P-2 under computer control – to repeat a desired cell growth pattern (*Expt. 4*) with cell density reduced by approximately half (*Expt. 5*). (Mou and Cooney 1983a)

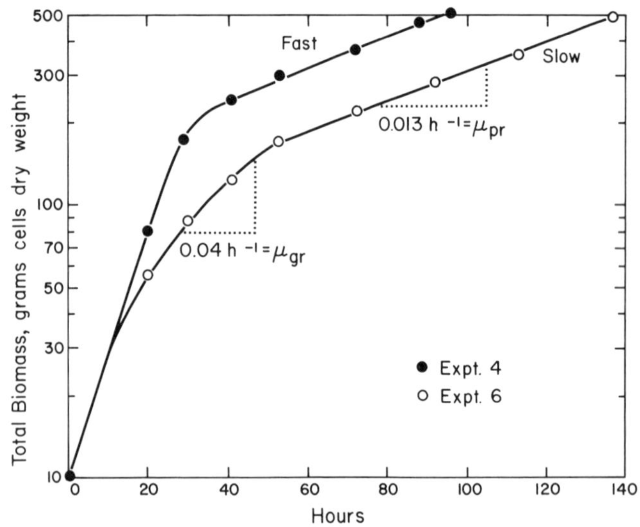

Fig. 8. Manipulation of the fast-growth-phase growth rate of *Penicillium chrysogenum* P-2 by computer-controlled feeding of glucose. Shown here is a comparison between *Expt. 4* and *Expt. 6*. (Mou and Cooney 1983a)

are ~ 0.04 and 0.013 h^{-1} during the growth and production phases, respectively. Again, they are in good agreement with the preselected growth-rate set points, and as desired, the culture enters the production phase at cell density comparable to that of Expt. 5.

Table 6 summarizes the various cell growth patterns made available by computer control for studying growth and production correlations. The successful use

Table 6. Summary of computer-controlled cell growth results for studying growth and penicillin production correlation in semidefined fermentation medium [a]

Expt. No.	$\mu_{gr}(h^{-1})$	X_{tr}(g/liter)	$\mu_{pr}(h^{-1})$
1	0.11	20	0.0
2	0.11	20	0.006
3	0.11	20	0.009
4	0.11	20	0.014
5	0.11	10	0.014
6	0.04	20	0.013

[a] μ_{gr}: specific growth rate in the fast-growth phase; X_{tr}: cell concentration at the end of logarithmic growth; μ_{pr}: specific growth rate in the penicillin production phase

of a computer to monitor and control cell growth is mainly due to the ability to recover >90% of the substrate carbon as CO_2, cell, and penicillin carbon.

D. Effect of Growth on Penicillin Production

The above success in controlling separately the various fermentation variables related to growth (see Table 6) enables us to examine directly and quantitatively the growth effect on production under the glucose fed-batch condition. Figure 9 shows

Fig. 9 a

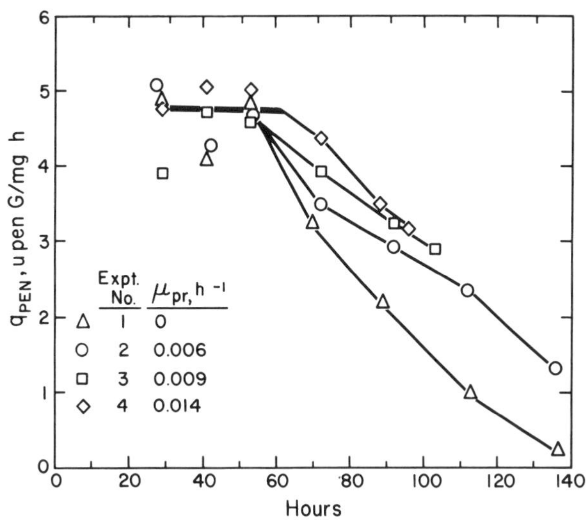

Fig. 9 a–c. Variations of specific penicillin production rate (q_{pen}) of *Penicillium chrysogenum* P-2 as a function of growth rate and cell concentration in the computer-controlled fed-batch fermentations using the semidefined medium. **a** Effect of production-phase growth rate ($\mu_{gr} = 0.11\ h^{-1}$); **b** effect of production-phase cell density; **c** effect of fast-growth-phase growth rate. 1 u = 0.6 μg pen G sodium salt. (Mou and Cooney to be published)

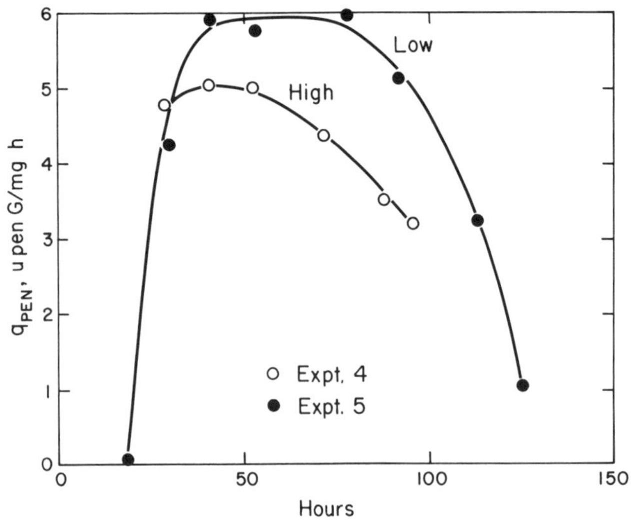

Fig. 9b

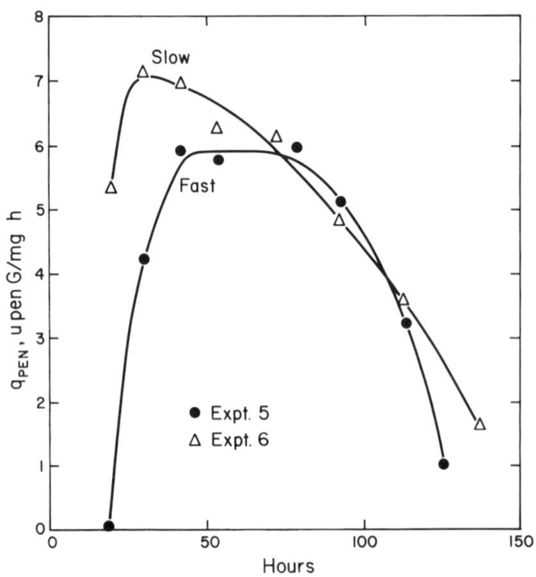

Fig. 9c

the variations of q_{pen} against fermentation time in these experiments. Despite a constant μ_{pr} as high as 0.014 h^{-1}, peak q_{pen} developed in the transition phase shown in Fig. 9a could not be maintained for more than 30 h. However, higher μ_{pr} does appear to slow the decay of q_{pen}. When bulk mixing and mass transfer were improved by reducing the cell density in the transition phase, peak q_{pen} was raised by 20% and also maintained longer (Fig. 9b). Except for the fact that high and constant μ_{pr} is not a sufficient condition for maintaining constant q_{pen} in the production phase, the rest of the results seem to agree with the continuous-culture observations (PIRT and RIGHELATO 1967; YOUNG and KOPLOVE 1972; RYU and HUMPHREY 1973). What is truly surprising is that a controlled slow growth (~ 1/

3 μ_{max}) in the growth phase could result in earlier penicillin production at a significantly elevated q_{pen} (Fig. 9c). These advantageous effects of slow growth plus the adverse effect of high cell density show the need to watch for unwarranted cell growth at the process development stage.

E. Effect of the Use of Corn-Steep Liquor

The use of complex nutrient ingredients at high concentrations in culture media is a widely accepted practice in the antibiotic fermentation industry. These are usually substances rich in organic nitrogen, e.g., amino acids, oligopeptides, proteins, and many known or unknown growth factors, and may include materials such as corn-steep liquor (CSL), peanut meal, soybean meal, cottonseed meal, dry yeasts, and fish meal. Despite their constant quality variation due to either nature's course or crude preparation and storage procedures, there is little doubt about their ability to enhance cell growth and stimulate antibiotic production. One example is the use of CSL in penicillin fermentation since the industry's infancy. High concentrations of CSL in the culture media not only serve as an emergency supply of readily utilizable carbon and nitrogen, but also help to maintain a high q_{pen} because of the ability of CSL to support a high growth rate in the fast-growth phase (PIRT and RIGHELATO 1967) and to supply the amino acid precursors for penicillin synthesis.

To study the non-growth-related effect of CSL on q_{pen}, the on-line method for growth monitoring and control was adapted to reproduce the cell growth curves in a medium containing ten times the CSL (MOU and COONEY 1983b). The cell growth rate data in three such experiments are summarized in Table 7, and the resulting q_{pen} profiles are plotted in Fig. 10 and 11. One obvious effect of high CSL concentration seen in Fig. 10 is its ability to reverse the adverse effect of high μ_{gr} on q_{pen} in the semidefined medium. Nevertheless, the beneficial effect of low μ_{gr} persists in the CSL-rich medium, as shown in Fig. 11; the culture started penicillin production earlier and also reached a slightly higher peak q_{pen}. In the semidefined medium, peak q_{pen} of 7.5 u/mg·h or more was attainable only under the low μ_{gr} condition.

Table 7. Summary of computer-controlled cell growth results for studying the non-growth-related effect of corn-steep liquor (CSL) on specific penicillin production rate[a]

Expt. no.	μ_{gr} (h^{-1})	X_{tr} (g/liter)	μ_{pr} (h^{-1})	CSL[b] (g/liter)
5	μ_{max}	10	0.014	6
7	μ_{max}	10	0.016	$\boxed{60}$
8	$\boxed{0.05}$	10	0.013	60

[a] μ_{gr}, specific growth rate in the fast-growth phase; X_{tr}, cell concentration at the end of logarithmic growth; μ_{pr}, specific growth rate in the penicillin production phase

[b] Concentration in the starting medium

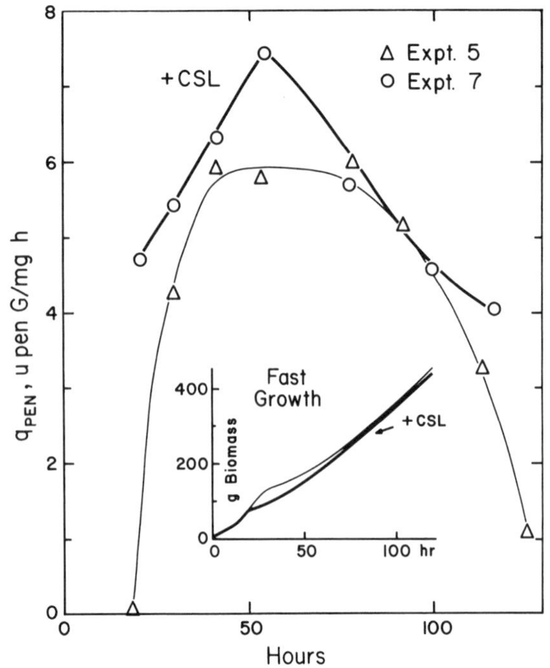

Fig. 10. Effect of a high concentration of corn-steep liquor (~ 60 g/liter) on specific penicillin production rate of *Penicillium chrysogenum* P-2 in the computer-controlled fed-batch fermentations with a maximized growth-phase growth rate. Insert shows the cell growth curves. 1 u = 0.6 μg pen G sodium salt. (MOU and COONEY to be published)

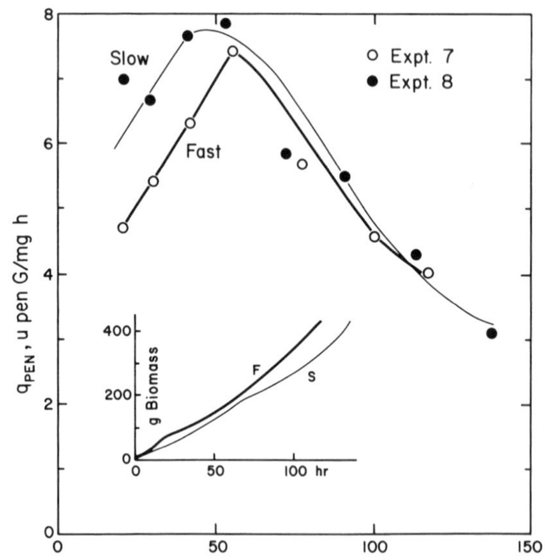

Fig. 11. Effect of fast-growth-phase growth rate on specific penicillin production rate of *Penicillium chrysogenum* P-2 in the computer-controlled fed-batch fermentations using a high concentration of corn-steep liquor. *Insert* shows the cell growth curves. 1 u = 0.6 μg pen G sodium salt. (MOU and COONEY to be published)

F. Maintenance Demand as a Fermentation Variable

Since most of the carbon-energy substrate consumed in a fed-batch penicillin fermentation is used to support cell growth and maintenance, increase of the specific penicillin production rate q_{pen} can improve the overall conversion yield of carbon-energy substrates to penicillin, $\bar{Y}_{P/S}$ (g penicillin/g glucose equivalent), by decreased carbon-energy demand for growth and the subsequent cell maintenance. Other independent means of lowering the maintenance demand, m (g glucose/g cells·h), can also increase $\bar{Y}_{P/S}$. All these improvements can be brought about by either strain or process improvement.

I. Calculation of Maintenance Demand for Sugar

Considering the thousandfold increase in penicillin broth potency during the past three decades, the contribution of strain improvement to the improvement of q_{pen} can easily be appreciated. However, few reports have dealt with the possible reduction of cellular maintenance demand as a result of strain and/or process improvements. To obtain this information, one needs a generally applicable method to calculate the maintenance demand in the antibiotic production phase. One method is by the use of the CO_2 balancing equation:

$$\text{CO}_2 \text{ production resulting from cell maintanance}$$
$$= \frac{\{\text{total CO}_2 \text{ production}\} - \{\text{CO}_2 \text{ production resulting from cell growth}\}}{\text{total [g cells} \cdot \text{h] maintained}},$$

$$m_{CO_2}(\text{mol CO}_2/\text{g cells} \cdot \text{h}) = \frac{\int_{t_1}^{t_f} [CPR]dt - (X_{t_f} - X_{t_1})/Y_{CO_2}}{\int_{t_1}^{t_f} X\,dt}, \tag{5}$$

where

t_1 = time at the end of the fast-growth phase (h);
t_f = time at the end of fermentation (h);
$[CPR]$ = CO_2 production rate (mol/h);
X = dry cell weight (g);
Y_{CO_2} = maximum CO_2 growth yield observed (g cells/mol CO_2).

In this calculation one assumes that the CO_2 production resulting from penicillin synthesis is negligible when compared to that from growth and maintenance (COONEY 1979). By measuring cell growth and CO_2 production throughout the fermentation, one can estimate the maintenance production of CO_2 by using the graphic integration method reported earlier (MOU and COONEY 1976). The equivalent glucose consumption can then be calculated by using the stoichiometric constant of complete glucose combustion to CO_2:

$$m(\text{g glu/g cells} \cdot \text{h}) = \frac{m_{CO_2}\left[\frac{\text{mol CO}_2}{\text{g cells} \cdot \text{h}}\right]}{6\left[\frac{\text{mol CO}_2}{\text{mol glu}}\right]} \cdot 180\left[\frac{\text{g glu}}{\text{mol glu}}\right] = m_{CO_2} \cdot 30\,. \tag{6}$$

Table 8. Average maintenance demand of *Penicillium chrysogenum* for sugar – as a function of strain type, carbon-energy source, and temperature

Strain type	Major carbon-energy source [a]	Temperature (°C)	Y_{CO_2} [b] (g/mol)	t [c] (h)	m_{av} [d] (g glu equiv/g cells · h)	Penicillin titer (u/ml) [e]
Wis. 54-1255	Lactose	25	60	59	0.019	930
Mou and Cooney	Lactose	25	58	70	0.025	1,320
unpublished work	Glucose	25	51	74	0.028	1,670
	Glucose	25	59	60	0.027	1,420
P-2 Mou and Cooney unpublished work	Glucose	26	35	154	0.020	12,200
ICI? [f]	Lactose + sucrose	19	55	190	0.010	8,700
McCann and Calam	Lactose + sucrose	22	63	150	0.011	9,500
(1972)	Lactose + sucrose	25	72	150	0.015	10,000
	Lactose + sucrose	27	63	145	0.013	11,200
	Lactose + sucrose	30	48	160	0.015	6,700
	Lactose + sucrose	30	42	170	0.017	9,700

[a] The two lactose experiments were batch fermentations; all others were fed-batch ones
[b] Calculated from the growth-phase data by assuming zero maintenance activity
[c] Time when penicillin titer leveled off
[d] Calculated by the integration method of Mou and Cooney (1976) using the CO_2 production data
[e] 1 u = 0.6 µg pen G
[f] Calculated from experimental data of McCann and Calam (1972)

II. Reduction of Maintenance Demand Through Strain Improvement

Calculated results from fermentations using the Wis 54-1255 strain and Panlabs' P-2 strain (Mou and Cooney unpublished work) and another strain (McCann and Calam 1972) are shown in Table 8. The Panlabs' strain improvement program did introduce new strains with reduced maintenance demand for sugar. With pH controlled at 6.5, the P-2 strain has an average maintenance demand of 0.020 g glu/g cells h – nearly 30% less than that of the Wis. 54-1255 strain under the same condition, 0.028 g/g h. The high-yielding strain used by McCann and Calam (1972) had an even lower maintenance demand for sugar, 0.015 g glu/g cells h at 25 °C. Because of the reduction of cellular maintenance demand for sugar and consequently oxygen, high-yielding strains with improved q_{pen} can be cultivated to and maintained at an even higher cell density in the production phase before entering the O_2-limited condition. This trend is evident in Table 3 and is likely characteristic of modern industrial strains. These strains therefore meet the primary objectives of an industrial screening program, i.e., higher volumetric productivity and overall conversion yield of the fermentation substrate(s).

III. Reduction of Maintenance Demand Through Process Improvement and Its Implication

The same process variables that affect growth also affect the maintenance demand (Pirt 1975). Maintenance demand was reduced and penicillin production was im-

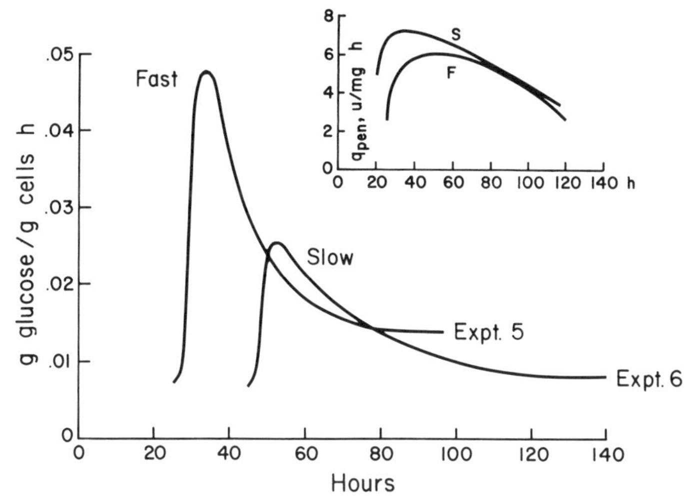

Fig. 12. Effect of the fast-growth-phase growth rate on the instantaneous maintenance demand for sugar in fed-batch penicillin fermentation using the semidefined medium. Expt. 5 – $\mu_{gr}=0.11\ h^{-1}$; $\mu_{pr}=0.014\ h^{-1}$ and Expt. 6 – $\mu_{gr}=0.04\ h^{-1}$; $\mu_{pr}=0.013\ h^{-1}$. *Insert* shows its effect on the instantaneous specific penicillin production rate. (MOU and COONEY to be published)

paired under oxygen- and/or sugar-limited growth, such as in a batch lactose fermentation (MOU and COONEY unpublished work). Maintenance demand is also substantially reduced when the fermentation temperature is lowered (see Table 8).

The implication of maintenance demand in the fed-batch penicillin fermentation can be unveiled further with knowledge of the instantaneous maintenance demand, m_t (MOU and COONEY to be published c), which can be calculated by either of the following two equations:

$$m_t = q_S - \frac{\mu_t}{Y_{X/S}} - \frac{q_{\text{pen}}}{Y_{P/S}}, \tag{7}$$

$$m_t = \left(q_{CO_2} - \frac{\mu_t}{Y_{CO_2}}\right) \cdot 30\,, \tag{8}$$

where q_S is the instantaneous specific rate of sugar consumption (g/g cells h) and q_{CO_2} is the instantaneous specific rate of CO_2 production (mol/g cells h). Equation (8) is more useful when complex fermentation media are used. With a zero maintenance demand assumed in the fast-growth phase, the on-line calculated (every 30 min) instantaneous maintenance demands in Expts. 5 and 6 are plotted versus time in Fig. 12. The instantaneous maintenance demand for glucose quickly reaches a peak after the step-down of cell growth rate and then decays slowly to a steady-state value. This so-called non-growth-associated metabolic demand is apparently influenced by the growth history of the culture as demonstrated by the present calculation.

One can hypothesize that the high turnover rate of biomass resulting from the shift-down of growth rate causes the surge in cell maintenance demand. This rate slows down and so does the maintenance demand when a reduced but constant growth rate is established and a new balance between catabolic and anabolic activities is again created. This speculation is consistent with the experimental observations of TRINCI and RIGHELATO (1970). They found that extreme change in protein metabolism occurs when a *P. chrysogenum* culture grown at 0.051 h^{-1} is carbon starved by medium feed stoppage. Cellular protein content fell exponentially at a rate of 0.057 h^{-1} during the first 6 h of starvation, and the rate of fall became slower after that. This loss in cellular protein alone can account for the rate of decrease in cell dry weight, ~ 0.011 h^{-1}, in their experiment. If a constant cell mass is to be maintained, this loss in cell mass through endogenous energy metabolism must be compensated by new cell growth supported by exogenous carbon-energy source. The amount of glucose needed to maintain constant cell mass in the above condition would be close to the peak maintenance demand of Expt. 6 shown in Fig. 12.

One may therefore assume that the cellular maintenance demand also reflects the extent of protein turnover during the transitionary and production phases of penicillin fermentation. Hence, accelerated maintenance demand could indicate accelerated degradation of the penicillin-synthesizing enzymes. Such a correlation does exist, as suggested by the time courses of q_{pen} and m_t shown in Fig. 12. Higher maintenance demand due to faster initial growth resulted in lower peak q_{pen} in Expt. 5. Because complex nitrogen-containing substances can ease protein breakdown and/or enzyme inactivation by their ability to slow the shrinkage of the amino acid pools during the growth rate step-down (BERNLOHR and GRAY 1969; GOLDBERG 1971; ST. JOHN et al. 1978), the non-growth-related beneficial effect of CSL on q_{pen} shown in Fig. 10 is not so surprising after all.

G. Overall Conversion Yield of Glucose to Penicillin-$\bar{Y}_{P/S}$

It is of interest here to examine the overall effects of cell growth and CSL concentration on the volumetric productivity and overall conversion yield of carbon-energy sources to penicillin in the computer-controlled experiments discussed above. Table 9 summarizes the growth conditions and production results at the time of maximum volumetric productivity in Expts. 4–9. To include the CSL consumption, $\bar{Y}_{P/S}$ is expressed here as grams of penicillin nucleus (6-aminopenicillanic acid) carbon produced per gram of substrate carbon consumed. The high cell density in Expt. 4 may have the growth curve typical of what is adopted in industry (QUEENER and SWARTZ 1979), but its $\bar{Y}_{P/S}$ is the poorest among all runs. Comparison of Expt. 5 with 7 and 6 with 8 shows that the main advantage of using CSL lies in its potential to prolong the penicillin-production. The beneficial effects of lowered fast-growth-phase growth rate in increasing q_{pen} and reducing m_t are reflected on the improved overall substrate conversion yields in fermentations with and without a high concentration of CSL. Further improvement in $\bar{Y}_{P/S}$ is possible if the production-phase growth rate can be properly optimized. A 29% increase of $\bar{Y}_{P/S}$ was achieved in Expt. 9 by lowering the μ_{pr} from 0.013 to 0.006 h^{-1}. This, however, was accompanied by a volumetric productivity reduction of more than 20%. This trade-off between the conversion yield and tank productivity also exists in the other experiments. Fast buildup of cell mass, essential for high volumetric productivity, usually resulted in raised maintenance demand for sugar. By growing the

Table 9. Effect of cell growth pattern and the use of complex medium on penicillin fermentation performance – data taken at time of maximum productivity

Expt. no.	4	5	6	7	8	9
(Growth condition)						
Medium	S.D.[a]	S.D.	S.D.	C[b]	C	C
$\mu_{gr}(h^{-1})$	0.11	0.11	0.04	0.12	0.05	0.05
$\mu_{pr}(h^{-1})$	0.014	0.014	0.013	0.016	0.013	0.006
(Pen G production)						
Time (h)	96	120	124	117	137	160
Broth titer (u/ml)	9,100^{+}[c]	11,000	11,000	11,000^{+}	12,000^{+}	12,100^{+}
Total production (g pen G)	60	72	71	71	76	71
(Objective functions)						
Maximum productivity (g pen G/day)	14.9^{+}	14.4	13.7	14.6^{+}	13.3^{+}	10.5
Overall conversion yield ($\bar{Y}_{P/S}$):						
in g pen G/g glucose	0.040	0.053	0.058	(0.060)[d]	(0.064)[d]	(0.085)[d]
in $\frac{\text{g 6-APA carbon}}{\text{g substrate carbon}}$[e]	0.027	0.036	0.039	0.036	0.038	0.049

[a] S.D., semidefined medium (~6 g/liter CSL)
[b] C, complex medium (~60 g/liter CSL)
[c] + Indicates the potential of having higher titer or productivity, had the fermentation been continued
[d] Calculation does not include the use of CSL
[e] Calculation includes the use of CSL

cells more slowly and letting them produce longer, conversion efficiency was improved by decreased demand of cell growth and maintenance for glucose. Furthermore, it may also allow a more efficient use of the existing agitation and aeration power, i.e., increase in kg product/kW h, when the compromise of volumetric productivity can be properly compensated for.

H. Summary

I. New Insight into Fermentation Kinetics

New process information has been derived after analyzing the computer-controlled fed-batch experiments for correlations among cell growth, maintenance, and penicillin production. Controlled cell growth rate and cell concentration in both the fast-growth and production phases were essential for reduction of glucose consumption. In the medium containing CSL in low concentration (~ 6 g/liter), maximized growth-phase growth rate resulted in elevated maintenance demand and reduced specific penicillin production rate. High CSL concentration (~ 60 g/liter) could reverse these effects, and so could a reduced growth-phase growth rate. What results from all these observations is a trade-off between the overall conversion efficiency of carbon-energy sources to penicillin and the overall volumetric productivity. From this interpretation, a fermentation process engineer can objectively choose between substrate economy and volumetric productivity in dealing with a new manufacturing cost structure. The strain P-2 fermentation results show that high CSL concentration is not essential for a realistic penicillin production. It can nevertheless boost the broth titer by promoting the longevity of the fermentation.

With the intrinsic relationships among penicillin titer, productivity, and overall conversion efficiency characterized, it is hoped that an objective criterion for optimizing penicillin fermentation under a totally different condition, e.g., change in production strain or major substrate, can be established quickly by the use of computer-aided on-line monitoring and control of cell growth. Besides being practical for this research and development role, fed-batch fermentation would continue to be the process of the future for the production of many secondary metabolites. Along with increased understanding of the fermentation, more and more external control of the production process would become desirable. Controlled feeding instead of batching of the carbon-energy source could let the operator instead of the culture have more control over the key metabolic events.

II. Proposal of a Working Methodology for Process Improvement

Based on the new methodology for quantitative interpretation of growth and production, a fermentation development routine for industrial application is proposed in Fig. 13. Since what really counts is improvement at the manufacturing stage, laboratory scientists should not be baffled by the end fermentation results in the shake

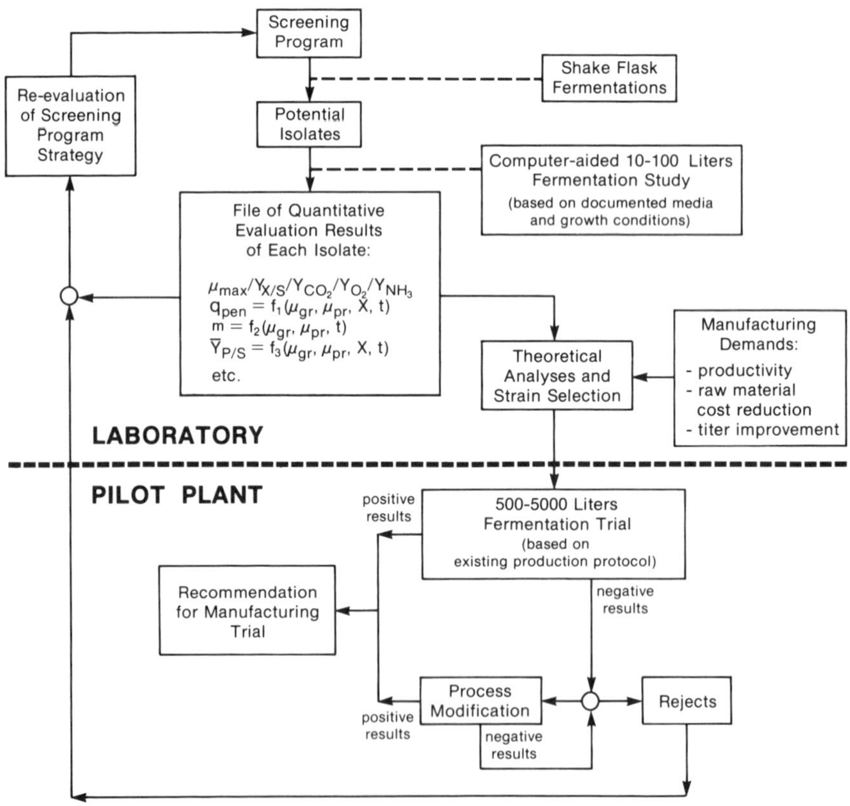

Fig. 13. Proposal of an engineering strategy for strain and process improvement in industry

flasks and laboratory fermentors in their efforts to uncover potential production strains. Instead, good judgement should be exercised in compromising between reality and interpretability of media and fermentation conditions to gain insight into their intrinsic fermentation behavior. Once a culture is transferred to the pilot plant for production trial, this knowledge becomes essential for the resolution of unexpected process difficulties. A straight empirical trial-and-error approach is lengthy and laborious and complicates the already perplexing fermentation conditions. The present scheme is expected to improve the effectiveness of the fermentation development effort and enhance scientific understanding of the process, which in turn would be subjected to further simplification and tighter control.

With the recently available techniques of molecular biology and recombinant DNA, a new generation of superproducing microorganisms can be expected to steer the industry to a new dimension of biosynthetic efficiency and capability. Engineering contributions to fermentation bioenergetics, process control, genetic reconstruction, and culture screening are needed if we are to meet this challenge.

References

Anderson RF, Whitmore Jr LM, Brown WE, Peterson WH, Churchill BW, Roegner FR, Campbell TH, Backus MP, Stauffer JF (1953) Penicillin production by pigment-free molds. Ind Eng Chem 45:768–773

Aiba S, Humphrey AE, Millis NF (1973) Biochemical engineering, 2nd edn. Academic Press, New York London

Bernlohr RW, Gray BH (1969) Enzyme inactivation during initiation of sporulation. In: Gerhardt P, Costilow FN, Sadoff HL (eds) Spores, vol IV. Am soc microbiol, international spore conference, East Lansing, 1968. American Society for Microbiology, Bethesda, MD, p 186

Brown WE, Peterson WH (1950) Factors affecting production of penicillin in semi-pilot-plant equipment. Ind Eng Chem 42:1769–1774

Calam CT (1976) Starting investigational and production cultures. Proc Biochem 11:7–12

Calam CT, Russell DW (1973) Microbial aspects of fermentation process development. J Appl Chem Biotechnol 23:225–237

Chaturbhuk K, Gopalkrishnan KS, Ghosh D (1961) Studies on the feed rate for precursor and sugar in penicillin fermentation. Hind Antibiot Bull 3:144–151

Cooney CL (1979) Conversion yields in penicillin production: theory vs. practice. Proc Biochem 14:31–33

Cooney CL, Acevedo F (1977) Theoretical conversion yields for penicillin synthesis. Biotechnol Bioeng 19:1449–1462

Cooney CL, Wang HY, Wang DIC (1977) Computer-aided material balancing for prediction of fermentation parameters. Biotechnol Bioeng 19:55–67

Davey VF, Johnson MJ (1953) Penicillin production in cornsteep media with continuous carbohydrate addition. Appl Microbiol 1:208–211

Demain AL (1973) Mutation and production of secondary metabolites. Adv Appl Microbiol 16:177–202

Donovick R (1960) Some considerations of bioengineering from a microscopic viewpoint. Appl Microbiol 8:117–122

Elander RP, Aoki H (1982) β-Lactam-producing microorganisms: their biology and fermentation behavior. In: Morin RB, Gorman M (eds) β-Lactam antibiotics, chemistry, and biology, vol III. Academic Press, New York, p 83

Giese AC (1973) Cell physiology, 4th edn. WB Saunders, Philadelphia London Toronto

Goldberg AL (1971) A role of aminoacyl-tRNA in the regulation of protein breakdown in *Escherichia coli*. Proc Natl Acad Sci USA 68:362–366

Hockenhull DJD (1963) Changing approaches to antibiotic production. In: The chemistry and biochemistry of fungi and yeasts, proceedings of the symposium on the chemistry and biochemistry of fungi and yeasts, 18–20 July 1963. Butterworth, London, p 617

Hosler P, Johnson MJ (1953) Penicillin from chemically defined media. Ind Eng Chem 45:871–874
Mason HRS, Righelato RC (1976) Energetics of fungal growth: the effect of growth-limiting substrate on respiration of *Penicillium chrysogenum*. J Appl Chem Biotechnol 26:145–152
McCann EP, Calam CT (1972) The metabolism of *Penicillium chrysogenum* and the production of penicillin using a high yielding strain, at different temperatures. J Appl Chem Biotechnol 22:1201–1208
Mou DG (1979) Toward an optimum penicillin fermentation by monitoring and controlling growth through computer-aided mass balancing. Ph. D. thesis, Massachusetts Institute of Technology
Mou DG, Cooney CL (1976) Application of dynamic calorimetry for monitoring fermentation processes. Biotechnol Bioeng 18:1371–1392
Mou DG, Cooney CL (1983a) Growth monitoring and control through computer-aided on-line mass balancing in a fed-batch penicillin fermentation. Biotechnol Bioeng 25:225–255
Mou DG, Cooney CL (1983b) Growth monitoring and control in a complex medium – a case study employing fed-batch penicillin fermentation and computer-aided on-line mass balancing. Biotechnol Bioeng 25:257–269
Mou DG, Cooney CL (to be published) Effect of growth on the maintenance demand and penicillin production of a high yielding strain of *Penicillium chrysogenum*. Biotechnol Bioeng
Pan CH, Hepler L, Elander RP (1972) Control of pH and carbohydrate addition in the penicillin fermentation. Dev Ind Microbiol 13:103–112
Pirt SJ (1975) Principles of microbe and cell cultivation. Blackwell, Oxford
Pirt SJ, Callow DS (1960) Studies of the growth of *Penicillium chrysogenum* in continuous flow culture with reference to penicillin production. J Appl Bacteriol 23:87–98
Pirt SJ, Righelato RC (1967) Effect of growth rate on the synthesis of penicillin by *Penicillium chrysogenum* in batch and chemostat cultures. Appl Microbiol 15:1284–1290
Queener S, Swartz R (1979) Penicillins: biosynthetic and semisynthetic. In: Rose AH (ed) Economic microbiology, vol 3. Academic Press, London New York, p 35
Righelato RC, Trinci APJ, Pirt SJ, Peat A (1968) The influence of maintenance energy and growth rate on the metabolic activity, morphology, and conidiation of *Penicillium chrysogenum*. J Gen Microbiol 50:399–412
Ryu DY, Humphrey AE (1972) A reassessment of oxygen-transfer rates in antibiotic fermentations. J Ferment Technol 50:422–431
Ryu DY, Humphrey AE (1973) Examples of computer-aided fermentation systems. J Appl Chem Biotechnol 23:283–295
St. John AC, Conklin K, Rosenthal E, Goldberg AL (1978) Further evidence for the involvement of charged tRNA and guanosine tetraphosphate in the control of protein degradation in *Escherichia coli*. J Biol Chem 253:3945–3951
Squires RW (1972) Regulation of the penicillin fermentation by means of a submerged oxygen-sensitive electrode. Dev Ind Microbiol 13:128–135
Swartz RW (1979) The use of economic analysis of penicillin G manufacturing cost in establishing priorities for fermentation process improvement. In: Perlman D (ed) Annual reports on fermentation processes, vol 3. Academic Press, New York London, p 75
Trinci APJ, Righelato RC (1970) Changes in constituents and ultrastructure of hyphal compartments during autolysis of glucose-starved *Penicillium chrysogenum*. J Gen Microbiol 60:239–249
Wang HY, Cooney CL, Wang DIC (1977) Computer-aided bakers' yeast fermentations. Biotechnol Bioeng 19:69–86
Wright DG, Calam CT (1968) Importance of the introductory phase in penicillin production, using continuous flow culture. Chem Ind (Lond) 1274–1275
Young TB, Koplove HM (1972) A systems approach to design and control of antibiotic fermentations. In: Proc IV int ferment symp 19–25 March 1972, Kyoto, p 163

CHAPTER 9

Screening for New β-Lactam Antibiotics

S. B. ZIMMERMAN and E. O. STAPLEY

A. Introduction

Although penicillin was the first antibiotic to be intensively developed for use in human medicine, there is still much to be learned about the β-lactam antibiotics. Reference to Fig. 1, which summarizes cumulative significant discoveries vs. time, will show that there was a long incubation period in the discovery of the wide variety of β-lactam molecules which are currently known from nature. In part, this lag phase may have resulted from the fact that the filamentous fungi, despite their primacy, have proven to be a relatively limited source of β-lactam molecules. Another factor was probably the wide variety of other types of antibiotics which were found in great profusion by determined and high-volume screening of the actinomycetes in many laboratories. The discovery that the actinomycetes also make β-

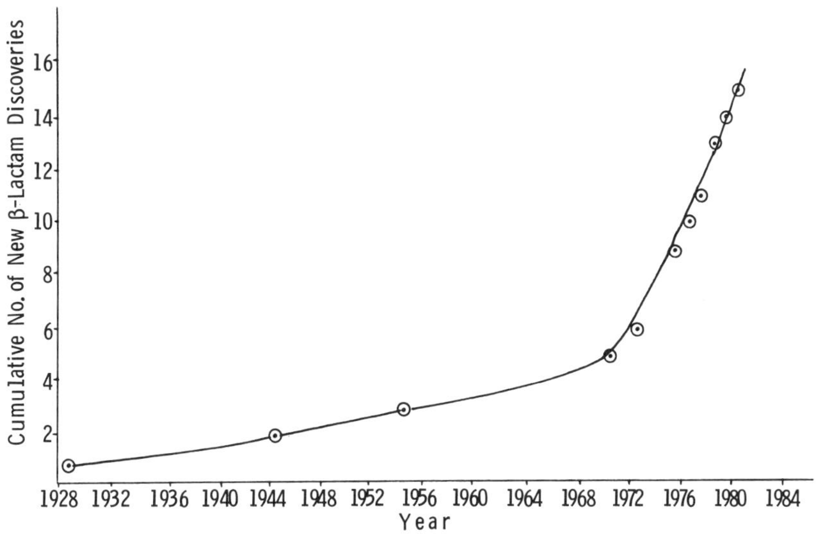

Fig. 1. Cumulative significant discoveries of β-lactam antibiotics vs. time. 1929: Penicillin (FLEMING 1929); 1948: cephalosporin, penicillin N from fungi (BROTZU 1948; NEWTON and ABRAHAM 1954, 1955); 1962: penicillin N from actinomycetes (MILLER et al. 1962); 1971: cephamycins (NAGARAJAN et al. 1971); 1976: nocardicins (AOKI et al. 1976); clavulanic acid (BROWN et al. 1976); thienamycin (KAHAN et al. 1976); 1977: epithienamycins (STAPLEY et al. 1977); 1978: PS-5 (OKAMURA et al. 1978); 1979: PS-6, PS-7 (OKAMURA et al. 1979b); 1980: carpetimycins (NAKAYAMA et al. 1980); 1981: sulfazecin, isosulfazecin (IMADA et al. 1981)

lactam compounds, although not considered earth-shattering at the time of its announcement, resulted in eventual realization that the actinomycetes were a specific source of a very wide variety of β-lactam compounds.

To this day, we are left with the question – why β-lactam antibiotics? The essential function, if there is one, of this interesting group of molecules is completely unknown. Indeed, if we but knew why β-lactam antibiotics were made, we might have the clue to a tool for finding many others as yet undiscovered. It seems possible that they are somehow related to filamentation since with one exception (IMADA et al. 1981) they have so far been found only as products of filamentous organisms. It is attractive to speculate that β-lactam compounds are ubiquitous among the filamentous microorganisms and that we call those cultures which are recognized as positive producers of β-lactam antibiotics positive because they overproduce a compound, or group of compounds, which may be essential at a concentration so low as to be undetectable.

The essential elements for finding new antibiotics of whatever type are very similar. To find β-lactam antibiotics, it is essential to develop a selective methodology which is based on the characteristics of the molecules sought. Selective methodology can be based on the chemistry of the compounds or the biology of the compounds. In the search for new antibiotics, if we accept the suggestion that new agents are likely to occur at very low concentrations, the biological tools will be the most useful since they are generally more sensitive and selective than chemical procedures. In the search for new β-lactam antibiotics, there is nothing that can be taken for granted. All the factors of a screening program are important. It is obvious that one must have a culture capable of making the new antibiotic that is going to be discovered. The second factor is that this culture must be grown under conditions where it will elaborate a detectable quantity of said antibiotic. The third factor is that we must have a detection system sensitive enough to determine the presence of the antibiotic and selective enough to tell us that it is likely to be a β-lactam antibiotic. The fourth requirement is that some type of identification program, as a next step or built into the detection system itself, must differentiate the β-lactam from the large number of compounds already known.

The testing of a large number of sources and potentially new substances and a "weeding process" are essential elements in the screening program for new β-lactam antibiotics. A typical program has been described by WOODRUFF and coworkers and is exemplified in Fig. 2 (WOODRUFF et al. 1979). In order to shortcut this process, it would be very desirable to build all of the initial steps of production, detection, recognition, and differentiation into the first screening process itself. Unfortunately, many of the β-lactam antibiotics occur in mixtures which must be separated in some fashion or subjected to a variety of sophisticated biological questions in order to determine whether a member of such a mixture is new. Anyone familiar with the literature on the discovery of new antibiotics is well aware that the exact methodology utilized for the original detection of new substances is seldom discussed in detail. In fact, the amount of information presented in detection papers which deals with details of the method for detection is very likely to be inversely proportional to the importance, or imagined importance, of a particular discovery; i.e., the most interesting discoveries always appear as the most mysterious. This is quite natural because of the competitive nature of the search for valu-

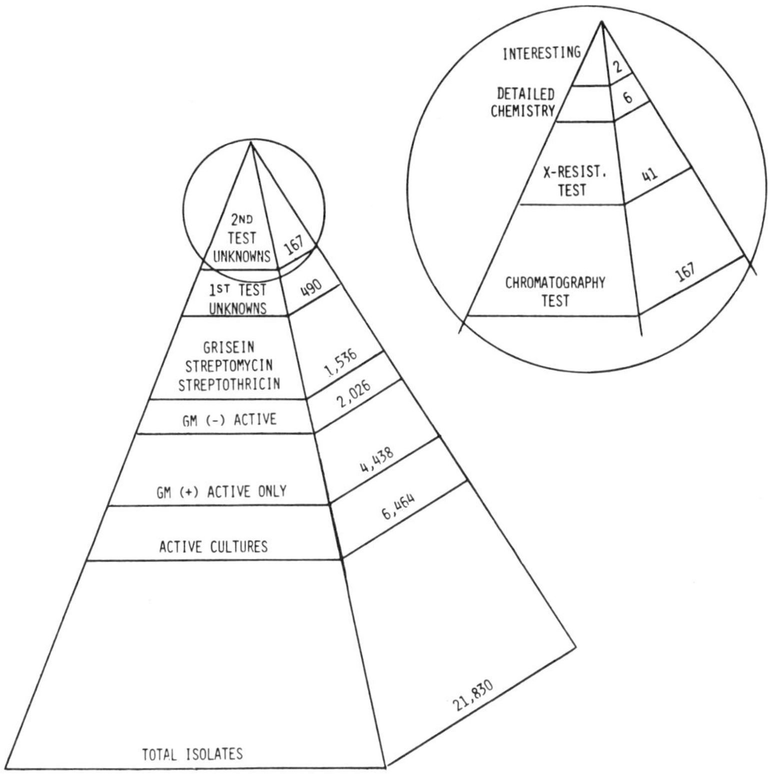

Fig. 2. Operation of a 1957 Antibiotic Screening Program in which 21,830 soil isolates were reduced to six cultures studied actively by chemists. (WOODRUFF et al. 1979)

able new microbial products, but it makes the task of reviewing screening methodology a difficult one. Despite this difficulty, there is a considerable literature on screening for β-lactam antibiotics which we will review before trying to construct a generalized strategy for such a screening program.

B. Rationale for Screening of β-Lactam Antibiotics

β-Lactam antibiotics make particularly attractive targets for screens because of their desirable mode of action, general lack of toxicity, intrinsic potency and/or breadth of spectrum, feasibility for enhancement of efficacy by derivatization and, by virtue of β-lactamase inhibitory properties, the capability of acting as synergists in combination with other β-lactam antibiotics.

I. Mode of Action

Many clinically useful β-lactam antibiotics have been shown to act as inhibitors of bacterial cell wall (peptidoglycan) synthesis (LEDERBERG 1956; STROMINGER et al. 1967; STAPLEY et al. 1972; ONISHI et al. 1974; SPRATT 1975; ZIMMERMAN and STAP-

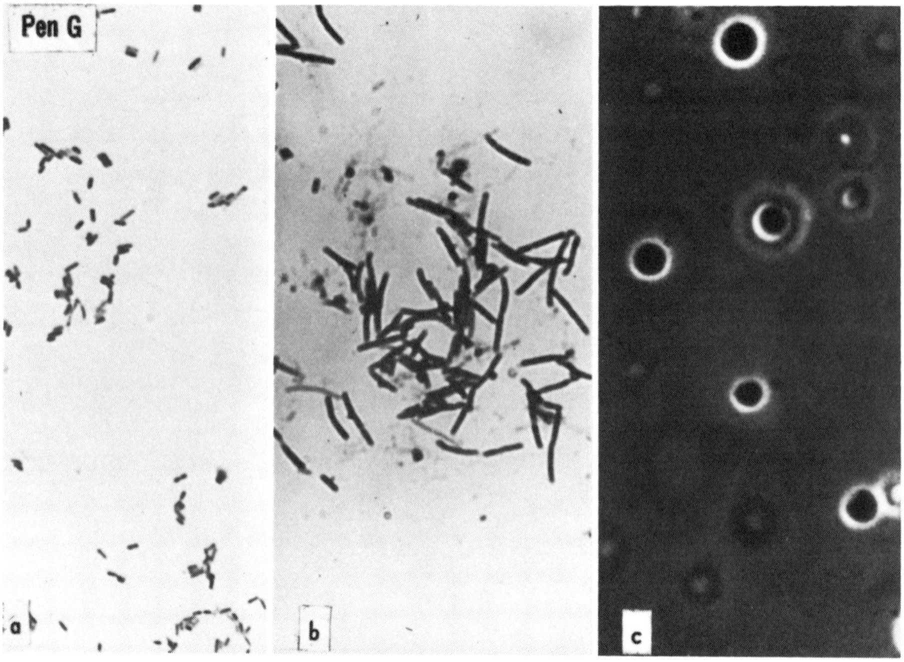

Fig. 3. Morphological changes induced in *Enterobacter cloacae* by penicillin G at **a** noninhibitory concentrations; **b** at subinhibitory concentrations in which filament formation is evident; and **c** at inhibitory concentrations showing spheroplast formation. Photomicrographs of **a** and **b** are gentian violet strains; **c** is a wet mount as observed by phase contrast microscopy. (ONISHI et al. 1974)

LEY 1976) (Fig. 3). Since peptidoglycan synthesis is essentially a prokaryotic function, peptidoglycan inhibitors would be expected to yield agents of comparatively low toxicity to mammalian systems. Extensive clinical experience has indeed confirmed this expectation.

II. Potency and Spectrum

Intrinsic potency and/or breadth of spectrum of many naturally occurring and semisynthetic β-lactam antibiotics have inspired intensive screening programs for these agents. Examples of such agents include the cephamycins (NAGARAJAN et al. 1971; STAPLEY et al. 1972), the epithienamycins (STAPLEY et al. 197), olivanic acids (HOOD et al. 1979), thienamycin (KAHAN et al. 1976, 1979), and the carpetimycins (NAKAYAMA et al. 1980).

III. Chemical Alterability

Many naturally occurring β-lactam molecules are capable of chemical alteration to improve potency, spectrum, oral absorption, resistance to enzymatic inactivation, or achievement of higher serum, urine, and tissue levels. Semisynthetic derivatives of the natural product 6-aminopenicillanic acid, have yielded many clinically useful antibiotics. The cephamycin derivatives cefoxitin, cefmetazol, and SKF-

73678 are semisynthetic β-lactams which have demonstrated greater clinical efficacy than the natural product from which they were derived. MK-0787, which is the *N*-formimidoyl derivative of the natural product thienamycin (LEANZA et al. 1981) has been reported to show greater potency and chemical stability than the natural product (KROPP et al. 1980). MK-0787 appears promising for clinical use in human medicine. Deacetoxycephalosporin C, a natural product, can be altered chemically to produce cephalexin and other cephalosporin derivatives (HIGGENS et al. 1974).

IV. Potentiation of Other Antibiotics

Clavulanic acid (BROWN et al. 1976), a naturally occurring oxypenicillin, is finding clinical use as a potent inhibitor of β-lactamases. Although clavulanic acid by itself is a relatively weak antibiotic, low concentrations synergize lactamase-sensitive β-lactams by protecting the latter from inactivation by a broad range of β-lactamases. Augmentin, a combination of clavulanic acid and amoxycillin, is planned for use in human medicine. Other potent β-lactamase inhibitors found in nature include the olivanic acids (BUTTERWORTH et al. 1979; HOOD et al. 1979), MC 696-SY2-A and -B (MAEDA et al. 1977), thienamycin (HUANG et al. 1980), PS-5 (OKAMURA et al. 1978, 1979 a), PS-6, and -7 (OKAMURA et al. 1979 b), and the carpetimycins (NAKAYAMA et al. 1980).

C. Finding β-Lactam-Producing Microorganisms

I. Discovery of Fungi as Producers of β-Lactams

The great discoveries of the activities of penicillin by FLEMING (1929) and of the cephalosporins by BROTZU (1948) dramatically demonstrated the production of potent β-lactam antibiotics by fungi. FLEMING's discovery was made by observing an area of lysis on a staphylococcal plate in the vicinity of an airborne contaminant of *Penicillium notatum*. FLEMING isolated the fungus in pure culture and showed that the culture fluid exerted high activity against certain bacteria (ABRAHAM 1974). Brotzu took samples of seawater near a sewage outlet in Sardinia and isolated a strain similar to *Cephalosporium acremonium* which inhibited several gram-positive and gram-negative organisms. The choice of a sewage outlet was based on the rationale that the self-purification of the water might be attributable to bacterial antagonism (ABRAHAM and LODER 1972). BROTZU's approach combined a culture isolation technique and a nonspecific mode of action, leading to the subsequent isolation of penicillin N (cephalosporin N; synnematin B) (NEWTON and ABRAHAM 1954) and of cephalosporin C (NEWTON and ABRAHAM 1955).

II. Discovery of Actinomycetes as Producers of β-Lactams

Following the pioneering soil culture isolation studies of Dubos, which were aimed at discovering microorganisms which would lyse capsules of pneumococci (DUBOS 1939), isolation of streptomycetes from soil samples by Waksman and Woodruff soon demonstrated the remarkable abilities of these organisms to elaborate antibiotics. Their work on the study of actinomycetes from soils promptly led to the discoveries of actinomycins and streptothricin (WAKSMAN and WOODRUFF 1940,

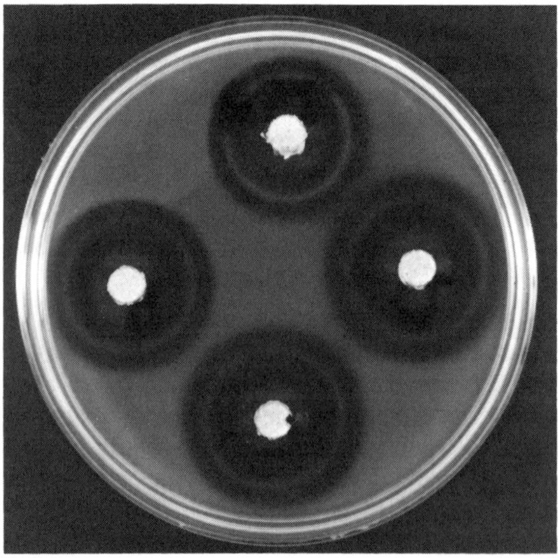

Fig. 4. Demonstration of antibiotic activity by *Streptomyces* spp. cultures on a normal antibiotic-sensitive test bacterium. Zones of inhibited bacterial growth surround agar plugs selected from four different strains of *Streptomyces*. (WOODRUFF et al. 1979)

1942), streptomycin (SCHATZ et al. 1944), grisein (REYNOLDS et al. 1947), and a host of other broad-spectrum antibiotics. Later, with the rediscovery of penicillin N (MILLER et al. 1962) and the cephamycins (NAGARAJAN et al. 1971; STAPLEY et al. 1972) it became apparent that actinomycetes were a source of potentially useful β-lactam antibiotics.

1. World-Wide Search for Antibiotic-Producing Microorganisms

Soil samples collected from a wide variety of geographical locations led to the screening of hundreds of thousands of microorganisms (WOODRUFF and McDANIEL 1958; WOODRUFF et al. 1979). Antibiotics were detected from agar plugs of the producing organism placed on media seeded with test bacteria (Fig. 4).

2. Development of Culture Isolation Techniques

Selective isolation of actinomycetes was aided by the addition of antibiotics to plating media (DULANEY et al. 1955; HAMILL 1977; GAUSE 1974) in order to detect a wide variety of antibiotic-producing strains. Streptomycin-containing agar plates are reported to eliminate many redundant, commonly occurring *Streptomyces* species and preferentially give rise to the *albus* and *helvolus* strains as well as the genus *Nocardia* (GAUSE 1974). Daunomycin (rubomycin) and polyene macrolide antibiotics have also been used to increase selectivity of antibiotic-producing cultures (LAVROVA et al. 1972; TSAO and THIELEKI 1966). Aerobic actinomycetes were found to proliferate from $CaCO_3$-treated soil samples when plated on arginine-glycerol-salts medium (EL-NAKEEB and LECHEVALIER 1963). Isolation of *Microbiospora* and *Streptosporangium* strains were favored when soil samples were air dried, ground and dry-heated to 120 °C before being placed on chemically defined agar containing an antifungal substance (NONOMURA and OHARA 1969; OKAMURA et al. 1979a). The latter procedures led to the isolation of cultures which produced PS-5, a potent carbapenam antibiotic related to thienamycin.

III. Discovery of Bacteria as Producers of β-Lactams

Recently, the first report was made of bacterially produced novel monocyclic β-lactam antibiotics, sulfazecin, and isosulfazecin (IMADA et al. 1981). These are true antibiotics, produced by *Pseudomonas aeruginosa*, unlike the β-lactam-containing wild-fire toxins reported to be produced by phytopathogenic bacteria (STEWART 1971; TAYLOR et al. 1972).

D. Screening Systems Which Detect β-Lactams

I. Biospectrum and Physicochemical Data Comparisons

Comparisons of data obtained from activity spectra, chromatography (Fig. 5), electrophoresis, etc., can be used either as a primary screen (MILLER et al. 1962)

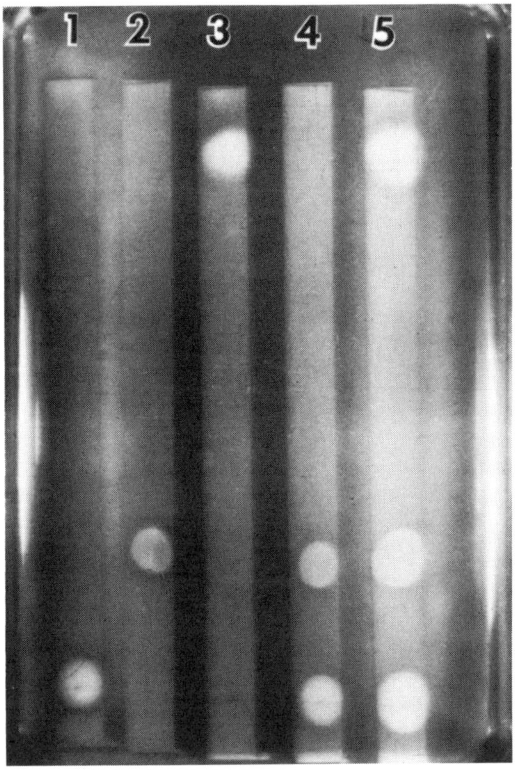

Fig. 5. Resolution of known antibiotics by paper chromatography and bioautography. *1*, streptothricin; *2*, cycloserine; *3*, chloramphenicol; *4*, streptothricin + cycloserine; *5*, streptothricin + cycloserine + chloramphenicol. Solvent system: *n*-butanol (8) + H_2O(2) + acetic acid (1). Antibiotic applied at end opposite to numerals, developed by ascending technique. Visualized by bioautography with *Escherichia coli* on nutrient agar. (WOODRUFF et al. 1979)

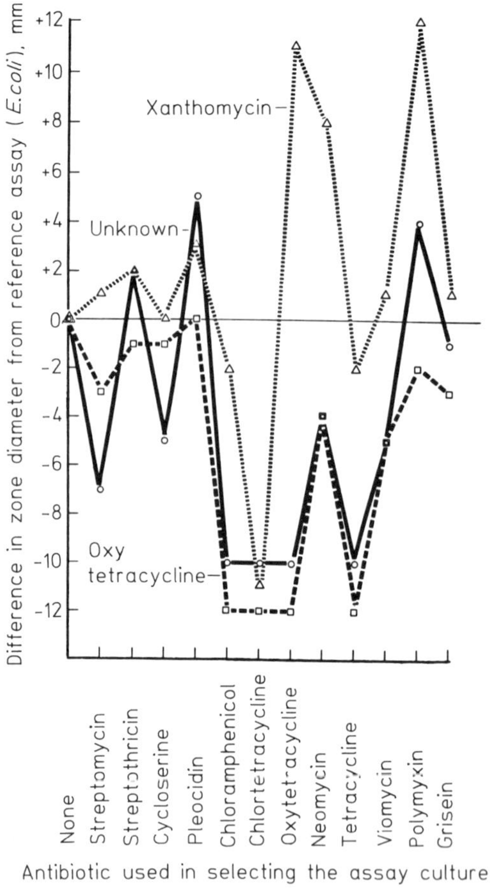

Fig. 6. Graphic comparison of the activity of an "unknown" antibiotic broth with the patterns of two different antibiotics. The tests are performed by agar diffusion plate assays against a series of antibiotic-resistant strains derived in the laboratory from the same parent "sensitive" *Escherichia coli* culture which serves as the base line or "zero" value for calculation of relative sensitivity. Such in vitro resistant cultures show characteristic patterns of hypersensitivity and/or cross resistance for different families of antibiotics. In the case shown here the "unknown" bears a superficial similarity, in some tests, to xanthomycin but is very similar to oxytetracycline and belongs to the tetracycline family. (WOODRUFF et al. 1979)

or as a secondary identification system following a primary screen (STAPLEY 1958; PERLMAN 1970). Integrated biospectrum patterns rather than individual pieces of data have been utilized (WOODRUFF et al. 1979) for both detection and identification (Fig. 6). Extensive reference data bases have been established with the purpose of comparing data from unknown antimicrobial substances with reference collections of known antibiotics. One such reference data base was compiled and coded on edge-punched cards (BERDY 1974). Characteristics in the Berdy data base are: spectrum of activity, mode of action, physicochemical properties, and chemical structure. Computerization and expansion of the Berdy system was used to identify

Table 1. Characteristics included in the Bostian–Berdy antibiotic database

Antibiotic name, synonyms	Chromatography
Chemical type[a]	Stability
Chemical formula	Test organisms
Elementary analysis	Toxicity data
Antibiotic code number[a]	Antitumor/antiviral effects[c]
Producing organisms	Isolation methods:
Molecular/equivalent weight	Filtration
Appearance-physical characteristics[b]	Extraction
Optical rotation	Ion-exchange
Ultraviolet spectra	Absorption
Solubility	Chromatography
Qualitative chemical reactions	Crystallization

[a] According to the Berdy classification system
[b] Color, crystal structure, etc.
[c] In vitro and in vivo characteristics

unknown antitumor agents (BOSTIAN et al. 1977). The Bostian system incorporates tolerance ranges for numeric values to compensate for variations between experiments. The expanded reference database contains over 5,000 compounds containing over 1.5 million characteristics of data with 110,000 individual values or value sets (Table 1).

1. Penicillin N

The first penicillin antibiotic found to be produced by actinomycetes, penicillin N (symnematin B), was detected and identified by examination of comparative data obtained from broth filtrates and their purified extracts (MILLER et al. 1962). Antimicrobial spectrum, inactivation by penicillinase, cross-resistance with penicillin (STAPLEY 1958), mobility in several paper chromatography systems, chemical identity of degradation products, and electrophoretic mobility were used to differentiate penicillin N from known reference antibiotics.

2. Cephamycins

Comparative biospectrum and physical–chemical characteristics contributed to the detection and identification of the cephamycins (STAPLEY et al. 1972).

II. β-Lactamase Inhibition

1. Clavulanic Acid

Clavulanic acid, discovered in a screen which was aimed specifically at finding β-lactamase inhibitors (BROWN et al. 1976) has shown clinical efficacy as a synergist for lactamase-sensitive β-lactams. A β-lactamase-producing strain of *Klebsiella aerogenes* NCTC-418 (ATCC 15380) was used in agar plates containing 10 μg/ml benzylpenicillin. Synergism, i.e., protection, of benzylpenicillin was detected by observing zones of inhibition around diffusible inhibitors of the *Klebsiella* β-lactamase.

2. Olivanic Acids

The olivanic acids (BUTTERWORTH et al. 1979; HOOD et al. 1979) were discovered in independent screening systems for β-lactamase inhibitors in two laboratories. The above-mentioned method (BROWN et al. 1976) which led to the discovery of clavulanic acid was used to detect olivanic acids MM 4450 and MM 13902 from *Streptomyces olivaceus* in the Beecham Laboratories. A second method (UMEZAWA et al. 1973) detected MC 696-SY2-A (identical to MM 4450) and MC 696-SYZ-B. MC 696-SY2-A and -B, produced by *Streptomyces fulvoviridis*, were found by applying the iodometric method for detecting inhibition of β-lactamase obtained from *Escherichia coli* K12 W3630 $R_{75}{}^{+1}$. An agar plate method was also used in which commercial β-lactamase and 10 units/ml of benzylpenicillin were incorporated into agar seeded with *Staphylococcus aureus* FDA 209P. Zones of inhibition signifying β-lactamase inhibition were interpreted in a manner similar to that used in the Beecham β-lactamase inhibition screen described above.

3. PS-5, -6, and -7

Enhancement of antimicrobial activity, by PS-5, of the activity of ampicillin or cephaloridine against a β-lactamase-producing strain of *Proteus vulgaris* was used to detect the β-lactamase inhibitory properties of PS-5 (OKAMURA et al. 1978, 1979a). *Comamonas terrigena* bioassay plates with and without β-lactamase from *P. vulgaris* P-5 or *Citrobacter freundii* E-9 were used in the screening method, which detected antibiotics PS-6 and PS-7 (OKAMURA et al. 1979b). Enhancement of benzylpenicillin and cephaloridine activities in the presence of the enzyme preparations was the criterion for selection of PS-6 and -7.

4. Carpetimycins

The carpetimycins (NAKAYAMA et al. 1980) demonstrated synergistic activity in combination with penicillins and cephalosporins against various β-lactam-resistant strains of bacteria. The synergistic mode-of-action was presumably via inhibition of β-lactamases produced by the tester strains.

III. β-Lactam Supersensitive Bacterial Mutants

1. The Nocardicins

The nocardicins were detected in fermentation broth by screening with a series of mutants of *E. coli* which were mutagenized to hypersensitivity to β-lactam antibiotics (AOKI et al. 1976, 1977; HOSODA et al. 1977). The β-lactam hypersensitivity of these mutants is probably attributable, at least in part, to alterations in membrane-bound penicillin-binding proteins (SPRATT 1975; CASSIDY 1981).

2. Deacetoxycephalosporin C

A *P. aeruginosa* mutant (Ps C) was used as the screening organism which detected deacetoxycephalosporin C (KITANO et al. 1975). Ps C was obtained by a three-step mutagenesis of strain IFO 3080. A new penicillin, KPN, and three other new cephalosporins, including C-43-219, were also found with the Ps C screen (KITANO et al. 1977).

3. PS-5

A cephalothin-hypersensitive strain (B996) of *C. terrigena* was the organism which detected antibiotic PS-5 (OKAMURA et al. 1979a), a broad-spectrum carbapenam antibiotic from a fermentation broth of *Streptomyces* sp (A271-ATCC 30358) isolated from a Japanese soil sample. PS-5 was also found active in a screen for β-lactamase inhibitors (OKAMURA et al. 1978).

4. Sulfazecin and Isosulfazecin

P. aeruginosa PsC^{33} and *E. coli* PG8, the latter lacking chromosomal β-lactamase and penicillin-binding protein (PBP)1B, were used to detect these novel β-lactam antibiotics of bacterial origin (IMADA et al. 1981).

IV. Screening for Bacterial Cell Wall Inhibitors

General screens which look for peptidoglycan inhibitors predictably can detect β-lactam antibiotics.

1. Cephamycin, Epithienamycins, and Thienamycins

An extensive collection of microbial strains, isolated from a world-wide collection of soil samples, which were tested for bacterial cell wall inhibition at the Merck Sharp and Dohme Research Laboratories led to the discovery of the cephamycins (STAPLEY et al. 1972; WOODRUFF et al. 1979) the thienamycins (KAHAN et al. 1976, 1979), and the epithienamycins (STAPLEY et al. 1977).

2. Azureomycin

Azureomycin is not a β-lactam antibiotic but was detected in a cell wall inhibition screen which did find several previously discovered β-lactam antibiotics (OMURA et al. 1979). The methods used in the primary screen include examination of culture broths of soil isolates for activity vs. *Bacillus subtilis* and for lack of activity vs. *Acholeplasma laidlawii*. In a secondary test, examination was made of prevention of incorporation of meso- (^{3}H) diaminopimelic acid without prevention of incorporation of L- (^{14}C) leucine into the acid-insoluble macromolecular fraction of growing cells of *Bacillus subtilis*. In a tertiary test, inhibitors of MW $\leqq 1000$ were selected using a Diaflow UM-2 membrane.

V. Screening of Penicillin N-Producing Cultures

1. Deacetoxycephalosporin C

Previous evidence that production of penicillin N by fungi and actinomycetes was associated with the production of cephalosporin compounds (NEWTON and ABRAHAM 1955; NAGARAJAN et al. 1971; STAPLEY et al. 1972) prompted the establishment of a screen (HIGGENS et al. 1974) for new cephalosporins from penicillin N–producing cultures in the culture collection of the Lilly Research Laboratories. Deacetoxycephalosporin C was discovered in 22 strains of fungi and two streptomycetes. Most of the organisms also produced deacetylcephalosporin C, cephalosporin C, and, less frequently, the lactone of deacetylcephalosporin C.

Deacetoxycephalosporin C, after chemical deacetylation to remove the aminoadipoyl side-chain to yield 7-aminoacetoxycephalosporanic acid, can be used to produce new antibiotics such as cephalexin (HIGGENS et al. 1974).

E. Future Trends

The success achieved in screening for naturally occurring β-lactam antibiotics leaves little doubt that such investigations will continue. Increased specificity and sensitivity of the screening tools will be essential factors for success. Since secondary metabolites are a rich source of new β-lactam antibiotics (ZAHNER 1977; OKA 1980), an intensified search should be made for such intermediates in fermentation broths. High-pressure liquid chromatographic techniques may prove to be useful in detecting such new molecules.

The clinical importance of β-lactamase-resistant β-lactams, e.g., the cephamycins, thienamycin, moxalactam, etc. demonstrates the importance of screens which seek such resistant molecules. A variety of β-lactamases should be isolated and used to detect resistant β-lactams, monitored perhaps with a chromogenic cephalosporin substrate (O'CALLAGHAN et al. 1972; MAHONEY et al. 1976).

Affinity of β-lactams for certain penicillin-binding proteins (PBP) could constitute a useful screen for β-lactam antibiotics. Since β-lactams which bind preferentially to PBPs 1 and/or 3 demonstrate lysis of *E. coli* K12 at lower concentrations than β-lactams which bind to other PBPs (SPRATT 1975), a screen is suggested which would seek β-lactams which bind preferentially to PBPs 1 and/or 3 (GEORGOPAPADAKOU and LIU 1980).

ZAHNER (1977) suggested several screening methods which could be fruitful in finding new β-lactams: (a) growth of test organisms on nonoptimal media at nonoptimal temperatures; (b) use of permeation-damaged organisms; (c) use of synergists to facilitate penetration, e.g., EDTA, detergents; (d) observation of differentiation and morphogenesis rather than cell death; (e) application of microbial transformation; (f) use of transport mechanisms for screening.

The recent proliferation of clinically useful β-lactam antibiotics provides many tools which could have an important role in the future search for new β-lactam molecules.

F. A Hypothetical Screening Model

Figure 7 represents a flow chart for a hypothetical screening system aimed at detecting β-lactam antibiotics. Its complexity emphasizes the myriad challenges in such an undertaking. The general procedures for the overall design of a screening program to detect β-lactam antibiotics are dictated by the nature of the search process and the objective itself. As shown in Fig. 7, the process is redundant after the initial detection step. It is necessary to have a detection step which does more than simply look for antibiotic activity. Having found an antibiotic activity which is presumptively β-lactam in nature, some type of comfirmatory test must be performed followed by a classification of the activity to eliminate obvious known β-lactam

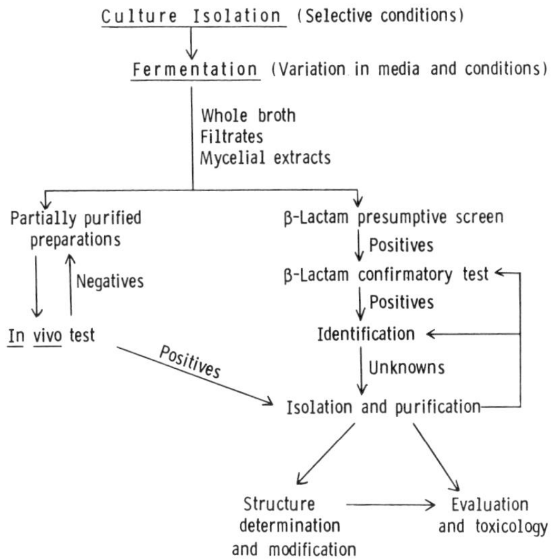

Fig. 7. A hypothetical screening model for β-lactam antibiotics from fermentation broths. (Adapted from HAMILL 1977)

antibiotics. Both chemical and biological data indicating factors which are novel about the crude activity must be reiterated at each depth of purification and testing, in order to be certain that with extraction and with modifications in fermentation conditions, etc., the activity of interest is not lost or masked by a known substance. In most programs, one would expect an evaluation of toxicity and small-scale in vivo activity to precede a full-scale evaluation and development program. However, in the case of a family of substances which has historically been as interesting as the β-lactams, it may be advantageous to purify and learn the structure of new members of this large family even though the original testing does not disclose the immediate practical potential.

References

Abraham EP (1974) Some aspects of the development of penicillins and cephalosporins. In: Murray ED, Bourquin AW (eds) Developments in industrial microbiology, vol 15. American Institute of Biological Sciences, Washington DC, p 3

Abraham EP, Loder PB (1972) Cephalosporin C. In: Flynn EH (ed) Cephalosporins and penicillins. Chemistry and biology. Academic Press, New York London, p 1

Aoki H, Sakai H, Kohsaka M, Konomi T, Hosada J, Kubochi Y, Iguchi E (1976) Nocardicin A, a new monocyclic β-lactam antibiotic I. Discovery, isolation, and characterization. J Antibiot 29:492–500

Aoki H, Kunugita K, Hosoda J, Imanaka H (1977) Screening of new and novel β-lactam antibiotics. Jpn J Antibiot 30:S207–S217

Berdy J (1974) Recent development of antibiotic research and classification of antibiotics according to chemical structure. Adv Appl Microbiol 18:309–406

Bostian M, McNitt A, Aszalos A, Berdy J (1977) Antibiotic identification: a computerized data base system. J Antibiot 30:633–634

Brotzu G (1968) Richerche su di nuovo antibiotics. Lav Ist Iqiene Cagliari:1–11

Brown AG, Butterworth D, Cole M, Hanscomb G, Hood JD, Reading C (1976) Naturally occuring β-lactam inhibitors with antibacterial activity. Jpn J Antibiot 29:668–669

Butterworth D, Cole M, Hanscomb G, Rolinson GN (1979) Olivanic acids, a family of β-lactam antibiotics with β-lactamase inhibitory properties produced by *Streptomyces* species I. Detection, properties, and fermentation studies. J Antibiot 32:287–294

Cassidy PJ (1981) Novel naturally occurring β-lactam antibiotics – a review. In: Underkofler LA (ed) Developments in industrial microbiology, vol 22. American Institute of Biological Sciences, Washington DC, p 181

Dubos RJ (1939) Studies on a bactericidal agent extracted from a soil bacillus. I. Preparation of the agent. Its activity in vitro. J Exp Med 70:1

Dulaney EL, Larsen AH, Stapley EO (1955) A note on the isolation of microorganisms from natural sources. Mycologia 47:420–422

El-Nakeeb M, Lechevalier HA (1963) Selective isolation of aerobic actinomycetes. Appl Microbiol 11:75–77

Fleming A (1929) On the antibacterial action of cultures of a *Penicillium* with special reference to the isolation of *B. influenzae*. Br J Exp Pathol 10:200–206

Gause GT (1974) Recent trends in the screening of new antibiotics. Postepy Hig Med Dosw 28:471–477

Georgopadakou NH, Liu FY (1980) Binding of β-lactam antibiotics to penicillin-binding proteins of *Staphylococcus aureus* and *Streptococcus faecalis:* relation to antibacterial activity. Antimicrob Agents Chemother 18:834–836

Hamill RL (1977) General approaches to fermentation screening. Jpn J Antibiot 30:S164–173

Higgens CE, Hamill RL, Sands TH et al. (1974) The occurence of deacetoxycephalosporin C in fungi and streptomycetes. J Antibiot (Tokyo) 27:298–300

Hood JD, Box SJ, Verall MS (1979) Olivanic acids, a family of β-lactam antibiotics with β-lactamase inhibitory properties produced by *Streptomyces* species. II. Isolation and characterization of the olivanic acids MM4550, MM13902, and MM17880 from *Streptomyces olivaceus*. J Antibiot (Tokyo) 32:295–304

Hosoda J, Konomi T, Tani N, Aoki H, Imanaka H (1977) Isolation of new nocardicins from *Nocardia uniformis* subspecies *tsuyamanensis*. Agric Biol Chem 41:2013–2020

Huang L, Jakubas K, Burg RW (1980) Easy method for evaluating the structure activity relationship of penicillinase and cephalosporinase inhibition by β-lactam antibiotics. In: Nelson JD, Grassi C (eds) Current chemotherapy and infectious disease. Proceedings of the 11th ICC and the 19th ICAAC, vol 1. American Society for Microbiology, Washington DC, p 744

Imada A, Kitano K, Kintaka K, Muroi M, Asai M (1981) Sulfazecin and isosulfazecin, novel β-lactam antibiotics of bacterial origin. Nature 289:590–591

Kahan JS, Kahan FM, Goegelman R et al. (1976) Thienamycin, a new β-lactam antibiotic I. Discovery and isolation, Abst 227. In: Abstract of the 16th interscience conference on antimicrobial agents and chemotherapy. American Society for Microbiology, Washington DC

Kahan JS, Kahan FM, Goegelman R et al. (1979) Thienamycin, a new β-lactam antibiotic I. Discovery taxonomy, isolation, and physical properties. J Antibiot (Tokyo) 32:1–12

Kitano K, Kintaka K, Suzuki S, Katamoko K, Nara K, Nakao Y (1975) Screening of microorganisms capable of producing β-lactam antibiotics. J Ferment Technol 53:327–338

Kitano K, Nara K, Nakao Y (1977) Screening for β-lactam antibiotics using a mutant of *Pseudomonas aeruginosa*. Jpn J Antibiot 30:S239–S245

Kropp H, Sundelof JG, Kahan JS, Kahan FM, Birnbaum J (1980) MK-0787 (N-formimidoylthienamycin): evaluation of in vitro and in vivo activities. Antimicrob Agents Chemother 17:993–1000

Lavrova NV, Preobrazhenskaya TP, Sveshnikova MA (1972) Isolation of soil actinomycetes on selective media with rubomycin. Antibiotiki (Mosc) 17:965–970

Leanza WJ, Wildonger J, Hannah J, Shih D, Ratcliffe RW, Barash L, Walton E, Firestone RA, Patel GF, Kahan FM, Kahan JS, Christensen BG (1981) Structure activity relationship in the thienamycin series. In: Gregory GI (ed) Recent advances in the chemistry of β-lactam antibiotics. Chemical Society. Special Publication No 38, London, p 240

Lederberg J (1956) Bacterial protoplasts induced by penicillin. Proc Natl Acad Sci USA 42:574–577

Maeda K, Takahashi S, Sezaki M, Iinuma K, Naganawa H, Kondo S, Ohno M, Umezawa H (1977) Isolation and structure of a β-lactamase inhibitor from *Streptomyces*. J Antibiot (Tokyo) 30:770–772

Mahoney DF, Koppel GA, Turner JR (1976) Substrate inhibition of beta-lactamases, a method for predicting enzymatic stability to cephalosporins. Antimicrob Agents Chemother 10:470–475

Miller IM, Stapley EO, Chaiet L (1962) Production of synnematin B by a member of the genus *Streptomyces*. Bacteriol Proc A49:32

Nagarajan R, Boeck LD, Gorman M, Hamill RL, Higgens CE, Hollin MM, Stark WM, Whitney JG (1971) β-Lactam antibiotics from *Streptomyces*. J Am Chem Soc 93:2308–2310

Nakayama M, Iwasaki A, Kimura S, Mizoguchi T, Tanabe S, Murakami A, Watanabe I, Okuchi M, Itoh H, Saino Y, Kobayashi F, Mori T (1980) Carpetimycins A and B, new β-lactam antibiotics. J Antibiot (Tokyo) 33:1388–1389

Newton GGF, Abraham EP (1954) Degradation, structure, and some derivatives of cephalosporin N. Biochem J 58:103–111

Newton GGF, Abraham EP (1955) Cephalosporin C, a new antibiotic containing sulfur and D-α-aminoadipic acid. Nature 175:548

Nonomura H, Ohara Y (1969) Distribution of actinomycetes in soil VI A culture method for both preferential isolation and enumeration of *Microbiospora* and *Streptosporangium* strains in soil. J Ferment Technol 47:463–469

O'Callaghan CH, Morris A, Kirby SM, Shingler AH (1972) Novel method for detection of β-lactamase by using a chromogenic cephalosporin substrate. Antimicrob Agents Chemother 1:283–288

Oka T (1980) New screening strategies for discovering useful microbial metabolites. In: Abstracts of the VI th international fermentation symposium and V th international symposium on yeasts, 20–25 July 1980. National Research Council, Canada, Ottawa

Okamura K, Hirata S, Okumura Y, Fukagawa Y, Ishikura T, Shimauchi Y, Kouno K, Lein J (1978) PS-5, a new β-lactam antibiotic from *Streptomyces*. J Antibiot (Tokyo) 31:480–482

Okamura K, Koki A, Sakamoto M, Kubo K, Mutoh Y, Fukagawa Y, Kouno K, Shimauchi Y, Ishikura T, Lein J (1979a) Microorganisms producing a new β-lactam antibiotic. J Ferment Technol 57:265–272

Okamura K, Hirata S, Okumura Y, Fukagawa Y, Ishikura T, Shimauchi Y, Kouno K, Lein J (1979b) New antibiotics PS-6 and PS-7 having β-lactamase inhibitory activity. European patent application 1567

Omura S, Tanaka H, Oiwa R, Nagai T, Koyama Y, Takahashi Y (1979) Studies on bacterial cell wall inhibitors VI Screening method for the specific inhibitors of peptidoglycan synthesis. J Antibiot (Tokyo) 32:978–984

Onishi HR, Zimmerman SB, Stapley EO (1974) Observations on the mode of action of cefoxitin. Ann NY Acad Sci 235:406–425

Perlman D (1970) Antibiotics. In: Burger A (ed) Medicinal chemistry, 3rd edn. Wiley-Interscience, New York, p 305

Reynolds DM, Schatz A, Waksman SA (1947) Grisein, a new antibiotic produced by certain strains of *Streptomyces griseus*. Proc Soc Exp Biol Med 64:50–54

Schatz A, Bugie E, Waksman SA (1944) Streptomycin, a substance exhibiting antibiotic activity against gram-positive and gram-negative bacteria. Proc Soc Exp Biol Med 55:66–69

Spratt BG (1975) Distinct penicillin-binding proteins involved in the division, elongation, and shape of *Escherichia coli* K12. Proc Natl Acad Sci USA 72:2999–3003

Stapley EO (1958) Cross-resistance studies and antibiotic identification. Appl Microbiol 6:392–398

Stapley EO, Jackson M, Hernandez S, Zimmerman SB, Currie SA, Mochales S, Mata JM, Woodruff HB, Hendlin D (1972) Cephamycins, a new family of β-lactam antibiotics I production by actinomycetes. Antimicrob Agents Chemother 2:122–131

Stapley EO, Cassidy P, Currie SA, Daoust D, Goegelman R, Hernandez S, Jackson M, Mata JM, Miller AK, Monaghan RL, Tunac JB, Zimmerman SB, Hendlin D (1977) Epithienamycins: biological studies of a new family of β-lactam antibiotics. In: Abstracts of the 17th interscience conference on antimicrobial agents and chemotherapy. American Society for Microbiology, Washington DC

Stewart WW (1971) Isolation and proof of structure of wildfire toxin. Nature 229:174–178

Strominger JL, Izaki K, Matsuhashi M, Tipper DJ (1967) Peptidoglycan transpeptidase and D-alanine carboxypeptidase: penicillin-sensitive enzymatic reactions. Fed Proc 26:9–22

Taylor PA, Schnoes HK, Durbin RD (1972) Characterization of chlorosis inducing toxins from a plant pathogenic *Pseudomonas* sp. Biochim Biophys Acta 286:107–117

Tsao PH, Thieleki DW (1966) Stimulation of bacteria and actinomycetes by the polyene antibiotic pimaricin in soil dilution plates. Can J Microbiol 12:1091–1094

Umezawa H, Mitsuhashi S, Hamada M, Iyobe S, Takahashi S, Utahara R, Osato Y, Yamazoki S, Ogawara H, Maeda K (1973) Two β-lactamase inhibitors produced by a Streptomyces. J Antibiot (Tokyo) 26:51–54

Waksman SA, Woodruff HB (1940) Bacteriostatic and bactericidal substances produced by a soil actinomyces. Proc Soc Exp Biol Med 45:609

Waksman SA, Woodruff HB (1942) Streptothricin, a new selective bacteriostatic and bactericidal agent particularly against gram-negative bacteria. Proc Soc Exp Biol Med 49:207–210

Woodruff HB, McDaniel LE (1958) The antibiotic approach. Symp Soc Gen Microbiol 8:94

Woodruff HB, Hernandez S, Stapley EO (1979) Evolution of an antibiotic screening programme. Hind Antibiot Bull 21:71–84

Zahner H (1977) Some aspects of antibiotic research. Angew Chem Int Ed 16:687–694

Zimmerman SB, Stapley EO (1976) Relative morphological effects induced by cefoxitin and other β-lactam antibiotics in vitro. Antimicrob Agents Chemother 9:318–326

CHAPTER 10

High-Performance Liquid Chromatography of β-Lactam Antibiotics

R. D. MILLER and N. NEUSS

A. Introduction

Analytical procedures for β-lactam antibiotics were described in great detail in the early 1970 s in the monograph *Cephalosporins and Penicillins, Chemistry and Biology* by FLYNN (1972). These procedures included microbiological, chemical, chromatographic, and physical-chemical determinations of this important group of biologically active substances in pharmaceutical preparations, body fluids, and formulations subjected to long-term stability studies.

Since that time, however, the application of high performance liquid chromatography (HPLC), which was just beginning to be utilized in the early 1970 s, has been steadily growing. At present there is an enormous amount of information on this subject in the literature. In addition, the discovery of new types of β-lactam-containing fermentation products has had a renewed impact on research on β-lactam antibiotics leading to discoveries of natural products unrelated to penicillins and cephalosporins. The reference is made here to compounds such an clavulanic acid, thienamycin, olivanic acids, and nocardicins and their derivatives. The discovery of cephamycins and synthesis of oxygen-containing β-lactam antibiotics of the moxalactam type further enlarged the number of interesting, biologically active compounds containing a β-lactam moiety.

In almost every case, HPLC has now assumed an important role in determining the purity of compounds to be used in the treatment of disease, establishment of the nature of metabolites, and the study of antibiotic biosynthesis etc. We have chosen to list compounds separately with a short summary of available systems, giving very little consideration to microbiological, chromatographic, and physical-chemical determinations. These can be easily found in review articles on the chemistry and biology of these new compounds.

It is worthwhile to include here some basic terms used in HPLC (SNYDER and KIRKLAND 1974) in order to insure better understanding of conditions used and results obtained.

Capacity factor (k′) is a term describing the degree of retention of a compound in a particular system. The term is dimensionless so that other conditions are not required to describe its value. The general formula for capacity factor is:

$$k' = \frac{t_r - t_o}{t_o},$$

where t_r = time of retention for a specific peak and t_o = time of retention for an unretained component. This term is related to R_f in thin layer chromatography

(TLC) and paper chromatography (PC) by the following equation:

$$k' = \frac{1}{R_f}.$$

This relationship is valid only if the HPLC system used is identical with that of the TLC or PC in both stationary and mobile phase properties.

Column efficiency (N_{eff}). This quantity describes the ability of the column to prevent band spreading as a component travels through the column. Obviously, this value affects resolution especially of minimally separated components. The general expression describing this quantity is:

$$N_{eff} = 16 \left[\frac{t_r - t_o}{t_w}\right]^2,$$

where t_r = retention time of the specific peak
t_o = retention time of the unretained peak
t_w = retention width of the specific peak.

This value has great significance in the comparison of efficiencies of different columns. It is, in fact, the standard to which quality control of commercial column is related. Unfortunately, it can be misleading and sometimes does not bear a real relationship to experience in the laboratory. This is the result of the basic truth of the final goal in separation which only partly depends upon column efficiency. N_{eff} is also very dependent on mobile phase; so when final separation conditions are developed, one very often finds a much lower N value than that quoted for the particular column.

Separation or selectivity factor (α) is the reason that classic liquid chromatography (LC) endured over the many years prior to HPLC. It indicates that resolution can be achieved in the absence of high efficiency if selectivity factor is great enough. The formula for obtaining this factor is:

$$\alpha = \frac{k_2}{k_1},$$

where k_2 and k_1 are peaks of the separation at hand.

Resolution (R_s) is the term that describes the total observed chromatographic behavior. The combined equation for resolution is

$$R_s = 1/4 \left[\frac{\alpha - 1}{\alpha}\right] \sqrt{N} \left[\frac{k'}{k' + 1}\right].$$

This shows the relationship of each parameter previously described and indicates the effect on resolution that can be expected by increasing each of the controllable parameters.

B. Penicillin Antibiotics

All members of this important class of therapeutic agents contain 6-aminopenicillanic acid (6-APA). It is obvious that this type of chromophore will have a weak sensitivity to UV absorption. However, since the important antibiotics of this type contain relatively strong absorbing chromophores in the acyl function at C-6, their detection becomes much easier. We shall describe individually each antibiotic including the nucleus, 6-APA, itself.

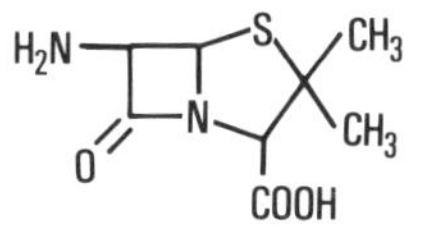

I. 6-Aminopenicillanic Acid (6-APA)

This compound is a true secondary metabolite and occurs as such in the broth of *Penicillium chrysogenum*. It exhibits weak antibacterial activity. It is acylated enzy-

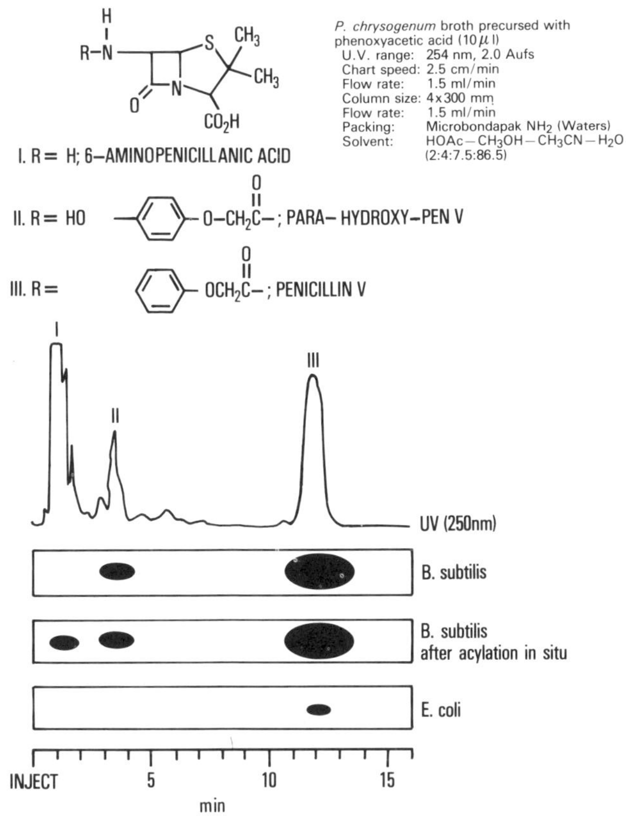

Fig. 1. HPLC/bioautography of 6-APA, *p*-hydroxypenicillin V and penicillin V. (Miller and Neuss 1978)

matically with a variety of acids which can be added to the fermentation in order to yield a product with an expanded antibacterial spectrum. The HPLC of 6-APA has been described by several authors. Thus, NACHTMANN (1979) described a reversed phase (RP) system on Lichrosorb RP8 eluting with a phosphate buffer (pH 7.0). He observed $k' \simeq 1$ using 220 nm absorption for detection. We were able to achieve a slight retention of 6-APA using μBondapak NH_2 with a mobile phase of $HOAc:CH_3OH:CH_3CN:H_2O$ (2:4:7.5:86.5). Detection was achieved by UV at 254 nm and was followed by a biological overlay technique (MILLER and NEUSS 1978) (Fig. 1). In the process of direct comparison of UV detection sensitivity of 6-APA with that of 7-ACA (7-aminocephalosporanic acid), 7-ACA revealed a 20-fold greater sensitivity than 6-APA (Fig. 2).

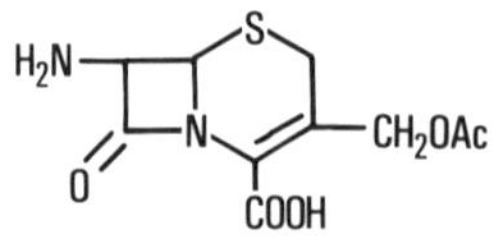

7-Aminocephalosporanic Acid (7-ACA)

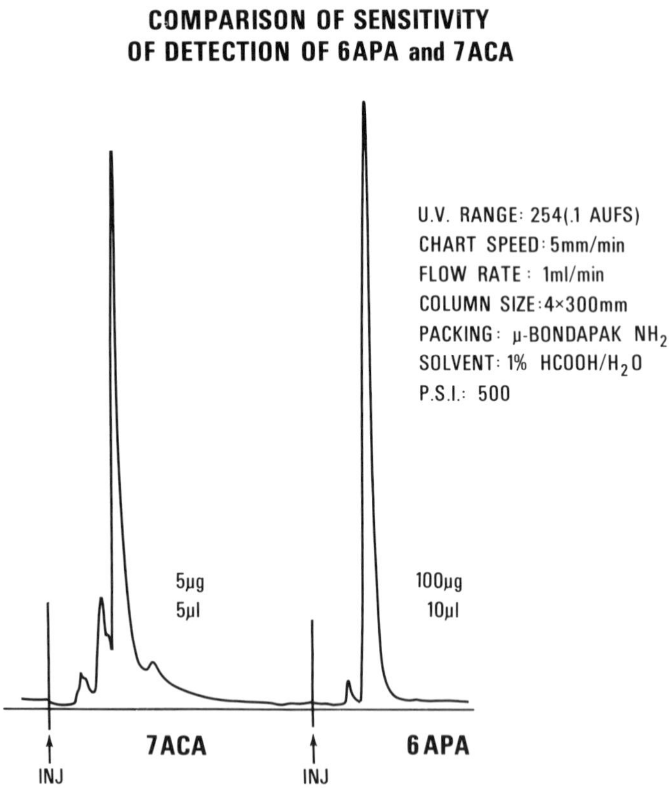

Fig. 2. HPLC of 6-APA and 7-ACA: sensitivity of UV detection at 254 nm

II. Amoxicillin (Clamoxyl)

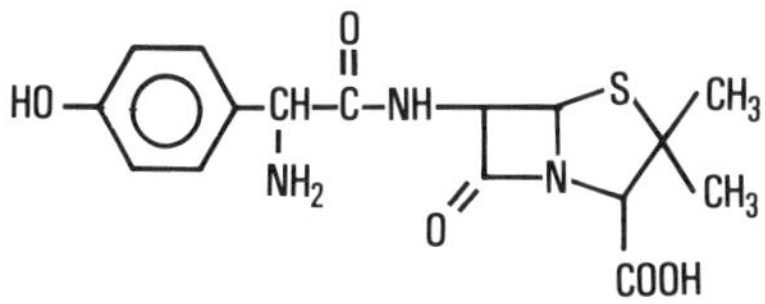

In most of the literature references pertaining to the analysis of amoxicillin by HPLC, authors used RP (reversed phase) chromatography for the support. It has been shown by VREE et al. (1978) that sensitivity of detection of amoxicillin in biological fluids can be as low as 0.5 μg/ml. KINGSTON (1979) also described this methodology in his review of HPLC methods. The support used was Lichrosorb RP8 with a mobile phase of dihydrogen phosphate buffer (pH 4.6). UV absorption at 225 nm was used for detection. LEE et al. (1979) made use of RP18 coupled with postcolumn derivatization to observe minimum detection at 2.5 μg/ml in biological fluids. His mobile phase was HOAc:CH_3OH:H_2O (0.5:15:85). YAMANA et al. (1977) also utilized RP18 with a mobile phase of aqueous ammonium chloride and methanol to analyze this drug. This detection was at 254 nm in the UV.

III. Ampicillin (Penbritin)

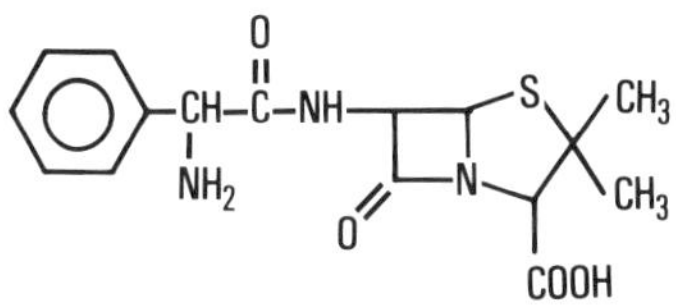

VREE et al. (1978) and KINGSTON (1979) have mentioned the use of Lichrosorb RP8 with a mobile phase of 15% CH_3OH in KH_2PO_4 buffer (pH 4.6). This system, using UV absorption at 225 nm, gives sensitivity of analysis at 0.5 μg/ml in biological fluids. WHITE et al. (1977) used Lichrosorb RP8 with 35% MeOH in phosphate buffer and obtained excellent retention. SALTO (1978) has demonstrated resolution of ampicillin diastereomers using RP18 and aqueous phosphate as mobile phases. YAMANA et al. (1977) also retained ampicillin on Lichrosorb (RP18) with aqueous ammonium chloride. Ampicillin polymers in clinical preparations can be detected by HPLC using a gradient of CH_3CN with aqueous phosphate on RP18 as shown by LARSEN and BUNDGAARD (1978).

IV. Carbenicillin

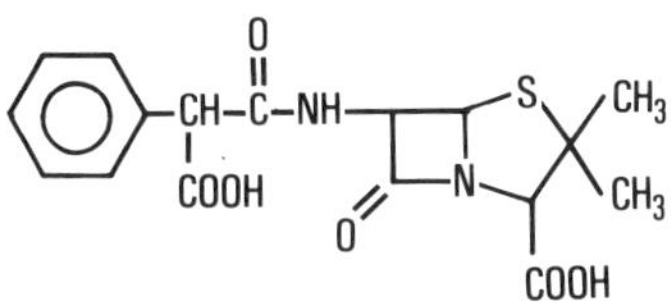

The assay of carbenicillin is complicated by the possibility of the presence of diastereomers arising through racemization of the side-chain carbon bearing the carboxyl group. The compound also can decarboxylate to form another bioactive impurity. HPLC can be used to quantitate all three of these compounds even in the presence of a complex matrix. YAMAOKA et al. (1979) has examined this compound in serum and found that ion-pair RP chromatography permits the resolution required. He used a μBondapak C18 column with a mobile phase of tetrabutyl ammonium bromide modified with methanol. This system using UV detection at 254 nm gave a linear response down to 0.2 mg/ml. Yamana et al. (1977) used Lichrosorb RP18 with aqueous ammonium chloride as mobile phase.

V. Penicillin G

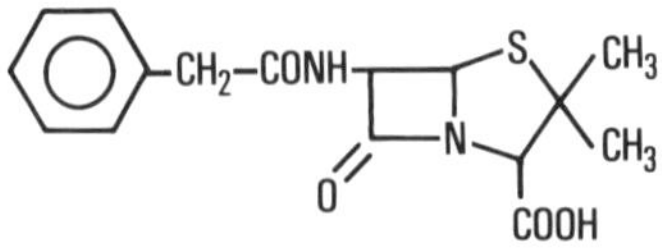

Penicillin G is very unstable as the free acid but can be chromatographed in a number of HPLC systems. KINGSTON (1979) cited two separate ion-exchange systems. One utilized Vydac P150/Ax with a sodium nitrate/borate buffer at pH 9.1 as mobile phase. The other used Bondapak Ax/corasil with a citric acid/phosphate buffer at pH 3.8. We have used the bonded ion-exchanger, μBondapak NH_2, for the retention of penicillin G with a mobile phase of $HOAc/CH_3OH/CH_3CN/H_2O$ (2/4/7.5/86.5) (unpublished data). More recently, the use of RP chromatography has overshadowed these earlier techniques. WHITE et al. (1977) described the use of RP8 with a phosphate/methanol mobile phase for this compound. YAMANA et al. (1977) used RP18 with an aqueous ammonium chloride, methanol mobile phase. Some clinical preparations make use of benzathine salts; these are chromatographed on RP8 resins with phosphate/methanol mobile phases as described by LE BELLE et al. (1979).

VI. Penicillin V[1]

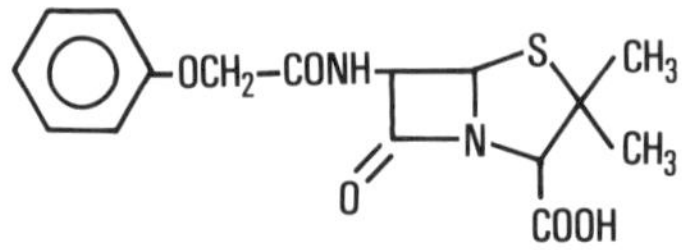

Penicillin V is one of the most widely used penicillin derivatives and is easily chromatographed by HPLC. Ion-exchange techniques were mentioned by KINGSTON (1979) using a stationary phase of Vydac P150AX and a mobile phase of 10% methanol in a sodium nitrate/borate buffer at pH 9.1. Most other references indicate that RP chromatography is the most frequently used method. WHITE et al. (1977) and YAMANA et al. (1977) used RP18 while NACHTMANN (1979) used RP8. These authors made use of ammonium phosphate or acetate and an organic modifier solvent such as methanol. We have successfully used HPLC to examine Pen V broth directly with the μBondapak NH_2 column (MILLER and NEUSS 1978), as described in Fig. 1. The importance of this technique will be discussed in detail later in this chapter. Although 6-APA, p-hydroxy Pen V and Pen V are present in

1 V-CILLIN K (penicillin V potassium, Lilly)

different concentrations, all are present in sufficient concentration to be detected biologically with suitable bacteria. This example also points out the option of acylation in situ to enhance the biological activity of certain components; in this case 6-APA has no activity versus *Bacillus subtilis* until acylation has occurred. This step is used to confirm the presence of the penicillin nucleus.

VII. Sulbenicillin

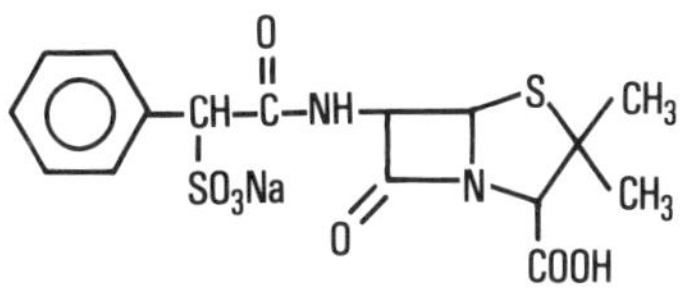

RP ion-pair chromatography of sulbenicillin has been reported by YAMAOKA et al. (1979). The column used was μBondapak C18 and the mobile phase was aqueous tetrabutyl ammonium bromide with methanol as a modifier. YAMANA et al. (1977) retained sulbenicillin on RP18 and eluted it with aqueous ammonium chloride and methanol as mobile phase.

VIII. Concluding Remarks

Chromatographic procedures of penicillins can be divided into two groups; the first makes use of ion-exchange and the second employs RP as a support. The choice of supports is largely a function of the problem to be solved. Ion-exchange resins are less expensive and more commonly used in isolation procedures. RP supports are mostly used in the analytical mode since they are more efficient and easier to handle in re-establishing equilibrium conditions. RP supports are being constantly shifted toward the preparative mode but as of now are only suitable for laboratory scale work. Our modification of microbiological monitoring of effluent after detection by UV or increase in refractive index (ΔRI) is especially useful in the direct analysis of fermentation broth, body fluids, or in cases where there is no UV absorption and the ΔRI cannot be used due to the scarcity of biologically active components (MILLER and NEUSS 1978). In addition, the use of μBondapak NH_2 has special advantages. The stationary phase is much more polar than the octadecyl function. This allows a better retention of metabolites that are not extractable into organic solvents. The amine function also acts as a weak anion exchanger at low pH giving access to an additional selectivity feature.

C. Cephalosporin Antibiotics

This class of compounds contains a nucleus of 7-aminocephalosporanic acid (7-ACA). Unlike 6-APA this derivative has to be prepared by chemical cleavage (MORIN et al. 1962) of cephalosporin C (7-α-aminoadipoyl derivative of 7-ACA) and then chemical acylation to prepare the appropriate derivatives. A number of these derivatives constitute an important class of therapeutic agents and will be discussed individually.

I. 7-Aminocephalosporanic Acid (7-ACA)

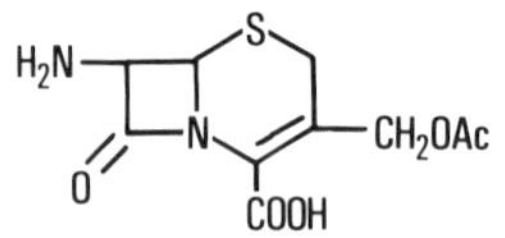

The cephalosporin nucleus (7-ACA) does not occur in fermentation broths except where it is formed by degradation of cephalosporin C. It contains a strong chromophore and can be detected at a much lower concentration than 6-APA (Fig. 2).

CHROMBEZ et al. (1979) described the use of ion pairing HPLC for this derivative; using tetrabutyl ammonium counter ion and 7.5% methanol on a Vydac RP column. WHITE et al. (1977) showed that 7-ACA can be retained on Lichrosorb C18 with an aqueous NaH_2PO_4 mobile phase. We have retained 7-ACA as well as other derivatives on μBondapak NH_2 utilizing a mobile phase of 2/4/7.5/86.5 HOAc/MeOH/MeCN/H_2O (MILLER and NEUSS 1976).

II. Cefaclor[2]

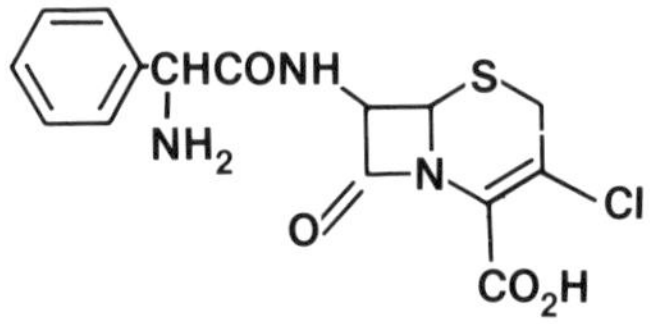

We have found good retention of this compound on μBondapak C18 with a mobile phase of 1/10/89 HOAc/CH_3CN/H_2O (unpublished data). This system provides enough resolution to observe the presence of the 3-chloro nucleus.

III. Cefamandole[3]

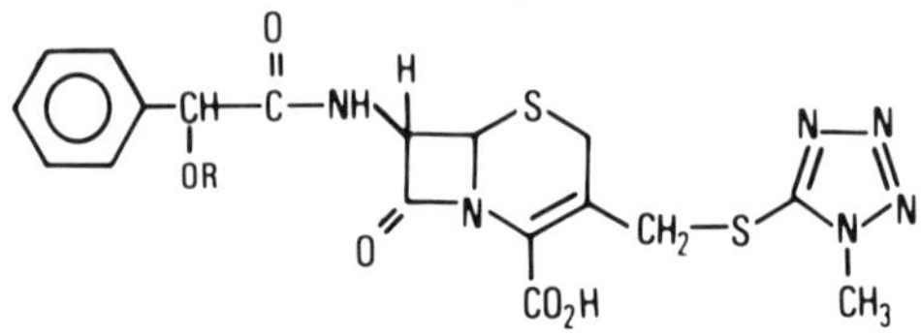

R = H cefamandole

R = CH(=O) cefamandole nafate[3]

In our study we used the μBondapak NH_2 as stationary phase with a mobile phase of HOAc/CH_3OH/CH_3CN/H_2O (2/4/50/44). This system gave good resolution of products expected to be formed by hydrolysis of the compound, namely cefamandole, des-[thiotetrazole]-cefamandole and thiotetrazole (see Fig. 5).

2 CECLOR (cefaclor, Lilly)
3 MANDOLE (cefamandole nafate, Lilly)

IV. Cefazolin

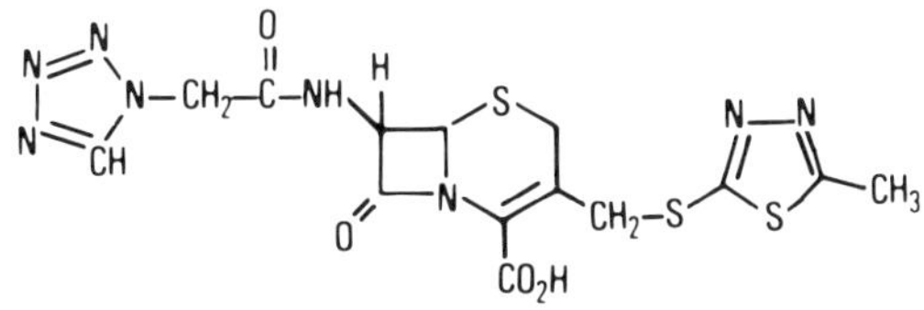

The chromatography of cefazolin is generally carried out on RP supports with either ion-suppression or ion-pairing. CROMBEZ et al. (1979) showed retention on Vydac RP using tetrabutyl ammonium ion and 7.5% methanol in an aqueous mobile phase. WHITE et al. (1977) and YAMANA et al. (1977) used NaH_2PO_4 and NH_4Cl salts, respectively, to retain cefazolin on C18 stationary phases. They also used methanol as a modifier in an aqueous system.

V. Cefoxitin

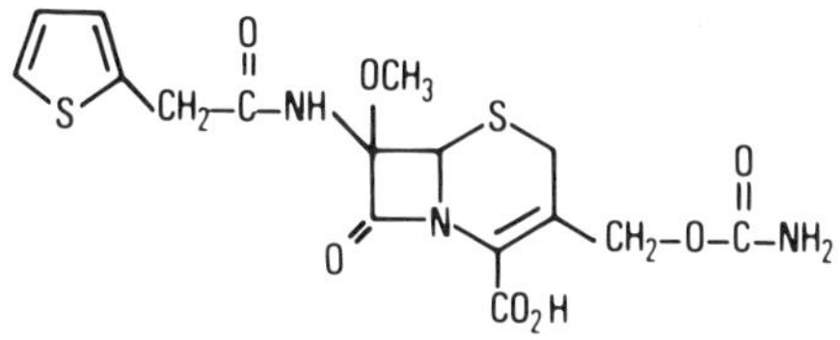

The presence of the 3-carbamoyl group in the antibiotic cefoxitin greatly influences the polarity and thereby the retention on RP resins. KINGSTON (1979) has reported good retention on ion exchange supports such as Zipax SAX using an aqueous acetic acid solution at pH 5.0. We have used μBondapak C18 with a mobile phase of acetic acid, acetonitrile, and water to analyze cefoxitin and its degradation products.

VI. Ceftizoxime

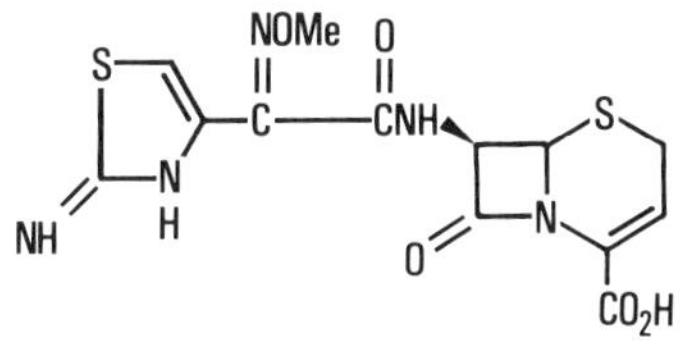

Very recently, SUZUKI et al. (1980) reported on the HPLC assay of ceftizoxime in rat serum, bile, and urine. The structural differences from most other cephalosporin antibiotics consist of the absence of a substituent at the 3-position and the presence of 7-aminothiazole oxime moiety. The separation was accomplished on a μBondapak phenyl column, eluting with acetic acid and phosphate buffers at low pH (2.6) and 11%–13% concentrations of acetonitrile. A variety of mobile phases were used to insure resolution of peaks in the various biological fluids.

VII. Cephalexin[4]

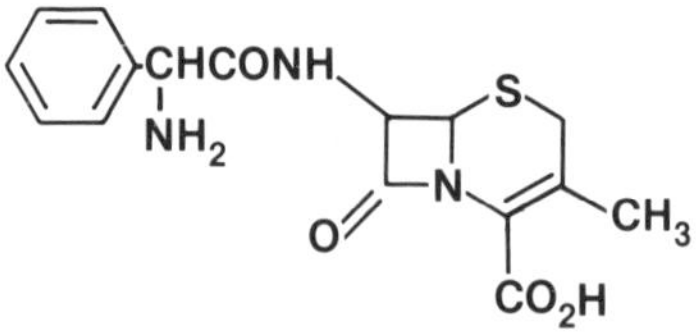

Cephalexin has similar chromatographic properties to those of ampicillin. All of the recent reports dealing with HPLC of this compound mention use of RP supports. NAKAGAWA et al. (1978) used C18 with acetic acid, methanol, and water. WHITE et al. (1977) and SALTO (1978) used phosphate buffer and methanol in Lichrosorb C18. Salto described separation of diastereomers created by the use of racemic phenylglycine. KINGSTON (1979) described the use of micropak CH with a phosphate buffer and methanol. Other references on C18 are that of YAMANA et al. (1977) using NH_4Cl buffer and CARROLL et al. (1977) using $(NH_4)_2CO_3$ buffer. We (MILLER and NEUSS 1976) have used μBondapak NH_2 with acetic acid, methanol, acetonitrile, and water (see Figs. 4 and 5).

VIII. Cephaloglycin[5]

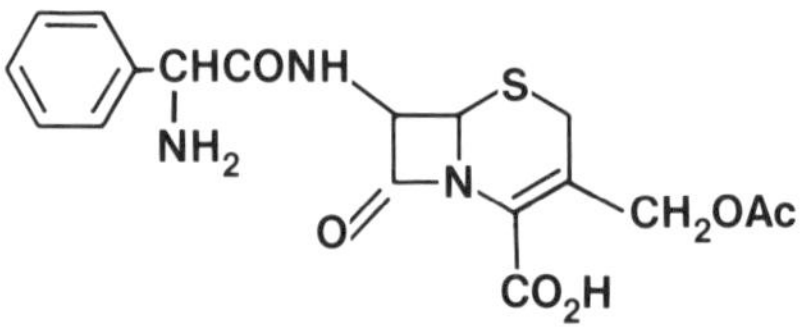

Chromatographically this compound behaves almost identically to cephalexin. Therefore most of the systems used for cephalexin apply to cephaloglycin. WHITE et al. (1977) and YAMANA et al. (1977) both cited HPLC of this compound. We have found good retention on the μBondapak NH_2 column reported in cephalexin section (see Figs. 4 and 5).

IX. Cephaloridine[6]

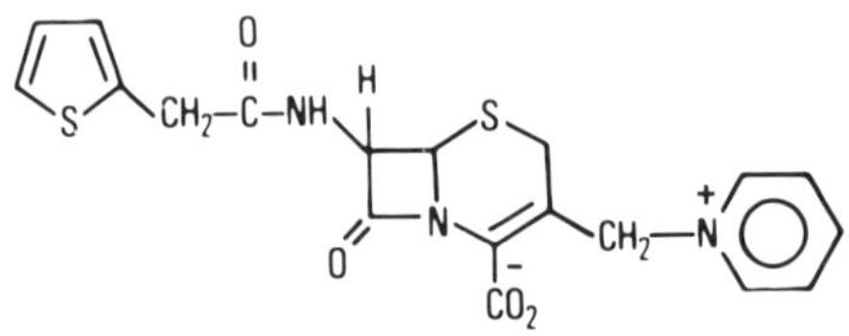

Cephaloridine also has zwitterionic properties that make retention on reversed phase packing materials more difficult. We (MILLER and NEUSS 1976) have used ion exchanger μBondapak NH_2 to retain the compound. KINGSTON (1979) described the use of μBondapak phenyl with ammonium acetate in aqueous methanol. YAMANA et al. (1977) used Zorbax ODS eluting with ammonium chloride in aqueous methanol (see Figs. 4 and 5).

4 KEFLEX (cephalexin, Dista)
5 KAFOCIN (cephaloglycin, Lilly)
6 LORIDINE (cephaloridine, Lilly)

X. Cephalosporin C

Cephalosporin C is the major product of *Cephalosporium acremonium* fermentations. Although its own spectrum of activity is low, when the 7-amino adipoyl side-chain is replaced with other acyl groups the spectrum of activity is significantly improved. Chromatography of this compound is generally related to fermentation development, mutation work, biosynthetic studies and its isolation. The 3′-acetoxy methyl group is easily hydrolyzed to form the 3′-desacetyl derivative. This impurity, in addition to other 3′-derivatives, is typical of a series of compounds that need to be resolved if one is to chromatograph cephalosporin C with reasonable certainty in quantitation (Fig. 3). In the early 1970 s the method of choice was ion exchange because of its selectivity. The use of ion exchange, as always, leads to difficulties concerned with re-equilibration of the system and satisfactory reproducibility. We have used the weak anion exchanger, namely μBondapak NH_2 (MILLER

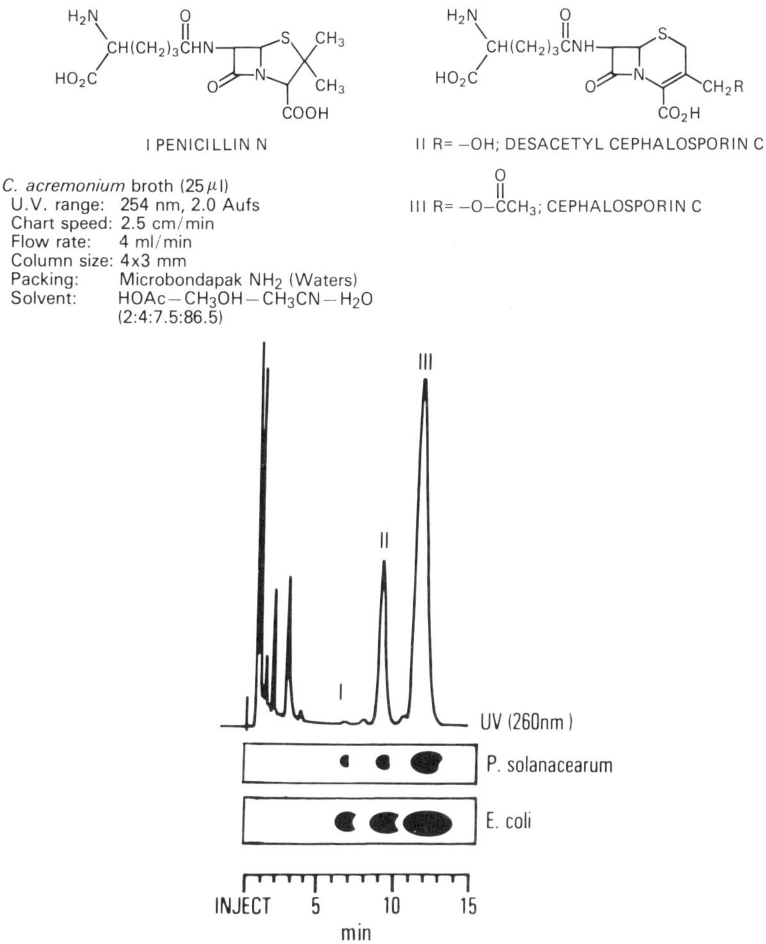

Fig. 3. HPLC/bioautography of *Cephalosporium acremonium* fermentation broth. (MILLER and NEUSS 1978)

and NEUSS 1976) to separate a wide variety of cephalosporin derivatives with minor structural variations. Later, WHITE et al. (1977) demonstrated the use of RP chromatography with NaH_2PO_4 in aqueous methanol on these types of compounds. We have also used ion pairing reagents tetrabutyl ammonium and *d*-10-camphorsulfonic acid to resolve various cephalosporin C derivatives (unpublished data).

XI. Cephalothin[7]

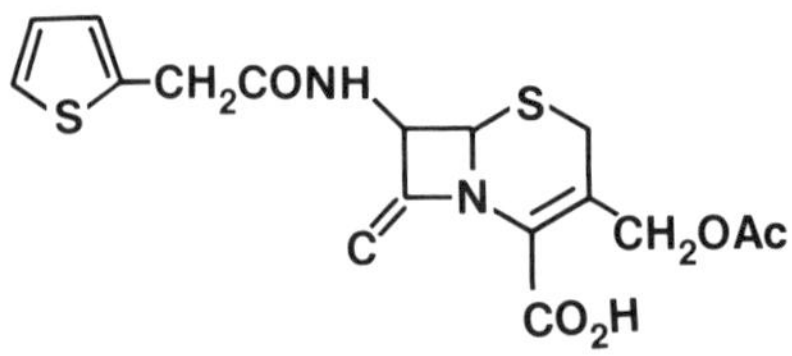

Cephalothin is very lipophilic and is therefore easy to retain on RP columns; however, pH control of the mobile phase improves the peak shape and thereby provides quantitation of the chromatograms. WHITE et al. (1977) and YAMANA et al. (1977) used C18 column with an ion-suppression mobile phase of phosphate and NH_4Cl, respectively. Ion-pair chromatography was used by CROMBEZ et al. (1979) on a Vydac RP column with tetrabutyl ammonium counterion. In addition to using the μBondapak NH_2 column (MILLER and NEUSS 1976) (Figs. 4 and 5), we have routinely analyzed cephalothin samples using μBondapak C18 with a mobile phase of 2/20/78 acetic acid/acetonitrile/water (unpublished data).

XII. Cephapirin

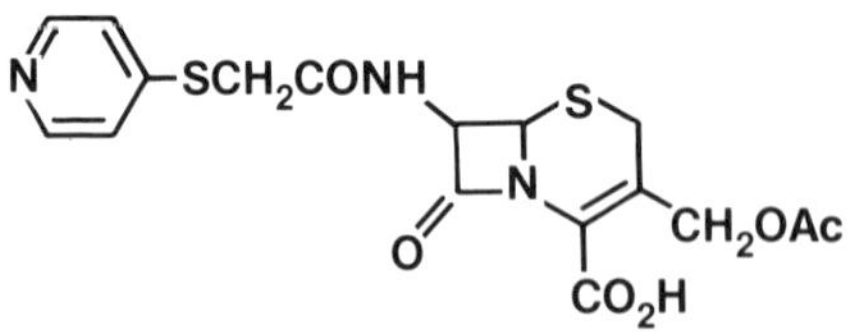

The cephalosporin antibiotic cephaphirin has an amphoteric nature due to the substituent containing the pyridinyl moiety. CROMBEZ et al. (1979) reported an analytical HPLC system using Vydac RP with a paired ion mobile phase with tetrabutyl ammonium hydroxide in aqueous methanol. We have also retained this compound in the amino column (MILLER and NEUSS 1976) (Fig. 5) and also on μBondapak C18 with an acetonitrile modifier (10%) at a low pH (unpublished data).

XIII. Cephradine

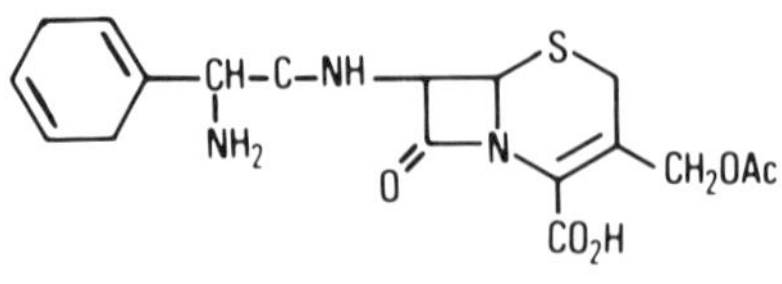

Cephradine differs only slightly from cephalexin in that it contains a cyclohexadienyl glycine substituent at the C_7. The HPLC conditions for both can be considered identical. However, specific citings of this compound were found in King-

7 KEFLIN (cephalothin sodium, Lilly)

ston's paper (KINGSTON 1979) using an ammonium carbonate aqueous methanol as mobile phase on μBondapak C18. WHITE et al. (1977), YAMANA et al. (1977), and CARROLL et al. (1977) also used C18 as a stationary phase with aqueous methanol buffers as mobile phases. The salts employed were NaH_2PO_4, NH_4Cl, and $(NH_4)_2CO_3$, respectively.

XIV. Concluding Remarks

The ease of separation of cephalosporin antibiotics, particularly using bonded phase supports, is illustrated in Figs. 4 and 5 (MILLER and NEUSS 1976). There is

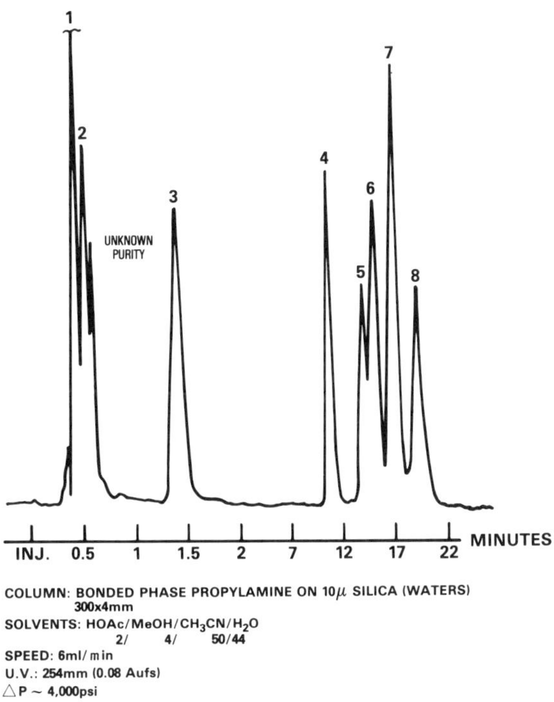

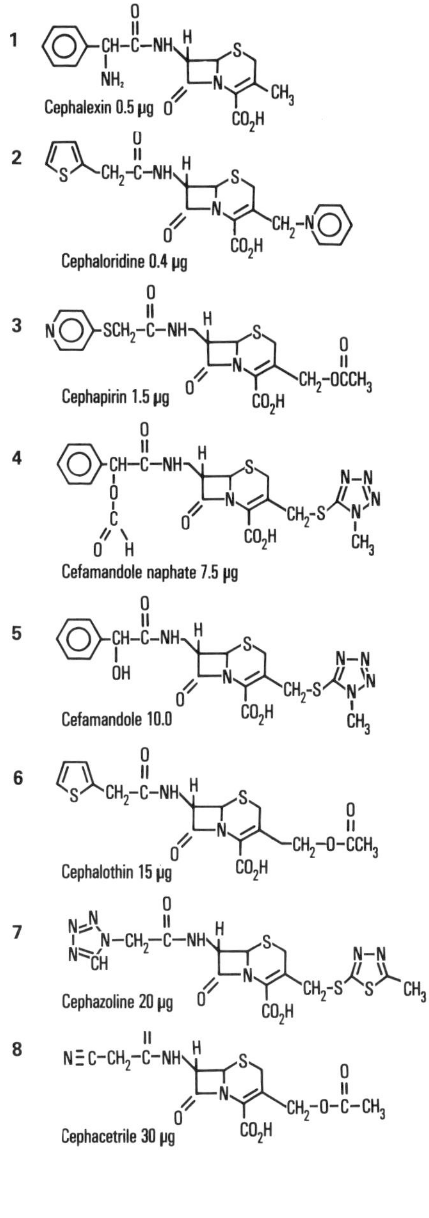

Fig. 4. HPLC of cephalosporin antibiotics I. (MILLER and NEUSS 1976)

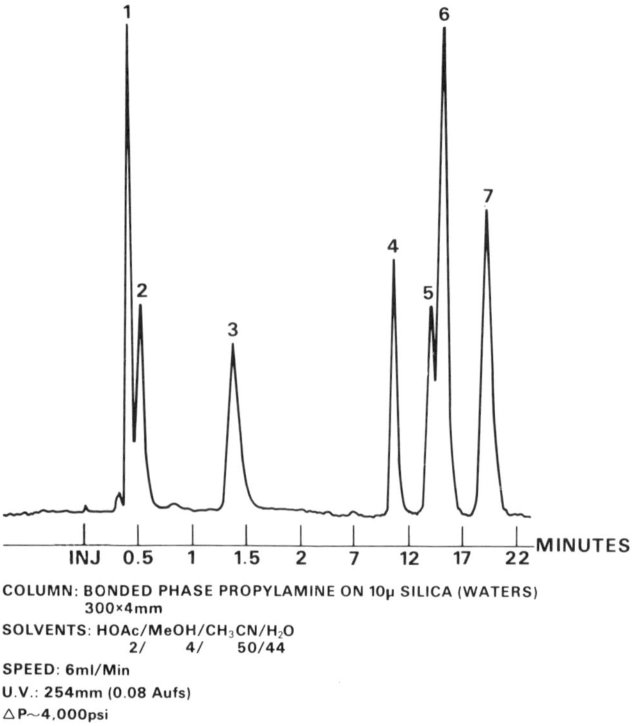

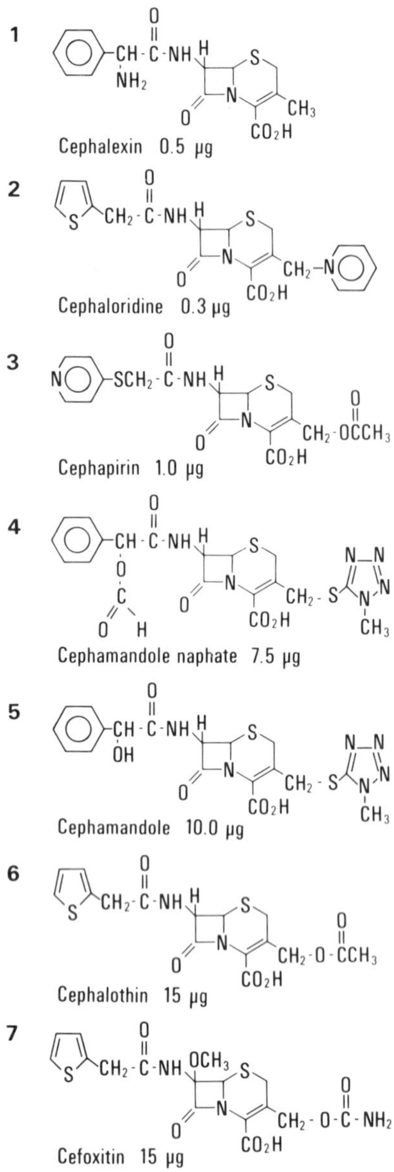

Fig. 5. HPLC of cephalosporin antibiotics II

no question that cephalosporin derivatives are particularly suited for this technique, partially due to their high degree of inherent lipophilicity; also, newly developed mobile phases effectively neutralize isolated polar functional groups of certain antibiotics. We refer here to ion-pairing chromatography as well as ion-suppression RP LC. The presence of a strong UV chromophore permits detection in the nanogram range with most commercially available 254 nm UV detectors.

A further example of the outstanding resolution of compounds with the cephalosporin nucleus is shown in Fig. 6. This type of result permitted the use of the

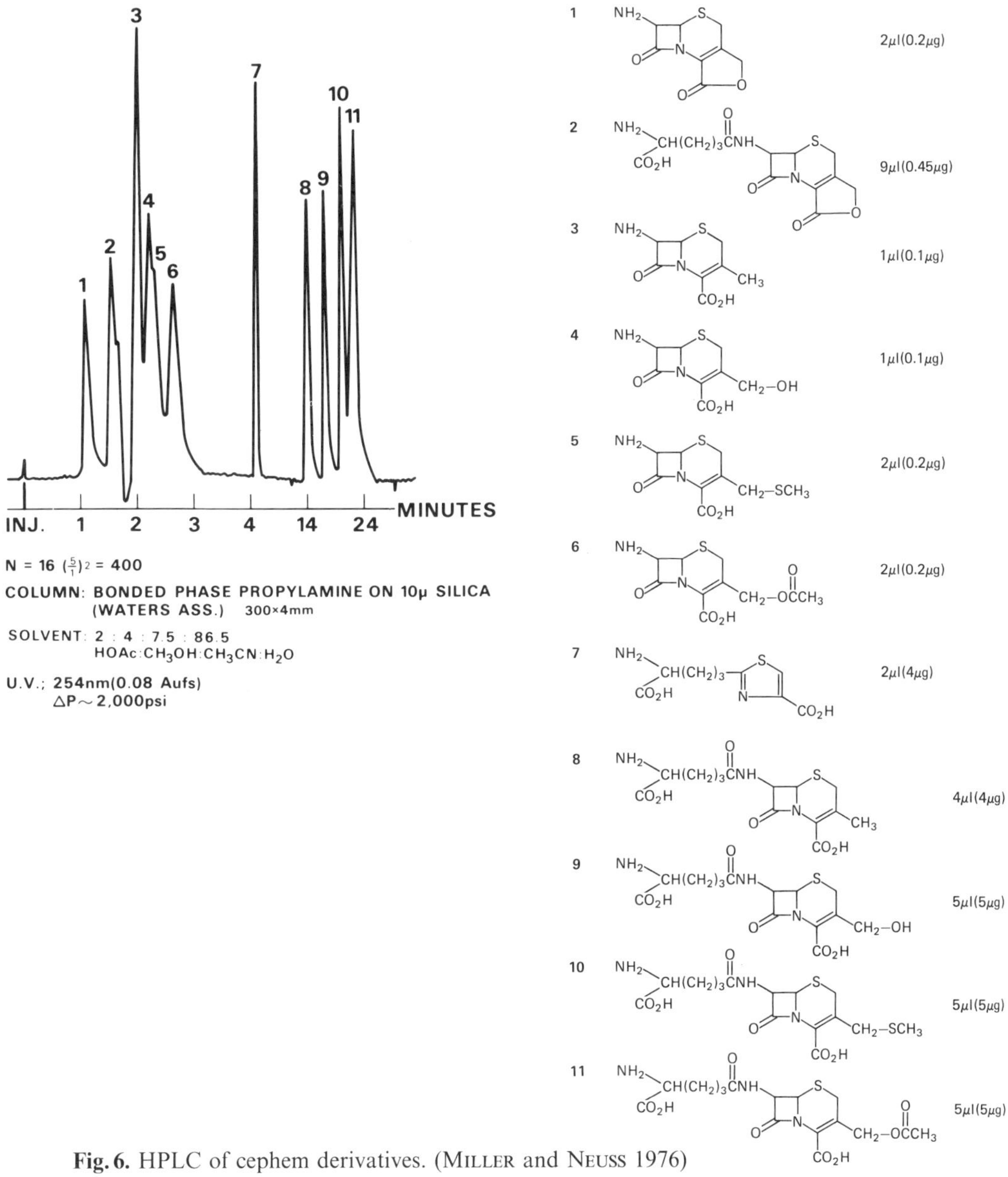

Fig. 6. HPLC of cephem derivatives. (MILLER and NEUSS 1976)

same system in the preparative isolation of cephalosporin C directly from filtered fermentation broth. Of course, a slightly larger μBondapak NH_2 column is required for this application (Waters, 8 × 600 mm). We first established the peak position by spiking with authentic cephalosporin C. Then in our preparative run we injected broth several times in the 0.5–1.5 ml range, collecting the peak corresponding to cephalosporin C. Our yield was 55%–70% based on microbiological assay. Identity of the compound was established by TLC and NMR spectroscopy

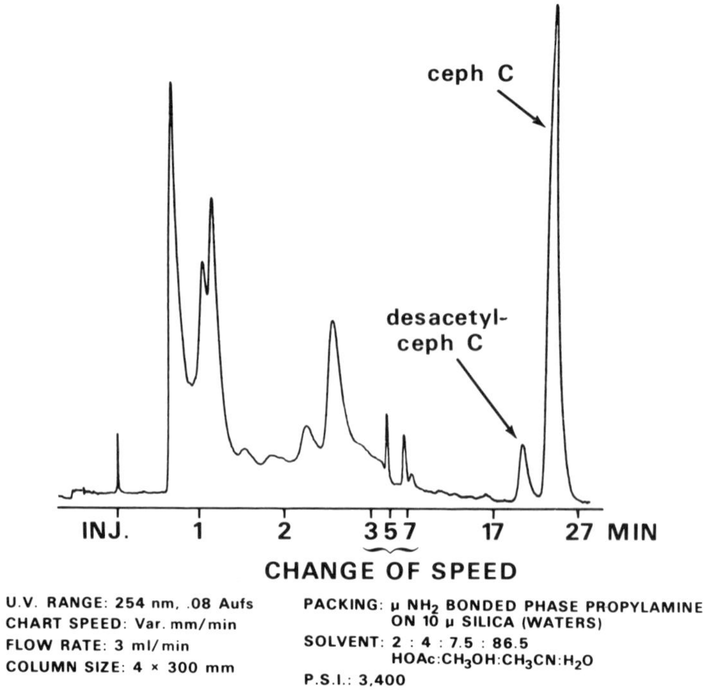

Fig. 7. HPLC of *Cephalosporium acremonium* filtered broth (2 μl). (MILLER and NEUSS 1976)

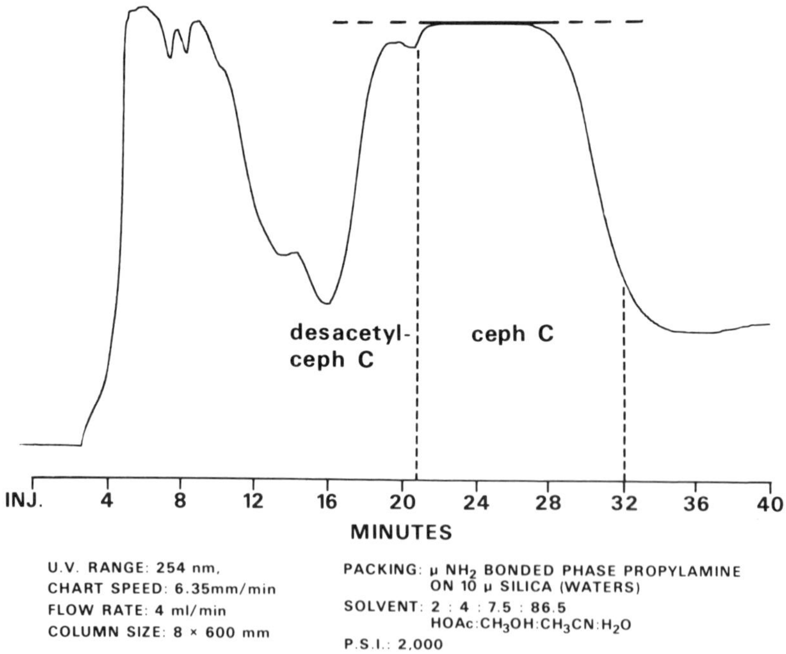

Fig. 8. Preparative HPLC of cephalosporin C from *Cephalosporium acremonium* filtered broth (1.3 ml). (MILLER and NEUSS 1976)

in comparison with data obtained on an authentic specimen (MILLER and NEUSS 1976) (Figs. 7 and 8).

D. Other β-Lactam Compounds

The original observation of AOKI et al. (1976) on nocardicin A, a monocyclic β-lactam, marks the beginning of a new era of surprising discoveries in the field of biologically active β-lactams of great structural variety. We are referring here to naturally occurring fermentation products such as clavulanic acid, thienamycin, and olivanic acids. In addition, nuclear analogs of cephalosporins, both naturally occurring and synthetic, have shown enhanced or unique antibacterial activities and will be discussed below.

I. Nocardicin A and B

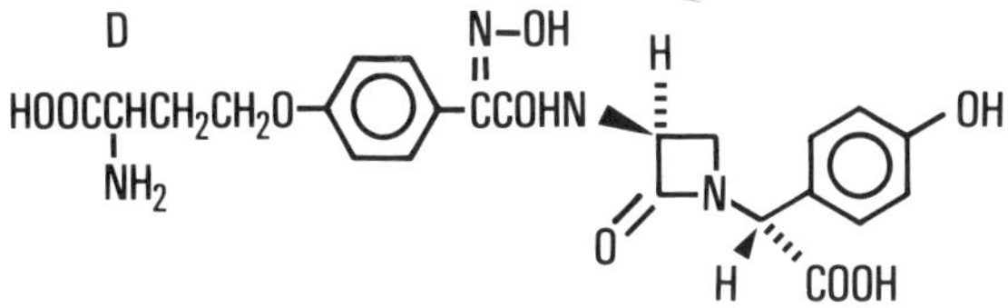

Nocardicin A

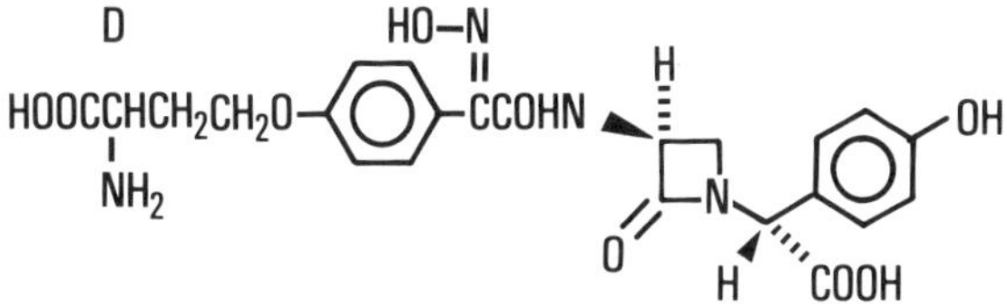

Nocardicin B

A – OH (anti)
B – OH (syn)

Nocardicin A and B were isolated from *Nocardia uniformis* and characterized by AOKI et al. (1976) and KURITA et al. (1976). They have moderate activity against a broad spectrum of gram-negative bacteria and relatively low toxicity. KURITA et al. (1976) reported TLC and HPLC of both A and B. TLC was performed on a cellulose plate developed with *n*-BuOH:AcOH:H_2O (4:1:2) giving R_f values of 0.46 for factor A and 0.54 for factor B. In HPLC, μBondapak C18/porasil B was used with a mobile phase of 0.01 *M* Na_2HPO_4:0.01 *M* KH_2PO_4:MeOH (95:95:10). Column dimensions were 8 × 1,200 mm and a flow rate of 5.5 ml/min gave a retention time of 10.8 min for factor A and 17.8 min for factor B. We have also examined nocardicin A in a system essentially identical to that reported for cephalosporin antibiotics (MILLER and NEUSS 1976). Excellent retention on the μBondapak NH_2 column was observed with a mobile phase of 2/4/7.5/86.5 HOAc/CH_3OH/CH_3CN/H_2O and a flow rate of 3.5 ml/min. A capacity factor of 6.0 for nocardicin A was obtained. Our stream splitting device was used in conjunction with the

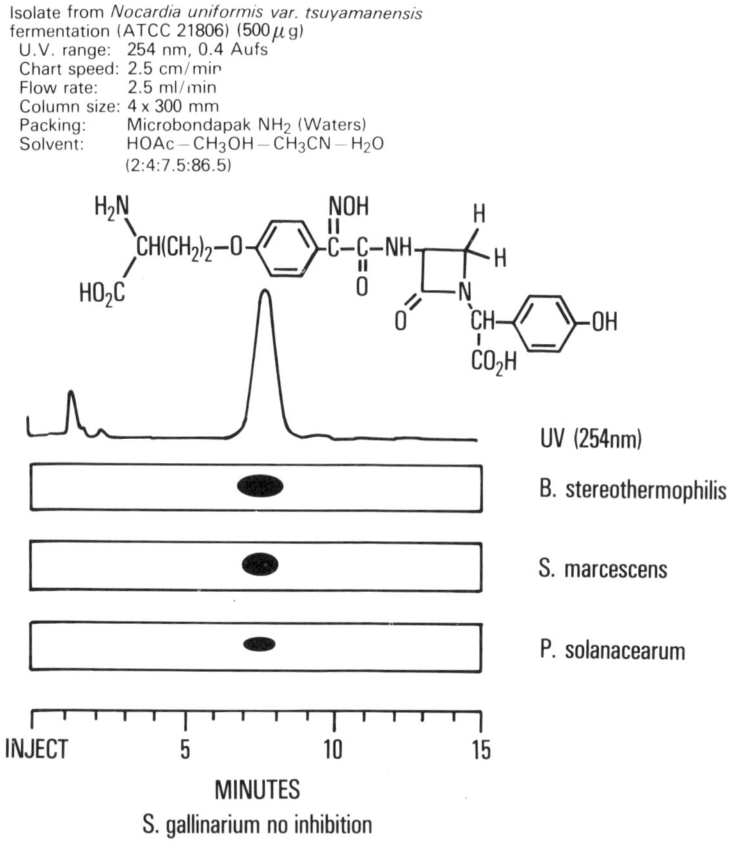

Fig. 9. HPLC/bioautography of nocardicin A. (MILLER and NEUSS 1978)

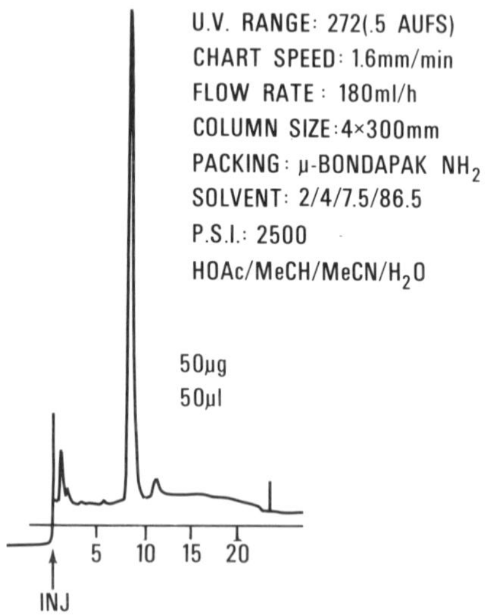

Fig. 10. HPLC of nocardicin A

isolation of this antibiotic. Figures 9 and 10 represent HPLC on a fermentation isolate demonstrating retention and sensitivity of the method.

II. Clavulanic Acid

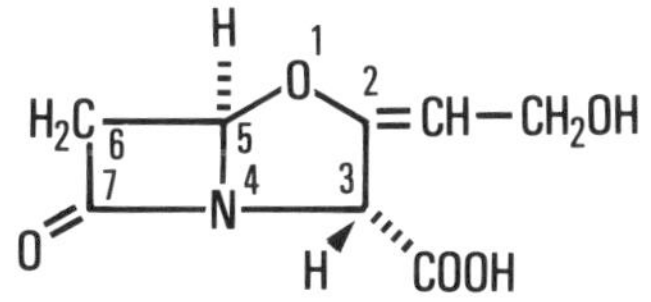

In 1976, HOWARTH (1976) published a note on the isolation and structural elucidation of clavulanic acid, a potent β-lactamase inhibitor. At that time some TLC and PC data were available. We (MILLER and NEUSS 1978) showed the presence of clavulanic acid in broth using the HPLC/bioautographic approach. Using a stationary phase of μBondapak NH_2 and a mobile phase of HOAc/MeOH/MeCN/H_2O (2/4/7.5/86.5), we ovserved a k′ value of ~ 15 for clavulanic acid. We have also used the pairred ion reagent tetrabutyl ammonium hydroxide in aqueous acetonitrile on μBondapak C18 (unpublished work). The instability of clavulanic acid makes quantitation by slower chromatographic methods less desirable. Figure 11 shows the HPLC data of the above system.

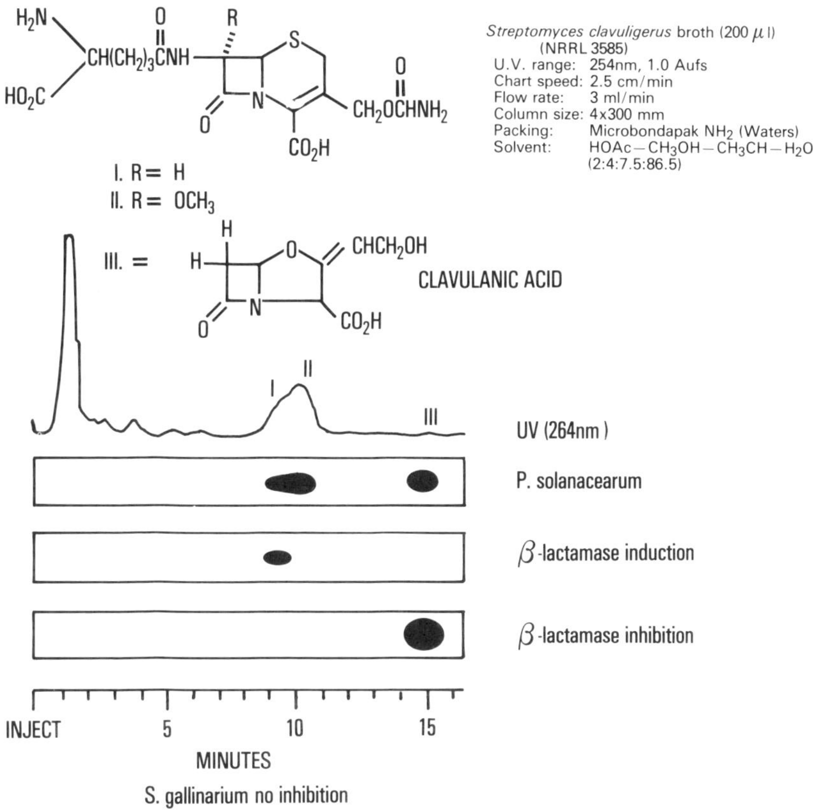

Fig. 11. HPLC/bioautography of clavulanic acid. (MILLER and NEUSS 1978)

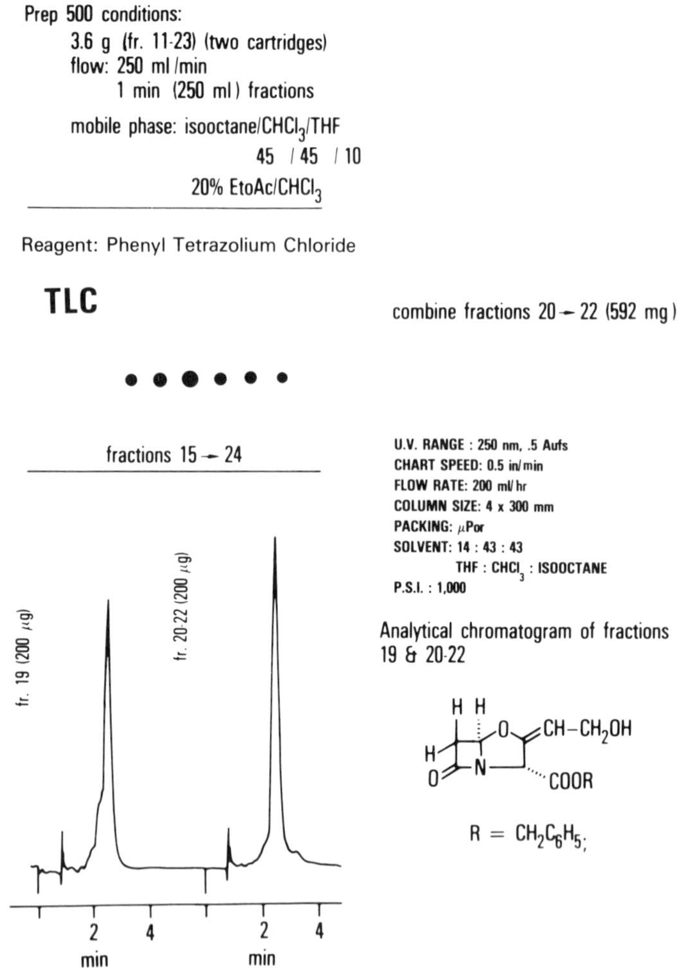

Fig. 12. Preparative HPLC of benzylclavulanate

The inherent instability of clavulanic acid can be overcome by derivatizing the compound to its benzyl ester:

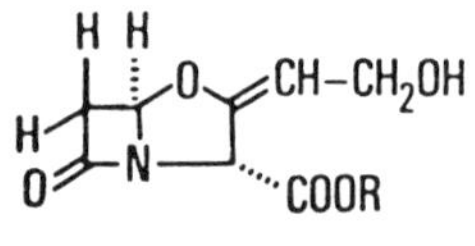

$$R = CH_2C_6H_5$$

This procedure, first reported in 1975 in a German patent (2,517,316 A1) issued to COLE et al. (1975) of the Beecham group in England, allows for isolation of the compound by silica column chromatography. In this form, however, it can also be handled by HPLC (Fig. 12) (MILLER and NEUSS 1980). After its isolation, the material can be hydrogenolized to the Na salt of the acid.

III. Thienamycin

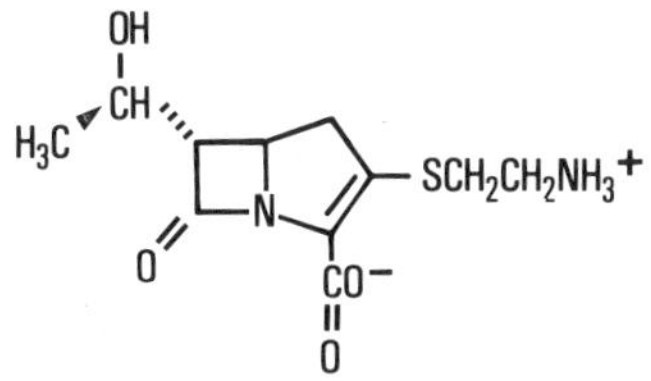

Thienamycin represents a new potent broad-spectrum antibiotic from *Streptomyces cattleya* where it occurs together with other related compounds (KAHAN et al. 1979; ALBERS-SCHONBERG et al. 1978). To our knowledge, there are no HPLC data in the literature on this particular metabolite. Using a standard sample, we have found that the antibiotic is eluted in a manner similar to cephalosporin nuclei in the system containing μBondapak NH_2. In a reversed phase ion-pair system it was not well retained (Fig. 13).

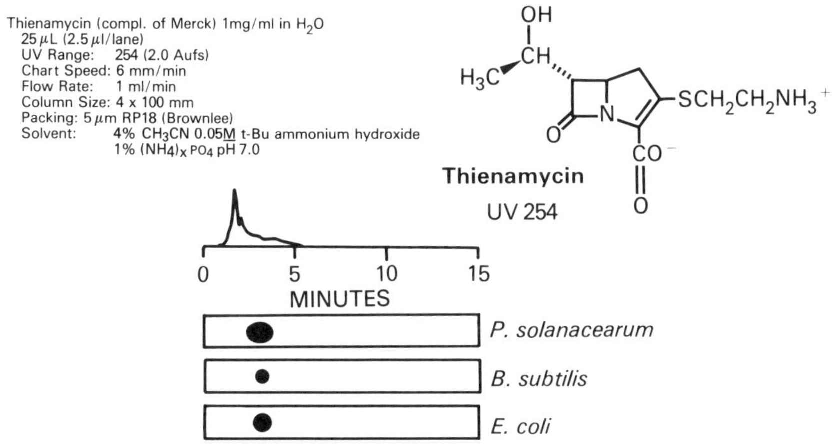

Fig. 13. HPLC/bioautography of thienamycin

IV. Olivanic Acids

Compound	R_1	R_2
MM4550	$-\overset{O}{\underset{\uparrow}{S}}-CH=CH-NH-\overset{O}{\overset{\|\|}{C}}\,CH_3$	$-SO_3H$
MM13902	$-S-CH=CH-NH-\overset{O}{\overset{\|\|}{C}}\,CH_3$	$-SO_3H$
MM17880	$-S-CH_2CH_2-NH-\overset{O}{\overset{\|\|}{C}}\,CH_3$	$-SO_3H$
MM22380	$-S-CH_2CH_2-NH-\overset{O}{\overset{\|\|}{C}}\,CH_3$	$-H$
MM22382	$-S-CH=CH-NH-\overset{O}{\overset{\|\|}{C}}\,CH_3$	$-H$

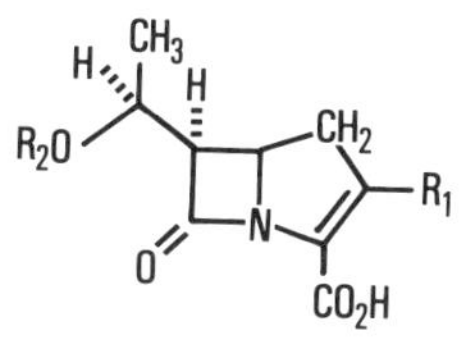

Compound	R
MM22381	$-S-CH_2CH_2NH-\overset{O}{\overset{\|\|}{C}}\,CH_3$
MM22383	$-S-CH=CH-NH-\overset{O}{\overset{\|\|}{C}}\,CH_3$

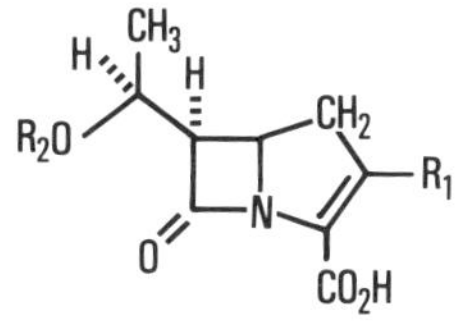

Japanese workers were the first to report on the isolation of these new metabolites from *Streptomyces fulvoviridis* (UMEZAWA et al. 1973). One of these was later shown to have the structure shown above for MM4550 (MAEDA et al. 1977). Independently, a group from Beecham reported on three new β-lactam antibiotics from *Streptomyces olivaceus*, MM4550, MM13902, and MM17880 (HOOD et al. 1979). Other olivanic acid derivatives were described by BOX et al. (1979) (MM22380, MM22381, MM22382, and MM22383). He described the use of RP HPLC in the isolation efforts. The stationary phase was C_{18}, and mobile phase was 0.05 *M* ammonium phosphate (pH 4.7) containing 5% CH_3CN (v/v). He used a procedure involving cysteine degradation of these compounds to identify potential olivanic acid derivatives during the isolation. We have examined one of these derivatives (MM13902) using out HPLC/bioautographic system. The data are given in Fig. 14.

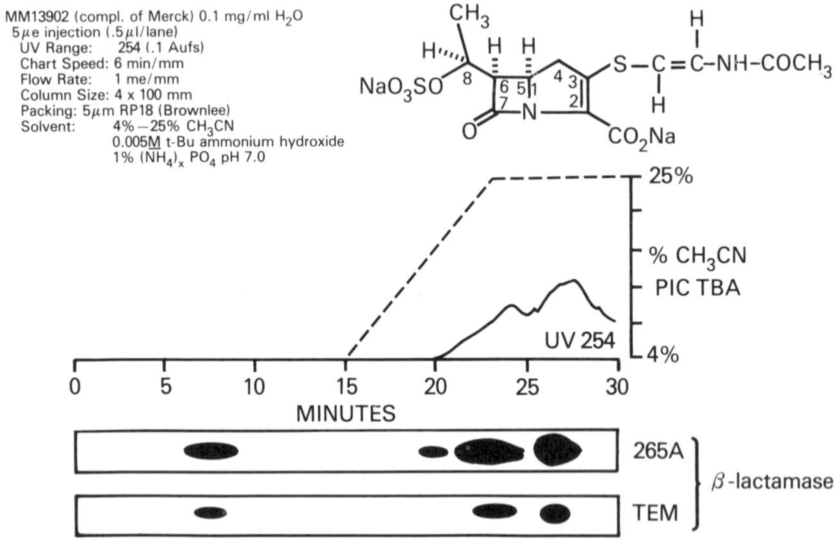

Fig. 14. HPLC/bioautography of an olivanic acid derivative (MM13902)

E. Oxy-β-Lactams

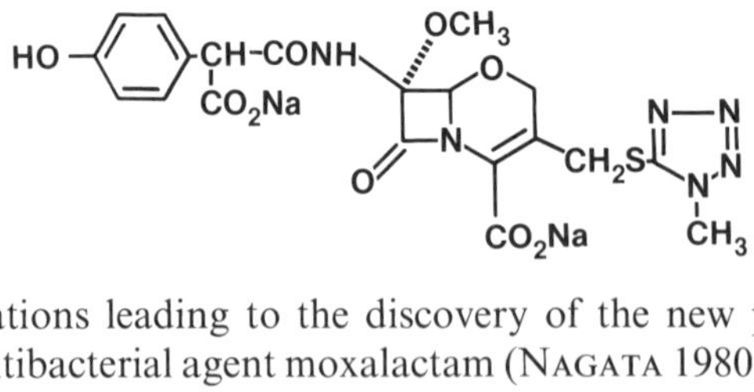

Chemical investigations leading to the discovery of the new parenterally useful broad-spectrum antibacterial agent moxalactam (NAGATA 1980; SENDO et al. 1982) (LY127935) necessitated comparisons with many other oxy-β-lactam derivatives. Some of the compounds examined are shown in Tables 1 and 2. The results of the direct comparison between the nuclear derivatives (sulfur- vs. oxygen-containing compounds) are summarized in Figs. 15 and 16 and Tables 1 and 2.

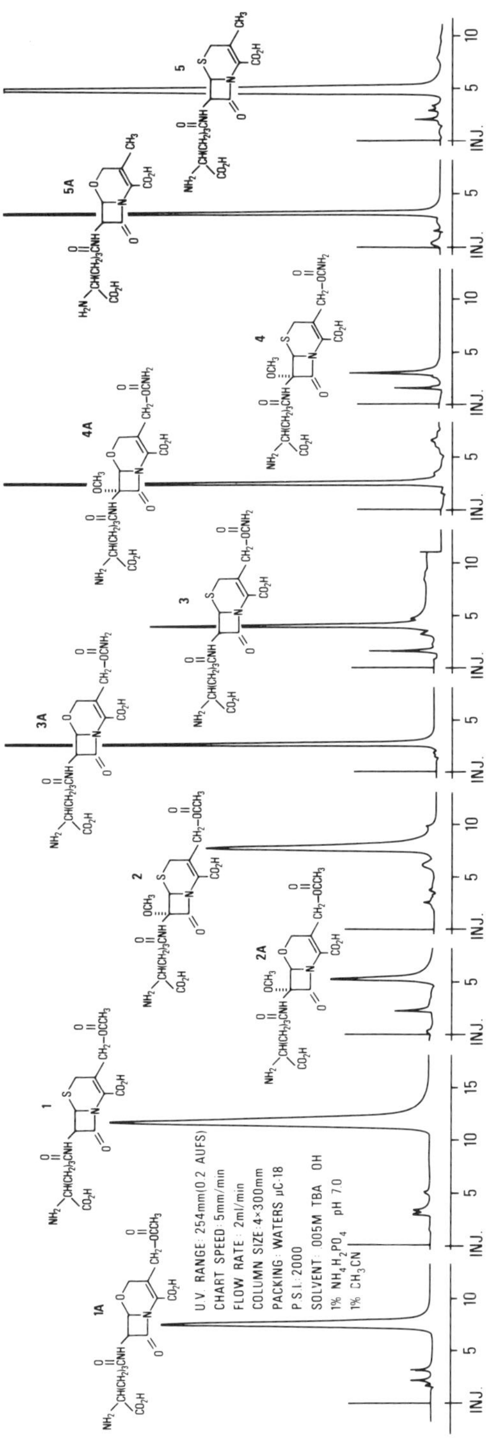

Fig. 15. HPLC comparison of 1-oxa and 1-thio-β-lactam derivatives (μBondapak C-18)

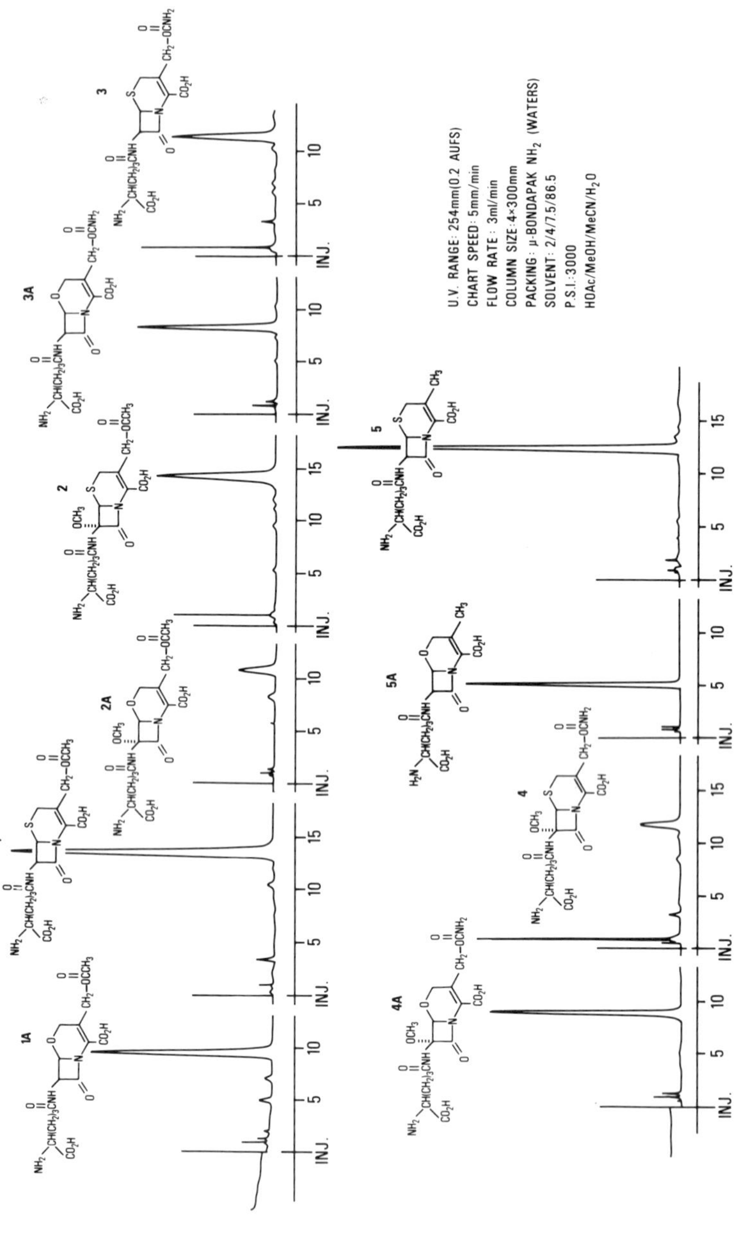

Fig. 16. HPLC comparison of 1-oxa and 1-thio-β-lactam derivatives (μBondapak NH_2)

Table 1. Comparison of cephalosporins and corresponding oxa-β-lactam derivatives

Paired ion chromatography (PIC) Tetrabutyl ammonium hydroxide (0.005 *M*) 1% CH_3CN		
k′O Cpds Nos. 1A–5A	k′S Cpds Nos. 1–5	k′S/k′O
1A 4.85	1 8.15	1.68
2A 2.23	2 5.15	1.59
3A 1.08	3 2.08	1.93
4A 0.92	4 1.31	1.42
5A 1.54	5 2.85	1.85

Table 2. Comparison of cephalosporins and corresponding oxa-β-lactam derivatives

μg NH_2 bonded phase propylamine on 10 μg silicia (Waters) 2/4/7.5/86.5 HOAc/CH_3OH/CH_3CN/H_2O		
k′O Cpds Nos. 1A–5A	k′S Cpds Nos. 1–5	k′S/k′O
1A 14.2	1 20.3	1.43
2A 16.2	2 21.3	1.31
3A 12.0	3 17.1	1.43
4A 13.2	4 17.6	1.33
5A 7.6	5 18.8	2.47

The data clearly indicate that a consistent trend in k′ values might be expected with the structural variation. In the case of the RP system, changing from the sulfur [S] to the oxygen [O] derivative gave rise to a nearly linear decrease in k′ values. The μBondapak NH_2 system also yielded a decrease in k′ in going from [S] to [O], but the data were not linear. It is obvious that the presence of the oxygen atom in place of the sulfur has significant impact on the polarity of the entire β-lactam compound, and if this property alone is used to consider chromatography of the derivative, a linear response could be expected. However, when the additional ion-exchange property is exploited with the μBondapak NH_2 column, nonlinearity indicates that the effect of hetero-atom replacement can have varied effects on the pK_a of the derivatives (Miller et al. 1981).

F. Concluding Remarks

Over the past 10 years analytical procedures for β-lactam compounds have shifted from PC coupled with microbiological assay to a physical chemical methodology. There are many reasons for this change of direction. Only the most significant will be mentioned. First, the presence of by-products in the fermentation broths and degradation products of metabolites have always created some uncertainty with microbiological assay results because of differences in activity between individual components and combinations on assay organisms. Physical properties such as chromatographic mobility, especially in multiple systems, give a more conclusive identity of the desired product.

Therefore, it is easy to understand the acceptance of HPLC as the most useful tool in analysis of purity or composition of the matter. On the other hand, many attempts have been made to couple HPLC to mass, infrared, or NMR spectrometry in order to achieve identification of compounds during the short time the new and often unknown substance is retained. Thus, most recently an analytical high-pressure liquid chromatograph has been coupled to a UV/visible spectrophotometer and a mass spectrometer and used for separation and subsequent identification of compounds in different plant extracts (Schuster 1980). This kind of operation becomes almost impossible to handle when one uses some of the extravagant solvents (Miller and Neuss 1976) necessary for the separation of different

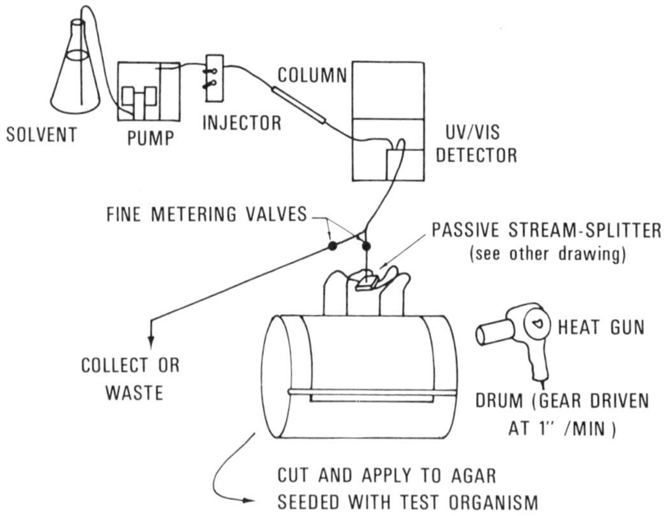

Fig. 17. Flow diagram of HPLC/bioautography system

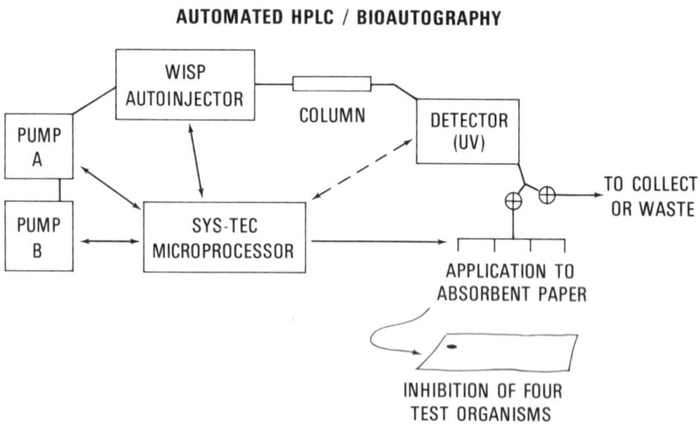

Fig. 18. Flow diagram of microprocessor-controlled HPLC/bioautography system

metabolites in the fermentation broth, particularly in the course of one passage through the system. We have succeeded in diverting a portion of the eluent from the column during LC of the fermentation broth and applying it to an adsorbent paper at the same rate as the recording of the UV absorption. The paper is then placed in the conventional manner over agar and the latter inoculated with an appropriate test organism. After incubation, the zones of antibacterial activity can be directly correlated with corresponding peaks in the UV recordings. In such a way, one can detect biological activity of pure components directly in the fermentation broth which can be particularly valuable when the compound of interest either does not have any UV absorption, e.g., clavulanic acid (Fig. 11) or very little absorption, as it is in the case of penicillin N (Fig. 3) (Miller and Neuss 1978).

Finally, it is obvious that the examination of many samples by HPLC suggests the use of automation. In Fig. 17, the schematic diagram shows the use of HPLC bioautography and, in Fig. 18, in conjunction with the Systec microprocessor, permitting unattended sample handling. Operations include gradient elution, as well as column washing procedures with two solvents. The inclusion in the system of a WISP (Waters) autoinjector provides programmable injection of 48 samples.

These applications as well as routine analytical procedures point out the necessity for data manipulation and storage. The enormous amount of data that can be generated by automatically injected HPLC systems simply requires such peripheral support in order to obtain maximum efficiency. Commercial computerization systems are available ranging from small dedicated data processors to large systems that can manipulate many LC inputs.

Acknowledgments. We gratefully acknowledge to following individuals: Dr. K. Koch and Mr. S. Nash of the Lilly Research Laboratories, Eli Lilly and Company, for a sample of nocardicin A; Dr. B. G. Christensen of the Merck, Sharp and Dohme Research Laboratories for the deblocking procedure of benzyl clavulanate; Drs. Yuji Sendo, Toshiro Konoie, Masayuki Murakami, and Mitsuru Yoshioka, Shionogi Research Laboratories, Shionogi and Co., Ltd., Fukushima-ku, Osaka, 553 Japan, for samples of -1-oxa analogs of naturally occurring cephalosporins and cephamycins; and Mrs. Barabara F. Albright of the Lilly Research Laboratories, Eli Lilly and Company, for expert handling and patience in preparing this manuscript.

References

Albers-Schonberg GA, Arison BH, Hensens OD, Hirshfield J, Hoogsteen K, Kaczka EA, Rhodes RE, Kahan JS, Kahan FM, Ratcliffe RW, Walton E, Ruswinkle LJ, Morin RB, Christensen BG (1978) Structure and absolute configuration of thienamycin. J Am Chem Soc 100/20:6491–6499

Aoki H, Sakai H, Kohsaka M, Konomi T, Hosoda J, Kubochi Y, Iguchi E, Imanaka H (1976) Nocardicin A, a new monocyclic β-lactam antibiotic: I. discovery, isolation, and characterization. J Antibiot 29/5:492–500

Box SJ, Hood JD, Spear SR (1979) Four further antibiotics related to olivanic acid produced by *Streptomyces olivaceus*: fermentation, isolation, characterization, and biosynthetic studies. J Antibiot 32/12:1239–1247

Carroll MA et al. (1977) The determination of cephradine and cephalexin by reverse phase high-performance liquid chromatography. J Antibiot 30/5:397–403

Cole M, Dorking S, Howarth T, Rudwick T, Reading C (1975) Ger. pat. 2,517,316A1

Crombez E, Van Den Bossche W, De Moerloose P (1979) Separation of some cephalosporin derivatives by ion-pair reversed phase high-performance liquid chromatography. J Chromatogr 169:343–350

Flynn EH (1972) Cephalosporins and penicillins: chemistry and biology. Academic Press, New York London

Hood JD, Box SJ, Verrall MS (1979) Olivanic acids, a family of β-lactam antibiotics with β-lactamase inhibitory properties produced by *Streptomyces* species II. Isolation and characterization of the olivanic acids MM4550, MM13902, MM17880 from *Streptomyces olivaceus*. J Antibiot 32:295–303

Howarth TT (1976) Clavulanic acid, a novel β-lactam isolated from *Streptomyces clavuligerus:* X-ray structure analysis. Chem Commun 1976:266–267

Kahan JS, Kahan FM, Goegelman R, Currie SA, Jackson M, Stapley EO, Miller TW et al. (1979) Thienamycin, a new β-lactam antibiotic. I. Discovery, taxonomy, isolation, and physical properties. J Antibiot 32:1–11

Kingston D (1979) High performance liquid chromatography of natural products. J Nat Prod 42:237–260

Kurita M, Joman K, Komori T, Miyairi N, Aoki H, Kuge S, Kamiya T, Imanaka H (1976) Isolation and characterization of nocardicin B. J Antibiot 29:1243–1245

Larsen C, Bundgaard H (1978) Polymerization of penicillins V. Separation, identification and quantitative determination of antigenic polymerization products in ampicillin sodium preparations by high-performance liquid chromatography. J Chromatogr 147:143–150

LeBelle M, Graham K, Wilson WL (1979) High performance liquid chromatographic analysis of penicillin V benzathine oral suspensions. J Pharm Sci 68:555–556
Lee TL, D'arconte L, Brooks MA (1979) High pressure liquid chromatographic determination of amoxicillin in urine. J Pharm Sci 68:454–458
Maeda K, Takahashi S, Sezaki M, Ilnuma K, Naganawa H, Kondo S, Ohno M, Umezawa H (1977) Isolation and structure of a β-lactamase inhibitor from *Streptomyces.* J Antibiot (Tokyo) 30:770–772
Miller RD, Neuss N (1976) High performance liquid chromatography of natural products I. Separation of cephalosporin C derivatives and cephalosporin antibiotics: isolation of cephalosporin C from fermentation broth. J Antibiot 29:902–906
Miller RD, Neuss N (1978) High performance liquid chromatography of natural products II. Direct biological correlation of components in the fermentation broth. J Antibiot 31:1132–1136
Miller RD, Neuss N (1980) Preparative high-performance liquid chromatography of natural products. Abstracts of the Pittsburgh conference, Atlantic City, 10–12 March 1980, paper 188
Miller RD, Affolder C, Neuss N (1981) HPLC of cephalosporins and their oxa-derivatives. Experientia 37:928–930
Morin RB, Jackson BG, Flynn EH, Roeske RW (1962) Chemistry of cephalosporin antibiotics. 1. 7-Aminocephalosporanic acid from cephalosporin C. J Am Chem Soc 84:3400
Nachtmann F (1979) Automated high performance liquid chromatography as a means of monitoring the production of penicillins and 6-aminopenicillanic acid. Chromatographia 12:380–385
Nagata W (1980) Straightforward synthesis of 7-methoxy-1-oxacephem from penicillin. In: Penicillin fifty years after Fleming, a royal society discussion organized by Sir James Baddiley FRS and EP Abraham, FRS, May 2 and 3, 1979. The Royal Society of Chemistry, London, p 225
Nakagawa T, Hakinaka J, Yamaoka K, Uno T (1978) High speed liquid chromatographic determination of cephalexin in human plasma and urine. J Antibiot 3:769
Salto F (1978) Separation of penicillin and cephalosporin diastereomers by reversed phase high-performance liquid chromatography. J Chromatogr 161:379–385
Schuster R (1980) Separation and positive identification of compounds in complex sample mixtures using on-line LC-UV/VIS and LC/MS, direct coupling. Chromatographia 13:379
Sendo Y, Konoike T, Murakami M, Yoshioka M (1982) Delta-3-delta-2 isomerizations in cephems and their 1-oxa congeners. Heterocycles 17:231–234
Snyder LR, Kirkland JJ (1974) Introduction to modern liquid chromatography. Wiley Interscience, New York
Suzuki A, Noda K, Noguchi H (1980) High performance liquid chromatographic determination of ceftizoxime, a new cephalosporin antibiotic, in rat serum, bile, and urine. J Chromatography 182:448–453
Umezawa H, Mitsuhachi S, Hamanda M, Iyobe S, Tokahashi S, Utahara R, Osata Y, Yamazaki S, Ogawara H, Maeda K (1973) Two β-lactamase inhibitors produced by *Streptomyces.* J Antibiot (Tokyo) 26:51–54
Vree TB, Hekster YA, Baars AM, Van der Kleijn E (1978) Rapid determination of amoxycillin (Clamoxyl) and ampicillin (Penbritin) in body fluids by HPLC. J Chromatogr 145:496–501
White ER, Carroll MA, Zarembo JE (1977) Reversed phase high speed liquid chromatography of antibiotics. J Antibiot 30:811–818
Yamana T, Tsuji A, Miyamoto E, Kubo O (1977) Novel method for determination of partition coefficients of penicillins and cephalosporins by high-pressure liquid chromatography. J Pharm Sci 66:747–749
Yamaoka K, Nariata S, Nakagawa T, Uno T (1979) High performance liquid chromatographic analysis of sulbenicillin and carbenicillin in human urine. J Chromatogr 168:187–193

CHAPTER 11

Strategy in the Total Synthesis of β-Lactam Antibiotics

B. G. CHRISTENSEN and T. N. SALZMANN

A. Introduction

The total syntheses of various β-lactam antibiotics have been discussed previously (HEUSLER 1972; SAMMES 1980). While existing reviews present in varying detail the chemistry employed in these total syntheses, the present account will instead discuss the strategies involved. Rather than attempting a comprehensive review, one example of each type of strategy used to date will be given. The strategies will be discussed by bond-forming type and the stereochemical strategies will be discussed concomitantly.

One paramount strategy is found in all synthetic efforts. The chemical reactivity of the final product dictates that the nucleus be constructed as near as is practicable to the end of the synthesis. This is somewhat less important in the cephalosporins, which are the most stable of all of the β-lactam antibiotics. Inspection of the various routes employed indicates that they all fit into the following schemes, based upon a classification utilizing the final bond-forming step as the key.

B. β-Lactam Closure

Those total syntheses in which closure of the amide bond of the azetidinone ring is the crucial step in the construction of the ring system are considered as part of this category. The Sheehan penicillin synthesis remains the classic example of this strategy.

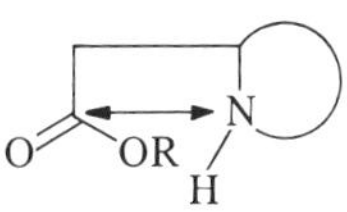

C. 2+2 Annelations

When the final step in the construction of the nucleus involves simultaneous formation of the bonds of the azetidinone, they may be regarded as 2+2 annelations. The acid chloride–imine reaction is the most often used example of this type and the Merck cefoxitin synthesis might be regarded as the first total synthesis of a β-lactam antibiotic using this approach:

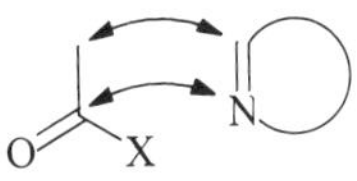

D. Monocyclic β-Lactam Antibiotics

Obviously, examples which contain a monocyclic β-lactam constitute a new class whenever the azetidinone synthesis involves a new method of construction not covered in the rest of the classification. Nocardicin is the only well-known example of a monocyclic β-lactam and so all examples of this type will be nocardicin syntheses.

E. Examples Involving Prior Construction of the Azetidinone

With the publication of the Woodward cephalosporin total synthesis, virtually all modern total syntheses of bicyclic β-lactams have been of this general type. This category may be divided into four different subclasses, depending upon the final bond-forming step of the nucleus construction.

1. Closure to C-4 of the Azetidinone. The only examples of this type involve attachment of a heteroatom (sulfur or oxygen) to the C-4 carbon of the azetidinone. The example chosen to represent this strategy is the Beecham clavulanic acid total synthesis.

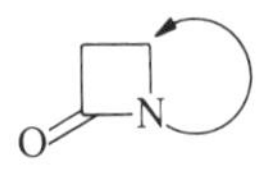

2. 1,2-Bond Formation. The Woodward cephalosporin total synthesis exemplifies the first example of total synthesis involving formation of a 1,2-bond by a Michael addition of a sulfhydryl group to a highly activated double bond. Another example, the Baldwin penicillin total synthesis, will be utilized to exemplify this type of closure as well as the use of stereocontrol in β-lactam syntheses.

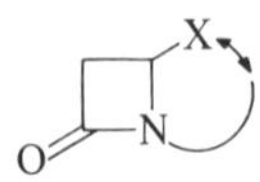

3. Carbon–Carbon Bond Formation. The most widely used example of this type of strategy is the method of forming a double-bond using a Witting-type closure. The initial Merck thienamycin total synthesis also involved carbon-carbon bond formation, but utilized a displacement reaction.

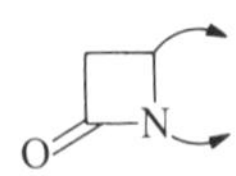

4. Closure to N-1 of the Azetidinone. The final category of this classification involves closure to the azetidinone nitrogen atom. The Merck stereocontrolled, chiral total synthesis of thienamycin involves a carbene insertion into the N-H bond of the azetidinone.

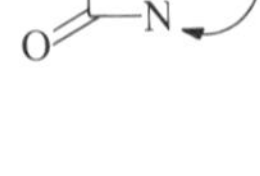

Historically, the first useful β-lactam total synthesis was that of penicillins achieved by SHEEHAN and HENERY-LOGAN in 1957. A further decade passed before WOODWARD (1966) reported his cephalosporin C total synthesis. The Woodward synthesis was stereocontrolled whereas the Sheehan synthesis was not, reflecting the advances in the art of organic synthesis that had occurred in the interim. It is the intent of this review to discuss these advances from the conceptual point of view, detailing the changes in strategy and stereocontrol that they exemplify.

F. Penicillin Total Synthesis – Sheehan

Three papers (SHEEHAN and HENERY-LOGAN 1957, 1959, 1962) present the total synthesis of penicillin V. Earlier, DUVIGNEAUD et al. (1946) reported an extremely low-yielding reaction forming benzylpenicillin *(3)* from the oxazolone *(1)* and penicillamine *(2)*. Conceptually, the Sheehan synthesis is related since both employ the 1,4-addition of the thiol group of penicillamine to an enol form of β-aldehyde-ester. The α-position of penicillamine also contributes the only stereocontrolled chiral center in the product in both syntheses. Because of the inherent instability of the penicillin nucleus, closure of the β-lactam was deferred until the penultimate step.

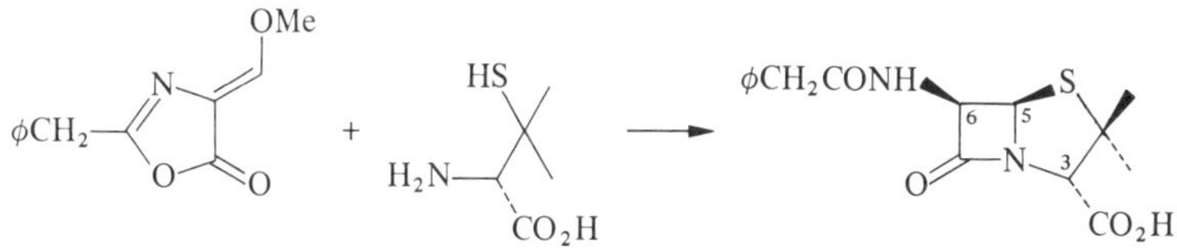

1 *2* *3*

One of the building blocks of the nucleus, *t*-butyl α-phthalimidomalonaldehyde *(5)*, was prepared by the condensation of *t*-butyl formate and *t*-butyl phthalimidoacetate *(4)* (SHEEHAN and JOHNSON 1954).

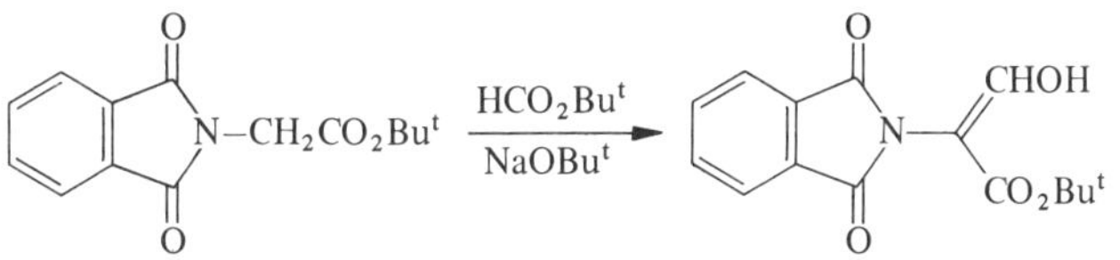

4 *5*

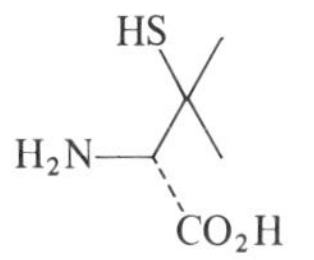

6

→ 7

D-Penicillamine *6* contains all of the remaining atoms of the penam nucleus and the α-carbon atom contains an asymmetric center of the same chirality as C-3 of penicillin. Condensation of *5* and *6* affords a mixture of penicilloic esters *(7)*. Although there are four possible stereoisomers that could be formed in this reaction, only two were isolated from the reaction mixture. Termed α and γ isomers, subsequent conversion of the α-isomer to penicillin V established its configuration as 5-*R*,6 *S*. The γ-isomer can be equilibrated to a mixture of α and γ isomers and additional α-isomer can be isolated. Acidic treatment produces a third isomer (as the acid). The lack of stereocontrol is the major deficiency of this synthetic approach.

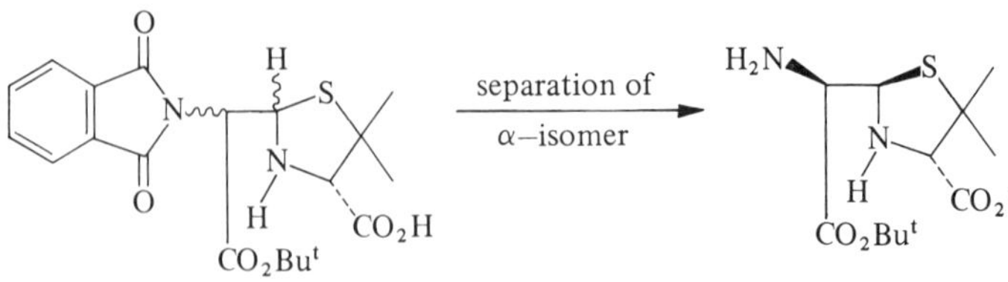

7 *8*

Penicillins are unstable to the reaction conditions necessary to remove the phthalimidoyl protecting group, so it was removed at this stage. Hydrazinolysis of the α-isomer of *7* afforded *8; 8* could be acylated with a variety of acyl functions giving versatility to the synthesis. Acylation with phenoxyacetyl chloride gave *9*, which could be deblocked to the penicilloic acid *(10)*. Previous efforts to cyclize penicilloates with the traditional acid halide- or anhydride-forming reagents had met with little success. These failures can most readily be ascribed to the instability of penicillins in the presence to these acidic reagents. An elegant synthetic solution to this problem was found by SHEEHAN and HESS (1955), who developed the use of organic carbodiimides to form amide bonds directly from amines and organic acids

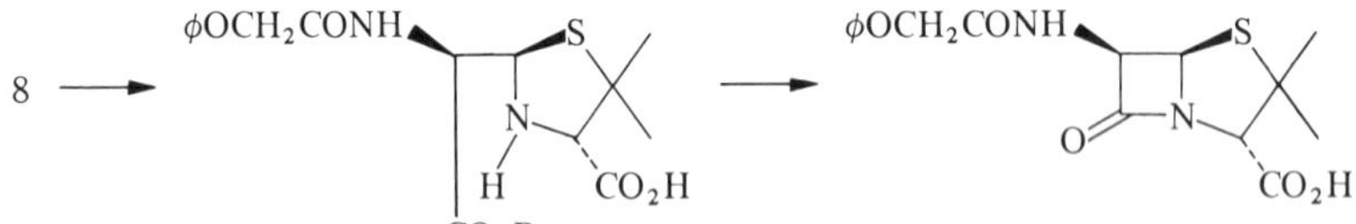

11

9 R=Bu^t
10 R=H

in aqueous solution. These mild conditions also worked well for the cyclization of penicilloic acids to penicillins. The use of *N,N'*-dicyclohexylcarbodiimide readily effected the transformation of *10* to *11*, completing the total synthesis of penicillin V.

Because of the low yield (5%) in the cyclization of *10* to *11* a higher yielding alternative route was explored. To prepare the crucial intermediate *(15)*, the α-isomer of *7* was converted to the benzyl ester *(12)*. Hydrazinolysis afforded the free amine *(13)*. The *t*-butyl ester was readily cleaved with dry HCl and the resultant product *(14)* was tritylated to give *(15)*. The carbodiimide mediated closure to *16* proceeded particularly well (67%). Catalytic debenzylation, followed by detritylation, afforded crystalline 6-aminopenicillanic acid *(18)*. Acylation of this intermediate gave penicillin V *(11)*. Acylation of *18*, prepared by fermentation or from side-chain cleavage of natural penicillins, is now the basic route to all semisynthetic penicillins.

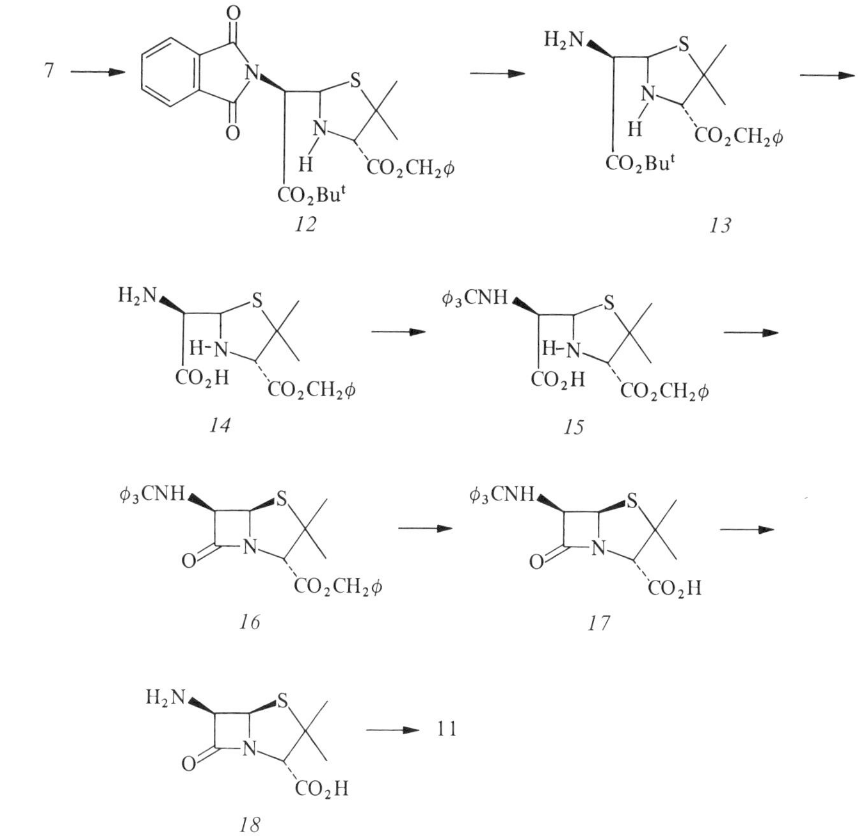

The Sheehan penicillin total synthesis was remarkable in several respects; indeed, several syntheses of cephalosporins were based upon his strategy of penultimate β-lactam closure (HEYMES et al. 1966, DOLFINI et al. 1968; GIROTRA and WENDLER 1972). The use of carbodiimides to form azetidinones was also pioneered by his group. The principal drawback of the Sheehan synthesis was the lack of stereospecificity, although nearly a decade passed before a stereocontrolled total synthesis was accomplished.

G. Cefoxitin Total Synthesis – Merck

One of the general methods for the synthesis of β-lactams developed by the Sheehan group was the reaction of an acid chloride with an imine in the presence of an organic base (SHEEHAN and RYAN 1951). While the acid chloride might be expected to form a ketene in the presence of an organic base and the resulting ketene undergo a 2+2 cycloaddition to an imine [the earliest known preparation of an azetidinone (STAUDINGER 1907)], this is apparently not the case. In order to introduce nitrogen α to the β-lactam carbonyl, phthalimidoylacetyl chloride was used, but as indicated earlier, the conditions necessary to deblock the phthalimidoyl groups are not compatible with the chemical reactivity of the β-lactam group. BOSE et al. (1967) introduced azidoacetyl chloride as the masked glycyl moiety as a way to circumvent this difficulty since hydrogenation is a preferred way to deblock a β-lactam intermediate.

Cefoxitin *(19)* is a β-lactam antibiotic, characterized by its broad spectrum and stability to β-lactamases (HAMILTON-MILLER 1974). The presence of the 7α-methoxy function confers β-lactamase stability upon the cephalosporin nucleus and structurally differentiates cefoxitin from the cephalosporins. Any synthesis of

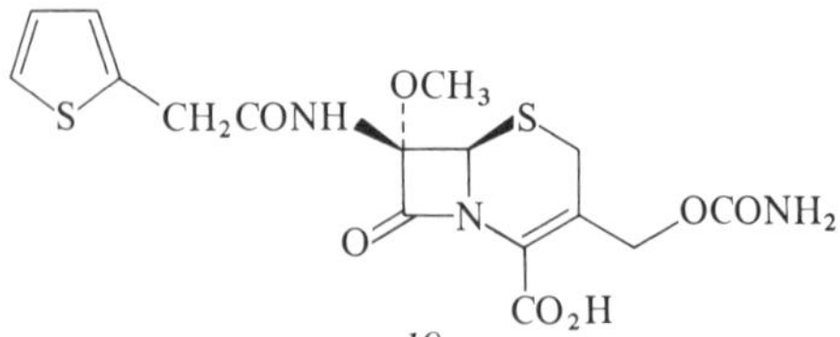

19

cefoxitin from the retrosynthetic point of view may be viewed as a cephalosporin total synthesis with the added complexity of stereospecifically adding the 7α-methoxy function. Since several direct insertions of the methoxy group were available from previous work, the strategy of attempting to use the acid chloride–imine annelation as a practical route to a cephem synthesis was adopted. This necessitated the synthesis of the appropriate imine, in this case, a thiazine. The key intermediates to these thiazines are α-thioformamidodiethylphosphonoacetates (RATCLIFFE and CHRISTENSEN 1973a).

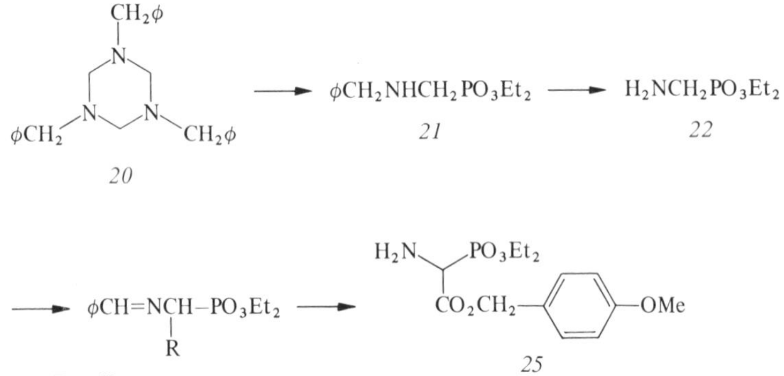

20 *21* *22*

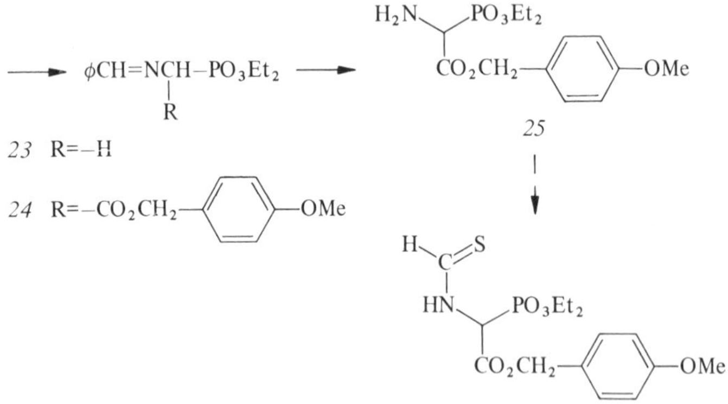

23 R=–H

24 R=–CO_2CH_2–C$_6$H$_4$–OMe

25

26

The 1,3,5-tribenzylhexahydro-3-triazine *(20)* gave the desired *N*-benzyl aminomethyldiethylphosphonate *(21)* and catalytic hydrogenolysis afforded *22*. The free amine was converted to the Schiff base *(23)* which could be acylated with

p-methoxybenzyl chloroformate to give *(24)*. The reverse procedure, phosphorylation of a glycyl ester Schiff base, afforded an O-phosphoryl product. After reversal of the Schiff base, thioformylation with ethyl thionoformate afforded the desired p-methoxybenzyl α-thioformamidodiethylphosphonoacetate *(26)*.

With the synthesis of the key synthon, attention was directed to its conversion to a thiazine. Alkylation of *26* with 1-chloro-3-acetoxy-2-propanone with excess K_2CO_3 in acetone gave the desired thiazine *(28)* directly (RATCLIFFE and CHRISTENSEN 1973b). Apparently the intermediate *(27)* undergoes cyclization

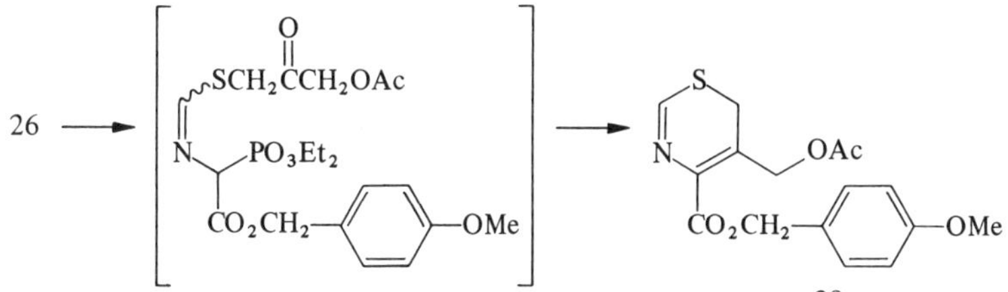

27 *28*

under the reaction conditions. Application of the acid chloride-imine annelation afforded the desired 3-cephem *(29)*. Choice of reaction conditions are critical since

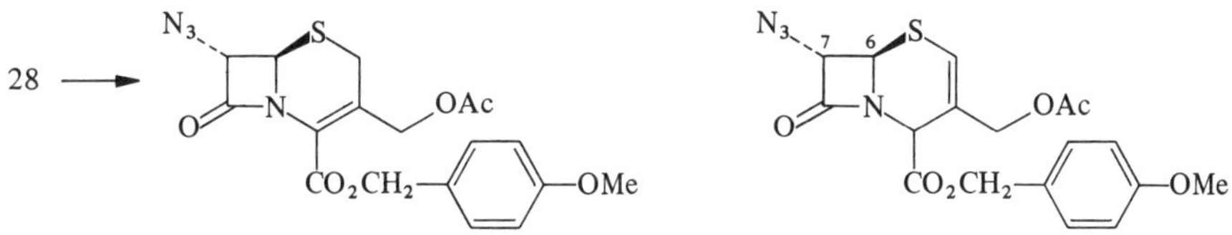

29 *30*

exposure to base affords the Δ^2 isomer *(30)*. It should be noted that the stereochemistry at C-7 is inverted from the natural or bioactive configuration. However, since it was intended to use the C-6 chirality in the introduction of the 7α group, this is of no consequence. Of course, the product is racemic.

Reduction of the azide, followed by Schiff base formation, afforded *32* (RATCLIFFE and CHRISTENSEN 1973c). Because of the chirality at C-6, the less-hindered

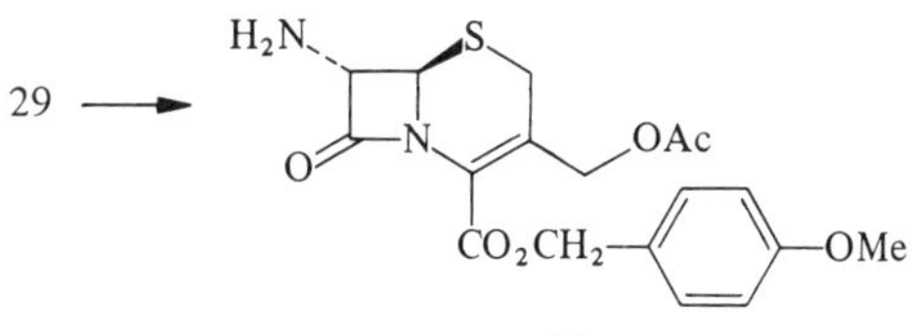

31

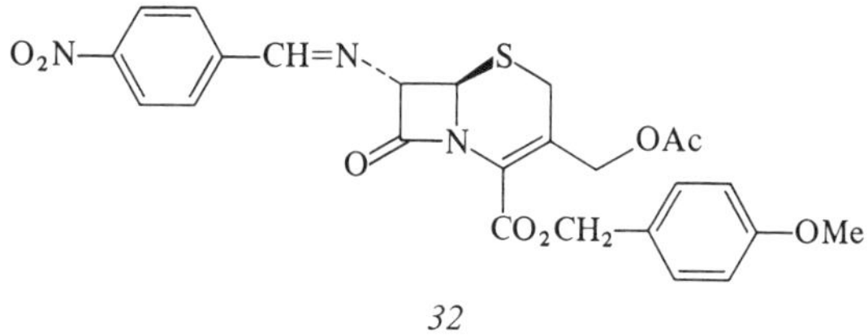

32

side at C-7 is α. Based upon this reasoning, it had been shown that methylation of a C-7 anion occurs from the α-face (FIRESTONE et al. 1972). Indeed, even protonation occurs from the α-face under kinetic conditions and this observation has enabled the completion of a penicillin (FIRESTONE et al. 1974) and a cephalosporin (RATCLIFFE and CHRISTENSEN 1973 b) total synthesis based upon a kinetically controlled epimerization of the C-6(7) anion. In the cefoxitin total synthesis, advantage was taken of this principle to introduce the methylthio group in a stereocon-

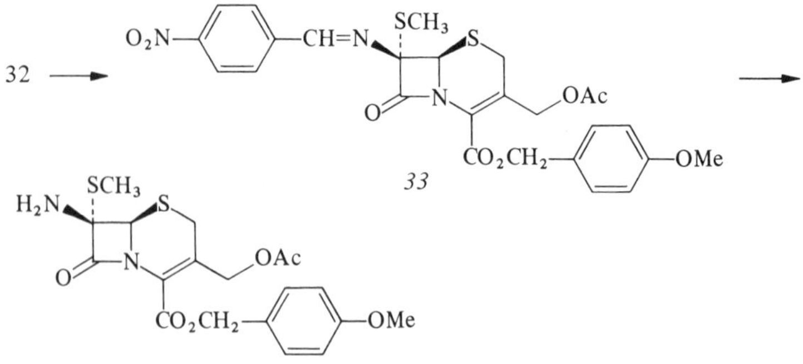

33

34

trolled manner to C-7. The anion of *32* readily reacts with methylsulfenyl chloride to afford only *33*. Removal of the Schiff base gave the amine *(34)* which was acylated to *35*. Treatment of *35* with thallium trinitrate in methanol again gave exclu-

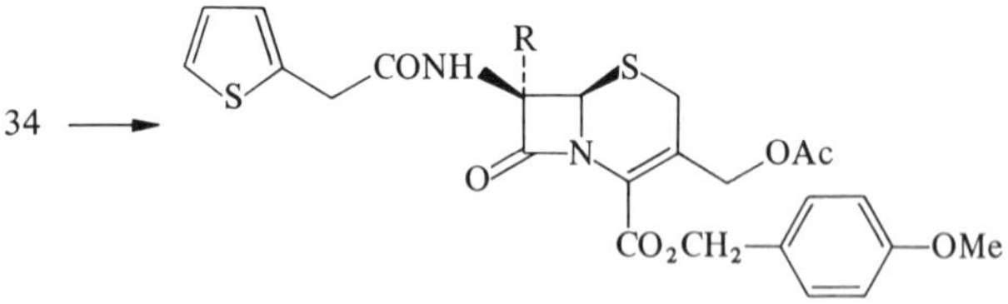

35 R=–SMe
36 R=–OMe

sively the 7α-methoxy derivative *(36)*. Presumably, the solvent reacts from the less-hindered α-face with either the carbonium ion derived by elimination of the methylthio group from *35* or the *N*-acylimine *(37)* to give *36*.

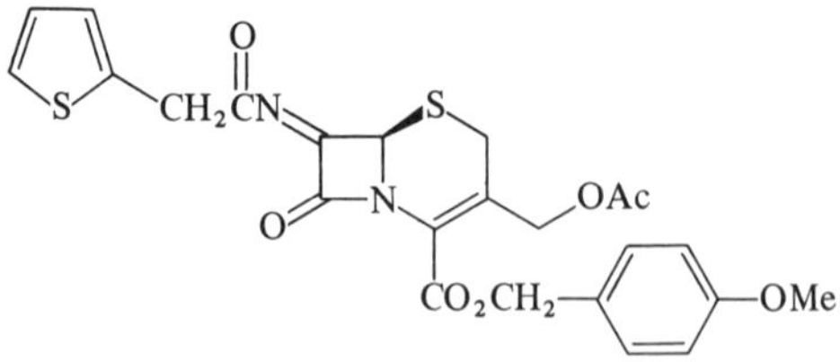

37

Compound *36* was deblocked to the free acid *(38)*. Deacetylation to *39*, followed by carbamoylation, completes the total synthesis of cefoxitin.

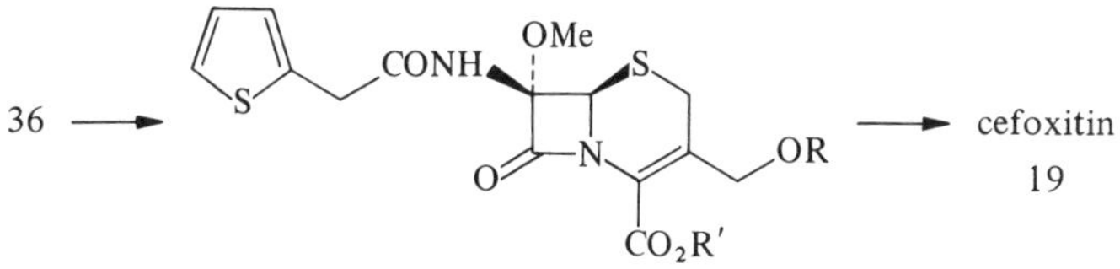

38 R=–Ac; R′=H
39 R=–H; R′=H

Besides its simplicity and the ready availability of starting materials, this synthesis is noteworthy for its use of the bridgehead chirality to control the C-7 stereochemistry and its versatility in the synthesis of analogs. Several analogs prepared by total synthesis have been synthesized by routes based upon the çefoxitin sequence.

H. Nocardicin Total Synthesis – Wasserman

The nocardicins (COOPER 1980) are a family of structurally related monocyclic β-lactam antibiotics that have been isolated recently. Primarily active against gram-negative bacteria, their structure stimulated a great deal of interest. According to the categories used in this chapter, any synthesis involving a new method of azetidinone formation would constitute a new scheme for inclusion in this review. Nocardicin has been totally synthesized (KAMIYA 1977; KAMIYA et al. 1978; KOPPEL et al. 1978; WASSERMAN and HLASTA 1978). The Wasserman total synthesis (WASSERMAN and HLASTA 1978) has been selected for inclusion since it employs β-lactam syntheses not used elsewhere in the total synthesis of natural products or analogs.

Since 3-aminonocardicinic acid (3-ANA) *(40)* had been converted to nocardicin A *(41)* (KAMIYA 1977), the strategy was to develop a novel and efficient

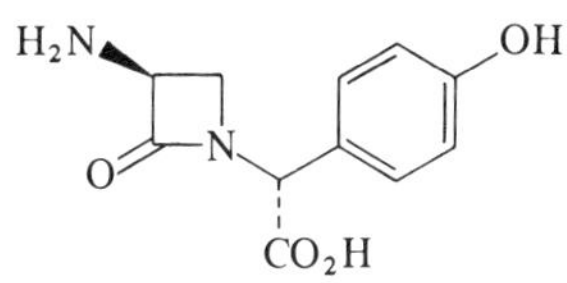

40

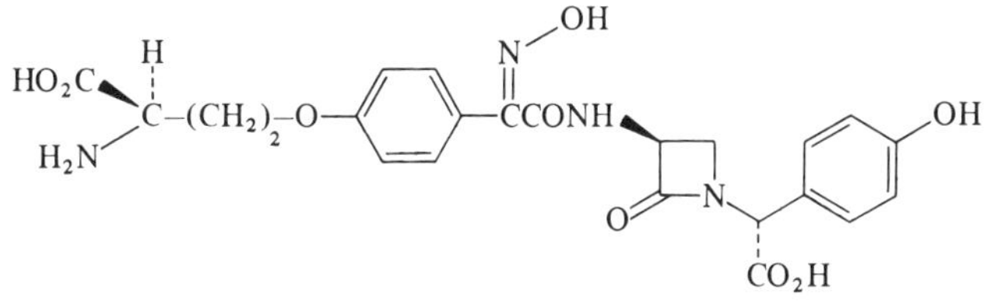

41

method to prepare 3-ANA. The key intermediate was *45*. Starting with methyl *p*-(benzyloxy)phenyl acetate, condensation with dimethyl carbonate, followed by introduction of the azido function with *p*-toluenesulfonyl azide and reduction, the desired compound, *45*, was readily prepared.

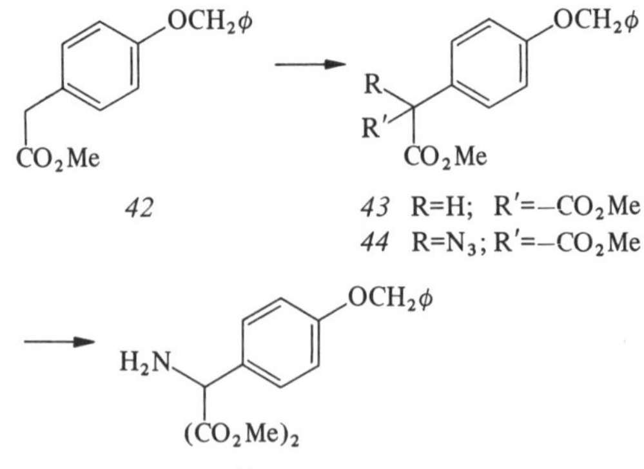

42

43 R=H; R'=–CO_2Me

44 R=N_3; R'=–CO_2Me

45

Two routes were used to prepare the nocardicinic acid analog *(48)*. When a solution of cyclopropanone (prepared from ketene and diazomethane) was added to *45*, *46* was formed in quantitative yield. *N*-chlorination and reaction with silver nitrate afforded *48*. A more convenient route to *48* involving acylation of *45* with 3-chloropropionyl chloride gave *49* and subsequent ring closure provided *48*.

Introduction of the 3-amino function was initiated by introduction of the 3-azido group. Hydrolysis, followed by acidification and spontaneous decarboxylation, gave *51* as a 1:1 mixture of diastereoisomers. Conversion to the benzyl ester and preparative HPLC separation afforded *52*. Reduction to the 3-ANA derivative *(53)* gave a product (KOPPEL et al. 1978) that had been previously converted to nocardicin A.

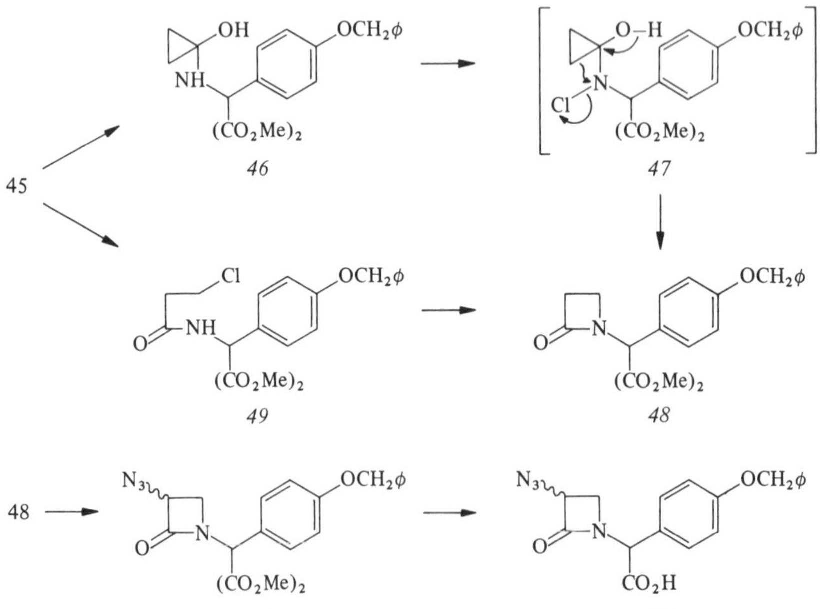

46 *47* *49* *48* *50* *51*

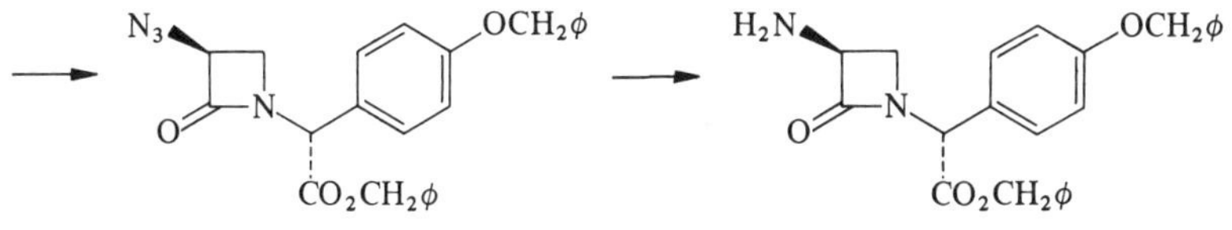

52 53

The Wasserman synthesis of nocardicin thus demonstrates the utility of two additional azetidinone syntheses in the total synthesis of natural β-lactam products.

I. Total Synthesis of (±)-Clavulanic Acid – Beecham

Clavulanic acid *(54)* is a naturally occurring β-lactamase inhibitor which has the novel oxapenam structure shown below.

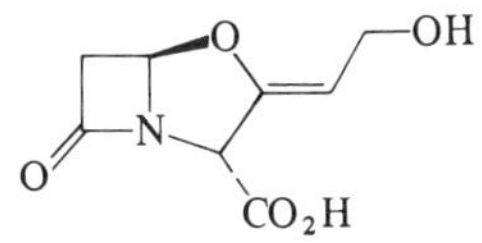

54

In addition to the obvious synthetic challenge of developing a method to construct the oxapenam ring nucleus, the important questions of the relative stereochemistry at positions *3* and *5* as well as the stereochemistry and regiochemistry of the double bond had to be addressed.

The Beecham group (Bentley et al. 1977) chose the known monocyclic azetidinone *(55)* as their starting material. Compound *55* was alkylated on nitrogen by reaction with dimethyl 2-bromo-3-oxaglutarate in the presence of two

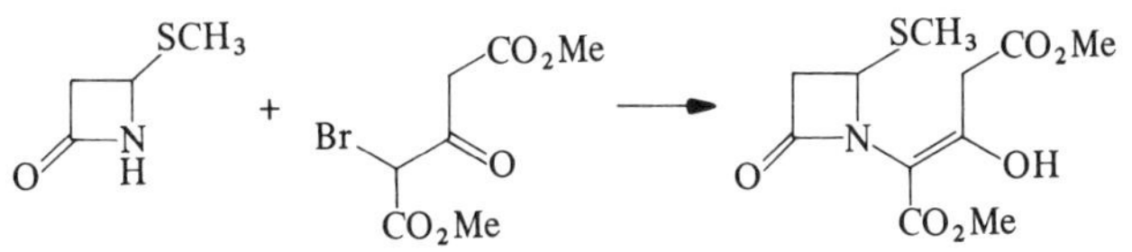

55 56

equivalents of sodium hydride. The resulting enolic product *(56)* was treated with a small excess of chlorine in carbon tetrachloride to give the chloro derivative *(57)*, which was not isolated but rather was treated directly with anhydrous potassium carbonate in dry dimethylformanide (DMF) to provide compound *58* as the only product in 34% overall yield.

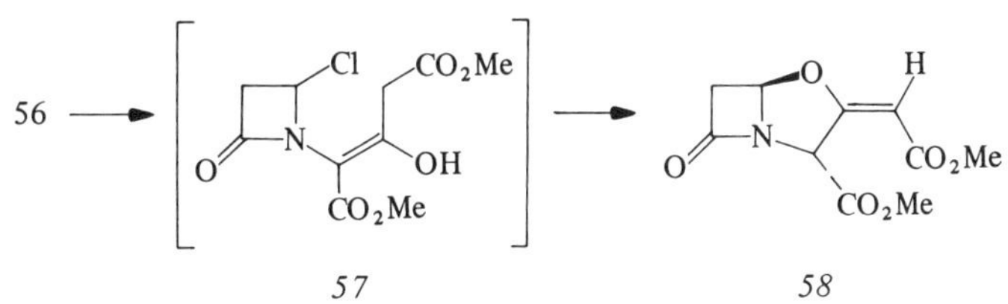

57 58

Although the basic cyclization conditions did provide the desired, thermodynamically more stable, relative configuration at C-3 and C-5, the trisubstituted olefin was produced exclusively in the "unnatural" E configuration. An alternate approach involving treatment of *57* with triethylamine in dry ether did provide a mixture of *58* and the corresponding *Z* isomer *(59)* in which *59* was predominant. However, in this case, compound *60* was also obtained in an amount approximately equal to that of *59*. Because both *58* and *59* were unstable to attempted chromatographic isolation, these workers decided to attempt to invert the olefin configuration of isomer *58*, which could be obtained in pure crystalline form.

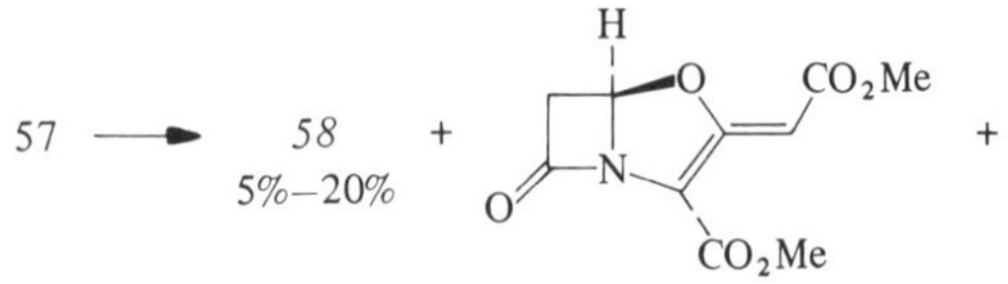

59

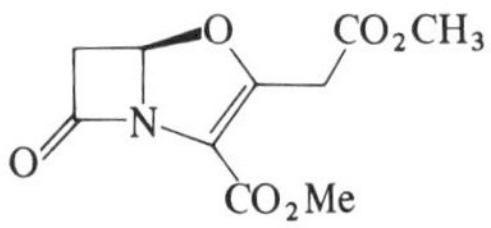

60

Irradiation of compound *58* in benzene solution gave a 3:2 mixture of *58* and *59* in quantitative yield. Reduction of this mixture with diisobutylaluminium hydride in toluene at −70 °C gave a low yield of a mixture of (±)-methylclavulanate *(61)* and (±)-methylisoclavulanate *(62)*. Since the corresponding optically active form of *61* had previously been deblocked to yield clavulanic acid, this route represents a total synthesis of (±)-clavulanic acid.

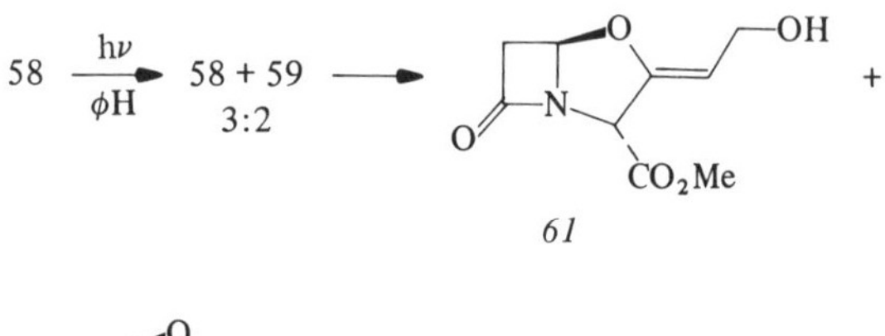

61

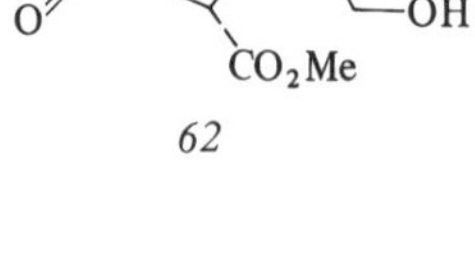

62

While the above route had the virtue of rapidly assembling the oxapenem nucleus from readily available starting materials, the problems of regio- and stereocontrol of the olefin were yet to be satisfactorily resolved. Subsequent work by the Beecham group (BENTLEY et al. 1979) has resulted in a new approach to the total synthesis of *54* which uses an analogous ring closure reaction but is much more stereocontrolled in the establishment of the exocyclic olefin.

J. Cephalosporin C Total Synthesis – Woodward

The report of the first total synthesis of cephalosporin C *(63)* by Woodward and coworkers marked a significant milestone in the historical development of synthetic strategy in the β-lactam field (WOODWARD et al. 1966; WOODWARD 1966). In contrast to the previous approaches to penicillin total synthesis, which invariably had postponed formation of the β-lactam ring until the end of the synthesis, Woodward constructed a fully functionalized β-lactam at an early stage in the scheme and utilized that group for subsequent elaboration of the dihydrothiazine moiety of *63*. In addition, for the first time, the important stereocenters at C-6 and C-7 were established both in the proper relative and absolute configuration by an ingenious combination of judicious choice of starting material and the use of constrained ring chemistry.

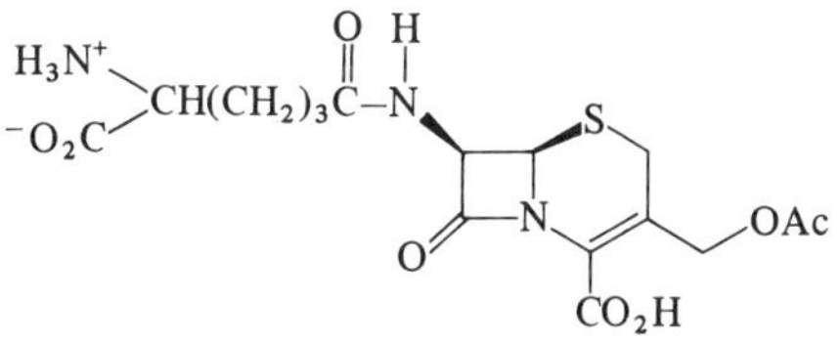

63

The starting material chosen for this approach was L-cysteine. The chiral center of L-cysteine, which ultimately becomes incorporated as C-7 in the final product, also serves as the directing force for the establishment of the chirality at C-6. Conversion of L-cysteine to the corresponding thiazolidine by reaction with acetone, followed by protection of the amino and acid moieties, gave compound *65*. In order to form the requisite β-lactam ring, it was necessary to effect an oxidation of the carbonbearing sulfur and thereby introduce an amino function. This oxidation was carried out by heating a solution of *65* and dimethyl diazodicarboxylate to 105 °C to produce compound *66* in essentially quantitative yield. Although this novel transformation produced only one isomer of the hydrazoester, i.e., that isomer with the methyl ester and hydrazo moieties in the less sterically hindered *trans* configuration on the five-membered ring, it was necessary to invert the configuration at the new center in order ultimately to form the desired lactam bond.

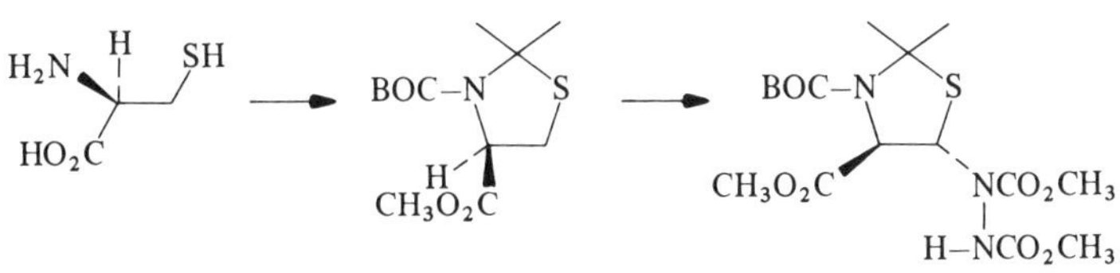

64 *65* *66*

The required inversion was accomplished in a multistep sequence which involved initial oxidation of *66* with lead tetraacetate to yield the acetoxy derivative *(67)* as a mixture of isomers. Hydrolysis of the acetate function of *67* with methanolic sodium acetate gave only the isomer in which the ester and the hydroxyl groups were *trans*, i.e., *70*, presumably via the ring opened tautomer *(69)*. Introduction of the desired nitrogen group in the proper stereochemistry was effected by conversion of *70* to the corresponding mesylate *(71)* followed by S_N2 displacement with azide ion to provide azido ester *(72)*. Dissolving metal reduction of *72* gave the amino ester *(73)* which served as the immediate precursor for the cyclization reaction.

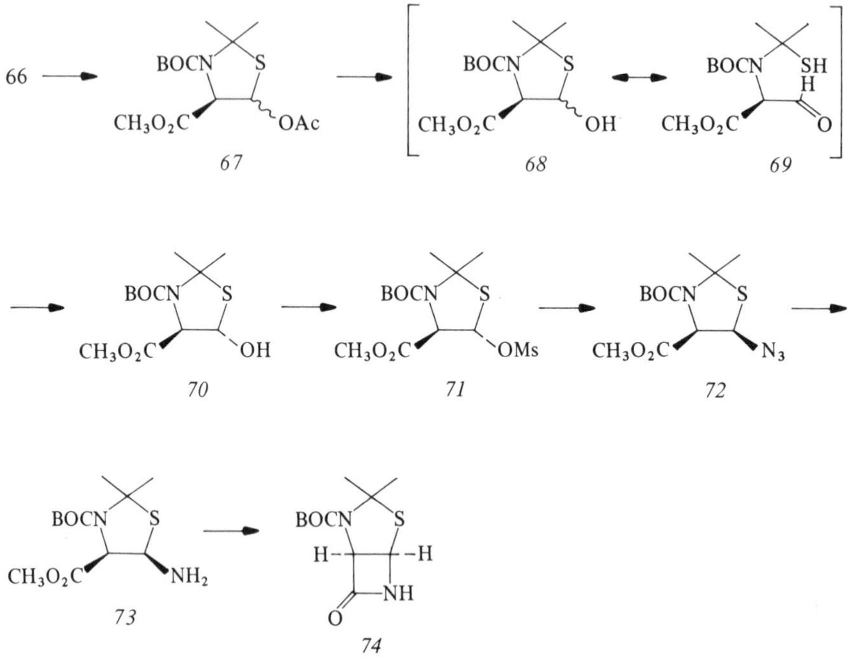

The cyclization of amino ester *(73)* to the bicyclic β-lactam derivative *(74)* was accomplished by treatment with tri-isobutylaluminum in toluene. This reaction was greatly facilitated by the *cis* disposition of the amino and ester moieties on the relatively rigid five-membered ring. In fact, x-ray analysis had revealed that the distance between the amino nitrogen and the carbonyl carbon in compound *73* was only 2.82 Å.

The remaining carbon atoms necessary for the formation of the dihydrothiazine ring were introduced by Michael reaction of *74* with the highly activated dialdehyde system *(75)* to yield the enolic addition product *(76)*. The use of the β,β,β-trichloroethyl ester for protection of the carboxylic acid function in compound *66* was an important strategic feature of this synthetic approach. Woodward recognized from the outset that the fragile nature of the cephalosporin C functionality required a judicious choice of protecting groups which could ultimately be removed under mild conditions at the penultimate step in the synthesis. The use of trichloroethyl esters, which are readily cleaved by reduction with zinc dust at or below room temperature, proved to be a good choice.

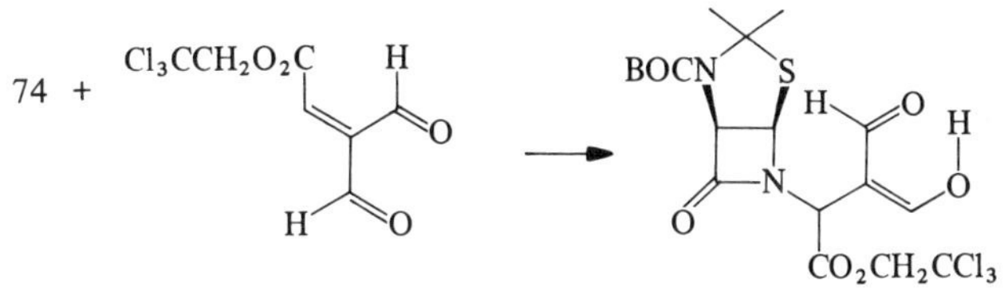

75 *76*

Treatment of compound *76* with trifluoroacetic acid results in the acid-catalyzed removal of both the *N-t*-butyloxycarbonyl and isopropylidene protecting groups as well as cyclization of the sulfur atom into the activated dialdehyde system to yield the bicyclic system *(77)*, wherein the double bond occupies the "unnatural" 2,3 position. Condensation of the amino group of *77* with *N*-β,β,β-trichloroethyloxycarbonyl-D-(−)-α-aminoadipic acid under DCC catalysis followed by esterification with β,β,β-trichloroethanol/DCC gave the tri-protected isocephem derivative *(78)*. Reduction of the aldehyde moiety of *78* followed by acetylation of the resulting allylic alcohol provided triprotected Δ-2 cephalosporin C *(79)*.

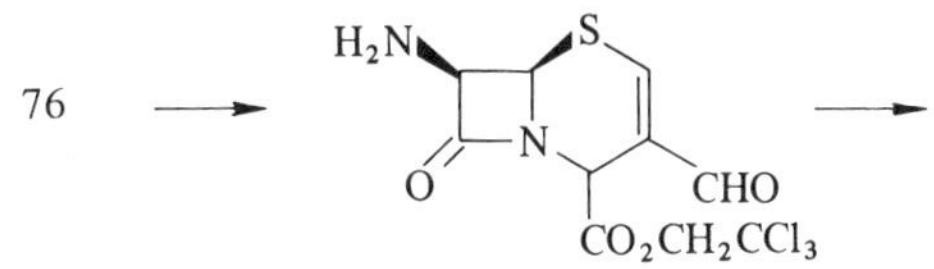

77

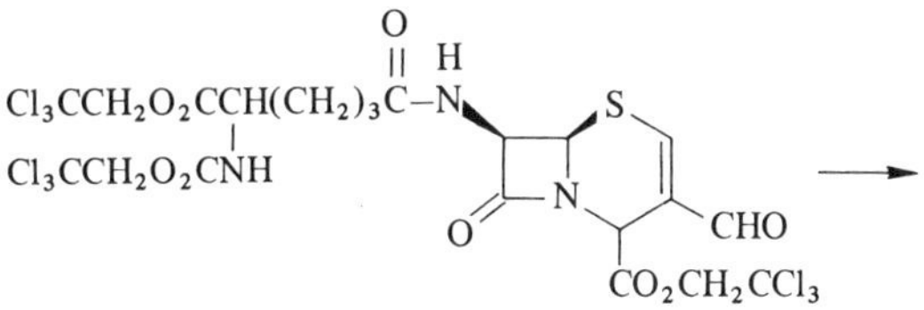

78

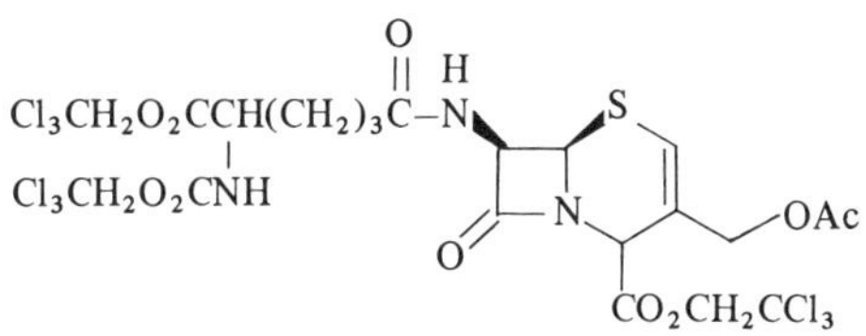

79

Attempts to isomerize the double bond of compound *79* into conjugation with the ester by treatment with pyridine at room temperature for 3 days provided a 4:1 ratio of *79* and the desired Δ-3 product *(80)*. The two isomers were readily separated by silica gel chromatography and *80* was treated with zinc dust in 90%

aqueous acetic acid at 0 °C to produce totally synthetic cephalosporin C which was identical to the natural product in all respects.

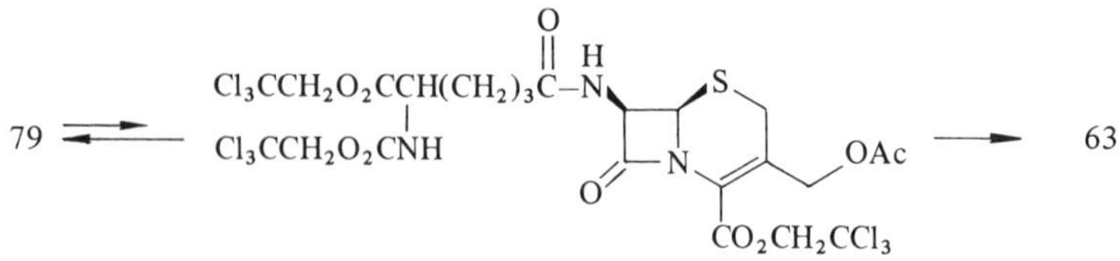

80

In summary, the synthesis of cephalosporin C is historically very significant for at least three reasons. First, it marked the first time that both the chirality and the carbon atoms of an amino acid were utilized to construct an appropriately substituted β-lactam derivative. Second, it was the first recognition that monocyclic or 3,4-fused azetidinones were sufficiently stable to allow such moieties to be established early in the synthetic sequence. Finally, the use of trichloroethyl esters and carbamates as protecting groups for carboxylic acids and amines respectively proved to be of general utility not only in subsequent β-lactam syntheses but also in synthetic approaches to other sensitive molecules. The one weakness in this otherwise highly controlled and specific synthesis is the unfavorable equilibrium ratio of the Δ-2 and Δ-3 double bond isomers.

K. Penicillin Total Synthesis – Baldwin

The pathways involved in the biosynthesis of penicillin and cephalosporins have prompted several suggestions regarding synthesis. Baldwin's penicillin total synthesis is based upon such biomimetic considerations. To convert the tripeptide *(81)* postulated in penicillin biosynthesis into penicillin, it is necessary to effect an

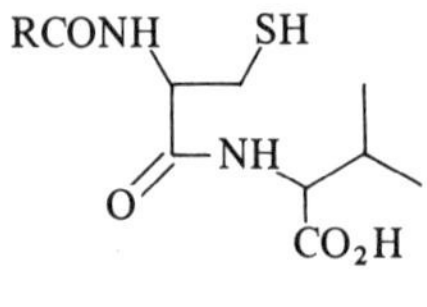

81

oxidative ring closure of N-4 to C-5 and subsequently to form the S-C-2 bond. The latter closure is well known in several variations and the Baldwin penicillin total synthesis (Baldwin et al. 1976) is primarily noted for the N-4 to C-5 closure and its stereocontrol.

D-Isodehydrovaline *(84)* was chosen as the thiazolidine ring precursor since it contains the correct stereochemistry and has the prerequisite functionality for oxidative ring closure with sulfur. It was prepared from methyl 2-nitrodimethyl acry-

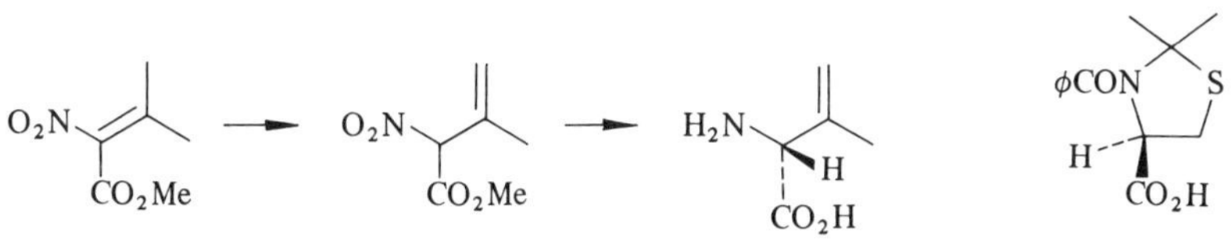

82 83 84 85

late *(82)*. Deconjugation afforded *83* which upon reduction gave *84*. Resolution of the *N*-chloroacetyl derivative with hog acylase *1* yielded resolved *84* after hydrolysis. The methyl ester of *84* was coupled with *85* to give the dipeptide *(86)*. Functionalization of *86* was achieved by treatment with benzoyl peroxide to give *87*. Presumably, an intermediate sulfurane undergoes a [2,3] sigmatropic rearrangement of the corresponding ylid. Stereoselectivity is achieved because the bulky dihydrovaline residue shields the α-face of the thiazolidine ring. Solvolysis of *87* to *88* was readily achieved with hydrogen chloride. Sodium hydride ring closure afforded the desired β-lactam *(89)*. The stereochemical portion of the synthesis is now complete since *89* possesses the same chirality at all asymmetric centers as natural penicillins.

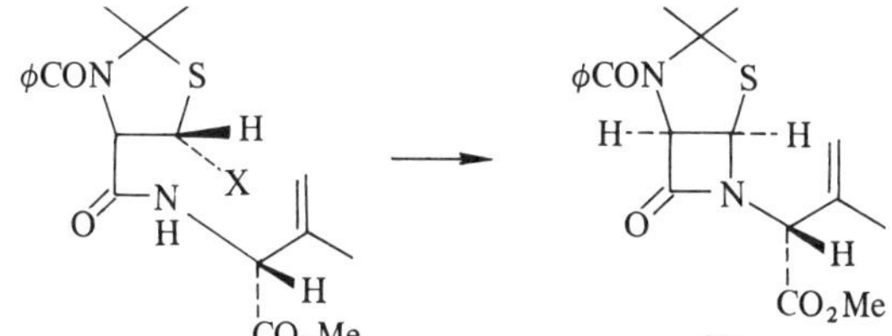

89

86 X=H
87 X=OCOϕ
88 X=Cl

To convert *89* to penicillin, it is necessary to effect an oxidative ring closure; *89* was oxidized to a single epimer, presumably *90*. Acidic ring opening gave the ketosulfide *(91)*. To generate the appropriate sulfenic acid, *91* was converted to

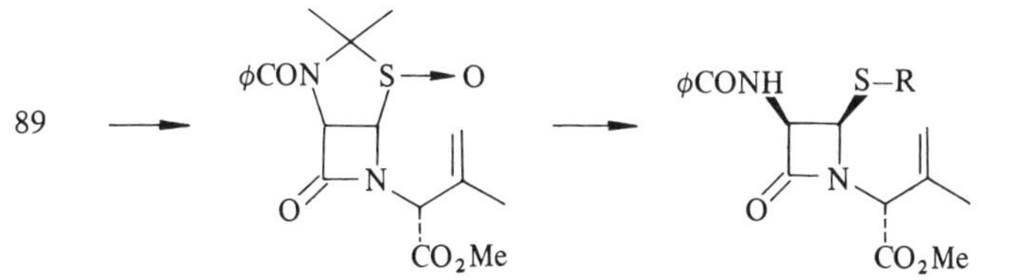

90

91 R=$-CH_2COCH_3$
92 R=

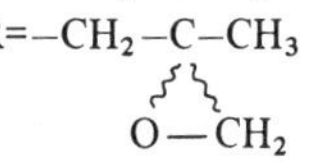

93 R=

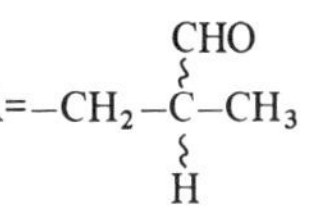

the epoxide epimer *(92)* and then rearranged to *93*. Oxidation of the aldehyde pair *(93)* gave the desired sulfoxide as a diastereoisomer mixture. Thermal syn-elimination of either sulfoxide can give only a single sulfenic acid. Thermolysis of the sulfoxide mixture gave the penicillin sulfoxide *(94)* and deoxygenation yielded methyl 6β-benzamidopenicillanate *(95)*, thus completing the total synthesis.

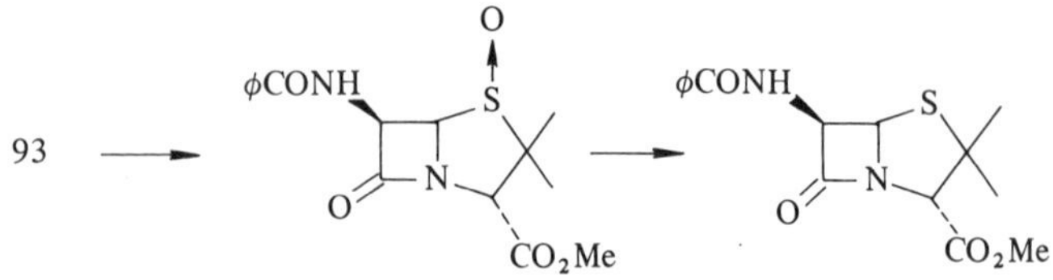

94 *95*

The Baldwin total synthesis was based upon biosynthetic considerations. The key reaction is the stereoselective functionalization of *86* and the stereocontrol throughout the synthesis. The Lilly nocardicin total synthesis (KOPPEL et al. 1978) and the Kishi 6(7)-substituted penicillin-cephalosporin total synthesis (NAKATSUKA et al. 1975) both employ similar procedures to form the azetidinone.

L. Synthesis of the Penem Nucleus – Woodward

The internal Wittig cyclization reaction which was pioneered by workers at the Woodward Institute as a route to partially synthetic penicillin and cephalosporin analogs (SCARTAZZINI et al. 1972a, b) has recently been widely utilized in the construction of such highly reactive systems as penems and carbapenems (SAMMES 1980; COOPER 1980; LANG et al. 1979; ERNEST et al. 1978, 1979; PFAENDLER et al. 1979, 1980). The success of the Wittig reaction in the preparation of such sensitive ring systems derives in large part from the relatively mild, neutral conditions which can be used to effect the cyclizations. The use of the Wittig approach can be illustrated by the recent total synthesis of the parent penem *(96)* (PFAENDLER et al. 1979).

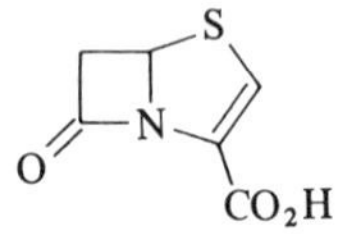

96

Reaction of 4-acetoxyazetidinone *(97)* with the sodium salt of methyl *cis*-β-mercaptoacrylate *(98)* in aqueous solution at −10 °C provided the displacement product *(99)* in 80% yield. Condensation of *99* with acetonyl glyoxylate, *(100)* in toluene-DMF at room temperature provided a mixture of the epimeric alcohols

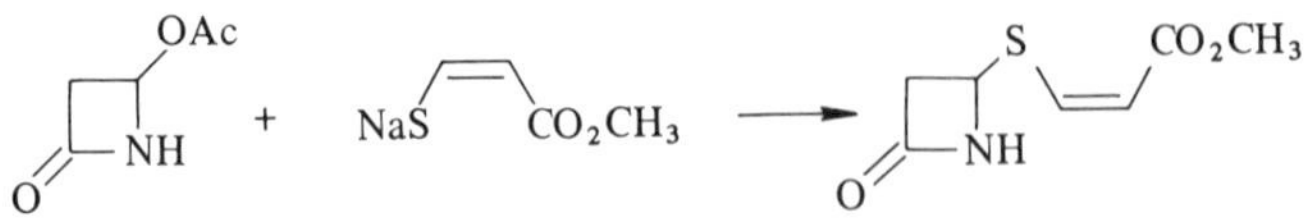

97 *98* *99*

(101). As is so often the case in β-lactam synthesis, the choice of protecting groups, in this instance the acetonyl ester, proved to be a crucial factor in the success or

failure of the entire route. The present workers found the acetonyl esters to be easily crystallized, stable to chromatography on silica gel and to acidic reagents but readily cleaved by mild alkaline hydrolysis.

The epimeric alcohols *(101)* were converted to the corresponding chlorides *(102)* by treatment with thionyl chloride and triethylamine. Subsequent reaction with tripenylphosphine in tretrahydrofuran gave a single phosphorane *(103)*.

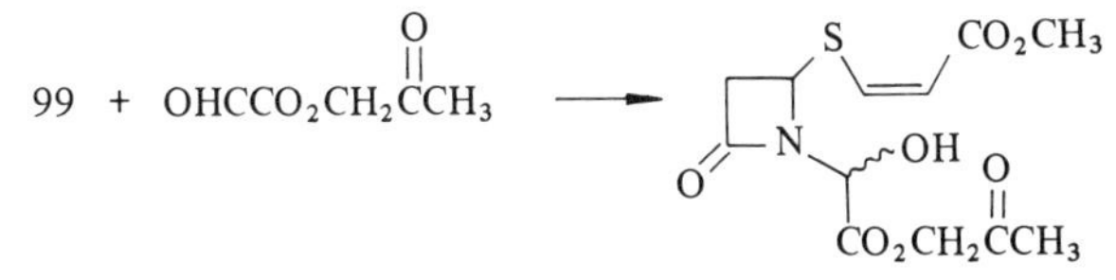

100 *101*

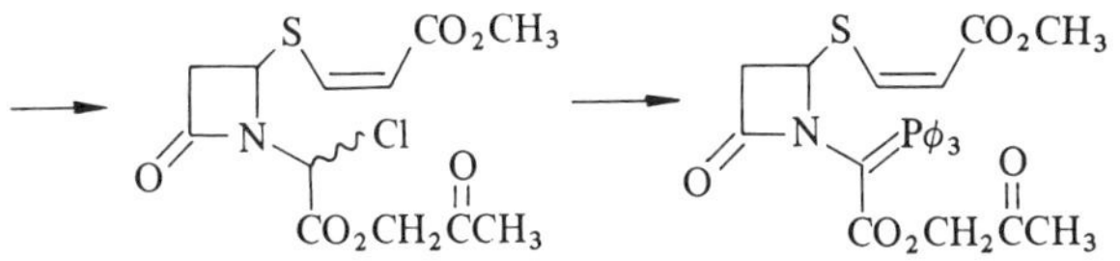

102 *103*

Ozonolysis of compound *103* was carried out in the presence of trifluoroacetic acid, which protected the otherwise ozone-sensitive phosphorane moiety by converting it in situ to the stable phosphonium salt *(104)*. After reductive workup, the resulting product *(105)* was deprotonated with sodium bicarbonate to give *106*, which was subsequently cyclized in refluxing methylene chloride to yield the protected penem *(107)*. The acetonyl protecting group was removed by hydrolysis with one equivalent of sodium hydroxide at 0 °C to yield the desired penem *(96)*.

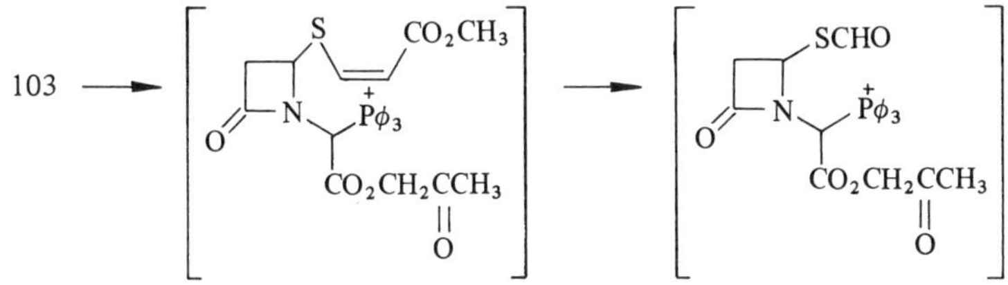

104 *105*

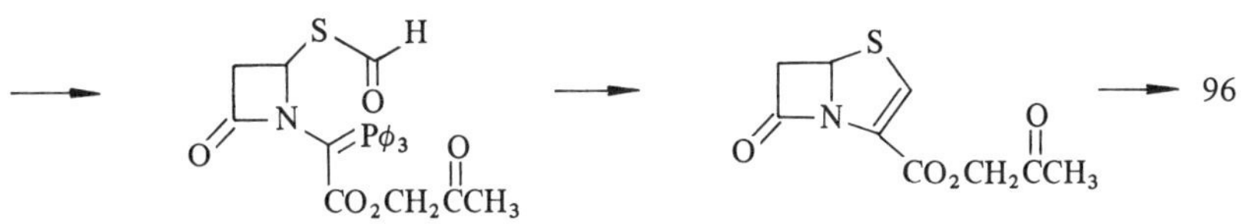

106 *107*

Although the sequence outlined above produced *96* in racemic form, the same workers have devised a minor modification whereby both enantiomers of *96* can be isolated in pure form (PFAENDLER et al. 1979). This approach involved reacting

97 with the β-mercaptoacrylate ester of (−)-menthol *(108)* to yield a 1:1 mixture of diastereomers *109* and *110*, which were separated by fractional crystallization. Each diastereomer was then converted independently by sequences exactly analogous to that previously oulined. In that manner, both the *R* and *S* configurations of *96* were isolated in pure form. Interestingly enough, the 5-*R* isomer which corresponds to the configuration of the naturally occurring β-lactams was determined to be approximately twice as biologically active as racemic *96*, while the 5-*S* isomer was totally inactive.

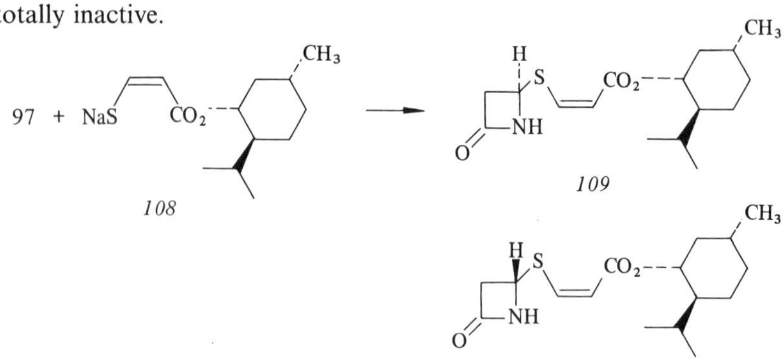

108 *109* *110*

M. Total Synthesis of (+)-Thienamycin – Merck

The recent discovery of thienamycin *(111)* and other related carbapenem-based natural products (COOPER 1980) presented the β-lactam chemist with new and unique challenges in synthesis. Whereas the cephalosporins are in general signifi-

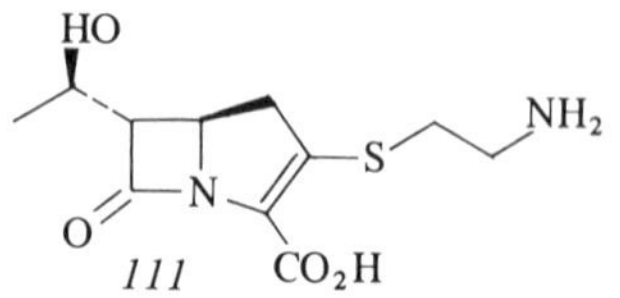

111

cantly more stable than the penicillins, thienamycin is even more labile in concentrated solution than the most sensitive penicillin derivatives currently in clinical use. This instability, which is related to the presence of the highly strained carbapenem ring nucleus in thienamycin, requires that potential routes of synthesis postpone the elaboration of the bicyclic nucleus until as late as possible in the sequence.

In addition to the requirement for the development of a route to the bicyclic nucleus, new methodology had to be designed for the elaboration of the cysteaminyl and hydroxyethyl side-chains. Related to the elaboration of the hydroxyethyl side-chain was the problem of the establishment of the three contiguous stereocenters at C-5, C-6, and C-8 in the appropriate R,S,R configuration. The fact that thienamycin possessed such unprecedented potency and spectrum of biological activity made it highly desirable to develop an approach to synthesis which could be subsequently modified to allow for the preparation of analogs necessary to study structure–activity relationships in the new series.

The first chiral, stereocontrolled synthesis of (+)-thienamycin was published by the Merck group in 1980 (SALZMANN et al. 1980). In this approach the key bicyclic ring system was formed via an internal carbene insertion reaction. Stereocontrol was achieved by a combination of the proper choice of an optically active starting material followed by the use of that chiral center to establish the configuration of adjacent positions.

The key chiral starting material in this synthesis was L-aspartic acid *(112)* which provides all the atoms necessary for formation of the β-lactam ring of *111* as well as the appropriate absolute chirality at the carbon which will ultimately become C-5 in thienamycin. The cyclization reaction to form the β-lactam ring was carried out by converting *112* to its dibenzyl ester *(113)* followed by monosilylation at nitrogen to yield the monosilyl derivative *(114)*. This compound was treated with *t*-butyl magnesium chloride in ether to provide the desired azetidinone *(115)* in about 70% yield. The optical purity of *115* was assayed by hydrogenolysis of the benzyl ester followed by hydrolysis of the resulting azetidinone acid *(116)*

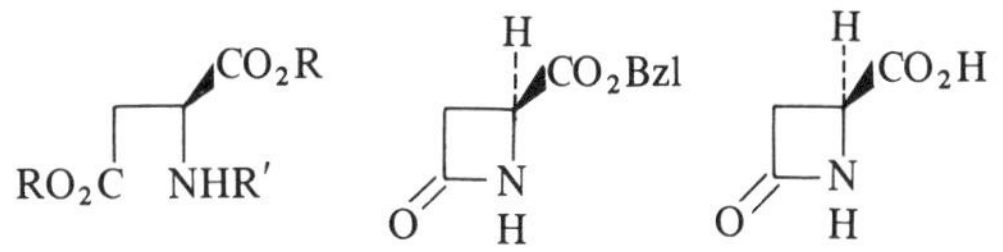

112 R=H, R′=H
113 R=Bzl, R′=H
114 R=Bzl, R′=TMS

115 *116*

to give aspartic acid. The product obtained in this manner had 97%–100% of the original rotation of the starting aspartic acid which indicated that the cyclization had indeed been stereospecific.

The conversion of ester *115* into an alkylating agent was accomplished by the four-step sequence shown below. Reduction of *115* with excess sodium borohydride gave a quantitative yield of azetidinone alcohol *(117)*. Conversion of *117* to mesylate *(118)* and subsequently to iodide *(119)* followed by silylation of the amide nitrogen with *t*-butyldimethylchlorosilane, gave the active alkylating agent *(120)* in about 50% overall yield from L-aspartic acid.

Prior to the elaboration of the hydroxyethyl side-chain, iodide *(120)* was reacted with 2-lithio-2-trimethylsilyl-1,3-dithiane to provide the disubstituted dithiane derivative *(121)* in 70%–80% yield. The use of the 2-trimethylsilyl-1,3-dithiane moiety as a latent carboxylic acid equivalent was pioneered in this sequence, where it was chosen because of the ease of reaction with *120*, its large steric bulk, which aids in the establishment of stereochemistry at C-6, and its ultimate easy conversion to the carboxylic acid.

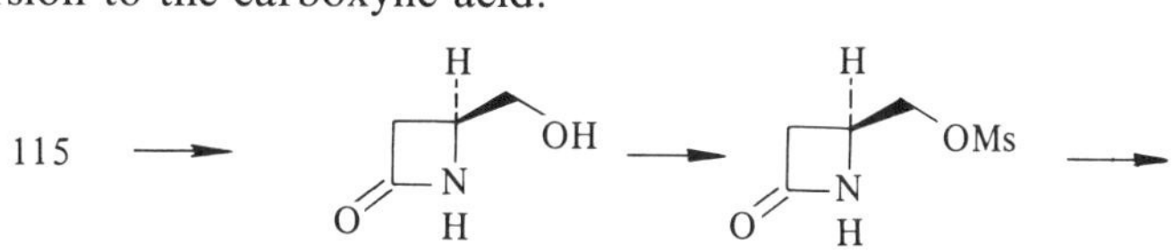

117 *118*

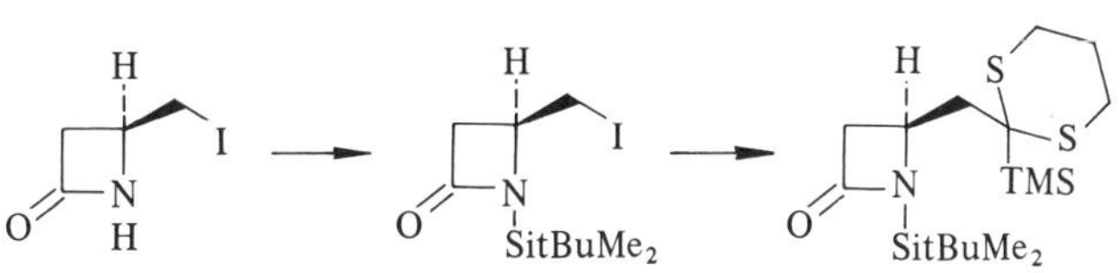

119 *120* *121*

Formation of the enolate ion of *121* by treatment with two equivalents of lithium diisopropylamide followed by inverse quench with acetyl imidazole gave the acetyl derivative *(122)*, which was exclusively the desired *trans* isomer as evidenced by its 300 MHz NMR spectrum. The exclusive formation of the *trans* isomer had been predicted based on the expected large steric hindrance which would be present in the corresponding *cis* isomer.

121

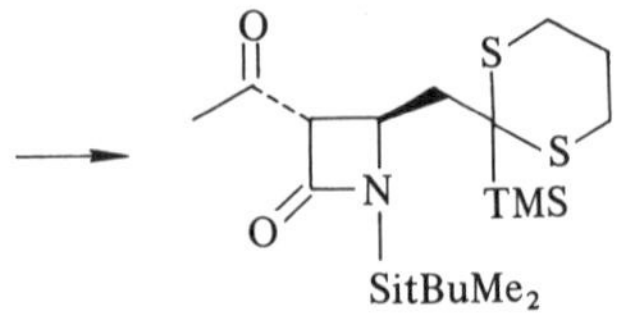

122

Examination of molecular models of compound *122* suggested that reduction of the acetyl moiety with a very bulky hydride reducing agent should, according to Cram's rule, provide a predominance of the required 8-*R* (thienamycin numbering) epimer. Treatment of *122* with potassium tri-sec-butylborohydride in ether gave an 85% yield of a 9:1 mixture of the desired 8-*R* isomer *(123)* and the 8-*S* epimer. Compound *123* incorporates all three of the required chiral centers of thienamycin in the correct absolute configuration.

Conversion of compound *123* to the corresponding carboxylic acid *(125)* was accomplished in two steps. Initial treatment of *123* with mercuric chloride–mercuric oxide provided silylketone *(124)* in 93% yield. Subsequent treatment of *124* with 30% hydrogen peroxide effects a Baeyer–Villiger type rearrangement to an intermediate silyl ester which hydrolyzes to the acid *(125)* in situ.

122

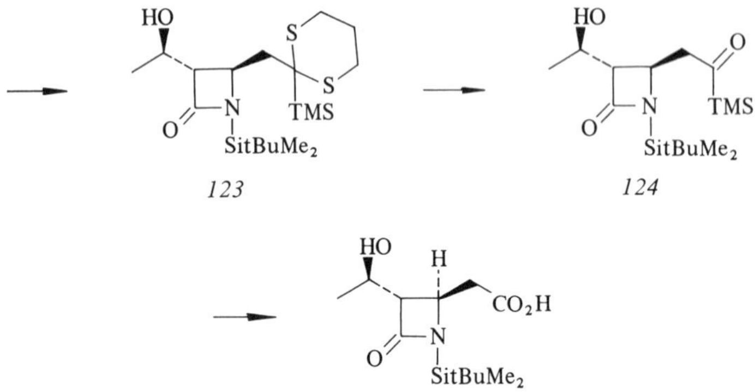

125

Elaboration of the remaining carbon atoms necessary to construct the carbapenem nucleus was accomplished in a one-pot reaction which involved activation of the carboxylate system as the corresponding imidazolide by treatment with diimidazole carbonyl, followed by addition of the magnesium salt of the half *p*-nitrobenzyl ester of malonic acid. After acidic workup, the desired keto ester *(126)* was isolated in 86% yield. As has already been shown to be the case in other examples, the choice of protecting groups was critical to the ultimate success of this route. Sensitivity of final product, i.e., thienamycin itself, necessitated the use of *p*-nitrobenzyl ester protection due to the fact that such esters are readily removed by hydrogenolysis under essentially neutral conditions.

Hydrolysis of the silyl protecting group of *126* gave the free NH compound *(127)* which was subsequently converted to the desired diazo derivative *(128)* on treatment with *p*-carboxybenzenesulfonyl azide and triethylamine.

Heating a toluene solution of *128* to about 80 °C in the presence of a catalytic amount or rhodium II acetate provided an essentially quantitative yield of the desired carbene insertion product, bicyclic ketoester *(129)*. Compound *129* was a single isomer at C-3 and the stereochemistry was assigned as shown based on model system work.

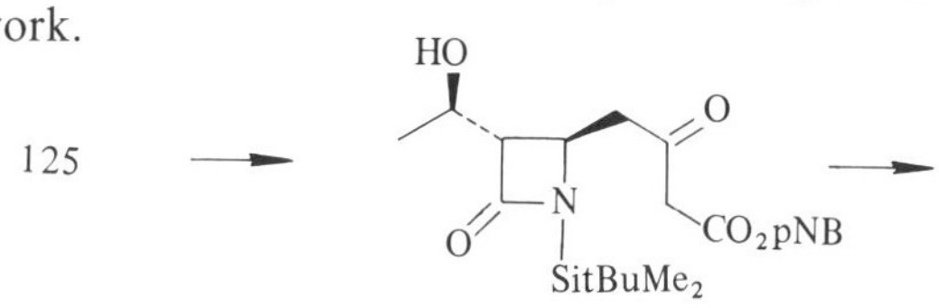

126

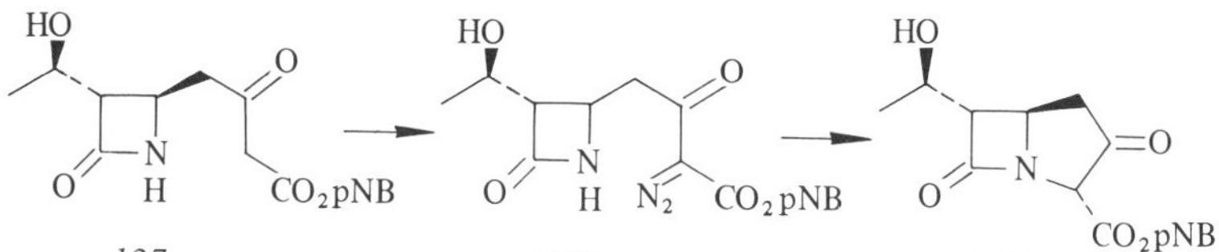

127 *128* *129*

The choice of conditions to be employed for the introduction of the cysteamine side-chain was critical to the success of the route since previous work had shown that both compound *129* and the ultimately desired product *(131)* were unstable in the presence of nucleophiles. In addition, studies on *131* obtained by derivatization of natural thienamycin had demonstrated that in the presence of tertiary amine bases, an equilibrium between the Δ-2 and Δ-1 double bond regioisomers was established, with the unnatural Δ-1 isomer predominating by a 4:1 ratio.

Treatment of *129* with diphenylchlorophosphate and diisopropylethylamine in acetonitrile at 0 °C provided the enol phosphate *(130)*. Although compound *130* could be isolated, it proved more convenient to treat in situ with *N*-*p*-nitrobenzyloxycarbonyl cysteamine and an additional equivalent of diisopropylethylamine to provide the *bis*-protected thienamycin derivative *(131)* in 70% overall yield. Hydrogenolysis of *131* provided thienamycin, identical in all respects to the natural product.

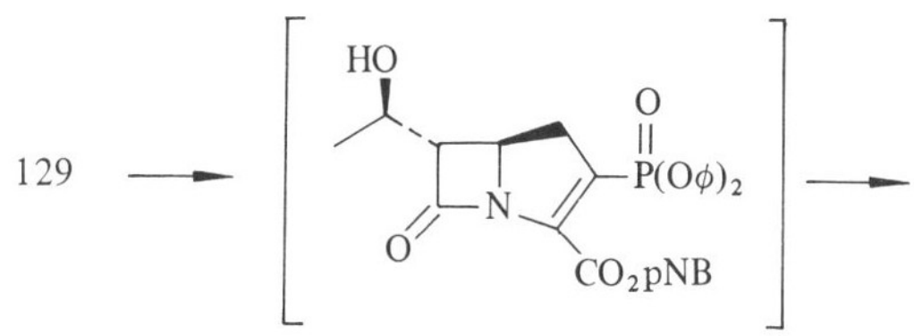

130

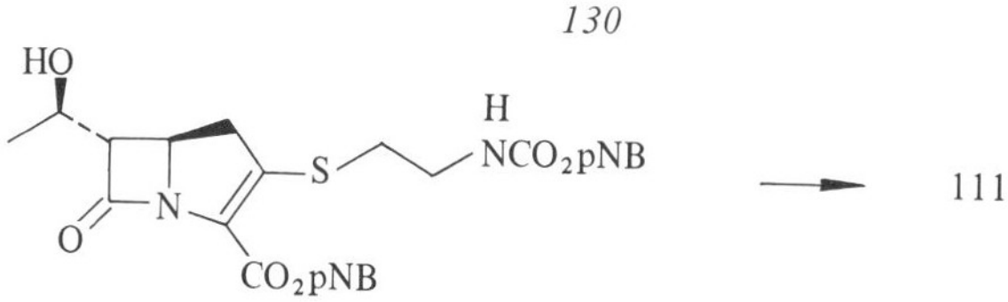

131

In summary, the total synthesis of (+)-thienamycin is noteworthy for its efficient construction of the carbapenem ring system and its achievement of stereocontrol in the establishment of the three chiral centers of *111*. In addition, the route was designed so that key intermediates such as compounds *121* and *129* could, with minor modification in strategy, allow for the preparation of a wide variety of thienamycin analogs with varying C-2 and/or C-6 substituents.

An alternate and potentially commercially viable total synthesis of (±)-thienamycin has also recently been developed at Merck (MELILLO et al. 1980). This approach utilized significantly different methodology for the production of the racemic form of compound *127*, from which point the sequence parallels that described above for the optically active compound.

N. Conclusion

It is abundantly clear that the art of total synthesis of β-lactam antibiotics has made great progress since the early and tentative attempts when the structure of penicillin was first determined. The difficulties involved are primarily stereocontrol, the usually high degree of substitution of the carbon atoms comprising the nucleus, and the instability of the final product. The increasing number of β-lactam total syntheses during the last few years is ample testimony that these challenges have been met. The progress is due in large part to an increasing maturity of the strategic considerations involved in their construction and this chapter has attempted to detail those strategies. The coming years will see new strategies evolve, and as a consequence, novel and more eloquent syntheses of these challenging targets will emerge.

References

Baldwin JE, Christie MA, Haber SB, Kruse LI (1976) Stereospecific synthesis of penicillins. Conversion from a peptide precursor. J Am Chem Soc 98:3045–3047

Bentley PH, Berry PD, Brooks G, Gilpin ML, Hunt E, Zumaya II (1977) The total synthesis of (±)-clavulanic acid. J Chem Soc Chem Commun 748–749

Bentley PH, Brooks G, Gilpin ML, Hunt E (1979) A new total synthesis of (±)-clavulanic acid. J Chem Soc Chem Commun 1889–1890

Bose AK, Anjanevulu B, Bhatlachary SK, Mankos MS (1967) Studies on lactones-V. 3-azido-2-azetidinones. Tetrahedron Lett 4769–4776

Cooper RDG (1980) New β-lactam antibiotics. In: Sammes PG (ed) Topics in antibiotic chemistry, vol 3. Ellis Horwood, Chichester, England

Dolfini JE, Schwartz S, Weisenborn F (1968) Synthesis of dihydrothiazines related to desacetylcephalosporin lactones. An alternate total synthesis of desacetylcephalosporin lactones. J Org Chem 34:1582–1586

duVigneaud V, Carpenter FH, Holley RW, Livermore AH, Rachele JR (1946) Synthetic penicillin. Science 104:431–433

Ernest I, Gostdi J, Greengrass CW, Hulick W, Jackman DE, Pfaendler HR, Woodward RB (1978) The penems, a new class of β-lactam antibiotics: 6-acylaminopenem-3-carboxylic acids. J Am Chem Soc 100:8214–8218

Ernest I, Gosteli J, Woodward RB (1979) The penems, a new class of β-lactam antibiotics. 3. Synthesis of optically active 2-methyl-(5R)-penem-3-carboxylic acid. J Am Chem Soc 101:6301–6305

Firestone RA, Schelechow N, Johnston DBR, Christensen BG (1972) Substituted penicillins and cephalosporins II. C-6(7)-alkyl derivatives. Tetrahedron Lett 375–378

Firestone RA, Maciejewicz NS, Ratcliffe RW, Christensen BG (1974) Total synthesis of β-lactam antibiotics IV. Epimerization of 6(7)-aminopenicillins and -cephalosporins from α to β. J Org Chem 39:437–440

Girotra NN, Wendler NL (1972) An efficient new synthesis of 7-phthalimido-8-t-butoxy-5,8-seco-desacetylcephalosporonic acid lactone, a key intermediate in a total synthesis of the cephalosporins. Tetrahedron Lett 5301–5304

Hamilton-Miller JMT, Kerry DW, Brunfitt W (1974) An in vitro comparison of cefoxitin, a semi-synthetic cephamycin, with cephalothin. J Antibiot 27:42–48

Heusler K (1972) Total synthesis of penicillins and cephalosporins. In: Flynn EH (ed) Cephalosporins and penicillins. Academic Press, New York, p 255

Heymes R, Amiard G, Nomine G (1966) A synthesis of the D,L-desacetyl-cephalothin-lactone (in French), CR Acad Sci [D] (Paris) 263:170–172

Kamiya T (1977) Studies on the new monocyclic β-lactam antibiotics, nocardicins. In: Elks J (ed) Recent advances in the chemistry of β-lactam antibiotics. The Chemical Society, London, p 281

Kamiya T, Oku T, Nakagushi O, Takeno H, Hushimoto M (1978) A novel synthesis of nocardicins and their analogues. Tetrahedron Lett 5119–5122

Koppel GA, McShane L, Jose F, Cooper RDG (1978) Total synthesis of nocardicin A. synthesis of 3-ANA and nocardicin A. J Am Chem Soc 100:3933–3935

Lang M, Prasad K, Hulick W, Gosteli J, Ernest I, Woodward RB (1979) The penems, a new class of β-lactam antibiotics. 2. Total synthesis of racemic 6-unsubstituted representatives. J Am Chem Soc 101:6296–6301

Melillo DG, Shinkai I, Liu T, Ryan K, Sletzinger M (1980) A practical synthesis of (±)-thienamycin. Tetrahedron Lett 21:2783–2786

Nakatsuka S-I, Tammo H, Kishi Y (1975) Biogenetic type synthesis of penicillin-cephalosporin antibiotics. II. An oxidative cyclization route to β-lactam thiazolidine derivatives. J Am Chem Soc 97:5010–5012

Pfaendler HR, Gosteli J, Woodward RB (1979) The penems, a new class of β-lactam antibiotics. 4. Syntheses of racemic and enantiomeric penem carboxylic acids. J Am Chem Soc 101:6306–6310

Pfaendler HR, Gosteli J, Woodward RB (1980) The penems, a new class of β-lactam antibiotics. 5. Total synthesis of racemic 6α-hydroxyethyl-penemcarboxylic acids. J Am Chem Soc 102:2039–2043

Ratcliffe RW, Christensen BG (1973a) Total synthesis of β-lactam antibiotics. I. α-Thioformamido-diethylphosphonates. Tetrahedron Lett 4645–4648

Ratcliffe RW, Christensen BG (1973b) Total synthesis of β-lactam antibiotics. II. (±)-Cephalothin. Tetrahedron Lett 4649–4656

Ratcliffe RW, Christensen BG (1973c) Total synthesis of β-lactam antibiotics. III. (±)-Cefoxitin. Tetrahedron Lett 4653–4656

Salzmann TN, Ratcliffe RW, Christensen BG, Bouffard FA (1980) The total synthesis of (+)-thienamycin. J Am Chem Soc 102:6161–6163

Sammes PG (1980) Total synthesis of penicillins and cephalosporins. In: Sammes PG (ed) Topics in antibiotic chemistry; vol 4. Ellis Horwood, Chichester, England

Scartazzini R, Peter H, Bickel H, Heusler K, Woodward RB (1972a) New β-lactam antibiotics. The preparation of 7-aminocephalosporanic acid (in German). Helv Chim Acta 55:408–417

Scartazzini R, Gosteli J, Bickel H, Woodward RB (1972b) New β-lactam antibiotics. The preparation of 8-β-phenylacetaminodihomoceph-4-em-5-carboxylic acid (in German). Helv Chim Acta 55:2567–2672

Sheehan JC, Henery-Logan KR (1957) The total synthesis of penicillin V. J Am Chem Soc 79:1262–1263

Sheehan JC, Henery-Logan KR (1959) The total synthesis of penicillin V. J Am Chem Soc 81:3089–3094

Sheehan JC, Henery-Logan KR (1962) The total and partial general synthesis of the penicillins. J Am Chem Soc 84:2983–2990

Sheehan JC, Hess GP (1955) A new method for forming peptide bonds. J Am Chem Soc 77:1067–1068
Sheehan JC, Johnson DA (1954) The synthesis of substituted penicillins and simpler structural analogs. VIII. Phthalimidomalonaldehyde esters: synthesis and condensation with penicillamine. J Am Chem Soc 76:158–168
Sheehan JC, Ryan JJ (1951) The synthesis of substituted penicillins and simpler structural analogs. I. Alpha amino monocyclic β-lactams. J Am Chem Soc 73:1204–1206
Staudinger H (1907) On the reactions of ketene (in German). Justus Liebig's Ann Chem 356:41–123
Wasserman HH, Hlasta DJ (1978) A synthesis of (±)-3-aminonocardicinic acid (3-ANA). J Am Chem Soc 100:6780–6781
Woodward RB (1966) Recent advances in the chemistry of natural products. Science 153:487–493
Woodward RB, Heusler K, Gosteli J, Naegeli P, Oppolzer W, Ramage R, Ranganathan S, Vorbruggen H (1966) The total synthesis of cephalosporin C. J Am Chem Soc 88:852–853

Subject Index

Handbook of Experimental Pharmacology

Continuation of "Handbuch der experimentellen Pharmakologie"

Springer-Verlag
Berlin
Heidelberg
New York

Handbook of Experimental Pharmacology

Continuation of "Handbuch der experimentellen Pharmakologie"

Volume 44
Heme and Hemoproteins

Volume 45: Part 1
Drug Addiction I

Part 2
Drug Addiction II

Volume 46
Fibrinolytics and Antifibrinolytics

Volume 47
Kinetics of Drug Action

Volume 48
Arthropod Venoms

Volume 49
Ergot Alkaloids and Related Compounds

Volume 50: Part 1
Inflammation

Part 2
Anti-Inflammatory Drugs

Volume 51
Uric Acid

Volume 52
Snake Venoms

Volume 53
Pharmacology of Ganglionic Transmission

Volume 54: Part 1
Adrenergic Activators and Inhibitors I

Part 2
Adrenergic Activators and Inhibitors II

Volume 55
Psychotropic Agents

Part 1
Antipsychotics and Antidepressants I

Part 2
Anxiolytis, Gerontopsychopharmacological Agents and Psychomotor Stimulants

Part 3
Alcohol and Psychotomimetics, Psychotropic Effects of Central Acting Drugs

Volume 56, Part 1 + 2
Cardiac Glycosides

Volume 57
Tissue Growth Factors

Volume 58
Cyclic Nucleotides
Part 1: **Biochemistry**
Part 2: **Physiology and Pharmacology**

Volume 59
Mediators and Drugs in Gastrointestinal Motility
Part 1: **Morphological Basis and Neurophysiological Control**
Part 2: **Endogenis and Exogenous Agents**

Volume 60
Pyretics and Antipyretics

Volume 61
Chemotherapy of Viral Infections

Volume 62
Aminoglycosides

Volume 64
Inhibition of Folate Metabolism in Chemotherapy

Volume 65
Teratogenesis and Reproductive Toxicology

Springer-Verlag
Berlin
Heidelberg
New York